The Trauma Manual

P9-DNK-359

Second Edition

The Trauma Manual
Second Edition

Andrew B. Peitzman, M.D., F.A.C.S.
Professor & Chief
Division of General Surgery
Department of Surgery
University of Pittsburgh School of Medicine;
Vice Chair for Clinical Services
Department of Surgery
University of Pittsburgh Medical Center, Presbyterian Hospital
Pittsburgh, Pennsylvania

Michael Rhodes, M.D., F.A.C.S.
Professor of Surgery
Thomas Jefferson University;
Chairman
Department of Surgery
Christiana Care Health Services
Wilmington, Delaware

C. William Schwab, M.D., F.A.C.S
Professor of Surgery
Department of Surgery
University of Pennsylvania School of Medicine;
Chief
Division of Trauma & Surgical Critical Care
University of Pennsylvania Medical Center
Philadelphia, Pennsylvania

Donald M. Yealy, M.D., F.A.C.E.P.
Professor
Department of Emergency Medicine
University of Pittsburgh;
Attending Physician and Vice Chair
Department of Emergency Medicine
University of Pittsburgh Medical Center
Pittsburgh, Pennsylvania

Timothy C. Fabian, M.D., F.A.C.S.
Professor & Chairman
Department of Surgery
University of Tennessee Health Science Center;
Attending Surgeon
Department of Surgery
Regional Medical Center
Memphis, Tennessee

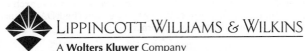

LIPPINCOTT WILLIAMS & WILKINS
A **Wolters Kluwer** Company
Philadelphia • Baltimore • New York • London
Buenos Aires • Hong Kong • Sydney • Tokyo

Acquisitions Editor: Anne M. Sydor
Developmental Editor: Sonya L. Seigafuse
Production Editor: Emmeline Parker
Manufacturing Manager: Benjamin Rivera
Cover Illustrator: Patricia Gast
Compositor: Circle Graphics
Printer: Vicks Lithograph

Library of Congress Cataloging-in-Publication Data

The trauma manual / Andrew B. Peitzman ... [et al.]--2nd ed.
  p. ; cm.
Includes bibliographical references and index.
ISBN 0-7817-2641-7
  1. Traumatology--Handbooks, manuals, etc. 2. Wounds and injuries--Handbooks, manuals, etc. 3. Surgical emergencies--Handbooks, manuals, etc. I. Peitzman, Andrew B.
  [DNLM: 1. Wounds and Injuries--Handbooks. 2. Emergency Medicine--Handbooks. 3. Traumatology--Handbooks. WO 39 T777 2002]
RD93 .T6895 2002
617.1--dc21

                                                                    2001050690

Care has been taken to confirm the accuracy of the information presented and to describe generally accepted practices. However, the authors, editors, and publisher are not responsible for errors or omissions or for any consequences from application of the information in this book and make no warranty, expressed or implied, with respect to the currency, completeness, or accuracy of the contents of the publication. Application of this information in a particular situation remains the professional responsibility of the practitioner.

The authors, editors, and publisher have exerted every effort to ensure that drug selection and dosage set forth in this text are in accordance with current recommendations and practice at the time of publication. However, in view of ongoing research, changes in government regulations, and the constant flow of information relating to drug therapy and drug reactions, the reader is urged to check the package insert for each drug for any change in indications and dosage and for added warnings and precautions. This is particularly important when the recommended agent is a new or infrequently employed drug.

Some drugs and medical devices presented in this publication have Food and Drug Administration (FDA) clearance for limited use in restricted research settings. It is the responsibility of the health care provider to ascertain the FDA status of each drug or device planned for use in their clinical practice.

10 9 8 7 6 5 4

This book is dedicated to those who have given their lives, and those who daily risk their lives, in the care of the injured.

CONTENTS

CONTRIBUTING AUTHORS

Louis H. Alarcon, M.D.
Fellow, Department of Surgical Critical Care, University of Pittsburgh, Pittsburgh, Pennsylvania

Harry L. Anderson, III, M.D., F.A.C.S., F.C.C.M.
Clinical Associate Professor, Department of Surgery, University of Pennsylvania School of Medicine, Philadelphia; Attending Surgeon, Department of Surgery and Trauma, St. Luke's Hospital, Bethlehem, Pennsylvania

Randall L. Beatty, M.D.
Assistant Professor, Department of Ophthalmology, University of Pittsburgh; Chief, Orbital and Oculoplastic Surgery, University of Pittsburgh Medical Center, Pittsburgh, Pennsylvania

Tiffany K. Bee, M.D.
Assistant Professor, University of Tennessee Health Science Center; Attending Surgeon, Department of Surgery, University of Tennessee, Memphis, Tennessee

Steven L. Bernard, M.D.
Assistant Professor of Surgery, Division of Plastic and Hand Surgery, School of Medicine, Case Western Reserve University; Department of Surgery, MetroHealth Medical Center, Cleveland, Ohio

Timothy R. Billiar, M.D.
George Vance Foster Professor of Surgery / Chairman, Department of Surgery, University of Pittsburgh Medical Center, Pittsburgh, Pennsylvania

Darrell C. Boone, M.D.
Assistant Professor of Surgery, Discipline of Surgery, Memorial University of Newfoundland; Attending Surgeon / Critical Care Physician, Health Sciences Centre, St. John's, Newfoundland, Canada

Marilyn J. Borst, M.D.
Henry Ford Hospital, Detroit, Michigan

Kimberly K. Cantees, M.D.
Director of Perioperative Services, St. Clair Hospital, Pittsburgh, Pennsylvania

Keith D. Clancy, M.D.
Medical Director, Trauma and Surgical Critical Care Services, York Hospital, York; Clinical Assistant Professor of Surgery, Pennsylvania State College of Medicine, Hershey, Pennsylvania

John S. Cole, M.D., F.A.C.E.P.
Assistant Professor, Department of Emergency Medicine, University of Pittsburgh, Pittsburgh; Medical Director, STAT Med Evac, West Mifflin, Pennsylvania

Martin A. Croce, M.D.
Professor and Chief, Trauma and Critical Care, Department of Surgery, University of Tennessee Health Science Center, Memphis, Tennessee

G. Paul Dabrowski, M.D.
Assistant Professor, Department of Surgery, Division of Trauma and Surgical Critical Care, Hospital of the University of Pennsylvania, Philadelphia, Pennsylvania

Joseph M. Darby, M.D.
Associate Professor, Department of Anesthesiology and Critical Care, University of Pittsburgh; Medical Director, Trauma Intensive Care Unit, University of Pittsburgh Medical Center, Presbyterian Hospital, Pittsburgh, Pennsylvania

Kimberly A. Davis, M.D.
Assistant Professor, Department of Surgery, Loyola University Medical Center, Maywood, Illinois

Theodore R. Delbridge, M.D., M.P.H.
Assistant Professor, Department of Emergency Medicine, University of Pittsburgh School of Medicine; Director of Emergency Services, University of Pittsburgh Medical Center, Presbyterian Hospital, Pittsburgh, Pennsylvania

J. Christopher DiGiacomo, M.D.
Associate Professor, Department of Surgery, State University of New York–Stony Brook School of Medicine, Stony Brook; Associate Director of Trauma, Associate Program Director, Department of Surgery, Nassau University Medical Center, East Meadow, New York

William F. Donaldson, III, M.D.
Chief, Division of Spinal Surgery, Associate Professor, Departments of Orthopaedic & Neurological Surgery, University of Pittsburgh Medical Center, Presbyterian Hospital, Pittsburgh, Pennsylvania

Timothy C. Fabian, M.D., F.A.C.S.
Professor and Chairman, University of Tennessee Health Science Center; Attending Surgeon, Department of Surgery, Regional Medical Center, Memphis, Tennessee

Kevin Farrell, M.D.
Assistant Professor, Department of Surgery, Emory University School of Medicine; Co-Director of the Burn Unit, Department of Surgery, Grady Memorial Hospital, Atlanta, Georgia

Michael P. Federle, M.D., F.A.C.S.
Professor, Department of Radiology, University of Pittsburgh; Chief, Abdominal Imaging, University of Pittsburgh Medical Center, Pittsburgh, Pennsylvania

Henri R. Ford, M.D.
Chief, Department of Pediatric Surgery, Children's Hospital of Pittsburgh; Benjamin R. Fisher Professor, Department of Surgery, University of Pittsburgh School of Medicine, Pittsburgh, Pennsylvania

Heidi L. Frankel, M.D.
Associate Professor, Yale University School of Medicine; Surgical Intensive Care Unit, Department of Surgery, Yale New Haven Hospital, New Haven, Connecticut

Paul T. Freudigman, M.D.
Director of Orthopaedic Trauma, Department of Orthopaedic Surgery, Baylor University Medical Center, Dallas, Texas

Gerard J. Fulda, M.D.
Director of Surgical Critical Care and Associate Director, Department of Trauma, Christiana Hospital, Newark, Delaware; Associate Professor, Department of Surgery, Jefferson Medical College, Philadelphia, Pennsylvania

Fredrick Giberson, M.D.
Clinical Assistant Professor, Department of Surgery, Jefferson Medical College, Philadelphia, Pennsylvania; Attending Physician, Department of Surgery, Christiana Care Health Services, Newark, Delaware

Gary Goldberg, M.D.
Visiting Associate Professor, Department of Physical Medicine and Rehabilitation, University of Pittsburgh; Director, Department of Brain Injury Rehabilitation, University of Pittsburgh Medical Center Rehabilitation Hospital, Pittsburgh, Pennsylvania

Michael D. Grossman, M.D.
Assistant Professor of Surgery, Department of Surgery, University of Pennsylvania, Philadelphia; Chief, Division of Traumatology and Surgical Critical Care, St. Luke's Regional Trauma Center, Bethlehem, Pennsylvania

Gary S. Gruen, M.D.
Vice Chairman and Associate Professor, Department of Orthopaedic Surgery, University of Pittsburgh School of Medicine; Chief, Orthopaedic Trauma, Department of Orthopaedic Surgery, University of Pittsburgh Medical Center, Pittsburgh, Pennsylvania

Linwood R. Haith, Jr., M.D.
Clinical Associate Professor, Department of Surgery, Temple University Hospital, Philadelphia; Director, Burn Treatment Center, Crozer Medical Center, Upland, Pennsylvania

C. William Hanson, III, M.D., F.C.C.M.
Professor of Anesthesia, Surgery and Internal Medicine, University of Pennsylvania School of Medicine; Medical Director, Surgical Intensive Care Unit, Section Chief, Critical Care Medicine, Department of Anesthesia, Hospital of the University of Pennsylvania, Philadelphia, Pennsylvania

Brian G. Harbrecht, M.D.
Professor, Department of Surgery, University of Pittsburgh; Director of Trauma Program, Department of Surgery, University of Pittsburgh Medical Center, Presbyterian Hospital, Pittsburgh, Pennsylvania

William S. Hoff, M.D., F.A.C.S.
Chairman, Department of Traumatology, Brandywine Hospital, Coatesville; Assistant Professor, Department of Surgery, Division of Traumatology and Surgical Critical Care, University of Pennsylvania, Philadelphia, Pennsylvania

John A. Horton, III, M.D.
Assistant Professor, Department of Physical Medicine and Rehabilitation, University of Pittsburgh; Director, Spinal Cord Injury Program, University of Pittsburgh Medical Center Rehabilitation Hospital, Pittsburgh, Pennsylvania

Jon W. Johnson, M.D.
Assistant Professor, Department of Surgery, University of Florida, Jacksonville; Surgeon, Department of Surgery and Trauma, Holmes Regional Medical Center, Melbourne, Florida

John M. Kane, III, M.D.
Assistant Professor, Department of Surgery, University of Pittsburgh Medical Center, Pittsburgh, Pennsylvania

Donald R. Kauder, M.D., F.A.C.S.
Vice Chief, Hospital of the University of Pennsylvania; Associate Professor, Division of Traumatology and Surgical Critical Care, University of Pennsylvania, Philadelphia, Pennsylvania

James Krugh, M.D.
Associate Professor, Staff Anesthesiologist, Department of Anesthesiology, University of Pittsburgh Medical Center, Pittsburgh, Pennsylvania

Ramon Llull, M.D.
Researcher, Department of Cell Biology, University of Barcelona Medical School, Barcelona, Spain

James M. Lynch, M.D., F.A.C.S.
Associate Professor of Clinical Surgery, Department of Pediatric Surgery, University of Pittsburgh School of Medicine; Attending Surgeon, Department of Pediatric Surgery, Children's Hospital of Pittsburgh, Pittsburgh, Pennsylvania

Ajai K. Malhortra, M.D.
Assistant Professor of Surgery, Department of Surgery, Virginia Commonwealth University Health Systems, MCV Hospitals & Physicians; Medical College of Virginia, Richmond, Virginia

Donald W. Marion, M.D., F.A.C.S.
Professor, University of Pittsburgh; Associate Chief, Department of Neurological Surgery, University of Pittsburgh Medical Center Presbyterian Hospital, Pittsburgh, Pennsylvania

Robert A. Maxwell, M.D.
Assistant Professor, University of Tennessee–Chattanooga Unit; Trauma Staff, Department of Surgery, Erlanger Medical Center, Chattanooga, Tennessee

Preston R. Miller, III, M.D.
Assistant Professor, Department of Surgery, Wake Forest University Baptist Medical Center, Winston-Salem, North Carolina

Gayle Minard, M.D.
Associate Professor, Department of Surgery, University of Tennessee Health Science Center; Attending Physician, Regional Medical Center, Memphis, Tennessee

Vincent N. Mossesso, Jr., M.D.
Assistant Professor, Department of Emergency Medicine, University of Pittsburgh; Medical Director, Department of Prehospital Care, University of Pittsburgh Medical Center Health System, Pittsburgh, Pennsylvania

N. Ake Nyström, M.D., Ph.D.
Hand Surgeon/Associate Professor, Department of Plastic and Reconstructive Surgery and Orthopedics, University of Nebraska Health Systems, Omaha, Nebraska

Juan B. Ochoa, M.D.
Associate Professor, Department of Surgery, University of Pittsburgh Medical Center, Pittsburgh, Pennsylvania

Mark W. Ochs, D.M.D., M.D.
Chair and Program Director, Department of Oral & Maxillofacial Surgery, University of Pittsburgh; Chief, Department of Hospital Dentistry, University of Pittsburgh Medical Center, Pittsburgh, Pennsylvania

Kevin S. O'Toole, M.D., F.A.C.E.P.
Associate Professor, Department of Emergency Medicine, University of Pittsburgh School of Medicine; Associate Director, Department of Emergency Services, University of Pittsburgh Medical Center, Presbyterian Hospital, Pittsburgh, Pennsylvania

Michael D. Pasquale, M.D.
Assistant Professor, Pennsylvania State University, Hershey; Chief of Trauma/Surgical Critical Care, Department of Surgery, Lehigh Valley Hospital, Allentown, Pennsylvania

Gary T. Patterson, M.D.
Assistant Clinical Professor, Department of Surgery, University of Pittsburgh School of Medicine, Pittsburgh, Pennsylvania

Andrew B. Peitzman, M.D., F.A.C.S.
Professor & Chief, Division of General Surgery, University of Pittsburgh School of Medicine; Vice Chair for Clinical Services, Department of Surgery, University of Pittsburgh Medical Center, Presbyterian Hospital, Pittsburgh, Pennsylvania

Louis E. Penrod, M.D.
Assistant Professor, Department of Physical Medicine and Rehabilitation, University of Pittsburgh School of Medicine, Pittsburgh, Pennsylvania

Michael J. Prayson, M.D.
Assistant Professor, Department of Orthopaedic Surgery, University of Pittsburgh Medical Center, Pittsburgh, Pennsylvania

John P. Pryor, M.D.
Assistant Professor of Surgery, Department of Surgery, University of Pennsylvania Health System; Faculty Member, Division of Traumatology and Surgical Critical Care, Hospital of the University of Pennsylvania, Philadelphia, Pennsylvania

James F. Reilly, M.D., F.A.C.S.
Clinical Assistant Professor, Department of Surgery, University of Pennsylvania, Philadelphia; Associate Director–Trauma Program, Department of Traumatology, St. Luke's Hospital, Bethlehem, Pennsylvania

Patrick M. Reilly, M.D., F.A.C.S.
Associate Professor of Surgery, Department of Surgery, Division of Traumatology and Surgical Critical Care, Hospital of the University of Pennsylvania, Philadelphia, Pennsylvania

Michael Rhodes, M.D., F.A.C.S.
Professor, Department of Surgery, Thomas Jefferson University; Chairman, Department of Surgery, Christiana Care Health Services, Wilmington, Delaware

Therese S. Richmond, Ph.D., C.R.N.P., F.A.A.N.
Associate Professor, Department of Trauma and Critical Care Nursing, School of Nursing, University of Pennsylvania; Researcher, Division of Traumatology and Surgical Critical Care, University of Pennsylvania Health System, Philadelphia, Pennsylvania

Kathy J. Rinnert, M.D., M.P.H.
Assistant Professor of Emergency Medicine, Department of Surgery, University of Texas Southwestern Medical Center; Emergency Medicine Faculty, Department of Emergency Services, Parkland Health and Hospital System, Dallas, Texas

Michael Rodricks, M.D.
Anesthesiologist and Intensivist, Department of Anesthesiology and Critical Care Medicine, Florida Hospital, Orlando, Florida

Ronald N. Roth, M.D., F.A.C.E.P.
Associate Professor, Department of Emergency Medicine, University of Pittsburgh; Chief, Division of Emergency Medical Services, Department of Emergency Medicine, University of Pittsburgh Health System, Pittsburgh, Pennsylvania

Michael F. Rotondo, M.D., F.A.C.S.
Professor and Vice Chair, Department of Surgery, Brody School of Medicine at East Carolina University; Chief, Department of Trauma and Surgical Critical Care, Pitt County Memorial Hospital, Greenville, North Carolina

James M. Russavage, M.D., D.M.D.
Assistant Professor, Department of Surgery, Division of Plastic and Maxillofacial Surgery, University of Pittsburgh, Pittsburgh, Pennsylvania

Michael Russell, M.D.
Assistant Professor, Department of Anesthesia, University of Pennsylvania; Staff Anesthesiologist and Intensivist, Department of Anesthesia and Surgical Critical Care, Hospital of the University of Pennsylvania, Philadelphia, Pennsylvania

Michael G. Scheidler, M.D.
Chief Resident, Department of General Surgery, Allegheny General Hospital, Pittsburgh, Pennsylvania

C. William Schwab, M.D., F.A.C.S.
Professor, Department of Surgery, University of Pennsylvania School of Medicine; Chief, Division of Traumatology and Surgical Critical Care, University of Pennsylvania Medical Center, Philadelphia, Pennsylvania

Michael B. Shapiro, M.D., F.A.C.S.
Assistant Professor, Department of Surgery, Division of Traumatology and Surgical Critical Care, Hospital of the University of Pennsylvania, Philadelphia, Pennsylvania

Bradley S. Taylor, M.D., M.P.H.
Chief Resident, Department of Cardiothoracic Surgery, University of Pittsburgh, Pittsburgh, Pennsylvania

Glen Tinkoff, M.D.
Medical Director of the Trauma Program, Christiana Care Health Services, Newark, Delaware; Clinical Associate Professor, Department of Surgery, Thomas Jefferson University Medical College, Philadelphia, Pennsylvania

Samuel A. Tisherman, M.D.
Associate Professor, Departments of Surgery and Anesthesiology / Critical Care Medicine, University of Pittsburgh, Pittsburgh, Pennsylvania

Ricard N. Townsend, M.D.
Associate Professor, Department of Surgery, University of Pittsburgh School of Medicine, University of Pittsburgh Medical Center, Presbyterian Hospital, Pittsburgh, Pennsylvania

Owen T. Traynor, M.D., F.A.C.S.
Instructor, Department of Emergency Medicine, University of Pittsburgh; Director of Emergency Medical Services, Department of Emergency Medicine, St. Clair Memorial Hospital, Pittsburgh, Pennsylvania

Rade B. Vukmir, M.D.
Clinical Associate Professor, Departments of Emergency Medicine, University of Pittsburgh, Pittsburgh; Director, Department of Emergency, Northwest Medical Center, Franklin, Pennsylvania

William C. Welch, M.D., F.A.C.S.
Associate Professor, University of Pittsburgh School of Medicine; Director of Spine Specialty Center and Neurological Spine Services, Department of Neurosurgery, University of Pittsburgh Medical Center, Presbyterian University Hospital, Pittsburgh, Pennsylvania

Donald M. Yealy, M.D., F.A.C.E.P.
Attending Physician & Vice Chair, Department of Emergency Medicine, University of Pittsburgh Medical Center; Professor, Department of Emergency Medicine, University of Pittsburgh, Pittsburgh, Pennsylvania

Bruce H. Ziran, M.D.
Assistant Professor, Department of Orthopaedic Surgery, University of Pittsburgh, Presbyterian Hospital, Pittsburgh, Pennsylvania

FOREWORD TO THE FIRST EDITION

The advent of another text in the important field of trauma care should prompt a careful examination of the motives of the editors and authors, their experience in this field, and their intentions in creating such a work. Their efforts should be weighed in a balance that measures the elements of the practical against the academic base upon which clinical care must be based: in short, the interplay of the art and the science of trauma care.

Underlying any manual outlining the clinical care of the injured patient should be a philosophy that defines the foundations of trauma care. Recognition of the multidisciplinary nature and breadth of trauma care—from prevention to rehabilitation and outcome measurement—and the basic philosophy of the "team approach" must be woven into the fabric of the work.

All this is not an easy task, and whether the intentions of the editors are achieved will depend heavily upon their experience in the actual provision of care, their exposure to students and of students to them, and the team that they have assembled to compose *The Trauma Manual*.

For these reasons we can expect much from this effort. The editors and authors here represent a young and vibrant cadre of clinicians who have been instrumental internationally in the definition and promotion of the art and science of trauma care. They are doers *and* thinkers who provide clinical care, and doers *and* dreamers who have a track record in the research that is so vital to the specialty.

This is perhaps the first comprehensive but concise trauma manual conceived during and based upon the significant strides made over the past decade in the management of patients in the "golden hour." The team assembled by the editors has been chosen with obvious care, representing clinicians who both do and teach. From beginning to end, the philosophy of a systems approach to the management of trauma and the importance of an efficient yet caring team approach are ever present in this work. The importance given to the recognition of patterns of injury reflects the clinical experience of the cadre of authors, as does the organized approach to diagnosis and early management. All this is presented against a background of applied anatomy and physiology woven into a clinical context. The prominence afforded to prehospital care and transport is testimony to the breadth of the view and experience of the editors, and reflects current thinking in this increasingly recognized field of care. The inclusion of an up-to-date review of pain management, social and family aspects of the critically injured patient, critical care, and rehabilitation illustrates the breadth of *The Trauma Manual* and its value to clinicians and students alike.

In its presentation and intention, *The Trauma Manual* reflects throughout a respect for students and clinicians at all levels of training and experience. *The Trauma Manual* demonstrates an economy of style that is fitting for the practical volume that it is designed to be. This is no small achievement by the editors.

If the measure of the value of a teaching manual is the achievement of a balance between accuracy and practicality, between the art and the science of clinical care, then this work is valuable indeed. It should evoke from students and clinicians admiration for a job well done on the part of the editors and authors, if not a sense of gratitude at the end of a long shift in the trauma center or from the clinician in a small hospital. This text can rest with dignity on the desk of the academic, or in the pocket of a first-year student in the late-night hours of a first night on call.

Ronald D. Stewart, o.c., b.a., bsc., m.d., f.r.c.p.c., f.a.c.e.p., dsc.
Professor of Emergency Medicine and Community Health and Epidemiology
Dalhousie University, Halifax, Nova Scotia, Canada
and Adjunct Professor of Emergency Medicine
University of Pittsburgh
Pittsburgh, Pennsylvania

FOREWORD TO THE FIRST EDITION

In 1966, two trauma centers were simultaneously formed in Chicago and San Francisco. Three years later, Dr. R.A. Cowley established the first statewide system in the state of Maryland. The development and maturation of trauma systems have yielded multiple positive by-products. The Optimal Resources Document of the American College of Surgeons Committee on Trauma requires that Level I Trauma Centers have a separate and identifiable trauma service. This in turn has led to the development of trauma and critical care fellowships. Residents and medical students now learn the principles of trauma care in a far more organized and scholarly manner.

The Trauma Manual is not just another book. It has been specifically crafted for the medical student, resident, and trauma fellow, and it has been designed specifically to be carried in their white jacket pockets. The editors have created a pragmatic, no-nonsense quick reference book for the people in the trenches. The editors have captured the principles of injury mechanisms, prehospital care, resuscitative care, operative priorities, and critical care. I predict that *The Trauma Manual* will be used often.

Donald Trunkey, M.D., F.A.C.S.
Professor and Chairman
Department of Surgery
Oregon Health Sciences University
Portland, Oregon

PREFACE

The goal of *The Trauma Manual* is to serve as a ready pocket reference for all who provide care for the trauma patient. The format of *The Trauma Manual* is that of a user-friendly pocket manual rather than a comprehensive textbook. With that said, this book contains a great deal of information covering all phases of trauma care. The major changes to the second edition of *The Trauma Manual* consist of updating information where necessary and making the book more compact to facilitate its use as a pocket reference.

The Trauma Manual is organized in a chronological fashion, following the usual events and phases of care after injury. As with the first edition, the chapters are written by authors within the appropriate specialties. The recommendations made are backed by the extensive clinical experience of these authors. Rather than listing every option in a clinical situation, a consensus recommendation is generally presented. Flow charts, sequential lists, and algorithms are used throughout as approaches to clinical problems. We have attempted to keep the content of *The Trauma Manual* practical and direct. The editors hope that this edition of *The Trauma Manual* again provides a clear, pragmatic approach to those providing care for the trauma patient.

Andrew B. Peitzman, M.D., F.A.C.S.
Timothy C. Fabian, M.D., F.A.C.S.
Michael Rhodes, M.D., F.A.C.S.
C. William Schwab, M.D., F.A.C.S.
Donald M. Yealy, M.D., F.A.C.E.P.

1. INTRODUCTION TO TRAUMA CARE

Michael D. Grossman

Trauma can be defined in terms of bodily injury severe enough to pose a threat to life or limb.

I. Epidemiology: The scope of trauma as a problem in the United States
   A. Trauma represents the leading cause of preventable death in persons under the age of 44 years in the United States. In 1998, accidental deaths—97,835—accounted for 4% of total deaths. Injury is the leading cause of productive life lost. Whether unintentional or intentional, most injuries are preventable.
   1. **Motor vehicle crashes** are the leading cause of unintentional and work-related death for all US citizens between the ages of 1 and 34 years. Annually, nearly 42,000 people die from motor vehicle-related injury, >3 million are injured, and 500,000 are hospitalized. Mortality rates are declining, however, because of comprehensive safety and prevention programs.
   2. **Falls** are second to motor vehicle crashes as a cause of unintentional death; 13,986 deaths were caused by falls in 1997. In children, falls are a common cause of head injury; the incidence is highest in infancy and declines steadily up to age 14 years.
   3. **Burn and fire-related injuries** in the home are declining in frequency, possibly because of the widespread use of safety devices such as smoke detectors. In 1997, burns caused 3,761 deaths; the incidence is highest in urban areas.
   4. **Intentional trauma** includes all aspects of violence: homicides, nonfatal assaults, and suicides. Most intentional trauma in the United States is caused by interpersonal violence; currently, most of this morbidity and mortality is related to firearms, the majority caused by handguns. Nearly 80% of the 40,000 deaths from penetrating trauma occur in the urban area, with 80% of these deaths caused by firearms. Of these firearm deaths, slightly less than half are homicides, the remainder are suicides.
   5. The trimodal distribution of deaths from trauma refers to the occurrence of death following trauma as a function of time. The three peaks of occurrence are immediate, early, and late. Massive head injury, brainstem injury, and major injury to the cardiovascular system cause immediate death. Half of all trauma deaths are immediate; most patients are unsalvageable. Early deaths occur within the first few hours. Major torso trauma and closed head injury, which account for most early deaths, are treatable in modern trauma centers. Deaths from multiple organ failure may represent 20% of all in-hospital deaths caused by trauma. Multiple organ failure following trauma has recently been described as occurring as an early and late consequence of injury. Early death from organ failure is more common in the patients with high injury severity score (ISS), greater transfusion requirement, and more severe hypoperfusion. Advanced age seems more important for late organ failure, which is commonly precipitated by infection.
   B. Trauma is the leading cause of disability in the United States. Approximately 50 million injuries occur each year, half of which require medical attention. Of those requiring medical attention, slightly >10% require hospitalization. Almost 20% of injured trauma victims sustain some form of disability; minor disability (e.g., a fractured extremity) occurs most often; major disability, including permanent neurologic impairment, affects 340,000 Americans per year.

    C. In the United States, in 1995, injury cost $260 billion. Cost is both direct, for healthcare expenditure, and indirect, lost productivity from death and disability.

        1. Nonfatal injury accounts for 69% of the total cost. Death occurs in only 1% of cases, but accounts for 31% of the costs.

        2. Spinal cord injury is the most expensive injury admission diagnosis in the United States: $56,800 per hospitalization, with a mean hospital stay of 16 days.

II. Trauma systems

    A. Trauma is a national health problem best dealt with by a coordinated system ensuring prompt access to optimal care and rehabilitation.

        1. Trauma systems have evolved that have been shown to:

            a. Equalize access of patients in both urban and rural environments to similar levels of care

            b. Reduce death and disability

            c. Create a formalized continuum from accident scene to rehabilitation

            d. Provide a mechanism for continuous quality improvement of the system

            e. Data collection and analysis of trends

III. Major components of a trauma system

    A. Prehospital care

        1. Discovery of injury. An "ordinary" citizen or a passerby may discover the injury, with varying periods of delay, depending on population density.

        2. Access and activation of prehospital care can occur through 911 or some alternative dispatch system that is hospital or municipal based.

        3. Life-saving prehospital medical care, including:

            a. Basic life support measures, including administration of oxygen, control of bleeding by direct pressure, and performance of cardiopulmonary resuscitation (CPR). In addition, provision of safe extrication and patient movement, as well as splinting and fracture immobilization.

            b. Advanced life support measures are provided by responders who have received advanced training in the assessment and treatment of the injured patient. Such responders provide basic life support (BLS) services, but also can perform airway intubation and chest decompression; establish intravenous (i.v.) lines; administer pharmacologic agents, and perform other sophisticated therapeutic maneuvers. These measures are done according to established protocol or standing orders directed by a medical command.

            c. Medical command is usually directed by the physician responsible for medical care given by the responding units in a given geographic area.

        4. Triage or injury assessment

            a. Triage determines severity of injury, injury to specific body parts, and special circumstances surrounding the mechanism of injury; it identifies "special populations" (i.e., the extremes of age and presence of significant comorbid medical conditions) and directs these patients at high risk to the most appropriate regional facility, usually a trauma center.

        5. Transport of these critically injured patients is by the most expeditious and efficient means possible.

            a. It is based on time and distance considerations, patient stability, and available skills of the prehospital providers. Both ground and aeromedical (usually helicopter) means are available.

    B. Acute hospital care

        1. Specialized, comprehensive acute care facilities called "trauma centers" are designated according to established criteria.

            a. Specialized personnel and services are available 24 hours a day.

                (1) Surgeons with special skills to treat injured patients facilitate an immediate diagnosis, surgery, and critical supportive care.

      (2) Operating rooms, anesthesia, blood bank, computed tomography (CT) scans, and so forth
      (3) Emergency physicians
      (4) Promptly available (within minutes): neurosurgeons, orthopedic surgeons, and other surgical and medical specialists
      (5) Trauma registries to facilitate continuous performance improvement (CPI) programs integrated with all components of the trauma system
      (6) Committed dedicated physician, nurse, and administrative leadership for the trauma program

  2. Each trauma center has its own trauma team activation system that responds to predetermined triage criteria, which single out those patients suspected of having sustained severe injury and ensure that they are met by a trauma team. Individuals on the trauma team have defined roles and responsibilities.

  3. Ideally, after the initial response, each hospital has a continuum of services to facilitate recuperation and rehabilitation of the trauma patient.
    a. Physical and occupational therapy, social work, physical medicine, and rehabilitation

  4. Each hospital has a mechanism in place to evaluate its professionals, and care and treatment services. This process is used for continuous performance improvement.
    a. The trauma system evaluates itself in the same fashion.

C. Long-term care and rehabilitation
  1. A dedicated link is in place between inpatient rehabilitation and acute care to ensure smooth transition to long-term recovery.

IV. Regional systems
  A. Regional systems are those that include prehospital provider agencies and hospitals.
  B. They are political in that they must determine how resources are allocated and where patients are taken.
  C. They must contain the following administrative components:
    1. Leadership (medical, political, economic, public health), usually located within a lead authority such as a Department of Health
    2. Continuous system development and planning for the future
    3. Legislation. Laws that assure that the trauma system functions as an integrated part of the Emergency Medical Services (EMS) system, but also as a larger comprehensive system to manage all aspects of injury care
    4. Finance: allocation of public funds
    5. Public education and injury prevention information (e.g., bicycle helmets, seatbelts, gun laws)
    6. Personnel
    7. Communications: 911, communication systems, access to system
    8. Hospitals and other facilities
      a. Trauma Centers designated and accredited by external objective review organizations using established national guidelines (e.g., American College of Surgeons and American College of Emergency Physicians)
      b. Ongoing periodic review to assure compliance with requirements for designation and accreditation
      c. Coordination with other system components to assure the needs of all injured patients

Axioms

- The care of the trauma patient requires a commitment to patient care that is independent of the circumstance of injury.
- Significant therapeutic interventions may be required with limited data to support them.
- Priorities for diagnostic and therapeutic procedures often compete, because of complex patterns of injury.

2. PATTERNS OF BLUNT INJURY

Michael D. Grossman

Mechanism Of Injury

Trauma is a severe physical injury resulting from dissipation of energy to and within the victim, caused by a penetrating or blunt mechanism. The anatomic injury and subsequent physical derangement depend on the location of the injury and the amount of energy dissipated. In general, widely used divisions are found in the pattern of injury: blunt versus penetrating; intentional versus unintentional; high energy versus low energy, and so on. In this manual, the division is between blunt and penetrating injury and emphasis is on the frequency of injuries associated with various mechanisms of injury.

As experience is gained in the care of trauma victims, patterns of injury associated with a particular mechanism of injury become apparent. Based on the report received from the crash scene, the injuries in the trauma victim should be anticipated.

Blunt Trauma
I. **Types**: motor vehicle crashes, motorcycle crashes, pedestrian–automobile impacts, falls, assaults
   A. **Chance of major injury increases 300% to 500% in a motor vehicle crash with ejection.**
      1. **Risk of spinal column injury is 1 in 13 when a victim is ejected** from the vehicle.
   B. Injuries are produced by a rapid decrease in velocity over a short distance (**deceleration**). Severity of injury depends on **energy transferred** during deceleration that occurs during the crash or fall.
   C. Motor vehicle crashes involve three separate collisions.
      1. Motor vehicle impacts another object—primary collision.
      2. Victim strikes internal parts of the car—secondary collision(s).
      3. Soft tissues versus supporting structures of the body.
         a. Deformation caused by deceleration causes differential movement of fixed versus nonfixed parts (e.g., shearing injury to the brain or transection of the thoracic aorta).
II. Motor vehicle collision: determinants of injury.
   A. Injury risk of occupant(s) inversely related to **size and weight** of car
   B. **Location of victim in the car**
      1. Injury patterns vary based on front seat versus back seat, driver versus passenger.
   C. **Use and type of restraint devices.** Restraining devices are effective if worn correctly. Improperly applied restraining devices can lead to unusual injuries. Injury risk is greater in unrestrained victims. Lap belts alone decrease mortality by 50% but increase the rate of abdominal injury. Three-point restraint plus airbag decreases mortality even further, especially in front-end collisions.
      1. Three-point restraint minimizes secondary collisions of occupant with vehicle; substantially decreases mortality; and prevents ejection. Driver's head may contact steering wheel (minor head injury) but most restraints prevent the passenger's head from contact with the car frame. Sternal and rib fractures are common. Extremity injuries are not prevented. **No effect on major injury patterns in side impact collisions.**
      2. Shoulder belt. Inadvisable to wear alone. Back seat passengers can "submarine" out from under the belt. The lap belt is designed to fit across the anterior superior iliac spines of the pelvis. **When applied over the abdomen, Chance fractures (hyperflexion) of the lum-**

bar spine can occur; hollow viscus injuries (particularly small bowel rupture) are also associated with improper use.
3. Air bag plays a principal role in frontal collisions. Gentler deceleration than three-point restraint, fewer rib and thoracic injuries, no head contacts with steering wheel. **Proportion and severity of lower extremity injuries increased relative to torso and head injuries.** Air bag can cause injuries to occupants who are "out of position": facing backward, leaning against steering wheel, leaning into passenger compartment.
D. **Direction of impact**
1. **Frontal impacts** are the most common direction of impact (64%). Victims are less likely to have been belted; they are more frequently intoxicated and have lower overall mortality than those of a lateral impact. Injury patterns associated with this direction of impact are shown in Table 2.1. Facial and chest injuries are most frequent. Lower extremity injuries are three times more common than in lateral impacts.
2. **Rear-end impact** collisions do not commonly produce injuries severe enough to warrant admission to a trauma center. Only 8% of crashes producing serious injury are rear impacts. Secondary front-end impacts can be produced from high-speed rear-end impacts. Cervical sprains or "whiplash" injuries are common.
3. **Rollover collisions** are difficult to model because force vectors vary. Kinetic energy of the car is often dissipated over a long distance as the car rolls, which can minimize injury to the occupants, particularly if the victim is restrained. Roof collapse can produce severe head injury. Compression fractures of the spine from axial load are common. Unrestrained occupants can be ejected or be crushed by the vehicle.
4. **Lateral crashes, or T-bone,** on the driver's side of the car cause direct impact between the victim and the colliding vehicle; neither space nor metal is present to slow the oncoming vehicle. Injury patterns associated with this direction of impact are shown in Table 2.1. **Lateral impact collisions are associated with twice the mortality of frontal impacts.** Thoracic and abdominal injuries are most prevalent. Victims tend to be older than victims of frontal impacts. If not restrained, the driver is projected into the passenger compartment.

Table 2.1 Injury patterns in frontal and lateral impact crashes

Injury	Frontal crashes No. (%) (n = 2,804)	Left lateral crashes No. (%) (n = 376)	P-value
Brain	488 (17.4)	68 (18.1)	NS
Face	1,268 (45.2)	102 (27.1)	<0.05
Thorax	680 (24.3)	137 (36.4)	<0.05
Abdomen (total)	693 (21.2)	138 (28.7)	<0.05
Liver	77 (2.8)	16 (4.3)	NS
Spleen	72 (2.6)	30 (8.0)	<0.0001
Pelvis	154 (5.5)	75 (20.0)	<0.05
Lower extremity (total)	508 (18.1)	26 (6.9)	<0.05
Femur	208 (7.4)	17 (4.5)	<0.05
Tibia/fibula	84 (4.5)	4 (1.1)	<0.001
Ankle/foot	138 (4.9)	4 (1.1)	<0.001

NS, not significant.
(Adapted from Dischinger PC, Cushing BM, Kerns TJ. Injury patterns associated with direction of impact: drivers admitted to trauma centers. *J Trauma* 1993;35:454, with permission.)

III. Pedestrian–automobile impact

A. Pedestrian–automobile impact accounts for 2% of traffic injuries and 13% of traffic-related deaths. This mechanism of injury is more common in children and elderly persons. Figure 2.1 depicts the common pattern of injury in pedestrian–automobile impacts. Musculoskeletal (35%) and intracranial injuries (27%) are most common. Torso injuries involving chest, abdomen, or pelvis occur in a few victims (6%).

    1. Initial contact is between bumper and lower extremity. A braking vehicle strikes low on the tibia as the front-end moves downward during rapid

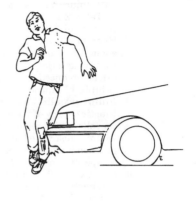

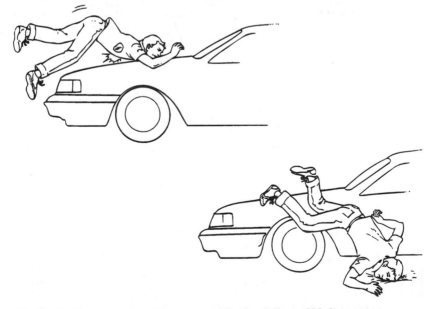

FIG. 2.1. Pedestrian–automobile impact. (©Baylor College of Medicine 1986. Modified from Feliciano DV, Moore EE, Mattox KL. *Trauma*, 3rd ed. Norwalk: Appleton and Lange, Englewood Cliffs, N.J., 1996:97, with permission.)

deceleration. The head, torso, or both strike the hood or windscreen, resulting in closed head injuries. Collision with the ground follows.

    a. Patients with this mechanism of impact may sustain **Waddle's triad** of injury: tibia-fibula or femur fracture, truncal injury, and craniofacial injury.

    b. Children tend to be "run-over."

    c. Adults tend to be struck in the lower legs by the car, again contact the car, then "run-under" or are thrown over the car with impact on the street. Contact between hip and fender can produce similar impact forces with lateral compression pelvic fractures.

IV. Motorcycle crashes. Victims in motorcycle crashes, unlike motor vehicle crashes, usually absorb all impact and kinetic energy. Injuries depend on motorcycle speed and the anatomic location of impact. Cranial injuries account for 75% of motorcycle deaths; risk decreases by one half when a protective helmet is worn. Spine, pelvis, including open pelvis, and extremity injuries are also common. Injuries to the tibia and fibula are often open or severe, with high risk of limb loss. Scapular fractures can be seen in victims following impact with the ground.

V. Falls. Two basic injury patterns occur after falls. Major, life-threatening unisystem injury can accompany falls from standing or low elevations. Such injuries are frequent in the elderly, with comorbid disease having a major impact on outcome. In the elderly, comorbid conditions (e.g., arthritis and visual disturbances) can also contribute to *causing* the fall. The elderly can fall while walking in the home, resulting in femoral neck fractures, and head and cervical spine injuries. Falls occurring from a height can involve a tumbling mechanism or "free fall." The elderly, infants, and toddlers can fall on stairs and tumble a distance of 10 to 15 feet. Multiple injuries—more common than in a fall from standing—include rib fractures and fractures of the thoracolumbar spine. Free falls imply a fall from a height directly to the ground. Mortality rates of 50% are associated with falls of 25 to 30 feet (three stories). Survival is rare in falls from above five stories.

    A. Injuries sustained in falls depend on distance of fall, surface struck, and position on impact.

    B. Energy at impact is the product of the victim's weight times distance of fall times gravitational forces.

        1. On impact, kinetic energy is dissipated throughout the skeleton and soft tissues of the victim.

        2. Duration of impact (i.e., how quickly the victim stops) is critical in determining injury severity.

            a. Impact force over a shorter time increases the magnitude of injury.

            b. Harder surface increases severity of injury because of immediate deceleration and transfer of all energy to the body (e.g., concrete versus grass or snow).

        3. **Falls are common in children under 5 years of age**. Head, the heaviest body part in young children, tends to impact first.

        4. Falls from a height above 10 to 15 feet have a variable injury pattern in adults (Fig. 2.2). Adults may try to land on their feet with a pattern of injuries that includes calcaneal fractures, lower extremity fractures, hip fractures, vertical shear injuries of the pelvis, and spine fractures (all segments). Renal injury is a common visceral injury. Energy dissipation can be greater with fewer injuries when a victim lands in a horizontal orientation. These injuries occur in a less predictable pattern and include craniofacial trauma, hand and wrist fractures, and abdominal and thoracic visceral injuries (particularly retroperitoneal structures, tear at aortic root).

        5. Falls down multiple stairs, which produce unpredictable injury patterns, are seen increasingly in the geriatric population. Significant energy can be imparted. Spine fractures should be suspected.

VI. Assaults (fist, kicking, stomping, baseball bat, pipe)

    A. Young men are most commonly affected. Injury patterns can be unpredictable, depending on weapon used, patient position, and intensity of the attack.

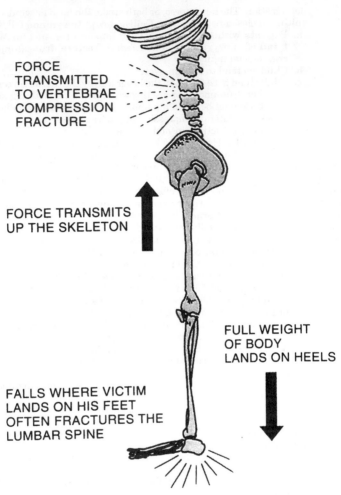

FORCE TRANSMITTED TO VERTEBRAE COMPRESSION FRACTURE

FORCE TRANSMITS UP THE SKELETON

FULL WEIGHT OF BODY LANDS ON HEELS

FALLS WHERE VICTIM LANDS ON HIS FEET OFTEN FRACTURES THE LUMBAR SPINE

FIG. 2.2. Injury patterns for falls. (From Campbell JE, ed. *Basic trauma life support*, 3rd ed. Prentice-Hall, 1988, with permission.)

  1. Injuries to head and face occur in 72%.
       a. Upper (5%) and lower extremity (4%) injuries can be seen from defensive wounds.
       b. Stomping or kicking injuries to supine or prone victims can result in severe torso injury. Pancreatic and hollow viscus injuries predominate in the abdomen.
       c. Intoxicated assault victims with depressed level of consciousness **have intracranial injuries until proved otherwise**.

Axioms
- Injuries are often predictable, based on vector and force involved on impact.
- Think injury patterns, rather than isolated injury.
- Lateral impacts cause twice the mortality to frontal crashes.

Bibliography

Daffner RH, Deeb ZL, Lupetin AR, et al. Patterns of high-speed impact injuries in motor vehicle occupants. *J Trauma* 1988;28:498.

Dischinger PC, Cushing BM, Kerns TJ. Injury patterns associated with direction of impact: drivers admitted to trauma centers. *J Trauma* 1993;35:454.

Feliciano DV, Wall MJ Jr. Patterns of injury. In: Moore EE, Mattox KL, Feliciano DV, eds. *Trauma*. Norwalk: Appleton & Lange, 1988:81–96.

Lowenstein SR, Yaron M. Carrero R, et al. Vertical trauma: injuries to patients who fall and land on their feet. *Ann Emerg Med* 1989;18:161–165.

Peng RY, Bongard F. Pedestrian versus motor vehicle accidents: an analysis of 5000 patients. *J Am Coll Surg* 1999;189:343.

Wladis A, Bostrom L, Nilsson B. Unarmed violence-related injuries requiring hospitalization in Sweden from 1987 to 1994. *J Trauma* 1999;47:733.

3. MECHANISMS OF INJURY/PENETRATING TRAUMA

J. Christopher DiGiacomo and James F. Reilly

Objects that penetrate the human body lacerate, disrupt, destroy, and contuse tissue. It is imperative that physicians have a detailed knowledge of how different projectiles cause injury. Management decisions are based on wound and location, trajectory, degree of tissue injury, and a thorough three-dimensional understanding of anatomy. In general, the aphorism for penetrating injury is: **Trajectory determination defines anatomic injury!**

FIREARMS: A firearm is defined as any weapon, especially a pistol or rifle, capable of firing a projectile and using an explosive charge as a propellant.

I. Gunshot wounds
   A. **Ballistics**. Ballistics strictly defined is the science of powder-propelled projectiles in motion. However, in medicine it has come to mean the study of wounding of the body by the projectile. The biomechanics of tissue damage is based on the **kinetic energy of the projectile** and the **density and elasticity of the tissue**. The wounding potential of a missile can be described by the permanent and temporary cavities that it produces, which is the wound profile.
      1. **Internal ballistics** refers to motion within the weapon.
         a. **Caliber** is the diameter of the bullet or gun barrel, designated in decimal fractions of an inch. Bullet caliber does not correlate to wound size.
         b. **Muzzle velocity** is the velocity of the bullet as it leaves the gun barrel. This is the maximal velocity the bullet attains and in general approximates the velocity of the bullet when it impacts its target.
         c. **Rifling** refers to the spiral grooves milled into the barrel of a firearm to stabilize the flight of a bullet and improve accuracy.
         d. **Barrel length**. Lengthening the barrel of a gun allows more time for the propellant powder to burn while it is in contact with the projectile. This typically increases the muzzle velocity of the projectile.
         e. **Cartridge**. A single round of ammunition is composed of the cartridge casing, propellant powder, primer, wads (shotguns), and projectile(s).
      2. **External ballistics** refers to motion of the projectile in the air.
         a. **Yaw** is the deviation of the longitudinal axis of the bullet from its line of flight. This is discouraged by rifling within the barrel of the firearm, which imparts spin and stabilizes the projectile in flight. This is analogous to the stable flight of a football when a long pass is thrown with a "perfect" spiral, as compared with the wobble when thrown imperfectly.
         b. **Tumbling** refers to yaw through 180°, at which point the projectile can stabilize in base-forward flight. This is also minimized by rifling.
         c. Because of resistance against air, the projectile starts to slow as soon as it exits the muzzle.
      3. **Terminal ballistics** refers to motion and effect of a projectile on striking a solid or liquid.
         a. **Kinetic energy**. Projectiles from firearms dissipate a tremendous amount of kinetic energy (KE) to the tissues through which they pass (Table 3-1). This energy is responsible for a significant degree of the damage caused by the projectile. Increasing the velocity of a projectile has a much greater effect on KE than increasing its mass.

         $$KE = 1/2 \ mv^2$$

         (KE = kinetic energy in joules; m = mass in grams; v = velocity in feet/second).

Table 3.1 Comparison of bullet weight, velocity, kinetic energy, and maximal temporary cavitation

Cartridge/ bullet	Weight (grains)	Velocity (m/sec)	Velocity (ft/sec)	Kinetic energy (joules)	Maximal temporary cavity (cm)
Handguns					
–.38	82–158	214–384	693–1,244	200–390	4.0–8.3
–9 mm	82–115	372–430	1,205–1,393	500–700	8.2–10.6
–.45	140–255	241–421	781–1,364	480–800	4.0–12.3
–.357	110–125	425–479	1,377–1,552	730–810	9.4–11.0
Shotguns					
–12g, #4 shot (27 pellets) @ 3 m	540	412	1,335	2,970	12.0
–12g rifled slug	437	461	1,494	3,018	11.0
Rifles					
–.22 long rifle	37–40	342–388	1,122–1,272	152–181	4.0–5.0
–30-30	170	615	2,017	2,089	18.0
–30 carbine	110	619	2,030	1,370	14.0
–223 center-fire	50–55	943–960	3,094–3,150	1,475–1,600	13.0–14.0
Military rifles					
–5.56 mm (M16)	50–55	853–1,000	2,800–3,250	1,350–1,670	13.0–14.0
–5.45 mm (AK-74)	53	935	3,029	1,486	14.0
–7.62 mm (AK-47)	150–170	615–891	1,993–2,887	2,010–3,850	14.0–23.0

    b. Tissue characteristics. In general, the greater the density of the tissue, the more energy transferred.

       (1) Permanent cavity—the hole or missile tract itself in which the projectile has destroyed tissue by crushing it as it moves through the tissue. Corresponds to the cross-sectional area of the projectile and is influenced by projectile deformation, yaw, and fragmentation (Fig. 3.1).

       (2) Temporary cavity is the maximal lateral displacement of the walls of the permanent cavity resulting from the dissipation of KE as the projectile interacts with the tissue. This is also influenced by projectile deformation, yaw, and fragmentation. Injury occurs in this area of *blast effect* as the result of tissues stretching; a function of the intrinsic elasticity of the tissue, its tolerance to stretch, and rate of energy dissipation (Fig. 3.1).

II. Gun types

    A. Handgun is a firearm that can be fired with only one hand. The barrel length is usually <8 inches and has no shoulder stock.

       1. Revolver is a handgun that uses a revolving cylinder to advance cartridges into line with the barrel for firing.

       2. Pistol can refer to any handheld firearm. The words handgun and pistol are often used synonymously. More commonly, the term pistol refers to semiautomatic handguns that use a spring-loaded magazine to "chamber" cartridges, which positions the next round into the firing chamber.

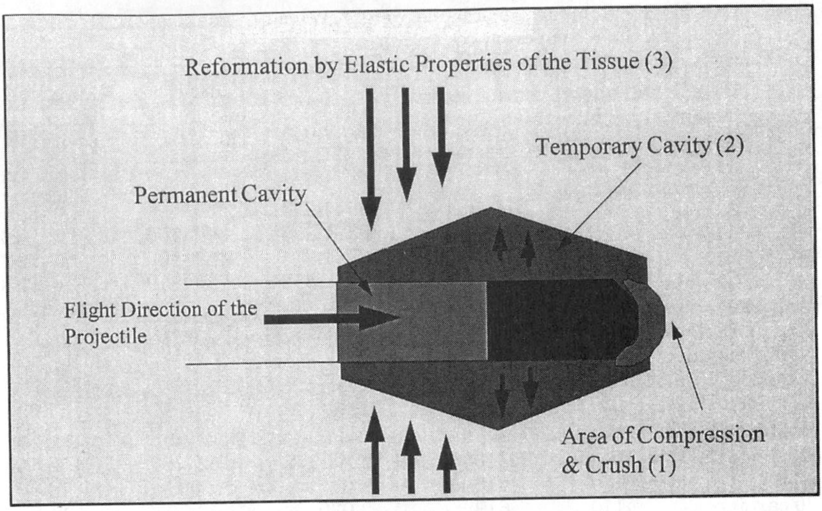

FIG. 3.1. Conceptual and graphic representation of the wound profile. As the projectile passes through the tissue, the permanent cavity is created by crushing. 1. The cavitation is created around the permanent cavity by stretching of the surrounding tissue. 2. This elastic property of the tissue recoils and closes the temporary cavity. 3. All this occurs in microseconds. (Modified from McSwain NE. Ballistics. In: Ivatury R, Cayton C, eds. *Textbook of penetrating trauma.* Philadelphia: Williams & Wilkins, 1996:105–120.)

      3. 22 Caliber. Low muzzle velocity. Tissue is disrupted by direct crushing and is greatest when the bullet is traveling sideways. Temporary cavitation is negligible.

      4. 38 Special. Common urban revolver. Produces most of its tissue destruction by direct crushing. Maximal temporary cavity occurs at a tissue depth of 20 to 25 cm, but remains too small to produce significant tissue injury through stretch.

      5. 9 mm Pistol. Popular urban pistol. Semiautomatic action (fires a single bullet as fast as the shooter can pull the trigger) allows more rapid firing of sequential rounds and has potential for an increased number of bullet wounds per patient as compared with revolvers. Wound profile similar to the .38 Special, but with larger temporary cavitation, resulting in stretch injury (radial splits) in less elastic tissues.

      6. 45 Caliber. Has a large bullet that produces tissue destruction by direct crushing.

      7. 357 Magnum. The term "magnum" refers to the addition of extra explosives in the cartridge of the bullet to increase muzzle velocity and KE of the bullet. These handguns are larger and heavier than most handguns.

   B. Long guns

      1. Shotgun is a long gun that can fire a shell containing multiple projectiles. Each shell can contain 8 to 400 or more spherical pellets (commonly referred to as "shot") or one rifled slug. Shotguns have one or two barrels, which can be shortened to 12 to 16 inches ("sawed-off") to increase the shot spread at close quarters. Cartridges are loaded with a manual, pump action, or semiautomatic loading mechanism. The size bore in the barrel is designated by gauge. Shotguns generate projectile KE in the range of high velocity and military rifles, although the energy of the shot pellets dissipates rapidly as the target distance increases. **At**

a range of <12 to 15 feet, the injury pattern is similar to high velocity rifle wounds with massive soft tissue destruction. At "close" ranges, multiple fragments of the shotgun shell, casing, and wadding are carried into and contaminate the wound. Most tissue destruction from temporary cavitation occurs within 5 to 10 cm of the skin surface and results from the pellets and expanding gases from the barrel, with deeper injuries resulting from crush injury by the pellets themselves. This typically results in massive destruction of the soft tissues with minimal bony injury. Given the extensive soft tissue injury, salvaging viable tissue is of the utmost importance and, therefore, extensive debridement at the initial operative exploration should be avoided. Instead, a limited initial washout and debridement to remove foreign bodies, bits of clothing, and so forth should be performed, followed by daily irrigation and debridement in the operating room. Reconstruction typically requires the skill of a plastic surgeon. These patients have the most expensive and longest length of stays in the hospital.

2. **Rifle** is a long gun with spiraling grooves, "rifling", milled into the inside of the barrel. Rifles usually discharge a single projectile using a manual bolt action, lever, pump, or semiautomatic mechanism for loading. Most bullets fired from rifles fall into a higher velocity range and will produce temporary cavities many times larger than the projectile itself. Injury from the stretching of tissues by the temporary cavity tends to begin within 5 to 10 cm of tissue depth (and may include the skin itself) and can extend to a depth of 40 to 45 cm.

3. A **machine gun** uses a fully automatic mechanism to load and fire rifle type cartridges. Machine guns can fire multiple shots per trigger pull. The weapon will continue to fire as long as the trigger is engaged and until the ammunition is spent.

4. A **submachine gun** uses a fully automatic mechanism to load and fire handgun caliber ammunition, making it easily fired by a single person.

5. An **assault rifle** can discharge rifle cartridges in either the fully automatic or semiautomatic mode. The full automatic mode allows the weapon to fire continuously while keeping the trigger depressed, as opposed to the semiautomatic mode, which automatically chambers the next round for firing, but requires the trigger to be depressed each time a round is to be fired. The automatic mode is restricted to use by only the military. The term "assault rifle" is commonly misused in the vernacular to refer to weapons that resemble military type guns, but that are, by law, only able to use a semiautomatic mode.

III. **Cartridges**. The term cartridge is used to describe a single round of ammunition used in a firearm. The basic elements of a cartridge include the cartridge casing, wads (shotgun), primer, propellant, and the projectile(s).

A. The **cartridge casing** is a metal casing that houses the propellant, primer, and bullet. The casing is the empty shell that is ejected from the firearm after the gun is fired.

B. A **bullet** is a single projectile fired from a firearm. In the case of shotguns, the projectiles are usually multiple spherical pellets.

C. The **jacket** is a harder metal coating on a lead bullet designed to enhance feeding into the firearm and control or prevent the bullet from deforming as it hits the target.

D. **Full metal jacketed bullet**. A metal jacketed bullet with no hollow point or exposed soft point typically does not deform on impact the target. This is the only type of bullet allowed by the Geneva Convention.

E. **Hollow point bullets** have a concave or hollow tip that allows the projectile to expand or flatten ("mushroom") as it hits the target. In some designs, the metal jacket can peel away from the tip of the bullet, forming talons or metal claws on the outer edge of the bullet.

F. A **soft point bullet** is partially jacketed, but has exposed lead at the nose to promote deformation or mushrooming on impact with the target.

    G. Core. The core of a jacketed bullet is usually made of lead.

    H. Bullet diameter. The United States system measures bullet diameter in hundredths or thousandths of an inch (e.g., .32, .357, .45), whereas the European system uses millimeters. A 9 mm bullet is about the same diameter as a .35 caliber bullet.

    I. Propellant powder is usually smokeless gunpowder, although black powder or various explosive charges are sometimes used. The term "magnum" refers to cartridges with increased amounts or higher quality powder used to increase bullet velocity.

    J. Wadding is material used in a shotgun shell to separate the powder from the projectile(s) and in firing to contain the powdered gases behind the shot pellets. Wadding is found in the shotgun shell between the propellant and the projectiles.

IV. Airguns, air rifles, and pellet guns are any type of gun that uses compressed air, gas, or springs to discharge the projectile. Typically, gas is released behind the projectile, which is then propelled down the barrel and out of the gun. Used primarily for sport and target shooting, or as toys for children, these weapons can generate muzzle velocities comparable to handguns. Projectiles can penetrate eyes, skin, calvarium, and torso, especially in children, causing visceral injury.

    A. Three types:

        1. Pneumatic. Two categories of pneumatic gun use either a single stroke or multiple strokes of a lever or pump to fill the reservoir with air. The air is released by a valve mechanism that is connected to the trigger. When the trigger is pulled, air escapes out the barrel, propelling the projectile. Produces muzzle velocities from 99 to 270 m/sec.

        2. Spring. The most common type and least expensive. The cocking mechanism retracts a piston inside a sealed cylinder. When pulled, the trigger releases the piston and forces compressed air against the base of the projectile. Produces muzzle velocities from 84 to 307 m/sec.

        3. Carbon dioxide cartridge. A valve mechanism is used to release CO_2 behind the projectile. In some designs, multiple rounds can be fired without the need for a manual lever action or reloading between shots. Produces muzzle velocities from 120 to 192 m/sec.

    B. Projectiles

        1. BB are spherical projectiles discharged from nonpowdered or air weapons. Most are made of steel with a copper coating. Lead BBs are less likely to ricochet; they weigh 5.5 grains (0.36 g).

        2. Pellets refers to any number of different projectiles that range in shape from spherical to cylindrical, conical, or hourglass shaped. They can be distinguished from bullets and shot, which are propelled via a powder charge. The most common size is .177 caliber (weight 15.3 grains or 0.99 g).

V. Stab wounds result from "hand driven" weapons, such as knives, needles, ice picks, and so forth.

    A. Slash type wounds, typically, are long laceration of relatively shallow depth. Wounds tend to gape, allowing easy visual inspection of their depth.

    B. Stab/impalement type. Weapon is usually plunged into victim along long axis of blade, resulting in small puncture wound of the skin and unknown depth. Wound size and history of type of weapon does not correlate to depth of wound or wound trajectory because victim's and witnesses' perceptions may not be accurate given the heightened emotional states at time of injury. "Stab" implies the use of a knife, whereas "impalement" connotes a larger object driven into the torso. If the wounding agent is still in the victim on arrival at the treatment facility, it should probably not be removed except in the operating room. Of stab wounds, 4% mortality rate is primarily from direct injury to great vessels or the heart.

VI. Impalement usually occurs secondary to a fall onto a piercing object or sustained from machinery or pneumatic tools (nail guns), but also includes low velocity non-firearm missiles such as arrows. An impaling object can be providing tamponade of major vessels and therefore **should be removed only in the op-**

erating room under direct vision after thorough dissection of the wound tract. The wound can be complicated by blunt deceleration from the fall, by secondary injuries resulting from extraction by untrained personnel, or unintentional shifts of the impaling object during transport.

VII. **Crossbows**. Usually used for hunting. Generates bolt velocity of 61–84.4 m/sec. Bolts are usually unable to pass through weight-bearing bone, but easily penetrate ribs, sternum, posterior vertebral elements, and calvarium. Should be treated as an impalement.

VIII. **Bows**. Archery and hunting bows can generate arrow velocities up to 74 m/sec. Arrow penetration is a function of arrow momentum (weight and velocity) and type of tip (target vs. hunting). These wounds should be treated as an impalement.

IX. **Forensics/wound description**. Because the medical record is a legal document that can be subpoenaed by the courts, it is essential that all wounds be accurately described in a precise and objective manner and evidence be preserved. Wound sizes should be measured—not estimated—and their positions related to recognized anatomic landmarks. **Drawings are especially useful**. Clothing represents important physical evidence and should be preserved. For example, bullet holes should not be disturbed when cutting through the patient's clothing. By destroying evidence, a physician or nurse is not acting as a victim's advocate and may jeopardize the ability of the justice system to convict the perpetrator or determine liability.

A. **Gunshot wounds**. The differentiation between entrance wounds and exit wounds is exceedingly difficult and not vital to the care of the patient. The incorrect documentation of a wound as an entrance or exit wound can undermine the ability to convict the perpetrator and, therefore, should be left to forensic experts. Indeed, two holes can represent two entrance wounds. **Documentation of wounds should only describe appearance and location**. Physicians should absolutely avoid using terms such as entrance or exit wounds. However, the dictated operative report should include descriptions of the organs injured and their injuries in the narrative; it can also include an assessment of trajectory and directionality if the intraoperative findings make such an opinion possible.

B. **X-rays**. When used in conjunction with the physical examination, x-ray films can often be used to determine trajectory. The caliber of the bullet, however, **cannot** be determined radiographically, and should not be attempted. No certainty exists that the radiodense object is in fact a bullet and not some other object shaped like a bullet. Further, it is not possible to ascertain the age of the bullet seen on the x-ray. It may, in fact, be a bullet from a previous and unrelated event and not be the "current" bullet. Therefore, documentation of the interpretation of the radiographs in the medical record should consist of terms such as "foreign body" or "bullet-shaped radioopaque object."

C. **Retrieved bullets**. Care should be taken not to damage any retrieved bullet because the markings on the side of the bullet are the gun's fingerprint and can be matched to the gun that fired it. Extraction from the body should be by rubber-shod instruments to prevent scratching and altering the bullet's signature. Mark the bullet on its base with the tip of a scalpel, with a simple mark such as X, +, =, or ++. The mark should be recorded in the brief operative note in the medical record and then must pass through a chain of evidence protocol, whether submitted to pathology or police. The caliber of the bullet should not be estimated for the same reasons as outlined above. However, any special or strange characteristics can be noted (i.e., four metal flanges on side.)

Bibliography

DiMaio VJM. Gunshot wounds: practical aspects of firearms, ballistics, and forensic techniques (CRC Series in Practical Aspects of Criminal and Forensic Investigation). Boca Raton, CRC Press, 1992.

Fackler ML. How to describe bullet holes. *Ann Emerg Med* 1994;23:386–387.

Fackler ML, Bellamy RF, Maliniwski JA. The wound profile: illustration of the missile-tissue interaction. *J Trauma* 1988;28(Suppl 1):S21–S29.

Karlson TA, Hargarten S. Reducing firearm injury and death: a public health source-book on guns. New Brunswick, NJ: Rutgers University Press, 1997.

McGonigal MD, Cole J, Schwab CW, et al. Urban firearm homicides: a five-year per-spective. *J Trauma* 1993;35:532–537.

Mendelson JA. The relationship between mechanisms of wounding and principles of treatment of missile wounds. *J Trauma* 1991;31:1181–1202.

Missile-caused wounds. In: Bowen TE, Bellamy RF, eds. *Emergency war surgery.* Washington, DC: United States Government Printing Office, 1988.

Nuzumlali ME, Kése H, Demirel D. Primary closure of gunshot wounds caused by high-velocity rifles. *Mil Med* 1993;158:563–565.

Rouse DA. Patterns of stab wounds: a six-year study. *Med Sci Law* 1994;34:67–71.

Swan KG, Swan RC. Principles of ballistics applicable to the treatment of gunshot wounds. *Surg Clin North Am* 1991;71:221–239.

4. THE PHYSIOLOGIC RESPONSE TO INJURY

Bradley S. Taylor and Brian G. Harbrecht

I. **Introduction.** Trauma results in significant physiologic changes in nearly all organ systems. The sympathetic nervous system and the neurohormonal response systems, acting locally and systemically, mediate the physiologic compensations that normally occur with traumatic injury. Fear, pain, hemorrhage, hypovolemia, hypoxemia, hypercarbia, acidosis, and tissue injury can contribute to the stress response to injury, which is designed to reestablish homeostasis. The response is proportional to the extent of injury. Critical illness and death can result when the stress response is sustained after severe trauma.
   A. **Stress response syndrome.** Psychological and physical perceptions of pain, injury, and shock can contribute to the stress response. Afferent impulses from the injury site are transmitted to the central nervous system where they are processed. Efferent signals mediate the physiologic response designed to correct the inciting event.
II. **Afferent stimuli (sympathoadrenal axis and hypothalamic-pituitary-adrenal axis).** Neural afferent signals via peripheral sensory nerves converge on the brain and activate the reflex arcs, which initiate the sympathetic nervous system output and hypothalamic stimulation. Epinephrine and norepinephrine are released from the sympathetic nervous system, resulting in an immediate increase in blood pressure, heart rate, myocardial contractility, and minute ventilation. Hypothalamic release of corticotropin-releasing hormone results in the production of corticotropin from the anterior pituitary gland, which stimulates the adrenal cortex to synthesize and release cortisol. The effects of hypercortisolism, designed to restore lost circulatory volume and provide energy substrates to sustain vital organ function, include gluconeogenesis, lipolysis, insulin resistance, sodium retention, and protein catabolism. The sympathoadrenal axis and hypothalamic-pituitary-adrenal axis are designed to initiate corrective responses to maintain essential organ perfusion and function.
   A. **Sensory neural input (pain).** The perception of pain and pain itself are important activators of the sympathetic nervous system and the hypothalamic-pituitary axis. Afferent signals from the injured tissue project to the thalamus via the spinothalamic tracts and result in activation of the hypothalamic-pituitary-adrenal axis and the subsequent release of cortisol. In addition, catecholamine release from the adrenal medulla is increased by direct neural stimulation.
   B. **Baroreceptor (hypovolemia).** Hemorrhage and intravascular hypovolemia stimulate baroreceptors in the aorta and carotid bodies and volume receptors in the atria, which signal to the central nervous system. Atrial baroreceptors are activated, first with low-volume hemorrhage, whereas arterial baroreceptors respond to more severe hemorrhage. Baroreceptors normally exert tonic inhibition of the autonomic nervous system. With hypovolemia, there is a reduction in baroreceptor impulses, which results in increased neural activity and centrally mediated vasoconstriction.
   C. **Chemoreceptor (hypoxemia, acidosis, hypercarbia, hypothermia).** Chemoreceptors located in the carotid bodies and aorta are activated by hypoxemia, acidosis, and hypercarbia, which activate the centrally mediated stress response systems. In addition, hypothermia is sensed by the preoptic area of the hypothalamus and triggers the hypothalamic-pituitary-adrenal axis.
   D. **Wound-mediated (cytokines).** Wounded and ischemic tissues produce a number of both locally and systemically acting mediators. The extent of these responses, which is dependent on the size and degree of ischemic injury at the tissue level, serves to initiate mechanisms important in coagulation, metabolism, and inflammation. These mediators are a less-rapid response to injury

than are the aforementioned neural inputs, and they frequently play a role in cell-to-cell communication (e.g., cytokines such as interleukin-6).

III. Efferent stimuli. The purpose of the efferent response is to reestablish homeostasis by restitution of the effective circulating plasma volume, to provide fuel, and to maintain vital organ function.

  A. Autonomic nervous system. Increased sympathetic output directly stimulates arteries and veins, producing vasoconstriction, decreased venous capacitance, and increased arterial resistance. These responses are rapidly initiated to correct hypovolemia and to maintain end-organ perfusion. In addition, sympathetic stimulation results in catecholamine release from the adrenal medulla, which produces a more sustained effect.

  1. Catecholamines. Tyrosine from the diet or by the endogenous conversion of phenylalanine serves as the substrate for catecholamine synthesis. Tyrosine is hydroxylated by tyrosine hydroxylase to form dihydroxyphenylalanine (Dopa), which undergoes decarboxylation to form dopamine. Norepinephrine is then converted by the hydroxylation of dopamine. Epinephrine is subsequently produced by the methylation of norepinephrine by phenylethanolamine-N-methyltransferase found in the adrenal medulla.

  a. Norepinephrine is released from neurons and diffuses into the circulation from the synapses.

  b. Epinephrine is released from the adrenal medulla.

  c. $\alpha 1$-mediated peripheral vasoconstriction is increased.

  d. $\beta 1$-mediated heart rate and contractility is increased.

  e. Glucose availability is increased by stimulating hepatic glycogenolysis, gluconeogenesis, and ketogenesis.

  f. Skeletal muscle glycogenolysis is increased and skeletal muscle glucose uptake is decreased.

  g. Glucagon secretion is increased.

  h. Insulin release is suppressed.

  i. Fatty acids are mobilized.

  B. Hormonal response. Traumatic injury initiates multiple endocrine responses.

  1. Corticotropin is released from the pituitary gland after stimulation by hypothalamic corticotropin-releasing hormone.

  a. Corticotropin stimulates adrenal release of cortisol, which stimulates hepatic gluconeogenesis and increases skeletal muscle amino acid release.

  2. Vasopressin (antidiuretic hormone). The posterior pituitary gland releases vasopressin in response to increases in plasma osmolality that occur with hemorrhage (major stimulus) and decreases in the effective circulating plasma volume.

  a. Increases peripheral vasoconstriction

  b. Increases water resorption in the distal renal tubule

  c. Increases hepatic gluconeogenesis and glycogenolysis

  d. Decreases hepatic ketogenesis

  3. Growth hormone. Growth hormone is released from the anterior pituitary gland in response to hypothalamic release of growth hormone releasing hormone.

  a. Increases amino acid uptake and hepatic protein synthesis

  b. Mediates the biologic activity of growth hormone by somatomedins

  c. Decreases hepatic glucose transport

  4. Thyroxine (T_4). Release of T_4 from the thyroid in response to thyroid-stimulating hormone from the anterior pituitary gland increases after injury. The conversion of T_4 to T_3 (more potent form) decreases following trauma.

  a. Increases oxygen consumption and sympathetic output.

  b. Increases glycolysis and gluconeogenesis.

5. **Renin, angiotensin, aldosterone.** The major regulator of aldosterone production is the renin-angiotensin system. Decreases in renal arterial blood flow and renal tubular sodium concentration, and increased β-adrenergic stimulation serve to stimulate renin secretion from the juxtaglomerular cells of the renal afferent arteriole. Renin release results in the enzymatic conversion of angiotensinogen from the liver to the inactive angiotensin I. Angiotensin-converting enzyme produced by the lung converts angiotensin I into angiotensin II. Besides acting as a potent vasoconstrictor, angiotensin II also stimulates the release of aldosterone.
   a. **Angiotensin II**
      (1) Increases peripheral vasoconstriction
      (2) Increases splanchnic vasoconstriction
      (3) Decreases renal excretion of salt and water
   b. **Aldosterone**
      (1) Is produced in the adrenal zona glomerulosa
      (2) Increases distal tubular sodium and chloride resorption
      (3) Increases potassium secretion
6. **Glucagon** is released from pancreatic αcells in response to α-adrenergic stimulation, hypoglycemia, and elevated circulating levels of amino acids.
   a. Increases hepatic glycogenolysis and gluconeogenesis
   b. Increases lipolysis
7. **Insulin** is released from pancreatic βcells in response to β-adrenergic stimulation, glucagon, elevated plasma glucose, and amino acid levels.
   a. Increases glycolysis and glycogenesis
   b. Increases protein synthesis
   c. Decreases gluconeogenesis
   d. The initial hyperglycemia seen following injury is secondary to an increase in the glucagon:insulin ratio and peripheral insulin resistance.
C. **Systemic mediators.** A variety of mediators are released after injuries that have both local and systemic effects. In addition, many of these mediators are released as a result of reperfusion and can lead to amplification of the inflammatory response. Many of these mediators are also released in infection, sepsis, and inflammation.
   1. **Complement.** Ischemia and endothelial injuries result in the activation of this cascade of plasma proteins, which initiates the inflammatory response and results in the destruction and lysis of invading organisms. Complement activation, which results in leukocyte adherence, activation, and degranulation, can contribute to tissue destruction and damage as seen in acute respiratory distress syndrome.
   2. **Oxygen radicals.** Highly reactive and short-lived oxygen species are produced by leukocytes and a variety of tissues in response to ischemia and hypoxia. The activation of endogenous xanthine oxidase by injury produces hydrogen peroxide (H_2O_2), superoxide (O_2^-), and hydroxyl radical (OH^-). Endogenous antioxidant defenses (superoxide dismutase, catalase, glutathione) serve to prevent cellular injury.
   3. **Cytokines.** Both local tissues and migratory inflammatory cells release a variety of polypeptide mediators that have paracrine effects and serve to amplify the inflammatory response and signal wound repair. Many of these substances reach the systemic circulation and initiate a systemic inflammatory response, stimulate fever production, and govern the acute phase response. These factors include the interleukins (IL-1, IL-2, IL-6), tumor necrosis factor, and the interferons.
   4. **Eicosanoids** are a group of lipid mediators (prostaglandins, thromboxanes, and leukotrienes) derived from plasma membrane phospholipids by phospholipase A_2 (PLA_2). PLA_2 produces arachidonic acid, which is further metabolized to the specific isoforms (prostaglandin [PGE]$_2$, PGE$_1$, prostacyclin [PGI]$_2$, Thromboxane A_2 [TxA_2], Leukotriene C_4 [LTC$_4$]).

Different compounds have vasoactive properties and induce vasodilation (PGI_2) or vasoconstriction (TxA_2). They can also influence leukocyte function (LTC_4). Some (PGE_2) are thought to modulate the immune response but their role in injury and hemorrhage are not fully known.

5. **Nitric oxide (NO).** Normally, constitutively produced NO from endothelial cells is a homeostatic regulator of blood pressure that provides second-to-second vasodilation. Inflammation produces increased NO from a variety of cells and may contribute to the profound hypotension typical of patients with decompensated hemorrhagic shock.

6. **Other mediators.** A variety of growth factors and other mediators are expressed after traumatic injury, which serve to regulate wound healing. These include platelet-derived growth factor, epidermal growth factor, transforming growth factors, bradykinins, endothelin, and platelet-activating factor.

IV. **Metabolic response.** The metabolic response to traumatic injury and hemorrhagic shock is directly related to the aforementioned neuroendocrine response. Oxygen consumption and carbon dioxide production increase secondary to increased catecholamine production from increased sympathetic activity and from increased expression of inflammatory mediators produced at the tissue level. The metabolic responses seen after trauma have traditionally been defined according to the definitions outlined by Cuthbertson.

A. **Cuthbertson's two phase**

1. **Ebb phase**, which occurs initially after traumatic injury, is characterized by physiologic responses designed to restore tissue perfusion and circulating volume.

2. **Flow phase** begins once the patient is successfully resuscitated.

   a. The flow phase can be further subdivided into catabolic and anabolic phases.

   (1) The catabolic phase, which is characterized by the hyperdynamic response to trauma, includes hypermetabolism, hyperglycemia, and sodium and water retention. This response can last from days to weeks.

   (2) The anabolic phase, beginning after wounds have closed, is characterized by the return of normal homeostasis.

B. The metabolic response to trauma can also be divided into the following four phases.

1. **Shock phase.** Characterized by hypoperfusion secondary to hemorrhage and tissue injury.

2. The **resuscitation phase** is seen with active volume resuscitation and operation to control hemorrhage. It is characterized by elaboration of many of the inflammatory mediators.

3. The **hypermetabolic phase (postinjury)**, similar to the catabolic phase described by Cuthbertson, is characterized by an increased sympathetic and adrenal response. The increased secretion of catecholamines, cortisol, and insulin causes increased protein catabolism, negative nitrogen balance, and lipolysis. Acutely, this response serves to protect the individual. However, with prolonged and sustained hypermetabolism, the patient can develop systemic inflammatory response syndrome (SIRS). Persistence of SIRS can lead to multiple organ dysfunction syndrome (MODS).

4. **MODS** can be caused by the sustained overexpression of injury-induced inflammatory mediators or the development of infectious complications. MODS is the most common cause of late death in the trauma intensive care unit. Mortality increases by approximately 20% to 25% per organ that fails.

V. **Summary of organ system response to stress.** The physiologic responses seen following trauma are designed to preserve organ blood flow and, if necessary, shunt cardiac output to the heart and brain.

A. **Cardiovascular system**

1. Increase cardiac output by increasing heart rate and contractility ($CO = HR \times SV$).

2. Maintain perfusion to the heart and brain by shunting blood from the skeletal and splanchnic vascular beds.
3. Increased peripheral vasoconstriction secondary to increased angiotensin II and vasopressin activity.
4. Preservation of effective circulating plasma volume by increasing transcapillary movement of fluid from the interstitium to intravascular space.

B. Renal system
1. Maintenance of glomerular filtration rate secondary to increased efferent arteriolar vasoconstriction.
2. Increased aldosterone and vasopressin expression results in increased sodium and water absorption.
3. Blood flow shunted from renal cortex to medulla.

C. Adrenal system
1. Regulates stress response through increased catecholamine, cortisol, and aldosterone production.

D. Pulmonary system
1. Increased minute ventilation from hyperventilation and increased tidal volume.
2. Produces angiotensinogen-converting enzyme.

E. Central nervous system
1. Physiologic responses to trauma are first interpreted and then initiate the physiologic responses.
2. Afferent stimuli are coordinated into a multisystem response.
3. Increased sympathetic nervous system activity
4. Governs neuroendocrine response

F. Splanchnic system
1. Decreased blood flow secondary to shunting of blood to preserve blood flow to the heart and brain
2. Provides glucose from hepatic glycogen and gluconeogenesis as well as from the conversion of amino acids and free fatty acids
3. Produces mediators secondary to the low blood flow state that can contribute to the inflammatory response

VI. Physiologic responses
A. Altered mental status. Belligerence, anxiety, immobilization, withdrawal, and antagonism are commonly seen after major trauma. It is important to be aware that this can signify severe hypovolemia, hypoxemia, or both.
B. Altered vital signs. Fever may be seen after fluid resuscitation, which can be caused by the sustained inflammatory response. It is critical to be vigilant for infectious causes.
C. Blood pressure may not become significantly decreased until the patient has lost 30% to 40% of circulating blood volume. Therefore, blood pressure correlates poorly with either blood volume or flow.
D. Tachycardia can persist after even after fluid resuscitation and pain is adequately controlled.
E. Increased minute ventilation secondary to both tachypnea and increased tidal volume is common.
F. Generalized edema is common secondary to increased total body salt and water within the interstitium. This is a result of increased sympathetic vasoconstriction, altered capillary permeability, and hypoproteinemia. Also, local inflammation at the wound site leads to edema formation secondary to the release of locally acting chemokines.
G. Increased cardiac output. Heart rate and contractility increase with trauma injury; however, with hypovolemia, preload may be decreased to a degree that significantly lowers cardiac output.
H. Hypermetabolism. Energy demands, oxygen consumption, and carbon dioxide production are all elevated following trauma.
I. Altered protein, glucose, and fat metabolism. Energy requirements are increased following injury, with the magnitude of the additional energy need dependent on the severity of injury, magnitude of tissue destruction, and lean body mass of the patient.

1. **Protein loss** is approximately 300 to 500 g/day of lean body mass, with visceral proteins spared at the expense of skeletal muscle proteins.
2. **Proteins** are broken down to constituent amino acids that are catabolized to ammonia (forms urea) and precursors of the tricarboxylic cycle (TCA).
3. **Carbohydrates** provide 4 kcal/g when oxidized. Muscle glycogen (storage form of glucose) is used only by skeletal muscle (i.e., not released systemically), whereas hepatic glycogen provides glucose for glucose-dependent tissues (brain, leukocytes).

   a. **Gluconeogenesis** can occur from amino acids, glycerol, lactate, or pyruvate via the TCA or Krebs' cycle.
4. **Lipids**, which are used by tissues that are not glucose dependent, are the largest source of energy (9.4 kcal/g) in the body. Lipids are catabolized to form ketone bodies in the liver along with CO_2 and energy from glycerol and fatty acids.

J. **Leukocytosis.** Elevation in the white blood cell count can be seen after traumatic injury.

VII. **Summary.** The physiologic effect of the stress response is to maintain perfusion and function of the heart and brain. Acutely, this results in a survival advantage; however, with prolonged activation of the inflammatory response, deleterious effects can be seen including SIRS, MODS, and even death.

Bibliography

Cuthbertson DP. Post-shock metabolic responses. *Lancet* 1943;433–442.

Demling R, Lalonde C, Saldinger P, et al. Multiple organ dysfunction in the surgical patient: pathophysiology, prevention and treatment. *Curr Probl Surg* 1993;30:345–424.

Guyton AC. *Textbook of medical physiology.* Philadelphia: WB Saunders, 1981.

Peitzman AB, Billiar TR, Harbrecht BG et al. Hemorrhagic shock. *Curr Probl Surg* 1995;32:925–1012.

Richardson JD, Rodriguez JL. The metabolic consequences of injury. In: Richardson JD, Polk HC Jr., Flint LM, eds. *Trauma: clinical care and pathophysiology.* Chicago: Year Book Medical Publishers, 1987.

Waxman K. Physiologic response to injury. In: Ayres SM, Grenvik AK, Shoemaker WC, eds. *Textbook of critical care.* Philadelphia: WB Saunders, 1995.

Wilmore DM. Homeostasis: bodily changes in trauma and surgery. In: Sabiston DC, Lyerly KH, eds. *Textbook of surgery: the biological basis of modern surgical practice.* Philadelphia: WB Saunders, 1997.

5. SHOCK

Brian G. Harbrecht and Timothy R. Billiar

Shock has been recognized as an important pathophysiologic element in surgery and trauma since the late 1800s. Pioneering studies by Wiggers and Blalock in the 1940s lay the foundation for current scientific studies in the field of shock research. Although the definition of shock may have changed greatly since these early investigations, the clinical syndrome and its profound impact on the care of injured patients remains essentially the same.

I. **Definition and classification.** Although the clinical syndromes responsible for shock can originate from a variety of causes, the different forms of shock have a number of common features.
   A. **Definition.** Shock is a condition of inadequate tissue perfusion sufficient to maintain normal cellular function and structure. Although cellular injury may become evident, its contribution to the sequelae of shock is unclear. Cellular dysfunction can become evident in a variety of ways. It cannot be emphasized strongly enough that shock **does not equal hypotension** and, conversely, a "normal" blood pressure **does not exclude** the presence of hypoperfusion.
   B. **Classification**
      1. **Hypovolemic shock** can be caused by decreased circulating volume from loss of red cell mass, plasma, and extracellular fluid, or a combination of these. The most common cause of shock in injured patients, hypovolemic shock, usually results from acute blood loss.
      2. **Cardiogenic shock** results from decreased peripheral perfusion because of ineffective pump function. Cardiogenic shock can result from direct cardiac injury (myocardial contusion) or intrinsic cardiac disease (myocardial infarction, dysrhythmia).
      3. **Vasogenic shock** is caused by changes in vascular resistance such that the normal blood volume fails to maintain adequate circulatory perfusion.
         a. **Neurogenic shock** is a form of vasogenic shock in which a high spinal cord injury (or spinal anesthesia) results in loss of sympathetic vascular tone, producing peripheral vasodilation. Bradycardia often accompanies it.
         b. **Septic shock** is a form of vasogenic shock in which proinflammatory mediator release results in peripheral vasodilation, decreased peripheral arterial resistance, and increased peripheral venous capacitance. Tachycardia often accompanies it.
      4. **Obstructive shock.** Mechanical obstruction to cardiac function (cardiac tamponade, tension pneumothorax) results in decreased peripheral perfusion.
      5. **Traumatic shock** includes components of the above mentioned causes that may not be sufficient to induce hypoperfusion in isolation, but markedly impair peripheral perfusion when combined. Generally, includes the sequelae of hypovolemia from blood loss and activation of proinflammatory mediators elaborated as a result of bony or soft tissue injury.
II. **Pathophysiology**
   A. **Cardiovascular response.** The body's normal response to maintain tissue perfusion is by adjusting peripheral arterial resistance, cardiac output, and heart rate to maintain perfusion to essential organs such as the heart and brain.
      1. **Peripheral arterial resistance** increases in response to decreased circulatory volume or impaired pump function and decreases as a contributor to shock in septic states and with loss of sympathetic tone.

2. **Cardiac output** will be intrinsically diminished because of pump failure in cardiogenic shock. May also be diminished by low circulatory volume or mechanical impediments (cardiac tamponade). Often increased in response to diminished peripheral arterial resistance in septic shock.

3. **Heart rate** is increased in response to decreased circulatory volume, decreased peripheral arterial resistance, and mechanical impediments to cardiac function. Often unchanged in neurogenic shock because of loss of sympathetic cardiac input. The normal reflexive change to hypovolemia can be absent or impaired in elderly patients with significant intrinsic cardiac disease or those taking selected medications (β-blockers). If shock is sustained, tachycardia can evolve into bradycardia as a preterminal event.

B. **Neuroendocrine response.** The neuroendocrine response to shock, which is similar to that of injury, is covered in detail in Chapter 4.

C. **Inflammatory mediators.** Proinflammatory mediators, which can be produced in response to bacterial products, lead to decreased arterial resistance and impaired tissue perfusion (septic shock). In addition, other forms of shock can result in the production of a variety of systemic and local mediators such as cytokines, eicosanoids, and radical species (see Chapter 4).

D. **Cellular response** to shock is a result of decreased oxygen delivery from hypoperfusion and direct changes in cell function caused by neural (adrenergic), humoral (corticotropin, vasopressin, glucagon), and proinflammatory (cytokine) mediators. Oxygen radicals, either intrinsically (i.e., xanthine oxidase) or extrinsically (i.e., neutrophils) derived, which are produced in shock, can alter cell function. Alterations in the local microcirculatory environment, metabolic derangements, and hypoxia at the cellular level lead to cell membrane depolarization, increased intracellular water and cell swelling, dysfunction of the Na-K-adenosine triphosphatase (ATPase) pump, increased anaerobic metabolism, uncoupling of oxidative phosphorylation, and increased intracellular calcium. Changes in cellular gene expression in response to shock have been described. The development of apoptosis in animal models of shock has been described but its significance is unknown.

III. **Diagnosis and treatment.** Whereas the end-organ manifestations of shock may be the same regardless of the specific cause, the treatment of shock depends on the specific cause leading to impaired perfusion.

A. **Hypovolemic shock**, which represents the most common cause of shock in injured patients, is caused by acute blood loss. Severity of shock insult depends on the depth and duration of shock. Mild shock of longstanding duration can be as lethal as acute, profound shock.

1. **Diagnosis.** Signs of inadequate end-organ perfusion depend on the degree of volume loss. Hypotension can be a relatively late manifestation of decreased circulating volume if compensatory mechanisms are adequate. Tachycardia, diminished urine output, decreased pulse pressure, restlessness and anxiety, and cold, clammy extremities can be manifestations of reduced circulatory volume. Lethargy and stupor caused by hypovolemia represent profound volume loss and can signal impending cardiovascular collapse. Hypotension is a sign that the compensatory mechanisms have been exceeded, but in itself may be a relatively poor predictor of the volume of blood loss. Patients in shock may not be hypotensive but patients who are hypotensive should always be considered to be in shock.

2. **Treatment.** Treatment of hypovolemia focuses on simultaneous restoration of circulatory blood volume and cessation of ongoing hemorrhage. Treatment for hypovolemia is usually instituted before a cause is identified.

a. **ABCs.** The airway should be secure and bilateral breath sounds present. Fluid resuscitation should be instituted with balanced crystalloid solution through two large-bore intravenous catheters. For adults who do not respond to 1 to 2 L of crystalloid, consider the use of blood and need for operative intervention. Patients who respond briefly or not at all to the above measures have a high likelihood of requiring operative intervention to control hemorrhage.

  b. Source. The source of blood loss in victims of penetrating injury depends on the nature, location, and path of the projectile. For blunt trauma victims, the potential sources of blood loss to be considered can be greater. For both, the search for sites of hemorrhage is identical. Four main sites of large volume blood loss exist.

  (1) Chest. May be identified by absent or reduced breath sounds or the presence of hemothorax on chest x-ray study.

  (2) Abdomen. Physical examination is a relatively insensitive method for detecting significant hemoperitoneum, which may be identified in the resuscitation area by ultrasound or diagnostic peritoneal lavage or in the operating room by laparotomy.

  (3) Retroperitoneum or pelvis. Usually because of associated pelvic fracture.

  (4) External. Visible on inspection, such as major vascular injuries from extremity wounds, large surface area wounds, or uncontrolled wounds in areas of increased vascularity (face, scalp).

  (5) Other sources of blood loss include long bone fractures and extensive soft tissue injury. If no bleeding site is identified, consider alternative causes of shock (cardiac tamponade, neurogenic, cardiogenic). Also consider repeating the assessment of the chest, abdomen, and pelvis to ensure that no possible sources have been overlooked.

B. Cardiogenic shock. In trauma patients, cardiogenic shock can be caused by either significant cardiac injury (myocardial contusion) or intrinsic cardiac disease (myocardial infarction, cardiac arrhythmia).

  1. Diagnosis. Suspicion of cardiogenic shock can be increased when hypovolemic shock has been excluded or risk factors are identified (elderly patient, known preexisting cardiac disease, dysrhythmias present on electrocardiogram (ECG) or monitor, presence of sternal fracture). The diagnosis of cardiac pump failure as a source of ongoing shock in injured patients requires exclusion of other causes and demonstration of diminished cardiac function (decreased cardiac output, echocardiographic evidence of cardiac dysfunction).

  2. Treatment of cardiogenic shock in trauma patients involves restoration of cardiac function in conjunction with the treatment of acute traumatic injuries.

  a. ABCs. The airway should be secure and bilateral equal breath sounds present. Fluid resuscitation should be instituted judiciously in patients with known cardiac dysfunction.

  b. Invasive hemodynamic monitoring. An arterial line and pulmonary artery catheter can help guide therapy and assess success.

  c. Inotropic agents. Selective use can be guided by the results of invasive hemodynamic monitoring.

  d. Circulatory support. Consider intraaortic balloon pump for refractory cardiac dysfunction.

C. Neurogenic shock, in trauma patients, is usually caused by injuries in the cervical or upper thoracic spinal column. Rarely, spinal cord injuries without bony abnormality (epidural hematoma of the cord) can result in neurogenic shock.

  1. Diagnosis. The classic description of neurogenic shock includes hypotension and bradycardia, with warm, perfused extremities and presence of a sensory or motor deficit consistent with cord injury. Tachycardia can be present. Hypovolemia, in addition to the neurogenic component, can contribute to hypotension. The diagnosis is often made once hypovolemia has been excluded and a vertebral fracture in the appropriate area identified.

2. Treatment
   a. ABCs. The airway should be secure and equal bilateral breath sounds present. Fluid resuscitation should be instituted and restoration of intravascular volume may be sufficient to restore blood pressure and perfusion.
   b. If the diagnosis of neurogenic shock is certain and hypotension persists, vasopressor support can be helpful. Phenylephrine or norepinephrine can be instituted as a continuous infusion. If vasopressor support is needed, its duration is typically brief (24–72 h). If vasopressor support is indicated, invasive hemodynamic monitoring (e.g., an arterial line, central venous pressure monitor, or pulmonary artery catheter) should be considered, based on patient age, associated injuries, and preexisting medical condition.
D. **Septic shock** in trauma patients, is an unlikely cause of shock in the emergency department or the early hospital stay. Septic shock can develop later in the hospitalization because of the development of infectious complications after injury.
   1. **Diagnosis.** A hyperdynamic hemodynamic profile is often present, with hypotension despite tachycardia and increased cardiac output. Fever, leukocytosis, and tachypnea are often present. Delirium or obtundation can also be present. Signs of localized infection (pneumonia, urinary tract infection, intraabdominal abscess, empyema, soft tissue infection) should be sought. Bacteremia can be present and secondary infection of monitoring devices (continuous venous pressure lines, intracranial pressure monitors) may need to be excluded.
   2. **Treatment**
      a. ABCs. The airway should be secure and proper ventilatory mechanics established. Intravascular volume should be restored initially. If hypotension persists, pharmacologic support may be necessary. Invasive hemodynamic monitoring should be considered to guide therapy. A pulmonary artery catheter can assist in deciding if inotropic or vasopressor support should be instituted.
      b. Treatment of the primary infection is essential. Systemic antibiotics should be instituted, purulent fluid collections should be drained (percutaneously or operatively), infected monitoring or prosthetic devices should be removed, and necrotic nonviable tissue should be debrided. Antibiotic therapy should be sufficient to cover the likely responsible organisms, based on the infectious cause, common organisms in the particular unit or institution, and the patient's previous history of infectious episodes. Antibiotics should be tailored to appropriate culture data when available and long-term empiric antibiotic usage should be discouraged to avoid the development of resistant organisms.
      c. The use of antiendotoxin strategies, cytokines, and anticytokine antagonists should be considered experimental. Their use has not been proved to be effective in clinical trials.
E. **Obstructive shock**. Mechanical obstruction to perfusion is usually caused by the development of tension pneumothorax or cardiac tamponade. The diagnosis of these entities is covered in detail in Chapter 26A and 26B. Correction of the primary cause should restore perfusion or additional causes should be sought.
F. **Traumatic shock** is usually caused by a combination of hypovolemic, cardiogenic, neurogenic, septic, and obstructive shock. Treatment of the contributing components can require rapid, coordinated medical decision-making. After securing the airway, prompt control of hemorrhage is generally the major objective.
IV. **Summary**. The term "shock" represents a state of abnormal tissue and cellular perfusion. Reliance on predetermined blood pressure criteria can lead to substantially underestimating the frequency of occurrence of shock states. In trauma patients, acute blood loss represents the most common form of shock but

other causes should be kept in mind. Often, treatment of the shock should be instituted before or in conjunction with steps to identify the underlying cause. Patients who are actively bleeding need prompt operative intervention and the need for operative treatment should be established early to avoid the potential end-organ dysfunction and death associated with continue tissue hypoperfusion.

Bibliography

Gutierrez G, Brown SD. Response of the microcirculation. In: Schlag G, Redl H, eds. *Pathophysiology of shock, sepsis, and organ failure*. Berlin: Springer-Verlag, 1993: 215–229.

Hierholzer C, Harbrecht BG, Meneze J, et al. Essential role of induced nitric oxide in the initiation of the inflammatory response following hemorrhagic shock. *J Exp Med* 1998;187:917–928.

Mullins RJ. Management of shock. In: Mattox KL, Feliciano DV, Moore EE, eds. *Trauma*. New York: McGraw-Hill, 2000:195–231.

Peitzman, AB, Billiar TR, Harbrecht BG, et al. Hemorrhagic shock. *Curr Probl Surg* 1995;32:925–1012.

6. MEASUREMENTS OF INJURY SEVERITY

Theodore R. Delbridge

I. **Introduction.** Emergency medical services (EMS) systems are charged with making rapid patient assessments at trauma scenes to effect appropriate triage decisions. Field personnel must determine extent of injuries in either individual patients or multiple casualty situations to maximize resource utilization and patient outcome. **Undertriage** occurs when a patient with severe injuries is transported to facilities without adequate care resources. **Overtriage** occurs when a patient with less severe injuries, who could be appropriately cared for at less resource-intense facilities, is transported to a trauma center when a closer adequate facility exists. The goal of triage is to get the patient to the appropriate facility in a timely fashion.

To facilitate the decision-making processes, several trauma severity scoring systems have been developed. Ideally, severity scales should be easy to use and require only readily available data. When applied in the field, these provide broad estimates of injury severity and should not be interpreted as absolute values.

These scoring systems also provide a more objective basis for comparing patients, pursuing quality improvement initiatives, and performing epidemiologic assessments. Scoring systems also enhance our ability to recognize distributions of injuries associated with segments of the population and identify their risk factors. Severity scores can be characterized by the type of information they require to be calculated. Current scoring techniques are based predominantly on anatomic or physiologic data.

II. **Physiologic scores**

   A. These scores depend on changes in blood pressure, heart rate, respiratory rate, and level of consciousness that occur in the presence of serious injuries. Information required for their calculation is routinely available to field personnel. In theory, physiologic scores are useful for prehospital measurement of injury severity and helpful during triage decision-making processes.

   1. **Glasgow Coma Scale.** The Glasgow Coma Scale (GCS) is a clinical index for assessing the degree of impaired consciousness.

      a. The GCS is calculated by determining the patient's best motor, verbal, and eye opening responses (Table 6.1). These parameters reflect the function of the central nervous system (CNS), its degree of integration, and brainstem function, respectively.

      b. Scores range from 3 to 15, increasing as the level of consciousness and integration capabilities improve. Scores ≤ 8 indicate coma.

      c. As initially described, the GCS did not account for the patient who was intubated or pharmacologically paralyzed. The patient with a GCS score of 3 because of head injury can be very different from the patient who was pharmacologically paralyzed and intubated for airway control, but who then has a GCS score of 3. In the latter circumstance, the GCS score should be recorded as 3TP, indicating that the patient was intubated (T) and pharmacologically paralyzed (P).

      d. The motor component is the most important value in the GCS. The motor component score correlates highly with the total GCS score.

   2. **Champion trauma score.** The Champion trauma score (TS) is based on assessments of respiratory rate and effort, systolic blood pressure, capillary refill, and the GCS. Scores range from 1 (most seriously injured) to 16 (least seriously injured). Similar to the GCS, the TS is derived from inpatient data and not as a prehospital tool. Nonetheless, it is widely used as a prehospital prediction rule to facilitate triage decisions.

   3. **Revised trauma score.** The revised trauma score (RTS) was developed to limit the need to assess certain ambiguous findings included in

Table 6.1 Glasgow Coma Scale

Eye opening	Spontaneous	4
	–To voice	3
	–To pain	2
	–None	1
Verbal response	Oriented	5
	Confused	4
	Inappropriate	3
	Incomprehensible	2
	None	1
Motor response	Obeys command	6
	Localizes pain	5
	Withdraws (pain)	4
	Flexion	3
	Extension (pain)	2
	None	1
Total score		3–15

the TS, such as respiratory expansion and capillary refill. Furthermore, the TS underestimated the effect of head injury on outcome. The RTS improves the accuracy of outcome predictions and requires assessment of fewer physiologic parameters. It incorporates the GCS, systolic blood pressure, and respiratory rate, using coded values ranging from 4 (normal) to 0 for each of the physiologic parameters. The final RTS ranges from 12 (normal) to 0 (Table 6.2). A lower than normal coded value (≤ 3) for any variable suggests the possible need for care at a Trauma Center.

    a. The RTS is limited in its ability to predict outcomes when used in the prehospital setting. However, it is often used to predict in-hospital outcomes, when the RTS components are weighted to emphasize changes in GCS score (RTS = [0.9368] GCS coded value + [0.7326] systolic BP coded value + [0.2908] respiratory rate coded value; maximal value = 7.8408).

  4. Other scores, such as the CRAMS scale (circulation, respiration, abdomen, motor, speech), *Prehospital Index*, and the *Trauma Triage Rule* are described and used in some areas of the country.

  5. Pediatric trauma score is discussed in the Chapter 47, *Pediatric Trauma*.

III. Anatomic scores. Anatomically based indices characterize injury severity within anatomic regions, either individually or collectively. The most commonly

Table 6.2 Revised trauma score

A Glasgow coma scale	B Systolic blood pressure (mmHg)	C Respiratory rate	Coded value (CV)
13–15	>89	10–29	4
9–12	76–89	>29	3
6–8	50–75	6–9	2
4–5	1–49	1–5	1
3	0	0	0

used anatomic scores are the **Abbreviated Injury Scale (AIS)**, which quantifies injury within individual body regions; and the **Injury severity score (ISS)**, which is derived from multiples of the AIS. Both require diagnosis of injuries, including those that are apparent only after definitive evaluation. Each serves as a tool for retrospective analyses of care, epidemiologic assessments, and outcomes evaluations.

A. The **AIS** is derived from a list of several hundred injuries, which are categorized according to their anatomic sites. Each injury is rated on a scale from 1 (minor injury) to 6 (maximal injury—usually fatal). Accurate AIS scoring requires recognition and full appreciation of the extent of all the injuries. Thus, it cannot be determined until the end of a patient's diagnostic evaluation. The AIS characterizes the severity of each injury individually and does not provide a summary of all injuries present in any given patient. For this purpose, additional scoring systems are required.

B. **Injury severity score**. The Injury severity score (ISS) summarizes multiple injuries in a single patient. ISS values range from 1 (minor injury with greatest probability for survival) to 75 (major injury with least probability for survival). The ISS is calculated by summing the squares of the three highest AIS scores in the different body regions: (a) head and neck, face, thorax, abdominal or pelvic contents; (b) extremities or pelvic girdle; and (c) external structures. For example, if the three highest AIS scores were in the face, thorax, and abdomen regions, each of those scores would be squared and then summed to arrive at the ISS. Additionally, if any AIS score is 6 (essentially a lethal injury), then the ISS is automatically 75. By convention, an ISS of >15 is felt to indicate the presence of significant injury that warrants care at the Trauma Center.

   1. Because the ISS is based on AIS scores, it suffers from limitations in terms of the timeliness with which it can be determined. That is, the ISS cannot be calculated until it is clear that all injuries have been identified. Furthermore, the ISS accounts for only the highest scores from each body region and treats equal AIS scores as injuries of equal severity. Thus, an ISS value can result from multiple combinations of injury patterns, and represent heterogeneous groups of patients with varying prognoses.

C. **International Classification of Diseases (ICD)**. The *International Classification of Diseases*, 9th revision (ICD-9) is a taxonomy system applied to nearly all hospitalized patients in the United States. The ICD-9 codes assigned to trauma patients have been used to predict mortality and, retrospectively, aid in AIS calculations. However, such predictions depend on determining mortality risk for each diagnostic code. ICD-9 codes are assigned at the time of discharge from the hospital.

D. **Penetrating Abdominal Trauma Index (PATI)**. The PATI anatomic scale has been applied to patients with penetrating wounds of the abdomen. The PATI sums the individual abdominal organ scores, which are calculated for the individual organs by multiplying the severity estimate for each organ (1–5) times the risk factor (1–5) for injury to that organ (Table 6.3).

E. **High-risk injuries**. Certain anatomic injuries can indicate a likelihood of significant trauma. These include penetrating injuries to the head, neck, torso, and extremities proximal to the elbow and knee; flail chest; combination of other trauma with burn; two or more proximal long bone fractures; pelvic fractures; limb paralysis; and amputations proximal to the wrist and ankle.

IV. **Applications of scoring in trauma care**

A. **Prehospital triage**. Despite the availability of scoring techniques, objective measurement of injury severity in the prehospital setting remains problematic. When severity scales are based on anatomic injuries, the data required to calculate them are often not available until after extensive in-hospital evaluation. Physiologic scores have a limited sensitivity in predicting the presence of major trauma. By nature, physiologic processes are dynamic and often overlapping. Thus, scoring systems function better with

Table 6.3 Calculation of the Penetrating Abdominal Trauma Index (PATI)*

Organ injured	Risk factor	Scoring
Duodenum	4	1. Single wall 2. ≤25% wall 3. >25% wall 4. Duodenal wall and blood supply 5. Pancreaticoduodenectomy
Pancreas	5	1. Tangential 2. Through-and-through (duct intact) 3. Major debridement or distal duct injury 4. Proximal duct injury 5. Pancreaticoduodenectomy
Liver	4	1. Nonbleeding peripheral 2. Bleeding, central, or minor debridement 3. Major debridement or hepatic artery ligation 4. Lobectomy 5. Lobectomy with caval repair or extensive bilobar debridement
Large intestine	4	1. Serosal 2. Single wall 3. ≤25% wall 4. >25% wall 5. Colon wall and blood supply
Major vascular	5	1. ≤25% wall 2. >25% wall 3. Complete transection 4. Interposition grafting or bypass 5. Ligation
Spleen	3	1. Nonbleeding 2. Cautery or hemostatic agent 3. Minor debridement or suturing 4. Partial resection 5. Splenectomy
Kidney	2	1. Nonbleeding 2. Minor debridement or suturing 3. Major debridement 4. Pedicle or major calyceal 5. Nephrectomy
Extrahepatic biliary	1	1. Contusion 2. Cholecystectomy 3. ≤25% wall 4. >25% wall 5. Biliary enteric reconstruction
Small bowel	1	1. Single wall 2. Through-and-through 3. ≤25% wall 4. >25% wall 5. Wall and blood supply or >5 injuries
Stomach	3	1. Single wall 2. Through-and-through 3. Minor debridement 4. Wedge resection 5. >35% resection

Table 6.3 *continued on next page*

Table 6.3 *Continued*.

Organ injured	Risk factor	Scoring
Ureter	2	1. Contusion 2. Laceration 3. Minor debridement 4. Segmental resection 5. Reconstruction
Bladder	1	1. Single wall 2. Through-and-through 3. Debridement 4. Wedge resection 5. Reconstruction
Bone	1	1. Periosteum 2. Cortex 3. Through-and-through 4. Intraarticular 5. Major bone loss
Minor vascular	1	1. Nonbleeding small hematoma 2. Nonbleeding large hematoma 3. Suturing 4. Ligation of isolated vessels 5. Ligation of named vessels

*Based on assigning a complication risk factor (x) to each organ system involved and grading each organ injury (1 = minimal, 2 = minor, 3 = moderate, 4 = major, 5 = maximal).
(Adapted from Moore EE, Dunn EL, Moore JB, et al. Penetration Abdominal Trauma Index. *J Trauma* 1981:21:439–445; Borlase BC, Moore EE, Moore FA. The Abdominal Trauma Index—a critical reassessment and validation. *J Trauma* 1990;30:1340–1344; with permission.)

repeated measurements or in cases of extreme deviations rather than when used to make a single measurement after an injury. The judgment of EMS providers (e.g., paramedics) plays an important role. The combination of EMS provider judgment and objective trauma scoring systems can improve the effectiveness of trauma triage criteria.

B. Outcome evaluation. More accurate predictions of outcome can be made by combining anatomic and physiologic criteria.

   1. TRISS (Trauma Related Severity Injury Score) is a combination of the ISS, RTS, mechanism of injury, and age. A probability of survival for any given patient can be predicted. More importantly, TRISS provides an objective evaluation that facilitates comparison of any particular institution's results against a standard or a norm. Performance monitoring or quality improvement programs can use TRISS to help identify unexpected survivors (those who survived but may have been expected to die) and unexpected deaths (those who died but should have been expected to survive).

   a. Probability of survival (Ps) is given by the formula:

   $$Ps = 1/(1 = e^{-b})$$

   where $b = b_0 + b_1(RTS) + b_2(ISS) + b_3(age)$; b_0, b1, b_2, and b_3 are coefficients derived from the Walker Duncan regression analysis from thousands of trauma patients enrolled in the Multiple Trauma Outcome Study (MTOS) (Fig. 6.1).

   2. A severity characterization of trauma (ASCOT). ASCOT was designed to improve on the predictive ability of TRISS. ASCOT combines the RTS, patient age, and a four-valued anatomic profile with values for

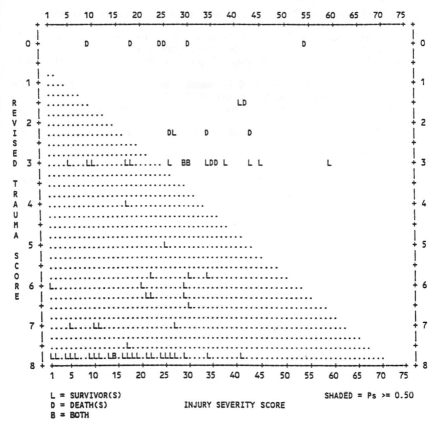

FIG. 6.1. TRISS (Trauma Related Severity Injury Score) diagram.

head and spinal cord (A), thorax and the front of the neck (B), other regions with AIS 3 to 5 (C), and other regions with AIS 1 to 2 (D).

Bibliography

The Abbreviated Injury Scale—1990 Revision. Des Plaines, IL: American Association for Automotive Medicine, 1990.

Baker SP, O'Neill B, Haddon W, et al. The injury severity score: a method for describing patients with multiple injuries and evaluating emergency care. *J Trauma* 1979;14:187–196.

Baxt WG, Berry CC, Epperson MD, et al. The failure of prehospital trauma prediction rules to classify trauma patients accurately. *Ann Emerg Med* 1989;18:1–8.

Baxt WG, Jones G, Fortlage D. Trauma triage rule: a new, resource-based approach to the prehospital identification of major trauma victims. *Ann Emerg Med* 1990;19: 1401–1406.

Boyd CR, Tolson MA, Copes WS. Evaluating trauma care: the TRISS method. *J Trauma* 1987;27:170–375.

Cayten CG, Stahl WM, Murphy JG, et al. Limitations of the TRISS method for interhospital comparisons: a multihospital study. *J Trauma* 1991;31:471.

Champion HR, Sacco WJ, Carnazzo AJ, et al. Trauma score. *Crit Care Med* 1981;9: 672–676.

Champion HR, Sacco WJ, Copes WS. A revision of the trauma score. *J Trauma* 1989; 29:623–629.

Champion HR, Sacco WJ, Copes WS. Trauma scoring. In: Moore EE, Mattox KL, Feliciano DV, eds. *Trauma*, 2nd ed. Norwalk: Appleton & Lange, 1991.

Gormican SP. CRAMS scale: field triage of trauma victims. *Ann Emerg Med* 1982; 11:132–135.

Koehler JJ, Baer LJ, Malafa SA, et al. Prehospital index: a scoring system for field triage of trauma victims. *Ann Emerg Med* 1986;15:178–182.

Moore EE, Dunn EL, Moore JB, et al. Penetrating abdominal trauma index. *J Trauma* 1981;21:439–445.

Sacco W, Copes W, Bain L, et al. Effect of preinjury illness on trauma patient survival outcome. *J Trauma* 1993;35:538.

Simmons E, Hedges JR, Irwin L, et al. Paramedic injury severity perception can aid trauma triage. *Ann Emerg Med* 1995;26:461–468.

Teasdale G, Jennett B. Assessment of coma and impaired consciousness: a practical scale. *Lancet* 1974;2:81–84.

7. PREHOSPITAL TRIAGE

Ronald N. Roth and Vincent N. Mossesso, Jr.

I. **Field triage** involves the sorting of patients based on the **severity of their injuries** and the **availability of resources**. Field triage becomes necessary when the number of casualties overwhelms the capabilities of the on-scene care providers or the resources of local receiving facilities.
   A. Two types of triage situations exist
      1. The first situation occurs when number of patients and their injuries **do not** exceed the resources of the field providers or local treatment facilities. In this situation, all injured patients are treated and transported immediately, and triage focuses on identifying the priority of treatment needs for each patient.
      2. When the number of patients and their injuries exceed the resources of the field providers or local treatment facilities, triage is required to identify potentially salvageable patients with life-threatening conditions that require immediate treatment and transport.
   B. **Field triage** is initiated by the first unit to arrive on scene. However, the responsibility for patient triage can be delegated to more experienced personnel when they arrive. Field triage works best when victims are limited to a small geographic area. Large disaster sites (e.g., earthquakes, floods) can require multiple triage sites.
   C. **Principles**. The most critically injured patients are transported first. However, triage must be a continuous process during a major event with constant monitoring of patient status. Changes in patient status can require a change in the initial categorization of patient.
   D. **Field triage guidelines**. Knowledge of injury, mechanism and existing comorbid factors is mandatory for all who participate in trauma triage. Unfortunately, no single factor exists that will guarantee triage success. The following issues must be incorporated in the triage decision-making process (Table 7.1).
      1. **Patient assessment**. The initial patient survey can often identify patients with immediately life-threatening injuries.
         a. **Abnormal physiologic signs** strongly suggest the need for rapid treatment and transport to an appropriate facility.
         b. **Anatomic location of injuries** can predict the need for emergent surgical or specialty care.
      2. **Mechanism of injury**. Although not as strong a predictor for the need to operate immediately or receive intensive care as the anatomic and physiologic criteria, analysis of injury mechanism at the scene can improve triage accuracy. This allows for the inferences of the forces involved and the kinetic energy transferred during the event.
      3. **Premorbid condition**. No formal scaling system exists for ranking premorbid conditions, however, their inclusion in triage decision-making is widely accepted.
      4. **Other issues** include medical and environmental resource factors that must be included in triage decision.
II. **Triage tools**. Several triage tools can assist the field provider with trauma triage decision-making. No universally accepted scoring system exists for the out of hospital triage of multiple trauma victims.
   A. **Trauma triage scoring**. Several trauma scoring techniques have been developed for determining the severity of injury of trauma victims both in the hospital and in the field (see Chapter 6). Accurate trauma scoring is dependent on diagnostic skills and can be limited by field conditions, patient intoxication,

Table 7.1 Field triage guidelines

Patient assessment
–Physiologic
 —Pulse <60 or >100/min
  –Respiratory rate <10 or >29/min
  –Systolic blood pressure <90 mmHg
  –Glasgow Coma Scale score <14
 —Revised Trauma Score <12
–Anatomic
 —Penetrating injuries to head, neck, torso, or extremities proximal to the elbow,
or:
  –Flail chest
  –Two or more proximal long bone fractures
  –Burns on >15% body surface area, face, or airway
  –Pelvic fractures
  –Paralysis
  –Extremity amputation
Mechanism of injury
–Ejection from automobile
 —Death of victim in the same passenger compartment
 —Extrication time >20 min
 —Fall >20 ft
 —Roll-over accident
 —High-speed vehicle crash
 —Auto versus pedestrian >5 mph
 —Motorcycle crash >20 mph or separation of rider from bike
Pre- or Comorbid conditions
 —Age <5 or >55 yr
 —Cardiac or respiratory disease
 —Diabetes mellitus (especially if using insulin)
 —Cirrhosis or liver disease
 —Active cancer/malignancy
 —Morbid obesity
 —History of bleeding disorder or anticoagulants
Other issues
–Potential for decline in patient condition
–Availability of resources
 —Personnel and level of training
 —Equipment and supplies
 —Transport vehicles (ground versus air)
 —Turnaround time for vehicles
–Local facilities and bed availability
 —Adult and pediatric trauma centers
 —Burn centers
 —Other specialized care centers (e.g., hazardous exposure decontamination,
  obstetric, psychiatric)
–Presence of ongoing hazards or environmental dangers

and compensatory physiologic mechanisms masking major injuries. Trauma scores tend to look at combinations of the following:
   1. **Cardiovascular system**
   2. **Respiratory system**
   3. **Central nervous system**
   4. **Type and location of injury**
   5. **Abdominal examination**
  B. **Simple triage and rapid treatment system (START)** is based solely on clinical presentation. Patients are categorized as immediate or delayed pri-

ority, based on the evaluation of three parameters: ventilation, perfusion, and mental status. An abnormality with any one parameter places the victim in the immediate transport category.

C. **Field provider judgment**. Without the use of formal trauma scoring techniques, field provider judgment has been shown to be sensitive but not specific in identifying patients with life-threatening injuries.

D. **Triage tags** are most effectively used in systems that use the tags routinely for large and small multivictim incidents.

1. **Problems** that can occur with triage tags include:
   a. Separation of the tag from the victim
   b. Contamination by blood or body fluids
   c. Limited space for documentation

2. **Color codes** identify patient categorization by injury severity and need for transport.
   a. **Red**. Most critically injured. Includes patients with major injuries to the head, thorax, and abdomen for which immediate surgical or specialty care is required.
   b. **Yellow**. Less critically injured. Includes patients who are less seriously injured, who still require surgical or specialty care, but not immediately.
   c. **Green**. No life- or limb-threatening injury identified.
   d. **Black**. Dead. Patients who are dead or with obviously fatal injuries.

III. **Limitations to triage**. Many factors affect triage; perfect triage is difficult to achieve. Overtriage of up to 50% may be necessary to achieve an undertriage rate of 10%.

A. **Overtriage** occurs when field teams overestimate the severity of a patient's injuries.

1. Overtriage can potentially burden existing resources with patients sustaining noncritical injuries.

2. Overtriage can prevent patients with serious injuries from receiving appropriate care.

B. **Undertriage** occurs when the field team underestimates the severity of a patient's injuries.

1. Undertriage can cause delays in treatment and transfer of patients with life- or limb-threatening injuries.

2. Undertriage can cause patients with life-threatening or complicated injuries to be sent to hospitals lacking the appropriate resources.

IV. **Traumatic arrest**. The term "post-traumatic arrest" refers to the end result of a variety of pathologic processes in response to injury and does not represent a singular entity. Although the term appears self-defining, subtle nuances within this category confer significant differences in prognosis. Physicians and healthcare workers involved in trauma care should approach trauma patients in cardiopulmonary arrest in an organized fashion to allow effective and rationale treatment and triage.

A. **Etiology**. Successful resuscitation of the patient in cardiopulmonary arrest after trauma requires identification and intervention for specific life-threatening processes. To achieve this, it is important to review the various causes that can lead to cardiopulmonary collapse after trauma.

1. **Airway. Loss of a patent airway is the most common reason for immediate cardiorespiratory collapse after trauma**. The following causes must be sought and treated:
   a. **Occlusion by tongue or epiglottis**
      (1) **Loss of tone** (Central nervous system [CNS] dysfunction caused by head trauma, hypoxia, drugs, stroke)
      (2) **Facial fracture**
   b. **Occlusion by foreign body** (especially consider blood, avulsed teeth or soft tissue, and emesis)
   c. **Direct traumatic disruption** (laryngeal fracture, tracheal collapse)

    2. Breathing. Even in the face of a patent upper airway, inadequate gas exchange can lead to rapid death. This can result from:
      a. Loss of respiratory effort, caused by:
        (1) Severe head injury
        (2) High spinal cord disruption (phrenic nerve roots exit C_{2-5})
        (3) CNS depression from toxins or drugs (including alcohol)
      b. Mechanical dysfunction
        (1) Tension pneumothorax
        (2) Large or bilateral open pneumothorax (sucking chest wound)
        (3) Flail chest
        (4) Thoracic crush or compression
        (5) Diaphragmatic rupture
        (6) Large hemothorax
      c. Other
        (1) Drowning
        (2) Systemic toxins (including drugs, alcohol, carbon monoxide, and cyanide from smoke inhalation)
    3. Circulatory. Impaired delivery of oxygenated blood to vital organs will similarly cause rapid clinical deterioration. This can occur from:
      a. Severe hemorrhage
        (1) External
        (2) Intrathoracic (includes disruption of great vessels)
        (3) Intraabdominal
        (4) Pelvis or retroperitoneal (pelvic fracture)
        (5) Multiple long bones
        (6) Not intracranial blood loss (except children <1 year of age)
      b. Obstruction of blood flow (prevents venous return to heart)
        (1) Tension pneumothorax
        (2) Pericardial tamponade
      c. Myocardial dysfunction
        (1) Contusion
        (2) Rupture
        (3) Infarction and ischemia
        (4) Dysrhythmia
          (a) Electrical shock
          (b) Commotio cordis (high energy blow to chest)
          (c) Hypoxemia or global ischemia (e.g., hemorrhagic shock)
    4. Although this list is lengthy, providers should be trained to **recognize the three most common treatable causes of cardiorespiratory collapse** in the **prehospital** setting:
      a. Airway obstruction
      b. Hypoventilation or hypoxemia
      c. Tension pneumothorax
B. Determination of viability
    1. Likelihood of survival. The research on this topic often includes a mixture of clinical conditions, making interpretation difficult. The papers include both blunt and penetrating trauma patients; those who arrest before and after EMS arrival at the scene and after arrival at the hospital; and patients with variable presence of other signs of life (e.g., pupil response or cardiac electrical activity). Although all studies report a dismal prognosis (with survival rates from 0 to 18%), only a few rules can be generated from the available data.
      a. Victims of penetrating trauma have a greater likelihood of survival from cardiac arrest than victims of blunt trauma.
        (1) Survival from arrest is more likely after stab wounds (15% to 40%) than after gunshot wounds (7% to 17%). Survival of patients in arrest following stab wounds to the heart approaches 40% in areas with aggressive prehospital care and trauma systems.

(2) Arrest before EMS arrival significantly decreases the likelihood of survival.

(3) Presence of recognized and quickly treated pericardial tamponade is a positive prognostic factor (i.e., associated with improved outcomes).

b. Victims of blunt trauma who suffer cardiopulmonary arrest have a low likelihood of survival (0 to 3%).

(1) Those found by prehospital personnel to be in arrest with no signs of life (absence of spontaneous movement or respirations, and absence of intact reflexes including pupillary) and no electrical activity on the electrocardiogram (ECG) have a negligible chance of survival. Prehospital resuscitation is **not** indicated for these patients.

(2) The presence of some life sign (eye movement, pupil reaction, corneal reflex, organized cardiac rhythm) in pulseless, nonbreathing patients confers a likelihood of survival of about 2% to 3%. Because aggressive interventions (e.g., intubation, ventilation, release of tension pneumothorax, and volume resuscitation) result in occasional long-term survival, resuscitation should be attempted. Persistence of pulselessness (especially asystole) on hospital arrival is uniformly fatal and further resuscitation is not warranted, other than to confirm absence of pulse and other signs of life.

(3) Deterioration into cardiac arrest after EMS arrival but before hospital arrival also has dismal prognosis but full resuscitative efforts should be undertaken. Some studies suggest no benefit to Emergency Department thoracotomy for prehospital blunt traumatic arrest.

C. Criteria for attempting resuscitation. Resuscitation should be attempted on **all** patients in arrest caused by major blunt or penetrating trauma **unless** one of the following criteria are met:

1. Injury obviously incompatible with life (e.g., decapitation, evisceration of thoracic contents)

2. Absent signs of life (no respiratory effort, no pupillary response or eye movement, no response to deep pain) and ECG rhythm of asystole

3. Documented, untreated pulselessness and apnea for >10 minutes (e.g., prolonged entrapment, hazardous scene) in a normothermic patient.

4. Rigor mortis

D. Special conditions

1. **Electrical shock or lightning.** Because arrest is usually caused by a cardiac dysrhythmia and is often reversible, aggressive resuscitation should be attempted on all patients. In cases of multiple casualties from an electrical incident, those in arrest should be given first priority.

2. **Drowning or hanging.** Arrest is usually caused by asphyxia in these situations. Although appropriate trauma care, such as spinal immobilization, should be instituted, the decision to resuscitate can be based on criteria for "medical" arrests. Hypothermia should be considered in drowning victims.

3. **Hypothermia.** The presence of hypothermia (core temperature <35°C) can result from or lead to a traumatic event. Hypothermia can make it difficult to detect signs of life. Patients who are severely hypothermic deserve active core rewarming before cessation of resuscitative efforts unless injuries are clearly incompatible with life. Refer to Chapter 42 for more detail on this illness and treatment.

4. **Arrest secondary to medical cause.** Caution should be taken to recognize patients who may have suffered arrest because of a medical condition, such as the driver of an automobile who develops ventricular fibrillation with the resultant crash. Unless strong evidence suggests a

fatal injury, these patients deserve resuscitative efforts similar to any other medical arrest.

E. **Management protocols**
1. **At the scene. Note**: Time on scene (excluding complicated extrication) should be <10 minutes.
   a. **Assure scene is safe before entry.**
   b. **Recognize cardiac arrest**:
      (1) Determine whether to initiate resuscitation (see Section III).
      (2) Assess for presence of special conditions such as hypothermia or a primary medical cause that might influence decision or course of resuscitation.
   c. **Maintain manual spinal immobilization.**
   d. **Open airway using jaw thrust without head tilt.** Inspect oral cavity; suction or manually remove debris.
   e. **Ventilate patient** at rate of 12 to 16 breaths/minute; use oxygen (100%) as soon as available.
   f. **Perform chest compressions at rate of 100/minute.**
   g. **Control severe external hemorrhage.**
   h. **Determine ECG rhythm**:
      (1) Defibrillate up to three times (200, 300, 360 J) for ventricular fibrillation.
      (2) Note presence of an organized rhythm (pulseless electrical activity [PEA]) as this confers a greater likelihood of a reversible condition.
   i. Attempt to perform endotracheal intubation (refer to Chapter 8).
      (1) If able to intubate, confirm proper tube position and carefully secure tube.
      (2) If unable to perform intubation, determine effectiveness of ventilation using basic techniques:
         (a) If able to ventilate adequately (chest rise and fall), continue ventilation with basic maneuvers.
         (b) If unable to ventilate adequately and rescuer is properly trained and qualified, perform cricothyroidotomy; otherwise, initiate rapid transport and continue to attempt ventilation with basic maneuvers.
   j. Check for tension pneumothorax.
      (1) Signs: unilateral (or bilateral) decreased breath sounds, poor or worsening lung compliance (especially with positive pressure ventilation), tracheal deviation, subcutaneous emphysema.
      (2) If pneumothorax suspected, perform needle decompression.
   k. Immobilize patient on long backboard with straps, rigid cervical collar, and head immobilization device.
   l. Transfer patient rapidly to vehicle and initiate transport.
2. **En route to hospital**
   a. Reconfirm endotracheal tube placement and ability to ventilate.
   b. Reassess for tension pneumothorax.
   c. Contact Medical Command and receiving facility, based on local protocol.
   d. Consider military antishock trousers (MAST).
   e. Initiate intravenous (i.v.) access and administer crystalloid i.v. fluid wide open (use pressure bag if possible):
      (1) Two large bore i.v. (≥16 g) is ideal.
3. **Advanced interventions** for **physicians and other advanced providers** may be indicated in some situations, especially when transport time is >15 to 20 minutes:
   a. **Surgical airway**
      (1) **Cricothyroidotomy**
      (2) **Translaryngeal jet ventilation**
   b. **Venous access**

(1) **Percutaneous puncture of central vein**
(2) **Cutdown on saphenous vein at groin or ankle**
(3) **Intraosseous puncture in children up to age 6 years**

c. **Tube thoracostomy**

   (1) Needle decompression can produce inadequate or only temporary decompression of pneumothorax and is inadequate for drainage of hemothorax.

   (2) Placement of bilateral chest tubes should be strongly considered before transfer from other medical facilities or during long transports (>20 minutes) from scene to Trauma Center in all patients in traumatic arrest.

Axioms

- The most critically injured patients are transported first.
- Physiologic abnormalities on patient assessment correlate with high risk of major injury → anatomic triage criteria → mechanism of injury.
- Overtriage, as much as 50%, is necessary to achieve acceptable rates of undertriage (10%).
- Loss of airway is the most common cause of cardiorespiratory arrest after trauma, followed by hypoventilation or hypoxemia, and tension pneumothorax.

Bibliography

Aprahamian C, Darin JC, Thompson, BM, et al. Traumatic cardiac arrest: scope of paramedic services. *Ann Emerg Med* 1995;14(6):583–586.

Baxt WG, Jones G, Fortlage D. The trauma triage rule: a new resource based approach to the prehospital identification of major trauma victims. *Ann Emerg Med* 1990; 19(12):1401–1406.

Committee on Trauma, American College of Surgeons. *Advanced trauma life support manual.* Chicago: American College of Surgeons, 1993.

Durham LA, Richardson RJ, Wall MJ, et al. Emergency Center thoracotomy: impact of prehospital resuscitation. *J Trauma* 1992;32(6):775–779.

Esposito TJ, Offner PJ, Jurkovich GJ, et al. Do prehospital trauma center triage criteria identify major trauma victims? *Arch Surg* 1995;130(2):171–176.

Fries GR, McCalla G, Levitt MA, et al. A prospective comparison of paramedic judgment and the trauma triage rule in the prehospital setting. *Ann Emerg Med* 1994; 24(5):885–889.

Lilja GP, Madsen MA, Overton J. Multiple casualty incidents. In: Kuehl AE, ed. *Prehospital systems and medical oversight.* St. Louis: Mosby, 1994.

Lorenz HP, Steinmetz B, Lieberman J, et al. Emergency thoracotomy: survival correlates with physiologic status. *J Trauma* 1992;32(6):780–788.

Maslanka AM. Scoring systems and triage from the field. *Emerg Med Clin North Am* 1993;11(1):15–27.

Priest ML, Campbell JE. The trauma cardiopulmonary arrest. In: Campbell JE, ed. *Basic trauma life support for paramedics and advanced EMS providers,* 3rd ed. Englewood Cliffs, NJ: Brady, 1995:292–300.

Rosemurgy AS, Norris PA, Olson SM, et al. Prehospital traumatic cardiac arrest: the cost of futility. *J Trauma* 1993;35(3):468–474.

8. PREHOSPITAL THERAPY

Kathy J. Rinnert and Kevin S. O'Toole

I. **Airway management**
  A. **Introduction.** Successful airway management is the most important skill to be mastered by field providers to have an impact on patient outcome. Special circumstances encountered by prehospital providers contribute to the challenge of establishing an airway, including adverse environmental conditions (rain, snow, darkness); limited patient access (entrapment); lack of personnel (often limited to two providers); concern for cervical spine injury (precluding certain airway maneuvers); and patients with full stomachs, head injury, or acute intoxication (each of which can increase complication rates).
  B. **Patient assessment.** The airway is assessed by simultaneous evaluation of several simple clinical features. These include level of consciousness, physical findings, and vital signs.
      1. **Level of consciousness.** The patient's general condition of wakefulness is the best predictor of the ability to protect the airway from aspiration or occlusion. Specific simple features are sought: Is the patient **awake**, eyes open, and conversing? Is the patient reacting to **verbal** stimuli? Is the patient arousable only to **painful** or noxious stimuli? Is the patient **unresponsive**? Abnormalities of mental status can have multiple causes: hypoventilation and hypoxemia are two common causes of altered consciousness, along with hypoperfusion, drug or alcohol intoxication, and head injury. If the patient's ability to maintain adequate oxygenation, ventilation, or airway patency is suspected to be impaired, airway interventions are required.
      2. **Physical findings.** Search for findings indicative of poor oxygen delivery to tissues: pale, cool, moist skin; delayed capillary refill (>2 seconds); noisy or labored respirations (too fast or too slow). These findings can result from decreased alveolar oxygen content (hypoxia), impaired blood oxygen content (hypoxemia), or poor delivery of oxygenated blood (hypovolemia and shock). Other physical findings more specific to a pure respiratory abnormality include asymmetric or shallow chest excursion, crepitus, thoracic ecchymosis, nasal flaring, scalene muscle use, abdominal breathing, or subcostal retraction.
      3. **Vital signs.** Abnormal vital signs must be addressed—abnormal respiratory rate and heart rate, blood pressure, and if available, pulse oximetry—and appropriate therapy instituted. It is important to note that **normal** findings do not guarantee adequate ventilation or airway protection; for example, a pulse oximetry reading of 99% in an unconscious patient requires intubation to ensure airway protection.
  C. **Resuscitation.** Airway resuscitation encompasses positioning and clearing the airway, delivering supplemental oxygen, using adjuncts or assist devices, and tracheal intubation techniques.
      1. **Positioning the airway.** Manual techniques for opening the airway include the head tilt/chin lift, jaw thrust, and jaw lift. Each acts to manually displace oropharyngeal soft tissues and the tongue away from the posterior portion of the throat, thereby allowing upper airway patency. In the trauma patient, presence of a cervical spine injury must always be suspected; therefore, the head tilt/chin lift is **contraindicated** in most trauma patients, aside from those with isolated extremity injuries.
      The **jaw thrust** is accomplished by placing two hands at the angles of the mandible and lifting the jaw forward. The **jaw lift** is performed by placing a thumb inside the mouth on the mandibular incisors and fingers under the tip of the chin. The jaw and its attached soft tissues are then

lifted forward. Semiconscious or combative patients may bite rescuers, precluding use of the jaw lift. Otherwise, when performed with cervical spine immobilization, jaw thrust and lift offer low-risk and good yield for patients requiring assistance in maintaining airway patency. These maneuvers are also adjuncts for more advanced interventions, including assisted ventilation and tracheal intubation.

2. **Supplemental oxygen.** To maximize alveolar oxygen concentration, supplemental oxygen should be administered to all trauma patients, which can be accomplished by numerous devices. Corresponding flow rates and estimated delivered F_{IO_2} are shown in Table 8.1.

The high flow devices, including the partial and non-rebreather masks, are best for delivering oxygen to the conscious, alert trauma patient. The F_{IO_2} delivery by nasal cannula is variable and limited by blood or secretions in the nares; for this reason, nasal cannula oxygen supplementation should not be used in place of high flow mask devices.

3. **Airway adjuncts** are devices or maneuvers that aid in maintaining airway patency.

   a. **Suctioning**. The clearing of secretions, mucus, blood, or vomitus is essential to establish airway patency; although carrying the appropriate equipment to perform this is often overlooked. Obstructive bodies (e.g., dentures, teeth, bone fragments, or foreign material) must be removed. Suctioning is performed with a plastic, rigid large-tip opening device (e.g., a Yankauer or tonsil tip) to allow rapid removal of materials without clogging of the device. Handheld pump-action devices or large-caliber suction tubing without a tip can also be used to clear the airway of debris. Care must be taken to avoid inducing or exacerbating oropharyngeal bleeding when using any suction device. Small-bore devices are not recommended for use in trauma patients.

   b. **Nasopharyngeal airway** is an aid to maintain airway patency in the semiconscious or unconscious patient. Nasal airways must be used in conjunction with manual positioning of the airway (jaw thrust or lift). The size of the patient's little finger can help guide choice of a nasal airway, and the most patent nostril should be used for insertion. The airway is an uncuffed, pliable rubber tube with a beveled tip and a funnel-shaped top. The device is inserted into the nose, extending from the nostril to the nasopharynx, coming to rest behind the base of the tongue. **Advantages** of the nasopharyngeal airway are ease of insertion; aid in maintaining airway patency behind the tongue; ability for repeated suctioning without intense stimulation; and usefulness in patients with a gag reflex or clenched teeth. **Disadvantages** include inability to isolate the trachea and obstruction by blood or secretions.

Table 8.1 Estimated delivered oxygen concentration of various delivery devices

Device	Flow rate (L/min)	F_{IO_2} (%)
Nasal cannulae	2	25
	4	35–38
	6	45
Simple mask	5–10	35–55
Mask with reservoir	10–15	60–70
Venturi mask	4	28
	8	40
Endotracheal tube (connected to demand valve device and bag)	NA	80–90

NA, not applicable.

   c. Oropharyngeal airway is a rigid, plastic, semicircular-shaped device with side ports for suctioning. **It is used in unconscious patients who lack a gag reflex.** Oropharyngeal airways must be used in conjunction with manual positioning of the airway. The device is placed into the mouth following the curvature of the tongue (while holding the tongue with a gauze pad or using a wooden depressor) with the tip resting behind the base of the tongue. Alternatively, the airway can be inserted with the open portion of the "C" facing cephalad or lateral, with the tip rotated to match the natural tongue curve after placement. The key with both methods of insertion is to enhance patency. Pushing the tongue posteriorly will occlude the airway. The size of the oropharyngeal airway is chosen based on the distance from the lip angle to the ear lobe distance. In addition to maintaining or restoring airway patency, the **major advantages** of an oropharyngeal airway include ease of suctioning and assistance of ventilation. **Disadvantages** are stimulation of the gag reflex in the semiconscious patient, inability to use in patients with clenched teeth, and inability to isolate the trachea.

   d. Esophagotracheal Combitube (ETC) (Fig. 8.1):

      (1) Similar to esophageal obturator airway (EOA) and esophagogastric tube airway (EGTA), the ETC is placed through the mouth without direct hypopharyngeal or glottic visualization. Normally, the tip resides in the upper esophagus and hypopharynx. After inflating the balloon to obstruct the flow of gases to the esophagus, the esophageal port is ventilated. Gas exits from holes above the esophageal cuff or balloon and is directed the short distance (compared with EOA/EGTA devices) toward the glottis, resulting in near normal tidal volumes delivered to the lungs, with attendant breath sounds and expired CO_2.

      (2) Approximately 10% to 15% of insertion attempts result in the glottis being entered rather than the upper esophagus; resultant ventilation of the esophageal port yields lack of chest ex-

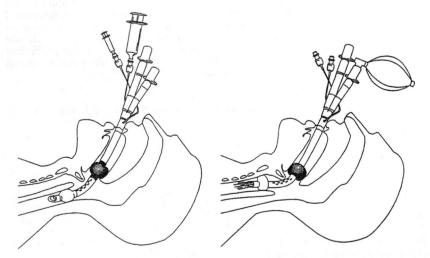

FIG. 8.1. Esophagotracheal Combitube (ETC). (Modified from the Sheridan Catheter Corporation, Argyle, NY, with permission.)

cursion or breath sounds. **This must be recognized**; in this situation, the second port should be ventilated. Similar to a standard endotracheal tube, this should provide direct oxygen to the trachea and produce symmetric breath sounds, CO_2 on exhalation, and a quiet epigastrium. Because the oropharyngeal cuff or balloon prevents loss of air seal, a face mask is not necessary. Clinical data show these devices to be superior to the EOA/EGTA in ease of use and adequacy of oxygen delivery. Additionally, little neck manipulation is needed with the blind insertion. The major disadvantages include lack of tracheal isolation in most cases and the need to identify the cases in which the glottis is entered (to allow ventilation through the correct port).

e. **EOA and EGTA** are large-bore, blind end tubes with attached face masks that are placed through the mouth, coming to rest in the esophagus. They are designed to occlude the esophagus with an inflated balloon.

   If encountered in the Emergency Department or Trauma Center, management consists of inserting an endotracheal tube while the EOA/EGTA device remains in place. After the airway is secured, the EOA/EGTA can be removed with large bore suctioning readily available. This sequence is important, because vomiting is a frequent complication of removal of these devices. Because of these risks and limits, the EOA/EGTA should not be used in trauma patients and are mentioned here only to familiarize personnel with their use.

f. **Laryngeal mask airway (LMA)** (Fig. 8.2). The LMA is a pliable, silicone "tear-drop" shaped diaphragm with an inflatable, cuffed rim

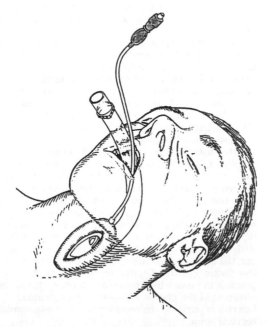

FIG. 8.2. Laryngeal mask airway (LMA). (Modified from The laryngeal mash airway: Its uses in Anesthesiology. *Anesthesiology* 1993;79:144–183, with permission.)

and a proximal ventilation tube. The diaphragm is placed through the oropharynx and rests above the glottis, with its tip in the esophagus. The diaphragm acts to isolate the posteriorly located esophageal structures from the anterior laryngeal opening. The proximal port is ventilated using a bag-valve device. **Advantages** of the LMA include rapidity and ease of placement, high success rates with training, and maintenance of in-line cervical positioning during insertion. Its ability to prevent aspiration is controversial. **Disadvantages** include initial training requirements, little data on its use outside of the operative suite or hospital, the requirement of an unconscious patient, and the necessity of "sizing" the device.

   g. Sellick's maneuver. Gentle pressure is placed on the cricoid cartilage, occluding the esophagus that lies directly behind it. When correctly performed, cricoid pressure limits the risk of aspiration by impeding gastric insufflation and the movement of vomited material into the hypopharynx and glottis (up to 15 cm H_2O force). It also can ease intubation by displacing anterior laryngeal structures into view during laryngoscopy. Care must be exercised as aggressive pressure can transmit forces to the underlying cervical spine. Otherwise, this maneuver offers little risk and great potential benefit. One common mistake is to put pressure on the thyroid cartilage rather than the cricoid cartilage, which does not alter the risk of aspiration and can tilt the glottis out of view during laryngoscopy.

4. Advanced airway skills in the field

   a. All advanced techniques, from direct oral intubation to surgical airways, require an investment in training, equipment, and retraining (to maintain facility). Each skill can be performed by physicians, paramedics, and nurses after proper training and with specific guidelines. It is unlikely that any one provider or system will master all options. More importantly, a plan with at least two options should be available and capable of being implemented. Chapter 14 discusses general trauma airway issues; here, we highlight those specific to the prehospital setting.

   b. Endotracheal intubation. This procedure is the placement of an open-end, cuffed (except for young children) tube into the trachea, providing a direct route for lung ventilation and bronchial tree suctioning and allowing protection from aspiration. **Orotracheal intubation** is the method of choice for most patients, with **nasotracheal intubation** an alternative method in certain spontaneously breathing patients with clenched teeth or inability to open their mouths. In the field, the success rate of nasal intubation is lower than with oral intubation (see Chapter 14).

   c. Digital intubation is useful when limited access to the patient or inability to directly visualize the airway structures exist. In the field, limited suction capabilities make this an attractive option for advanced providers. Digital intubation requires an unconscious patient and a "bite-block" (or other protective device) to prevent injury to the provider's fingers. The long finger of the nondominant hand is "walked" to the base of the tongue until a cartilaginous membrane (epiglottis) is encountered. While pushing the tongue downward with the long finger and elevating the epiglottis with the index finger, the endotracheal tube is guided blindly between the fingers into the glottic opening. Digital intubation has the advantage of being possible in cases where injury or foreign material limits direct visualization of the glottis. However, the technique requires dexterity, has risk of harming the provider, and causes uncertain motion of the cervical spine.

   d. Transillumination (lighted stylet) intubation. Newly developed intubation devices take advantage of fiberoptic technology to aid in tracheal intubation. A bright light introduced into the larynx will transmit through the anterior neck soft tissues to allow the operator to visualize correct stylet positioning and subsequent endotracheal intubation.

   (1) The procedure entails placing a malleable, plastic-coated stylet with a distal high-intensity light into the endotracheal tube. The stylet/tube assembly is bent in a "hockey stick" shape at the lower 3 to 4 cm, with the light at the tip (but not protruding). Using a scooping or "ladle" motion, while the nondominant hand gently pulls the tongue forward, the stylet/tube assembly is inserted through the mouth and into the hypopharynx and glottis. When the bright midline glow of the trachea is seen, the stylet is held in position while the tube is advanced into the trachea. If the esophagus is entered, no glow or a diffuse low intensity glow is seen; the stylet/tube assembly is withdrawn and reintubation attempted. Occasionally, intubation of the vallecula or lateral hypopharynx will produce a lateral glow, allowing midline repositioning.

   (2) **Advantages** of transillumination intubation include ability to intubate in patients with foreign material or other impediments to direct visualization, rapid tube placement, and minimal patient manipulation. **Disadvantages** include difficulties in confirming placement in high ambient light and training to gain and maintain facility.

 e. **Percutaneous translaryngeal catheter (jet) insufflation** is useful in either failed oral or nasal intubation or in those patients with incomplete upper airway obstruction unrelieved with standard maneuvers. It is discussed in Chapter 14.

 f. **Cricothyroidotomy**. Paramedics, flight nurses, and other providers can perform cricothyroidotomy for patients after failed intubation or with anatomic distortion that precludes other methods of gaining airway control. It is discussed in Chapter 14.

5. **Assist devices**. Prehospital personnel provide ventilatory assistance by multiple methods. These include rescue bag-valve ventilation, demand valve, and automatic ventilators.

 a. **Bag-valve devices**. The bag-valve is an oblong, self-inflating rubber bag with two one-way valves. The bag has a standard (15 mm) connection that can attach to a face mask or endotracheal tube for ventilation. When used with room air, delivered FIO_2 is 21%. High flow oxygen at 12 to 15 L/min provided by a supplemental oxygen inlet with a reservoir bag can deliver up to 90% to 95% oxygen. The bag-mask device can be used to assist spontaneous respirations or to ventilate apneic patients.

 b. **Demand valve devices**. The demand valve (manually triggered oxygen-powered breathing device) delivers 100% oxygen at high flow rates (40–60 L/minute). A push button valve allows oxygen to flow to the patient. **Advantages** include ease of use and high concentration of delivered oxygen. **Disadvantages** include lung barotrauma, inability to assess lung compliance, gastric distention, and inability to use in pediatric patients. Because of these disadvantages, demand valve use is discouraged in trauma patients requiring assisted ventilation.

 c. **Automatic ventilators** are time-cycled, constant-flow, gas-powered devices. These are portable and usually have at least two controls—one for ventilatory rate and one for tidal volume. A standard (15 mm) adapter allows use with an endotracheal tube.

D. **Field confirmation of tracheal tube placement**. Confirmation of proper endotracheal intubation is accomplished by multiple methods—**no singular method is infallible**.

1. **Physical assessment** includes **visualization** of the vocal cords and trachea during intubation and **auscultation** of bilateral breath sounds in the axillary lung fields. Lack of ventilatory sounds over the stomach (epigastrium) is also indicative of adequate placement. These are the first and easiest confirmatory methods for many patients.

2. **End-tidal carbon dioxide detectors** (electronic and colorimetric devices) are placed between the endotracheal tube and the ventilation device. These detect end-expiratory CO_2, with levels of 2% or greater indicating endotracheal placement. Semiquantitative CO_2 detectors may not be accurate in low pulmonary perfusion states such as cardiac arrest, massive pulmonary emboli, severe shock, or cardiac tamponade. Outside of these situations, expired CO_2 is very useful to confirm correct tube location.

3. **Bulb and suction devices** can be placed over the end of the endotracheal tube, creating negative expiratory pressure. Esophageal placement is indicated by the bulb device remaining flat, whereas rapid bulb reinflation indicates intratracheal location.

4. **Pulse oximetry** (oxygen saturation monitoring) is an adjunct to assess respiratory adequacy; however, arterial desaturation can be a late finding in respiratory failure. This, coupled with technical difficulties with sensing in the field, particularly with a hypotensive patient, limits the utility of this in rapid confirmation of tracheal tube placement, although it is valuable in identifying adequate arterial oxygenation.

II. **Other procedures and therapies**
  A. **Intravenous access and fluid therapy**
   1. Intravenous (i.v.) access allows the administration of crystalloids, blood products, and medications. Venous catheterization of trauma patients by paramedics is done routinely, even though outcome data supporting this practice are lacking. Currently, pragmatism suggests that i.v. access should be attempted while not delaying transport and other interventions (especially airway management and hemorrhage control). To limit the on-scene interval, attempts at i.v. placement should be made during extrication, while awaiting transport, or en route to the hospital. Two large-bore ($\geq$16 gauge) peripheral i.v. lines are optimal if rapid fluid therapy is needed or anticipated.

   2. **Failures**. It must be remembered that the paramedics are not working in ideal conditions. Starting an i.v. line in a combative patient in the back of a moving ambulance requires a great deal of skill. A number of trauma patients will arrive without i.v. access because of short transport times, technical difficulties, uncooperative patients, or other more pressing priorities (e.g., airway management, spine protection, or hemorrhage control).

   3. **Fluid therapy in the field**. Controversy exists over the composition, amount, and ultimate clinical goals of fluid therapy in trauma patients. Both under- and overtreatment are undesirable, and the specific heart rate or blood pressure targets to guide the amount of fluid are poorly understood. The issue does not appear to center on a "fluids: yes or no" question; rather, controlled resuscitation appears beneficial, although the endpoint and fluid makeup are still uncertain. In view of these uncertainties, treatment recommendation of presumed hemorrhagic shock is based on a simple algorithm (Chapter 4). These principles are discussed in detail in Chapter 4.

  B. **Military antishock trousers (MAST)**
   1. **Background**. MAST, also referred to as the pneumatic antishock garment (PASG) have been in use by civilian Emergency Medical Services for >20 years. Their use grew out of the experiences during the Vietnam War and documented clinical effects on blood pressure in the hypotensive trauma patient. However, little outcome data (especially with respect to mortality or morbidity) are available to support MAST use.

2. **Effects.** Several mechanisms of action are proposed for the elevated blood pressure seen with MAST inflation. The major effect is to increase peripheral vascular resistance, accomplished by decreasing the perfusion of the capillary beds of the lower extremities by the external pressure provided via the inflated MAST. This allows for increased blood flow to more vital organs, especially the heart and brain. MAST may help stabilize pelvic and femur fractures and limit blood loss.
3. **Indications**
   a. Hypotension associated with blood loss or loss of vascular tone (e.g., spinal cord injury) with transport times >20 minutes.
   b. Pelvic or lower extremity fractures as an aid to stabilize the fractures and decrease blood loss.
4. **Contraindications**
   a. Respiratory insufficiency or pulmonary edema
   b. Penetrating torso injuries
   c. Head injuries: MAST may increase intracranial pressure
   d. Pregnancy: if used in the second or third trimesters, inflate the leg sections only
   e. Suspected ruptured diaphragm
5. **Application and removal**
   a. The protocol for **applying** the MAST is straightforward. Remove any objects on the patients lower body that might cause the MAST or the patient to be punctured, especially glass, keys, or knives. The MAST is slid under the patient and the sections secured circumferentially. Often, the MAST is set onto the long spinal immobilization board before placing the patient onto it, allowing for efficiency with both procedures. After the MAST is secured with the Velcro strips, the leg sections are inflated first, using a foot pump. Inflation continues until the Velcro crackles or the MAST pressure gauge reads 100 mmHg. The abdominal section is then inflated in a similar manner. The patient's respiratory efforts should be observed closely because inflation of the abdominal section can limit pulmonary reserve. Large-bore suction should be available because the risk of vomiting is also increased with abdominal MAST inflation.
   b. The **removal** of the MAST **must** be done correctly; deflating prematurely can lead to hypotension that may not respond to reinflation of the MAST. **Each patient with an inflated MAST in place must be adequately volume resuscitated before attempting to remove the device.** When resuscitation is achieved, the abdominal section should be deflated first, in a slow and deliberate manner. A small quantity of air is removed and the patient's blood pressure is checked. If a fall of >5 to 10 mmHg occurs in the systolic blood pressure, deflation is halted and the patient is given more fluids. If no decrease in blood pressure ensures, deflation can proceed. Once the abdominal section is deflated, the leg sections are deflated, one at a time, in a similar fashion. Under no circumstances should the MAST be cut off of a patient. This is unnecessary and will render the MAST unusable.
6. **Complications.** The most common complication of MAST use is **interference with the physical examination** or gaining groin vascular access. Other complications include:
   a. Shock after inappropriate removal
   b. Compartment syndrome
   c. Lactic acidosis
   d. Myoglobinuria
   e. Ventilatory compromise
   f. Hyperkalemia
   g. Increased cerebral edema
C. **Needle thoracostomy**
   1. **Indications.** Needle thoracostomy should be performed when a tension pneumothorax has developed or is suspected, which can lead to

cardiovascular collapse within minutes. **Any trauma patient with severe respiratory distress should be evaluated immediately for tension pneumothorax**. The diagnosis is clinical and must be treated before arrival at the Trauma Center. Tension pneumothorax should be suspected in the trauma patient who is short of breath or hypotensive and with **any** of the following features:
   a. Decreased breath sounds
   b. Tracheal deviation (away from the involved side)
   c. Distended neck veins (this may not be seen in the patient who is hypovolemic)
   d. Hyperresonance to percussion of the chest (on the involved side)
   e. In the patient is intubated, increasing difficulty in bag-valve ventilation can be the earliest or sole indication of a developing tension pneumothorax.
2. Procedure. Treatment should proceed rapidly once the diagnosis is suspected; if incorrect, the only harm is creating the need for a formal tube thoracostomy in the receiving facility; whereas failing to recognize and treat can lead to death. Decompress the affected side of the chest by placing an i.v. catheter (12 or 14 gauge) into the hemithorax. Place the needle/catheter assembly perpendicular to the skin at the second or third intercostal space in the midclavicular line or the third or fourth interspace in the anterior axillary line; advance it until a rush of air occurs from the open distal port or until the hub reaches the skin. The large rush of air out the inserted needle and immediate improvement in the patient's cardiorespiratory status confirms the diagnosis. A common, potentially life-threatening mistake is to place the needle either too close to the sternum or cephalad to the second intercostal space, making heart or great vessel puncture likely. After placement, withdraw the needle, but leave the catheter in place to prevent reaccumulation of pleural gas. If the patient's condition worsens, suspect occlusion of the first catheter and place a second needle (Fig. 8.3).
3. Bilateral decompression. Occasionally, especially in the patient on positive pressure ventilation or with severe obstructive lung disease, bilateral tension pneumothorax can develop. The key is to recognize this potential, because the asymmetry described above with respect to tracheal and chest findings may not be present while an extreme threat to life exists. If uncertain, both hemithoraces should be decompressed.
4. Therapy after needle thoracostomy. At the Trauma Center or receiving facility, a chest tube is placed for definitive treatment once needle decompression is performed (whether or not clinical success occurred with the latter). Once the chest tube is in place, the catheter(s) can be withdrawn.
D. Splinting
   1. Indications. The purposes of splinting are to prevent further injury, decrease blood loss, and limit the amount of pain the patient will have with movement of that extremity. The extremity should be splinted in anatomic position, with the splint extending above and below the fracture site for stabilization. If the patient refuses or resistance to straightening exists, splint in a position of comfort. Dressings should be applied to any open wounds before splinting.
   2. Splint types. A large variety in design and sophistication of splints will appear on patients brought to a trauma center or an emergency department. They can be as simple as a rolled-up newspaper or as advanced as a vacuum or traction splint. A general list of splints is:
      a. Cardboard splints are made from heavy-duty cardboard and are meant for single use only.
      b. Board splints, which are common and durable, are made of straight pieces of wood, metal, or plastic cut to various lengths.

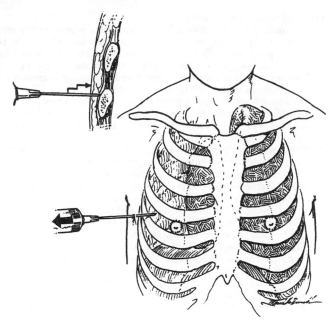

FIG. 8.3. Technique for needle thoracostomy. (Modified from Champion HR, Robbs JV, Trunkey DD. Trauma surgery. In: *Rob and Smith's operative surgery*. London: Butterworth, 1989:57, with permission.)

    c. Air splints, which encircle the injured extremity, are inflated with air to impart stiffness. They are usually clear to allow visualization of the underlying structures.

    d. Vacuum splints also encircle the injured limb. Instead of air being blown into them, it is withdrawn and a vacuum is produced, which stiffens the splint.

    e. Traction splints are used for femur fractures. Thomas half-ring splints and Hare® traction splints are those most commonly used. Their application requires specific training for proper placement.

    f. Ladder splints are made from heavy gauge wire in a ladder shape. They are useful for splinting extremities that cannot be straightened. Because they are bendable, these splints can be shaped to match the extremity, a quality unique to these devices.

  3. Complications. Although splinting is safe and effective in most patients, complications can develop, including:

    a. Neurovascular compromise. Whichever splint is used, distal neurovascular status must be checked before and after application of the splint. Also, if any patient movement has occurred, the patient reports more pain, or the extremity is noted to be cyanotic or edematous distal to the splint, reexamine the extremity. It is also advisable to periodically check the neurovascular status even without any of the above occurring. When impaired neurovascular status is seen distal to an injury, the splint should be loosened and the neurovascular status rechecked.

    b. Pain. When experienced, search for neurovascular compromise or malpositioning. Gentle repositioning should resolve this condition.

E. **Axial spine immobilization**
1. **Prehospital indications**. This is performed whenever the mechanism of injury, injury pattern, or physical examination indicate the **possibility** of spinal injury. Most trauma patients have experienced kinematic forces that warrant the precautionary application of spinal immobilization devices until definitive clinical and radiographic examinations can be performed in the Emergency Department. Patients with obvious physical findings (e.g., bony crepitation, palpable step-offs) or those with neurologic findings (e.g., paresthesia, weakness, paralysis) consistent with spine or cord injury should always receive complete immobilization before transport.
2. **Clinical "clearing" of the spine** often cannot and should not be performed by field personnel because of time, space, distracting injury, altered consciousness, and other concerns (e.g., airway, bleeding control, vascular access) that can preclude adequate infield evaluation to rule out spinal injury. The consequence of missed spinal injury and subsequent cord damage are often devastating and permanent. The rule in prehospital care is to maintain a high index of suspicion for such injuries and emphasis is placed on the liberal application of spinal immobilization.
3. **The need for spinal immobilization** occurs at the injury scene and continues through extrication (patient access), transportation, and stabilization in the Emergency Department. Immobilization is accomplished with the least allowable neck movement and ends only when physical and radiographic findings definitively rule out injury.
4. **Types of immobilization devices**. No single method or combinations of methods of immobilization consistently place the spine in neutral position or prevent all motion in the axial spine. Immobilization devices (cervical collars, cervical immobilization devices, and spine boards) will be discussed in a cephalad to caudad progression.
   a. **Cervical collars** (c-collars) are numerous in design and efficacy. These rigid, two-piece devices (e.g., Philadelphia Cervical Collar, Stifneck, Nec-Loc) encircle the cervical spine and soft tissues of the neck, effecting a snug fit between the tip the chin and the suprasternal notch of the anterior chest, and the occiput and a suprascapular region of the back. These collars limit movement of the head in the coronal and transverse planes, minimizing lateral and rotary motion. They do not, however, provide adequate immobilization in the sagittal plane (flexion-extension motion). For this reason, **a rigid cervical collar alone is inadequate for effective spinal immobilization** and is always used in conjunction with a cervical immobilization device (CID) and spine board (short or long). Soft neck collars (foam supports covered with loose weave material) are ineffective at limiting motion of the head in all planes and are not intended for use in spinal immobilization.
   b. **CID** are made of plastic, cardboard, or foam. They act to pad the lateral aspects of the head (limiting both lateral and rotary motion) and possess restraining straps that are positioned over the patient's forehead and chin, encircling the back of a short or long spine board. The CID affixes the patient's head and c-collar to a rigid spine board, limiting the head movements of flexion and extension. CID can be fashioned from blanket rolls, blocks, or sandbags placed alongside the head, with fixation to the spine board via wide (2″ to 3″) silk tape placed over the forehead and chin. Over the last several years, the use of sandbags has fallen into disfavor because of the weight exerted on the immobilized head and spine if emesis or secretion management requires turning the patient onto the side.
   c. **Spine boards** are termed "short" or "long," depending on the most distal portion of the patient immobilized. Short boards provide sta-

bility in the sagittal plane (limiting flexion and extension) from the head to the hips; they serve to minimize movement in all portions of the spine (cervical, thoracic, lumbar). Short boards are primarily used if patient access is limited (e.g., entrapment, confined space extrication) and stability in the axial spine is needed before and during the extrication process. Short boards utilize multiple straps crisscrossed at the mid thorax, abdomen, and groin to affix the patient to the board. Once extrication is performed and complete access to the patient is achieved, the short board and patient are secured to a long spine board. Long spine boards provide stability in the sagittal plane (limiting flexion and extension motions) from the head to the toes. Straps provide fixation points at the thorax, hips, and lower extremities (above the knees). It has been found that including the lower extremities in the immobilization process aids in stabilizing the lumbosacral spine and limits lateral motion of the torso if tilting of the board is needed to manage emesis. Padding between the lower extremities and under the knees enhances both stabilization and patient comfort.

  (1) **Secondary pain after immobilization**. With any of these devices in place, immobilization itself can produce symptoms or discomfort (e.g., occipital headache; neck, back, head, mandible pain) in otherwise healthy persons. This does not preclude the liberal application of spinal immobilization devices in most trauma patients. Padding behind the occiput and in the areas of a lordosis and kyphosis make intuitive sense and are especially important in the pediatric and elderly population, given their anatomic peculiarities.

Axioms

- Airway management is the most important skill to develop when managing trauma patients; plans should include the formulation and practice of both basic and advanced interventions.
- Never remove an EOA/EGTA before successfully intubating the trachea with a cuffed tube.
- No method of intubation or confirmation of intubation is infallible; be prepared for failure.
- Intravenous access should be attempted in all seriously injured patient in the field, but primarily during transport or extrication to prevent excessive delays in arrival to the Trauma Center.
- MAST has no role in penetrating torso trauma and a very a limited role in trauma care with short transport times.
- Field cervical and axial spine immobilization should be done with multiple devices in any patient suspected of having an injury and continued until clinical or radiographic clearance is complete.

Bibliography

Ali J, Qi W. Fluid and electrolyte deficit with prolonged pneumatic antishock garment application. *J Trauma* 1995;38(4):612–615.

Aprahamian C, Thompson B, Finger WA, et al. Experimental cervical spine injury model: evaluation of airway management and splinting techniques. *Ann Emerg Med* 1984;13(8):584–587.

Bledsoe BE, Porter RS, Shade BR. *Brady paramedic emergency care.* Englewood, NJ: Prentice-Hall, 1991:199–269.

Campbell JE. *Basic trauma life support: advanced prehospital care,* 2nd ed. Englewood, NJ: Prentice-Hall, 1988:42–90.

Cayten CG, Berendt BM, Byrne DW, et al. A study of pneumatic antishock garments in severely hypotensive trauma patients. *J Trauma* 1993;34(5):728–733.

Cline JR, Scheidel E, Bigsby EF. A comparison of methods of cervical immobilization used in patient extrication and transport. *J Trauma* 1985;25;649–653.

Dalton AM. Prehospital intravenous fluid replacement in trauma: an outmoded concept? *J R Soc Med* 1995;88(4):213P–216P.

Graziano AF, Scheidel EA, Cline JR, et al. A radiographic comparison of prehospital cervical immobilization methods. *Ann Emerg Med* 1987;16(10):1127–1131.

Huerta C, Griffith R, Joyce SM. Cervical spine stabilization in pediatric patients: evaluation of current techniques. *Ann Emerg Med* 1987;16(10):121–1126.

Jones SA, et al. *Advanced emergency care for paramedic practice*. Philadelphia: JB Lippincott, 1992:129–174.

Kaweski SM, Sise MJ, Virgilio RW. The effect of prehospital fluids on survival in trauma patients. *J Trauma* 1990;30(10):1215–1218.

Podolsky S, Baraff LJ, Simon RR, et al. Efficacy of cervical spine immobilization methods. *J Trauma* 1983;23(6):461–465.

Pollack CV. Prehospital fluid resuscitation of the trauma patient. An update on the controversies. *Emerg Med Clin North Am* 1993;11(1):61–70.

Sanders MJ. *Paramedic textbook*. St. Louis: Mosby Year Book, 1994:242–281.

Sasada MP, Gabbott DA. The role of the laryngeal mask airway in pre-hospital care. *Resuscitation* 1994;28:97–102.

Schriger DL, Larmon B, LeGassick T, et al. Spinal immobilization on a flat backboard: does it result in neutral position of the cervical spine? *Ann Emerg Med* 1991;20:(8) 878–881.

9. FIELD TEAMS: COMPOSITION, DIRECTION, AND COMMUNICATION WITH THE TRAUMA CENTER

Owen T. Traynor

I. **Introduction.** Trauma care begins with field providers at the trauma scene. In addition to their specialized training in the care of the trauma patient, Emergency Medical Services (EMS) field personnel can help improve the care delivered at the receiving facility by communicating with the trauma team members. The trauma facility must help maintain and support the prehospital providers and communication system to facilitate care and early notification for all trauma patients.

II. **EMS Providers**
   A. Although the United States Department of Transportation (DOT) has established national standard curricula for EMS training, each state has instituted its own EMS provider certification. Although many different certification levels and variability in types of procedures performed by these EMS personnel exist, provider training and capabilities can be grouped into some general classes.
      1. **First responder.** These EMS providers are often police officers or fire fighters. They have received approximately 40 hours of training to prepare them to deliver basic life-saving care. This includes teaching in cardiopulmonary resuscitation (CPR), basic first aid, supplemental oxygen use, and, in some select areas, automatic defibrillator use. First responders have basic familiarity with the equipment used by EMS technicians and paramedics.
      2. **Emergency medical technician (EMT).** Several levels of EMT certification exist. The terminology used to refer to these certifications can vary.
         a. **Emergency medical technician-ambulance or basic (EMT-A or EMT-B)** are similar levels of certification, with EMT-B replacing the older term. These are entry level providers and the only prehospital providers currently guided by a national training curriculum. The EMT-A/B has received approximately 100 hours of training in basic life support (BLS), use of airway adjuncts and supplemental oxygen, advanced first aid, and splinting. They have a basic understanding of some medical problems such as diabetes mellitus, chronic obstructive pulmonary disease (COPD), and heart disease.
         b. **Emergency medical technician-intermediate (EMT-I).** This level of training varies among states, requiring from 30 to 100 hours of training beyond the EMT-B level. In some states, these EMT are also known as advanced EMT (AEMT) or critical care EMT (EMT-CC). An EMT-I has all of the skill and training of the EMT-A/B, plus advanced airway management skills (e.g., endotracheal intubation), peripheral intravenous insertion skills, medication administration, interpretation of electrocardiograms, and training in defibrillation of patients.
         c. **Emergency medical technician-paramedic (EMT-P).** These EMS providers have an additional 350 to 1,000 hours of training beyond the basic EMT training. Paramedics have all of the skills of the EMT-A and EMT-I along with more advanced airway management skills, which can include surgical airway techniques; also, in some areas, the EMT-P can start central venous lines. The EMT-P has a greater understanding of anatomy and physiology than does the previously mentioned providers.

   3. **Other healthcare professionals.** In some systems, registered nurses
      and physicians serve as EMS providers. Most likely, they are part of an
      aeromedical transport crew.
III. **Medical control of field providers**
   A. Medical control is typically defined as the direction of patient care by a phy-
      sician who is not present at the location of the patient and the EMT. Medical
      control can take two general forms: direct and indirect. EMS systems use a
      mixture of both to direct patient care.
   B. **Direct medical control** is best defined as the real time, online direction of
      prehospital care by a physician or a physician surrogate. Direct medical con-
      trol is typically provided by radio from a local Emergency Department, where
      emergency physicians direct the care of patients who will be transported to
      their facility. A common alternative is the use of a centralized medical com-
      mand, where physicians direct the care of patients who will be transported
      to other facilities. In a few EMS systems, physicians respond to the location
      of the emergency and provide on-scene medical command.
   C. **Indirect medical control** is the sum of off-line activities that are used to
      direct care. These activities include EMS system design, training and certifi-
      cation of EMS providers, development of treatment protocols and guidelines,
      observation of prehospital care, and implementation of quality improvement
      programs. All programs use indirect control in some way.
IV. **Initial notification of the trauma team by field providers.** EMT at all lev-
    els should attempt initial notification as soon as it is known that a patient meets
    activation criteria for the trauma team. This initial notification should be brief
    to avoid delay or compromise patient care.
   A. **Important initial information** should include the mechanism of injury,
      number of patients, any requests for additional resources (EMS, fire or police
      department units), likelihood of prolonged extrication or prehospital inter-
      vals, and potential toxic exposures.
   B. **Coordination of resources** allows the EMS communication center to co-
      ordinate the emergency response and utilization of resources, including ac-
      tivation of the local disaster plan. This preliminary report can help the
      trauma team mobilize the hospital-based resources, radiology facilities and
      personnel, operating rooms, blood products, and so forth, thus saving valu-
      able time once the patient arrives.
   C. **Types of communication devices.** Several communication devices are
      commonly used by EMS systems.
      1. **Radio transmission** is the most widely used method because of ease
         of use and low cost. Specific UHF and VHF radio frequencies have been
         set aside for medical use. Although radio communication works well,
         signal quality can be poor in urban environments and remote moun-
         tainous terrain. Radio signals do not pass through metal walls or large
         land masses. In addition, a limited number of frequencies are available.
         Confidentiality is limited by the widespread availability of scanners.
      2. **Landline telephone.** Private telephones offer the least expensive and
         easiest way to communicate. Signal quality is excellent. Landline tele-
         phone use is limited by lack of portability and difficulty interfacing with
         portable electrocardiogram (ECG) units without additional equipment.
      3. **Cellular telephones** combine the ease of landline telephone use with
         the portability of radio communication. The equipment is relatively low
         in cost and easy to maintain. Arrangements must be made with local
         cellular carriers to grant EMS units priority access to cells.
      4. **Telemetry.** ECG data can be transmitted via radio, landline telephone,
         or cellular telephone. This capability is becoming a standard option on
         many of the newest ECG monitors. A recording device or fax is required
         to receive these data. In the future, other data or images may be trans-
         mittable using these technologies.

D. Patient report. A more thorough patient report should be given when practical. EMT and paramedics must be skilled in the transmission of pertinent information. Similarly, the receiving facility should have trained nursing or physician personnel who can assimilate the information and ask directed questions only when necessary to ensure adequate preparation without delaying care or transport. If not well controlled, online medical command use (physician or nurse interplay with verbal directives) can increase the on-scene interval for trauma patients. The typical patient care report should include the following:

1. **Patient description** is a headline sentence that includes the identifying data and the reason for the call (i.e., age, sex, chief complaint, and mechanism of injury).
2. **History of present illness** gives a brief history of the current event. For collisions involving motorized devices, whether the patient was wearing a seatbelt or an airbag was deployed, amount of vehicular damage, ejection from the vehicle, extrication time, and estimated speed of the vehicles involved; for falls, height and surface plus ambient conditions; for assaults or penetrating injuries, type of weapon, location of wounds, and nature of the event; and for fires or other exposures, the aforementioned data (if applicable) plus interval and intensity of exposure to fire, smoke, or toxic gas or fluid.
3. **Past medical history** lists significant major past medical history, current medication list, and drug allergies. Minor illnesses should not be reviewed at this time (e.g., upper respiratory infections, nonactive medical problems, and distant surgical procedures without physiologic sequelae).
4. **Physical examination findings** is a focused description of the primary and secondary survey, beginning with a description of the patient's appearance and vital signs, and then progressing through to a brief head-to-toe assessment. **Only pertinent positives and select pertinent negatives** (e.g., no jugular venous distention) should be presented.
5. **Presumptive diagnosis**. A one-sentence declarative statement discusses what injuries are presumed to be present.
6. **Therapeutic interventions** contain specific interventions given and response to therapy (e.g., needle thoracostomy for presumed tension pneumothorax with restoration of pulse and adequate breathing, fluids, and hemodynamic response).
7. **Receiving institution** names the receiving facility and estimated time of arrival (ETA).
8. **Additional orders** provides any additional orders for patient care.
E. Avoiding poor reports. The most common problems with oral case reports are poor organization and excessive length.
1. **Organization**. EMS providers can avoid these problems by developing a standard format for their reports. The opening statement provides an overview, orienting the listener to the remainder of the presentation.
2. **Brevity**. The EMS provider must select essential information from all available data and avoid a prolonged presentation. Information that is useful simply communicates illness or injury severity and what immediate resources are needed on arrival. On the receiving side, questions should be limited to those data needed to influence care or ensure adequate resources on arrival; other interplay should be limited not to interfere with care at the scene or transport.

Axioms

- The trauma team leaders should be familiar with the makeup and abilities of all field providers who deliver patients to the Trauma Center
- Physicians from all disciplines involved in trauma care should be involved with EMS teaching, design, and quality improvement

- Communication, brief but directed, should be practiced and rewarded to ensure continuity of trauma care

Bibliography

Coonan PR. Oral case presentations. In: Traynor OT, Coonan PR, Rahilly TJ, eds. *The streetmedic's handbook*. Philadelphia: FA Davis, 1996:379–382.

Erder MH, Davidson SJ, Cheney RA. On-line medical command. In theory and practice. *Ann Emerg Med* 1989;18:261–268.

Kuehl K, MacClean T, Pepe PE. Medical control. In: Schwartz GR, Cayten CG, Mangelsen, et al., eds. *Principles and practice of emergency medicine*, 3rd ed. Philadelphia: Lea & Febiger, 1992:3150–3154.

10. AIR MEDICAL AND INTERHOSPITAL TRANSPORT

John S. Cole

Air Medical Transport

Based on the experience of the Korean and Vietnam Wars, air medical transport has grown to become an integral part of trauma care in the United States. Approximately 300 private, hospital-based, public service and military air medical helicopter programs transport >250,000 patients annually. Two thirds of the transports are interhospital, with the remaining one third transported directly from the scene.

I. **Equipment**
   A. Most air medical transport today is accomplished with twin-engine helicopters specifically configured for medical missions. Some flight programs fly instrument flight rules (IFR) missions, allowing transport of trauma patients in weather conditions that previously prevented rotorcraft transport. Most aircraft with reconfiguration can transport two patients, in addition to two flight crew members and the pilot.
   B. The flight environment is noisy, making simple procedures such as auscultation of blood pressure and breath sounds difficult or impossible. Therefore, nonaudible-dependent monitoring is used. Most flight crews rely on noninvasive blood pressure monitoring, end-tidal CO_2, and pulse oximetry to monitor patients in flight. Rotorcraft rarely fly at altitudes above 2,000 feet above ground level (AGL). At these altitudes, pressure changes have only a minor impact on the volume of air-filled spaces such as a pneumothorax.
   C. The flight crew communicate with each other and the patient through headsets or helmets connected to internal communication systems. The crew must be able to communicate with the receiving hospital. Advance notification of patient assessment and changes in patient condition en route allow the receiving Trauma Center to be better prepared.

II. **Triage**
   A. The transport of trauma patients directly from the scene should be supported by online medical control or preapproved protocols based on the factors of time, distance, geography, patient stability, and local resources. Undue delay of transport from the scene to the closest hospital while waiting for a helicopter should be avoided. Rendezvous at the hospital's helipad would be more appropriate use of time.
   B. Interhospital transport of trauma patients usually involves moving a patient to a facility with a higher level of care. Multiple studies have shown that the skill of the flight crew is more important in patient outcome than the speed and size of the helicopter.
   C. The National Association of Emergency Medical Service Physicians (NAEMSP) has recommended triage guidelines for on-scene helicopter transport (Table 10.1).
   D. Weather, geography, logistics, or other factors determine flight suitability. The final decision to accept the mission should lie solely with the pilot. **Crew safety is paramount**.

III. **Flight crew**
   A. More than 70% of the medical flight crews consist of a nurse-paramedic team. Approximately 20% of programs use two nurses, and only 3% of programs use a flight physician. Respiratory therapists are also combined with nurses in a small percentage of programs.

IV. **Interventions**
   A. Most therapeutic interventions (e.g., endotracheal intubation, chest decompression, intravenous (i.v.) access, and control of hemorrhage) are completed before lift-off.

Table 10.1 On-scene helicopter triage

Trauma Center candidate based on triage criteria
>15 minutes to the Trauma Center by ground
>20 minute extrication time
Local ambulance out of service
Difficult patient access
Wilderness rescue
Multiple victims
No advanced life support available

B. Intravenous analgesia, sedation, and chemical paralysis, as well as administration of vasoactive substances and blood products can be done in flight. These interventions must be performed under strict online medical direction or predetermined approved protocols.

V. Helipad access team

A. A helipad team trained in helicopter safety is usually designated to assist the flight crew in unloading and transporting the patient from the helicopter to the Emergency Department. Helipads should be in close proximity to the resuscitation area, limiting the need for therapeutic interventions on the helipad.

B. When helipads are remote from the resuscitation area (e.g., rooftop with elevator and corridor transport), occasional therapeutic interventions may be required on the helipad. Only a limited number of resuscitative procedures should be performed on the helipad. Focus should be on identifying the need for immediate life-saving procedures; establishing an airway, decompressing a tension pneumothorax, applying direct pressure to an open bleeding wound, or administering resuscitative drugs and countershocks for dysrhythmias. Other interventions (i.v. catheter placement for volume resuscitation or thoracotomy) are best performed in the Emergency Department.

VI. Safety

A. The pilot's decision to complete a mission should be based on aviation factors alone and not influenced by patient criteria.

B. In general, a 500-foot ceiling and 1-mile visibility are required for daytime visual flight rules (VFR) flight. This may be geography-specific, depending on the presence of mountains and pockets of fog. Day-local is defined as <25 nautical miles from departure point to destination point, with generally the same terrain elevation.

C. Comprehensive safety orientation programs for local ground EMS personnel that include instruction covering helicopter communication, setting up landing zones, patient preparation, and conduct around the aircraft are an essential part of any EMS air medical program (Fig 10.1).

D. Table 10.2 outlines safety conduct around the helicopter.

Interhospital Transport

I. Introduction. Emergent interhospital transport usually occurs after initial stabilization of the trauma patient and determination by the referring facility that the patient's needs for definite care are beyond the scope of local capabilities. This practice is in response to evidence supporting the view that trauma outcome is enhanced if critically injured patients are cared for in facilities prepared for and dedicated to the needs of the acutely injured. A Trauma Center should have referral centers that facilitate transfers, outreach teams to provide referring facilities with continuing education, and public education programs about trauma systems and injury prevention.

A. Transfer of the trauma patient occurs with the expectation that care will continue en route to the receiving facility and that changes in patient status will be identified and treated. These goals frequently require specialized

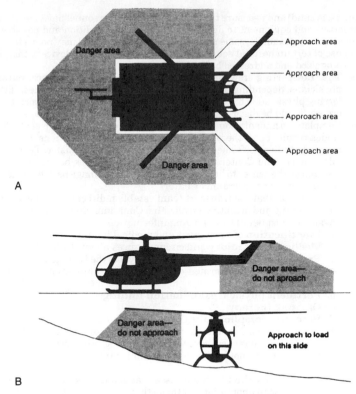

FIG. 10.1. Air view (**A**) and ground view (**B**) of safe approaches.

personnel and equipment. Coordination between referring and receiving institutions and medical direction during transport are fundamental to guarantee continuation of care.

II. Before transport. Interhospital transport can be performed by a transport team from the referring facility, the receiving facility, or by a third party. It is the responsibility of the **referring physician** to decide the best mode of transportation

Table 10.2 Safety around the helicopter

The same safety standards should be practiced whether the helicopter's engines are running or shut down.
- Do not approach the helicopter unless signaled to do so by a flight team member.
- Remain clear of the helicopter at all times unless accompanied by a flight team member.
- When approaching the helicopter, always approach from the front of the aircraft and move away in the same direction.
- When approaching the helicopter on a slope, **never** approach from the uphill side.
  –Always approach from the downhill side because the main rotor to the ground clearance is much greater. Always be aware of the blade clearance.
- **Never** walk around the tail rotor area.
- No unauthorized personnel within 100 feet of the aircraft.
- No intravenous devices or other objects should be carried above the head, and long objects should be carried parallel to the ground.

(air vs. ground) and to ensure that the transporting personnel have the necessary expertise and equipment to deal with the patient's condition and possible complications. For example, some nonhospital-based personnel may not be trained in the use of certain hospital equipment (drug pumps or other devices); this should be recognized and addressed before transport.

A. The transporting crew can be any combination of paramedics, nurses, or physicians, depending on the patient condition and local policies. If the referring physician is to provide medical direction during transport, transfer orders should be discussed before departure.

B. Complete documentation of all patient care records must be sent. This includes results of all therapeutic and diagnostic interventions, copies of all imaging studies performed, and patient consent for transfer. Teleradiology allows a Trauma Center to review a patient's studies before arrival. This also allows the center to help referring facilities manage patients who do not require transfer to a Trauma Center.

C. It is essential that the transport team establish direct communication with both referring and accepting physicians. Communication with the referring physician must detail the following information.

  1. Identification of the patient and medical history
  2. Mechanism of injury and circumstances about the incident
  3. Prehospital management before arrival to the Emergency Department
  4. Interventions performed during initial stabilization and patient's response
  5. Pertinent physical examination findings
  6. Ongoing therapy
  7. Potential complications that may occur during transport

D. The transport team should then perform their own directed evaluation, equivalent to a primary survey, without delaying transport. This evaluation should include, but not be limited to the following:

  1. Airway
    a. Recheck the airway or assess adequate position of endotracheal tube with appropriate methods that can include direct visualization, end-tidal CO_2, auscultation, esophageal detector device, or chest x-ray.
  2. Respiratory
    a. Document respiratory status before initiation of transport.
    b. Check for appropriate functioning of ventilatory equipment.
    c. Check or place nasogastric tube to prevent aspiration in obtunded or intubated patients.
    d. Check position of any tube or device (e.g., thoracostomy). Chest tubes ideally should have pleuravacs attached and placed on suction for transport.
  3. Cardiovascular
    a. Document heart rate, pulse, pulse oximetry, and blood pressure before initiation of transport.
    b. Control external bleeding and reevaluate bandages applied for bleeding control.
    c. Secure two large-bore i.v. catheters.
    d. Secure adequate supply of blood products for transfer.
    e. Invasive lines (e.g., arterial lines, central venous pressure [CVP] lines, and pulmonary artery catheters) should be connected to the transport monitor to allow continued hemodynamic monitoring during the transport.
    f. Connect patient to electrocardiograph monitor.
  4. Central nervous system
    a. Document neurologic examination and Glasgow Coma Scale (GCS) score before initiation of transport or administration of paralytic or sedative agents.
    b. Secure head, cervical, thoracic, and lumbar spine with immobilization devices, as needed.

III. During transport. The transport team must know before transport which physician is to be responsible for online medical direction. Responsibility for medical direction will vary, based on local practices and the policies of the transport service. The receiving physician, however, must always be made aware of changes in the patient's condition en route.

    A. Once the patient has been stabilized, the transport should be completed without delay. It is expected that care during transport be at the same level as received at the referring institution, within the obvious limitations of the out-of-hospital environment. Unstable patients should be accompanied by a provider capable of appropriate medical interventions; this may require a physician.

    B. The transporting unit must have the capabilities to continue cardiorespiratory support and blood volume replacement. Constant hemodynamic monitoring is necessary. Communication via radio or cellular telephone should occur to obtain medical direction and to provide updates to the receiving facility.

    C. When standing orders or protocols (the essential component of off-line medical direction) are given to the transport team, the referring physician must be sure that the orders match the team's capabilities and that the appropriate medications and equipment are present.

IV. After transport. On arrival at the receiving facility, the transport team must give a complete report to the receiving trauma team. This should include a brief summary of the initial history and treatments, followed by an update of any changes en route and any interventions. In addition, all documentation from the referring institution must be delivered to the receiving team leader. If the patient was transferred for diagnostic procedures and is to be transferred back to the original institution, the same transfer regulations apply now to the receiving hospital. If diagnostic procedures reveal new evidence of present or potential instability, the patient cannot be transferred back without appropriate stabilization.

V. Legal considerations. The transfer of patients from one institution to another is regulated by federal statute. The legislation that created the patient stabilization and transfer requirements for hospitals and physicians is the **Consolidated Omnibus Budget Reconciliation Act (COBRA) of 1985**, also known as the "antidumping law." This is the current legal standard. One of the main objectives of this resolution is to guarantee equal access to emergency treatment to all citizens regardless of their ability to pay.

    A. COBRA attributes responsibility for the patient's transfer to the referring hospital and physician.

        1. Violations can result in termination of Medicare privileges for the physician and hospital.

        2. A hospital can be fined between $25,000 and $50,000 per violation.

        3. A physician can be fined $50,000 per violation.

        4. A patient can sue the hospital for personal injury in civil court.

    B. The Emergency Medical Treatment and Labor Act (EMTALA) established by the COBRA legislation governs how patients can be transferred from one hospital to another. Hospitals cannot transfer patients unless the transfer is "appropriate," the patient consents to transfer after being informed of the risks of transfer, and the referring physician certifies that the medical benefits expected from the transfer outweigh the risks. Appropriate transfers must meet the following criteria:

        1. The transferring hospital must provide care and stabilization within its ability.

        2. Copies of medical records and imaging studies must accompany the patient.

        3. The receiving facility must have available space and qualified personnel and agree to accept the transfer.

        4. The interhospital transport must be made by qualified personnel with the necessary equipment.

Axioms

* The outcome of air medical transport for trauma patients is dependent on appropriate triage and the skill of the flight crew.
* Safety of crew and patient is paramount.
* Never approach a helicopter without the assistance of the flight crew.
* Transfers should be made for medical necessity and not financial reasons.
* The medical benefits anticipated from the provision of specialized trauma care at the receiving facility should outweigh the risks of transfer.

Bibliography

American College of Emergency Physicians (ACEP). *Appropriate utilization of air medical transport in the out-of-hospital setting.* Dallas: American College of Emergency Physicians, 1999.

American College of Surgeons (ACS). Stabilization and transport. In: *Advanced trauma life support (ATLS) student manual,* 7th ed. Chicago: American College of Surgeons, 2001.

Blumen IJ, Rodenberg H, eds. *Air medical physician handbook.* Salt Lake City: Air Medical Physician Association (AMPA), 1996.

National Association of EMS Physicians (NAEMSP). *Air medical dispatch: guidelines for trauma scene response.* Lenexa, Kansas: National Association of EMS Physicians, 1992.

Rau W. 2000 annual transport statistics and fees survey. *AirMed* July/August, 2000

Swor RA, Storer D, Domier R, et al. *Emergency medical services (EMS) committee policy resource and education paper: medical direction of interfacility patient transfers.* Dallas: American College of Emergency Physicians (ACEP), 1997.

11. TRAUMA TEAM ACTIVATION

Theodore R. Delbridge

I. **Introduction.** Healthcare facilities designated as Trauma Centers house the resources to provide initial definitive care, regardless of injury severity.
  A. As designated by the American College of Surgeons, **a level I trauma center** possesses the capabilities and physical resources necessary for comprehensive trauma care, including research, education, prevention, and rehabilitation components. **Level II centers** possess similar clinical resources, without requiring the research and education components. **Level III centers** can possess limited staff and resources for clinical care, providing care for many patients, and identifying those with more serious injuries who are better treated at a level I or II center.
  B. The **trauma team** is at the hub of the Trauma Center activities. Maintaining an available qualified trauma team represents a costly investment by the Trauma Center, indicating its commitment to providing quality trauma care for the community.

II. **Activation criteria**
  A. The trauma team is a resource that can be made available to all patients at the Trauma Center patients. However, it is important that the trauma team be activated for patients whose spectrum of injuries, as reported by Emergency Medical Service (EMS) personnel, are likely to demand multidisciplinary management, critical care, or an immediate operation.
  B. To some degree, "tiering," or grading of responses, occurs in all facilities that care for trauma patients. Not all injuries demand the attention of the entire trauma team (e.g., simple extremity fractures resulting from low force mechanisms of injury). To best match resource utilization and need, criteria for activation of varying levels of responses may be developed. These should be institution specific, based on resources, expertise, and needs.
  C. Many level I and II trauma centers currently employ triage criteria to guide the initial evaluation of trauma victims, including deployment of personnel and equipment. Development of such criteria follows recognition that primarily three categories of patients arrive at the Trauma Center.
    1. The trauma team should be activated before arrival at the center for **patients whose injuries are obviously severe** and demand an immediate multidisciplinary approach. These patients have clear evidence of life-threatening injury as evidenced by abnormal physiology (vital signs and sensorium) or penetrating truncal injury. Additionally, patients with less evidence of severe injuries, but who are arriving in numbers such that local resources would be overwhelmed, are often placed in this most serious category.
    2. **Patients whose injuries, or potential for injury, may not seem immediately life-threatening**, but deterioration is possible, may not require the immediate activation of the entire trauma team and are most appropriately evaluated immediately by qualified Emergency Department staff, together with some of the other trauma team members. They are treated where multidisciplinary resources are immediately available should they be needed. These are often patients with significant mechanisms of injury, but without obvious anatomic or physiologic abnormalities.
    3. **Patients who could be managed at most acute care facilities** by a qualified emergency department staff, including consultation with other providers as needed, require the resources similar to those used to evaluate and treat most other acutely ill, non-trauma patients.

D. Variations in activation criteria and responses

1. Trauma team activation criteria, in general, include components similar to those of the American College of Surgeons Triage Decision Scheme. Physiologic and anatomic factors, as strong predictors of the need for critical care or early operation, should be prominent components. Mechanism of injury information, by itself, is less predictive of the need for critical care or operation, but should be a consideration in the activation criteria.
2. Trauma team activation criteria reflect each institution's patient volume and resources. In general, activation criteria identify the resources and personnel assembled initially to care for a seriously injured patient. Some centers choose a singular response type ("all or none"), which eases implementation, but can expose the system to inefficient use of resources. A graded system of activation can help ensure prompt response without waste.
3. An example of trauma team activation criteria is in Table 11.1. **Full team activation** occurs for patients whose injuries, as reported by

Table 11.1 Sample trauma team activation criteria

Full response: Attending emergency medicine physician and trauma surgeon, trauma fellow or senior surgical resident, two junior residents, radiology technician, respiratory technician, three nurses (attending or resident anesthesiologist immediately available), blood bank personnel with blood.

Physiologic
–Respiratory distress
–Intubated or question of airway security
–Decreased level of consciousness at any time
–Systolic blood pressure <100 mmHg at any time

Anatomic
–Penetrating wound to the head, neck, chest, abdomen, or extremities proximal to the knee or elbow
–Amputation or degloving injury proximal to knee or elbow
–Multiple injuries
–Flail chest
–Suspected spinal cord injury
–Suspected pelvic fracture
–Two or more long bone fractures
–Multiple patients with significant injuries

Mechanism
–Pedestrian struck by a vehicle moving >20 mph
–Thrown from vehicle
–>20-minute extrication time

Partial response: Attending emergency medicine physician, trauma fellow or senior surgical resident, one junior resident, two nurses, radiology technician, notification of trauma surgeon attending; others called as needed.

Multiple patients without significant injuries

Mechanism of injury (not meeting level I criteria)
–Fall >15 feet
–Major vehicle deformity
–Vehicle passenger compartment intrusion
–Death of another vehicle occupant
–Roll-over vehicle crash

Helicopter scene flight

Emergency medical service personnel request (not meeting level I criteria)

EMS personnel, are or have potential to be severe. In such cases, the entire trauma team, including the attending trauma surgeon, responds to the Emergency Department. Partial team activations do not require anesthesiology, respiratory therapy, and certain surgical housestaff to respond. Furthermore, the attending trauma surgeon is notified immediately via the paging system, but is not required to respond initially for partial team activation. At any time, a partial response can be upgraded to a full response, if necessary.

4. **Results of tiered responses.** Level I trauma centers using tiered trauma team activations have reported that 52% to 57% of trauma patients meet the criteria for lesser responses. Furthermore, such guidelines have achieved 85% to 95% sensitivity in terms of requiring full trauma team response for those patients who require early operations or admission to a critical care unit. Patients initially met by a partial team who subsequently require a full team response have outcomes comparable to those met initially by the entire trauma team. Thus, trauma centers have reported that the immediate availability of multidisciplinary expertise and resources is crucial, but that their deployment during the initial evaluation of all trauma patients is not always necessary.

5. **Activation criteria and triage at other trauma centers.** For level II trauma centers, which are often community hospitals with the trauma surgeon on-call outside the facility, the issue of trauma team triage criteria is also important. Resources, including qualified surgeons, may not be as plentiful as at tertiary medical facilities. Their conservation for those situations when they are truly needed, while minimizing under-triage, is an important concern. When EMS personnel report that a trauma patient suffers respiratory compromise, altered mentation (e.g., Glasgow Coma Scale score <13), or hypotension, qualified emergency medicine and trauma surgery staff should be prepared to care for the victim on arrival. For other patients, evaluation by a qualified emergency physician and support staff, in consultation with an attending trauma surgeon, may be appropriate. When such guidelines have been used, no differences were found between observed and predicted mortality.

III. **Summary.** The trauma team brings the comprehensive multidisciplinary capabilities of the Trauma Center to the emergency evaluation and management of injured patients. Its activation is crucial if the Trauma Center is to effect favorable outcomes for critically injured patients. Judicious utilization of this resource is appropriate. As no standard criteria exist for trauma team activation, it is important for all centers to evaluate their trauma system components, quality and availability of resources, and prospectively create trauma team activation guidelines that are adequately dispersed and evaluated on an ongoing basis. Such efforts enhance the efficiency of care for the trauma patient.

Axioms

- Trauma team activation criteria must be developed locally, and consider the response capabilities and input of EMS, emergency medicine, trauma surgery, anesthesiology, and other related specialists.
- Grading of trauma team responses can help tailor resources, but guidelines should be planned, monitored, and adjusted, as needed.

Bibliography

Khetarpal S, Steinbrunn BS, McGonigal MD, et al. Trauma faculty and trauma team activation: impact on trauma system function and patient outcome. *J Trauma* 1999; 47(3):576–581.

Moore EE, Moore JB, Moore FA. The in-house trauma surgeon—paradigm or paradox. *J Trauma* 1992;32(4):413–414.

Phillips JA, Buchman TG. Optimizing prehospital triage criteria for trauma team alerts. *J Trauma* 1993;34(1):127–132.

Plaisier BR, Meldon SW, Super DM, et al. Effectiveness of a 2-specialty, 2-tiered triage and trauma team activation protocol. *Ann Emerg Med* 1998;32(4):436–441.

Shatney CH, Sensaski K. Trauma team activation for "mechanism of injury" blunt trauma victims: time for a change? *J Trauma* 1994;37(2):275–282.

Simon BJ, Legere P, Emhoff F. Vehicular trauma triage by mechanism: avoidance of the unproductive evaluation. *J Trauma* 1994;37(4):645–649.

Singh R, Kisson N, Singh N, et al. Is a full team required for emergency management of pediatric trauma? *J Trauma* 1992;33(2):213–218.

Terregino CA, Reid JC, Marburger RK, et al. Secondary emergency department triage (supertriage) and trauma team activation: effects on resource utilization and patient care. *J Trauma* 1997;43(1):61–64.

Thompson CT, Bickell WH, Siemens RA. Community hospital level II trauma center outcome. *J Trauma* 1992;32(3):336–343.

12. ORGANIZATION PRIOR TO TRAUMA PATIENT ARRIVAL

William S. Hoff

I. **The trauma response**
   A. **Institutional capability.** The ability of a hospital to respond to the needs of trauma patients is institution-specific. The American College of Surgeons Committee on Trauma has developed the following classification of trauma centers:
      1. **Level I.** Provides a 24-hour, in-house trauma team with the ability to fully resuscitate injured patients and provide definitive and comprehensive surgical care. These centers typically serve population-dense areas. The trauma team is usually led by an attending trauma general surgeon, emergency physician, trauma fellow, or a senior surgical resident. Level I centers demonstrate a commitment to education through physician training, research, and community prevention and outreach programs.
      2. **Level II.** Commitment to patient care is similar to level I centers. However, resources such as cardiac surgery, reimplantation surgery, and microvascular surgery may vary. Level II centers often provide trauma care to less population-dense regions. Research, education, and resident teaching programs are not required. The trauma team is not necessarily in-house, but must be available to meet the patient on arrival.
      3. **Level III.** Designation specific for hospitals in rural areas that are not accessible to level I or II centers. In-house surgical coverage is not required on a 24-hour basis, but must be available in a timely fashion. Availability of certain surgical subspecialties and advanced technology may be limited. Therefore, proper functioning requires formal transfer agreements to higher level centers.
      4. **Level IV.** Designed to provide initial evaluation and assessment of injured patients in more rural and remote areas, these centers may be located in a small hospital or clinic. Physicians with training in trauma resuscitation are usually available to manage patients. However, surgical coverage is not mandatory. Most patients will require transfer to higher levels of care.
      5. Most hospitals in the United States are not designated Trauma Centers. Many injured patients will arrive at nontrauma hospitals and require rapid initial evaluation, resuscitation, and potential transfer to a Trauma Center.
   B. **Levels of response.** An established response to injured patients is essential to all hospitals. In nontrauma centers, where a full trauma team may not be available, an established procedure (e.g., personnel, tasks) will facilitate resuscitation and optimize patient outcome. Many trauma centers use tiered levels of response based on field triage criteria. The composition of the trauma team varies, based on the level of trauma response:
      1. **Full response** ("trauma code," "code red," "level I trauma response") is designed for the patient who is physiologically unstable or who presents with life- or limb-threatening injuries (e.g., thoracic gunshot wound). The patient receives immediate evaluation by a full trauma team (i.e., trauma surgeon, anesthesiologist, and so forth).
      2. **Modified response** ("trauma alert," "level II trauma response") is intended for the patient with the potential for serious injury based on the mechanism of injury, but without physiologic or anatomic criteria defining a life- or limb-threatening injury. The composition of the trauma team will vary according to hospital resources, with emergency medicine physicians frequently providing a leadership role.
      3. **Trauma consultation** is designed for patients triaged to a Trauma Center based solely on mechanism of injury without physical signs of

significant injury. These patients are initially evaluated by the emergency physician and referred to the trauma service or an appropriate surgical subspecialist.

II. Trauma resuscitation area

A. Physical plant considerations

1. In hospitals that receive a significant volume of trauma patients, or where injured patients arrive without prior notification, a dedicated trauma resuscitation area (TRA) should be available in the Emergency Department. Although an exclusive TRA is impractical for most hospitals, every effort should be made to ensure that trauma resuscitation takes place away from the general Emergency Department workspace.
2. The TRA should be secure, with limited access to nonmedical personnel.
3. Convenient access to the operating room (OR), radiology suite, intensive care unit (ICU), and staff call-rooms are other important considerations in TRA design.
4. The TRA must be large enough to accommodate all members of the trauma team (approximately 5 to 10 people). Ample space must be provided to allow full resuscitation, basic radiographic evaluation, orthopaedic stabilization, and several emergency surgical procedures:
   - Rapid intubation
   - Cricothyroidotomy or surgical airways
   - Insertion of central venous catheters
   - Thoracostomy
   - Placement of urinary catheters
   - Resuscitative thoracotomy
   - Diagnostic peritoneal lavage (DPL)
   - Ultrasound (focused abdominal sonography for trauma [FAST])
   - Splinting of fractures
   - Emergency burr holes*
   - Placement of intracranial (ICP) monitoring devices*
   - Placement of pelvic external fixation devices*
5. **Other considerations relative to the TRA include:**
   a. **Lighting.** Sufficient lighting is important, but the light sources must allow free access to the patient and easy movement of personnel and equipment throughout the workspace.
   b. **Hypothermia** must be actively prevented during the resuscitative phase. Measures to prevent hypothermia (e.g., individual room thermostats, overhead heating elements) should be considered in the design of the TRA.
   c. **Multiple patients.** Each institution should have guidelines for resuscitation of multiple patients within the defined TRA or Emergency Department.

B. Barrier precautions in the trauma resuscitation area

1. **Bodily fluids** of all trauma patients are potential sources of transmissible disease. Therefore, barrier precautions should be mandatory for all members of the trauma team during resuscitation. Specifically, nonsterile gloves, an impervious gown, surgical mask, shoe covers, and protective eyewear are necessary for all team members who potentially can come in contact with the patient.
2. **Barrier precaution items** should be available in a designated area adjacent to the TRA, in full view of those who may enter the area. It is the responsibility of the trauma team leader or recorder to monitor and enforce compliance with barrier precautions.
3. **Arrival of trauma patients without sufficient prior notification is an unavoidable occurrence.** Therefore, guidelines should be developed for relieving personnel who have entered the TRA without barrier

---

* Appropriateness of these procedures depends on local protocols, available personnel, and access to the OR.

precautions. The goal should be to minimize the total number of unprotected individuals; protected team members should provide rapid relief for those who have not had the opportunity to don protective equipment.

C. **Equipment and placement.** The minimal amount of equipment and supplies necessary to effectively resuscitate should be stored in the TRA. Although frequent restocking may be necessary, eliminating superfluous inventory optimizes resuscitation space and facilitates standardization of care.

1. **Equipment trays should contain only those instruments and materials absolutely necessary to perform a given procedure.** Trays should be easily accessible, openly displayed, and clearly identified with simple, bold-faced labels. Equipment should be stored such that wasted effort is minimized during resuscitation. One logical approach is to arrange supplies in a head-to-toe configuration, such that airway equipment and cervical collars are stored near the head of the stretcher, thoracostomy trays near the midportion of the stretcher, and splinting materials at the foot of the stretcher.

2. A **resuscitation stretcher**, equipped with four-point restraints, should be oriented in the center of the workspace. Items ideally stored under the stretcher are outlined below:
   - Patient gowns
   - Blankets
   - Small oxygen tank
   - Nasogastric and orogastric tubes
   - Irrigation tray
   - Automatic blood pressure cuff
   - Electrocardiogram (ECG) leads
   - Pulse oximeter leads

3. Equipment necessary to manage immediately life-threatening conditions should be set-up close to the stretcher, in proximity to the trauma team member most likely to use it (Table 12.1; Fig. 12.1).

4. Additional equipment and materials listed below can be stored along the walls of the workspace. Large, portable equipment must be easily visible and accessible. Smaller items can be stored on shelves and counters or in designated trays. Cabinets are not recommended, as closed doors impede rapid identification and ease of access.
   - Mechanical ventilator
   - Fluid warmer: stocked with crystalloid solution
   - Rapid infusion–warming device
   - Central venous catheter, pulmonary artery (PA) catheter kits
   - Instrument trays (e.g., thoracotomy, surgical airway, basic surgical)

Table 12.1 Immediately accessible equipment and supplies

Head of stretcher	Equipment for airway management, including multiple endotracheal tubes, oxygen, suction devices, oral/nasal airways, Ambu bags and laryngoscopes
Tray #1	Equipment for intravenous access, intravenous tubing, phlebotomy, arterial blood gases
Trays #2 and #3	Thoracostomy trays, chest tubes (36 F, 40 F), appropriate suture material
Tray #4*	Diagnostic peritoneal lavage equipment
Foot of stretcher	Chest drainage system (e.g., Pleurovac®)
Left side	Manual blood pressure cuff, electrocardiogram wires, pulse oximetry monitor

*Ultrasound machine

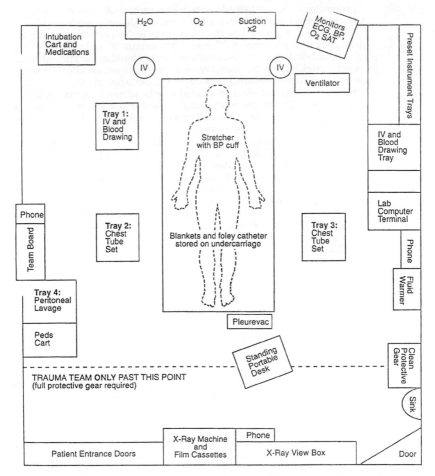

FIG. 12.1. Layout of the trauma resuscitation area. (From Committee on Trauma, American College of Surgeons. *Resources for the optimal care of the injured patient.* Chicago: American College of Surgeons, 1993, with permission.)

- Portable monitors
- Suture cart
- Traction devices (e.g., traction-splint)
- Preformed extremity splints
- X-ray view boxes

5. A modest inventory of equipment and supplies to replace items used from other areas (e.g., angiocatheters, intravenous tubing) should be readily available.

6. Equipment and supplies should be stocked in a portable carrier (i.e. "trauma kit") that can be transported with the patient outside of the TRA—to radiology, for example. Suggested contents include:
- Nasal airway, oral airway, bite block
- Cricothyroidotomy set

- Suction equipment and tubing
- Pulse oximetry probe
- Manual blood pressure cuff
- Angiocatheters (14, 16, 18 gauge)
- Intravenous tubing and adapters
- Syringes (3, 5, and 10 mL)
- Phlebotomy equipment and laboratory tubes
- Arterial blood gas (ABG) syringes
- Irrigating syringe (60 mL)
- Dressings, gauze, tape
- Medications (see II.E. below)
- Continuation forms for documentation
- Telephone and pager lists

7. Equipment and medications specific for pediatric resuscitation should be stored on a separate cart. The cart should be equipped with a Broselow tape for rapid calculation of dosages and selection of appropriately sized equipment.

D. **Communication in the trauma resuscitation area.** Reliable communication among members of the trauma team and throughout the institution is essential. Communication in the TRA can be facilitated by the following:

1. A podium provides a designated place to document the resuscitation events. In many designated trauma centers, one individual is primarily responsible for documentation (see III.D., below). A podium also serves as an area from which the general activity of the resuscitation can be observed.

2. Marker board or chalkboard can be useful to record history, physical findings, and test results as well as display pertinent pager numbers of on-call consultants and ancillary personnel.

3. Efficient communication to other areas of the institution is essential to facilitate the resuscitation. Dedicated extensions to the OR, computed tomography scan suite, blood bank, and the ICU should be available. Use of these extensions should be restricted to members of the trauma team. A laboratory computer terminal and digital x-ray station may be considered in a high volume Trauma Center.

4. Communication between the trauma team and the OR staff can be facilitated by a patient classification system. Such a system allows the OR and blood bank staffs to organize resources and allocate personnel. The trauma patient classification system described in Table 12.2 provides a template.

Table 12.2 Trauma patient classification system

Class A	Unstable patient: requires immediate surgical intervention; no further injury evaluation (e.g., x-ray or laboratory studies) required. Immediate access to the operating room is necessary. Initiate massive transfusion protocol for blood and blood products (e.g., fresh frozen plasma, platelets)
Class B	Unstable patient: high probability of surgical intervention within 15–30 minutes. Some injury evaluation in progress. Massive transfusion likely.
Class C	Stable patient: probability of surgical intervention within 2 hours. Complete injury evaluation (e.g., computed tomography scan) in progress. Crossmatched blood or type and screen sufficient.
Class D	Stable patient: minimal probability of surgical intervention (minor injuries).

E. **Medications in the trauma resuscitation area**. In addition to standard drugs stocked on the code cart, a small inventory of medications should be kept in the TRA.
  1. **Instantly available drugs** should include those for rapid sequence induction (e.g., succinylcholine, sodium thiopental, etomidate, vecuronium, midazolam), available at the time the patient arrives (see Chapter 14). Ideally, these agents are stored in labeled syringes for instant administration.
  2. Sedatives, analgesics, and antimicrobials that should be **immediately available** include lorazepam, morphine sulfate, fentanyl, naloxone, tetanus toxoid, cefazolin, and an aminoglycoside.
  3. Drugs that should be **readily available** include diphenylhydantoin, 50% dextrose, methylprednisolone (for blunt spinal cord injury), mannitol, thiamine, magnesium, and calcium.

III. **The trauma team**
  A. **Definition**. The trauma team is an organized group of professionals who perform initial assessment and resuscitation of critically injured patients. The composition of the trauma team, level of response, and responsibilities of each member are hospital-specific, and should be predetermined through established guidelines, policies, or procedures.
  B. **Trauma team members**. The actual composition of the trauma team varies, depending on the institution. Specific personnel typically include:
    1. **Trauma surgeon**—a general surgeon who has demonstrated interest, skills, and training in trauma care. In designated trauma centers, the trauma surgeon typically functions as the trauma team leader.
    2. **Emergency physician**—with demonstrated skills in evaluation and resuscitation of injured patients and advanced trauma life support (ATLS) certification. In many hospitals, the emergency physician functions as the trauma team leader or is in charge of airway management.
    3. **Anesthesiologist**—a physician with special skills in airway management, endotracheal intubation, sedation, and analgesia. In many institutions, this role is fulfilled by a certified registered nurse anesthetist (CRNA).
    4. **Trauma nurses**—Emergency Department nurses with specialized training and demonstrated interest in trauma care.
    5. **Resident physicians**. In hospitals with training programs, surgical or emergency medicine residents and trauma fellows assume active roles on the trauma team. In level I and II trauma centers, senior residents can function as trauma team leaders under the supervision of trauma attendings.
    6. **Respiratory therapist**—trained to anticipate the needs of the trauma patient—must be available to assist in the evaluation and management of the patient's respiratory status.
    7. **Radiology technologists**—with expertise in portable imaging techniques—are important to an efficient secondary survey.
    8. **Surgical subspecialists**. Although not typically involved in the initial assessment, surgical consultants (e.g., orthopaedic surgeons, neurosurgeons) are vital members of the trauma team.
    9. **Other personnel**. The trauma team can also include OR nurses, laboratory technicians, ECG technicians, chaplains, social workers, transport personnel, and case managers.
  C. During resuscitation of severely injured patients or during simultaneous resuscitation of multiple victims, some mechanism should be available to mobilize additional personnel from within the institution. In addition, appropriate on-call personnel must be available.
  D. **Roles and responsibilities**. Ideally, the trauma team can be organized and positioned before arrival of the patient. A generic scheme for **positioning** of the various trauma team members is illustrated in Figure 12.2. Specific responsibilities of each team member are outlined in Table 12.3.

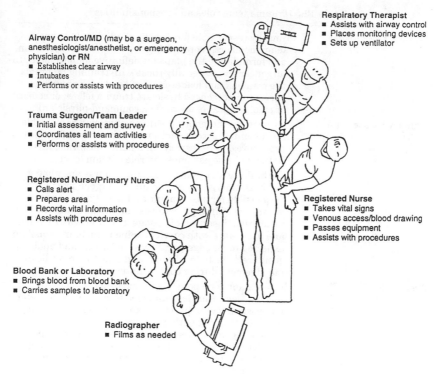

Respiratory Therapist
- Assists with airway control
- Places monitoring devices
- Sets up ventilator

Airway Control/MD (may be a surgeon, anesthesiologist/anesthetist, or emergency physician) **or RN**
- Establishes clear airway
- Intubates
- Performs or assists with procedures

Trauma Surgeon/Team Leader
- Initial assessment and survey
- Coordinates all team activities
- Performs or assists with procedures

Registered Nurse/Primary Nurse
- Calls alert
- Prepares area
- Records vital information
- Assists with procedures

Registered Nurse
- Takes vital signs
- Venous access/blood drawing
- Passes equipment
- Assists with procedures

Blood Bank or Laboratory
- Brings blood from blood bank
- Carries samples to laboratory

Radiographer
- Films as needed

FIG. 12.2. Positions and roles of the trauma team members. (From *Resources for the optimal care of the injured patient.* Chicago: American College of Surgeons, 1993, with permission.)

E. Multiple patient scenario

1. All hospitals must be prepared for the arrival of multiple trauma patients. This situation can overwhelm the resources of even the best-prepared Trauma Center. The definition of "multiple patients" is hospital-specific, based on Trauma Center designation, size, personnel, and other factors primarily related to resource availability.

2. The trauma team leader is responsible for assigning available personnel to assure effective resuscitation of each patient.

3. A triage plan for positioning patients and allocating resources and personnel should be formulated, based on the prehospital report and early clinical findings, for example:

   a. Position patients based on perceived needs (e.g., patients with severe head injury should be positioned near the mechanical ventilator).

   b. Assign a primary resuscitator for each patient. Each resuscitator must be directly supervised by the trauma team leader. Effective communication between these individuals is of the utmost importance.

   c. Recruit additional personnel to assist in resuscitation of the patients. Properly trained nurses, prehospital personnel, and technicians are potential in-house sources of personnel. Other on-call surgical personnel (e.g., orthopaedic surgeons) can also be mobilized to assist in the resuscitative phase.

   d. Reallocate personnel and resources, based on primary survey.

Table 12.3 Trauma team roles and responsibilities

Trauma team leader	Primarily responsible for directing individual trauma team members, coordinating events of the resuscitation, and formulating the plans for definitive management. In larger centers, especially those with training programs, the trauma team leader may be an attending trauma surgeon, emergency physician, trauma fellow, or senior or chief surgical resident (i.e., command-physician).
Primary resuscitator	A surgeon or emergency medicine physician responsible for the initial assessment and performance of surgical procedures, as necessary. In smaller hospitals, this individual also assumes the role of team leader.
Airway manager	Anesthesiologist, certified registered nurse anesthetist (CRNA), emergency physician, or surgeon primarily responsible for assessment and management of the airway. Required procedures can include endotracheal intubation, insertion of nasogastric or orogastric tubes, and assistance with cervical spine immobilization. Also expected to manage paralytics, sedatives, and analgesics relative to intubation and assist with medical management during code situations.
Assistant	The assistant is responsible for exposing the patient, placing electrocardiographic leads, and pulse oximeter, and assisting with patient transfers. In addition, may be asked to assist with any necessary procedures. Depending on the institution, the assistant may be a physician (e.g., surgical resident) or, in nonteaching hospitals, a trauma nurse or emergency medicine technician.
Trauma nurse	Prepares the trauma resuscitation area (TRA) for arrival of the patient. Serves as the patient's primary nurse during the resuscitative phase of care. Responsible for monitoring vital signs and performing select procedures (e.g., intravenous access, phlebotomy, urinary catheters). Assists with patient transfers, accompanies patient outside of TRA and reports to the receiving unit.
Recorder	Should be a nurse with extensive experience in trauma resuscitation. Responsible for documenting events of the resuscitation on an appropriate flowsheet. Facilitates communication and mobilization of additional resources (e.g., blood bank, operating room, consultants). May also assist in coordinating events of the resuscitation.
Respiratory technician	Responsible for assessment of the airway and breathing and placement of appropriate monitoring devices (e.g., pulse oximeter). Assists airway manager with intubation and ventilator setup.
Radiology technologist	Performs necessary radiographic studies. Assists with positioning the patient for the required studies. Processes films and returns completed radiographs to the TRA.
Laboratory technician	Draws blood samples and transports samples to the laboratory for processing. Delivers blood to the TRA before arrival of the patient. Transports additional blood and blood products to the patient as necessary.
Chaplain/Social worker Case manager	Assists with patient identification. Communicates between trauma team and patient's family.

e. Relocate stable patients out of the trauma resuscitation to other areas of the Emergency Department, based on rapid but thorough clinical assessment.

IV. Transfer of patient to the trauma team

A. A formal report at the time of patient arrival signifies the transition of care from prehospital provider to the trauma team. Ideally, the trauma team has assembled before arrival of the patient and received pertinent prehospital information from the individual providing medical command to the incoming unit.

B. With several exceptions (e.g., acute airway compromise), patients should be maintained on the transport stretcher until a prehospital report is completed. Once movement to the resuscitation stretcher is initiated, the trauma team cannot devote full attention to the report.

C. The prehospital report should be a concise (i.e., 30 to 45 seconds) summary given by a single prehospital provider, directed at the entire trauma team.

D. Following the report and transfer of the patient, a designated member of the trauma team (e.g., Recorder) should attempt to get a more detailed history from the prehospital providers.

Axioms

- Prior notification of patient arrival facilitates an organized response.
- Barrier precautions should be employed for all hospital-based providers in the TRA.
- Equipment and personnel placement in the TRA should be expedient and standardized.
- During trauma resuscitation, verbal communication among trauma team members should be minimized.
- The presence of an identified trauma team leader promotes efficiency and facilitates formulation of a definitive plan.
- The trauma team leader should attempt to maintain a panoramic view of the resuscitation.

Bibliography

American College of Surgeons Committee on Trauma. *Resources for the optimal care of the injured patient.* Chicago: American College of Surgeons, 1998.

Centers for Disease Control. Recommendations for prevention of HIV transmission in health-care settings. *MMWR* 1987;36(Suppl 2S):15–185.

DiGiacomo JC, Hoff WS. Universal barrier precautions in the emergency department. *Hospital Physician* 1997;33:11.

Driscoll PA, Vincent CA. Organizing an efficient trauma team. *Injury* 1992;23:107.

Fernandez L, McKenney MG, McKenney KL, et al. Ultrasound in blunt abdominal trauma. *J Trauma* 1998;45:841.

Hoff WS, Reilly PM, Rotondo MF, et al. The importance of the command-physician in trauma resuscitation. *J Trauma* 1997;43:772.

Maull KI, Rhodes M. Trauma center design. In: Feliciano DB, Moore EE, Mattox KL, eds. *Trauma*, Norwalk: Appleton & Lange, 1996.

Moore EE. Resuscitation and evaluation of the injured patient. In: Zuidema GD, Rutherford RB, Ballinger WF, eds. *The management of trauma.* Philadelphia: WB Saunders, 1985.

Morgan T, Berger P, Land S, et al. Trauma center design and the OR. *AORN J* 1986; 44:416.

Trauma Alert Policy, The Ohio State University Hospitals, May 22, 1984. In: Chayet NL, Reardon TM, eds. *Trauma centers and emergency departments.* Clifton, NJ: Law and Business, Inc., Harcourt Brace Jovanovich, 1985.

13. ADULT TRAUMA RESUSCITATION

Michael Rhodes

I. **Introduction**
   A. **Resuscitation is an intense period of medical care** in which initial and continuous patient assessment guides concurrent diagnostic and therapeutic procedures. As a dynamic period, resuscitation requires the trauma team to rapidly develop a differential diagnosis based on effectiveness of treatment and results of available diagnostic studies. When possible, the surgeon and emergency physician should direct this crucial activity. The supervising physician must ensure that the optimal resuscitation space, personnel, and equipment are present.
   B. Resuscitation of the trauma patient requires an organized, systematic approach using a well-rehearsed protocol. Advanced Trauma Life Support (ATLS) is a single-physician resuscitation course of the American College of Surgeons that describes the initial assessment approach to an unstable patient with life-threatening injury (Table 13.1). The principles of ATLS resuscitation are also applicable to a trauma center environment and should be supplemented by a **team approach** to the trauma patient. The approach of a trauma team should be multispecialty and protocol driven based on patient **"stability"** and mechanism of injury (blunt vs. penetrating) (Fig. 13.1). Definitive treatment of a patient's injuries will be dictated by the anatomic injury and the patient's physiology (stability). This chapter presents a team-oriented approach for trauma resuscitation.
II. **Patient stability**
   A. The term **"unstable"** has classically referred to physiologic parameters such as vital signs (pulse, blood pressure, respiratory rate, temperature). However, in the context of trauma resuscitation, the definition of unstable can be expanded to include some subjective, objective, or anatomic factors that may predict need for specialized trauma care in the Trauma Center. Criteria for the unstable trauma patient (Table 13.2) are liberal and refer to the potential need for operative intervention or admittance to the intensive care unit (ICU). Unstable patients who meet these expanded criteria usually have injuries that are life- or limb-threatening. A subcategory of unstable patients, those who present *in extremis* (sometimes referred to as "agonal"), requires a tailored approach.
   B. **Response to initial fluid challenge** is also a measure of stability. Hypotensive patients who sustain a normotensive response to the first 1 to 2 L of fluid are responders and considered stable. **Transient responders** and **nonresponders** are **unstable** and should be treated accordingly.
   C. **Significant injury may also be suspected** from interpretation of key phrases verbalized by patients.
      - "I'm choking": airway dysfunction
      - "I can't swallow": airway dysfunction
      - "I can't breathe": ventilatory dysfunction
      - "Let me sit up": ventilatory dysfunction, hypoxia, cardiac tamponade
      - "Please help me": blood loss, hypoxemia
      - "I'm going to die": blood loss, hypoxemia
      - "I'm thirsty": blood loss
      - "My belly hurts": peritoneal irritation
      - "I need to have a bowel movement": hemoperitoneum
      - "I can't move my legs": spinal cord injury
      - "Please do something for my pain": significant injury
III. **Management of the STABLE adult with blunt trauma**
   A. Assess for airway, breathing, circulation, and neurologic disability.
   B. Immobilize cervical spine.

Table 13.1 Phases of initial assessment

Primary survey (15 seconds)
–Airway with cervical-spine control
  Voice, air exchange, patency, cervical immobilization
–Breathing
  Breath sounds, chest wall, neck veins
–Circulation
  Mentation, skin color, pulse, blood pressure, neck veins, external bleeding
–Disability (neurologic)
  Pupils, extremity movement (site and type), voice
–Expose the patient
Resuscitation
–Generic: electrocardiographic leads, pulse oximetry, intravenous, draw fluid for
  laboratory studies
–Concurrent with life-threatening injuries identified on primary survey
–Include gastric and urethral catheters, or perform with secondary survey
Secondary survey
–Head-to-toe examination (including spine)
–AMPLE history (A = allergies, M = medications currently taken, P = past illness,
  L = last meal, E = events related to injury)
–Imaging
–Second survey may be delayed until after operating room in unstable patient
  or patient in extremis
Definitive care
–Surgery (may be in resuscitation phase)
–Splinting
–Medications (3 As): analgesics, antibiotics, antitetanus
–Consultants
–Transfer
Tertiary survey
–Repeat primary and secondary surveys within 24 hours for occult or missed injuries
–Create injury "problem" list with specific identification of physician handling each

(Modified from American College of Surgeons Committee on Trauma: *Advanced trauma life support
manual*. Chicago: American College of Surgeons, 2001, with permission.)

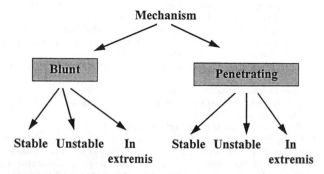

FIG. 13.1. Initial emergency department triage.

Table 13.2 Criteria for adult **unstable** trauma patient* (blunt or penetrating trauma)

Altered physiology
–Glasgow Coma Scale (GCS) score ≤14
–Pulse <60 or >120 beats/min
–Blood pressure <90 mmHg after 2 L fluid challenge
–Blood pressure >190 mmHg systolic
–Respiratory rate <12 or >24 breaths/min
–Poor gas exchange (e.g., SaO_2 <90%)
–Temperature <92°F (33°C)

Altered physical findings
–Paralysis
–Hoarseness/inability to talk
–Labored respirations
–Severe pain
–External hemorrhage site(s)
–Combative

Anatomic
–Severe deformity(ies): spine, neck, chest, extremities
–Penetrating wound from head to popliteal fossa

*Increased index of suspicion
–Age >55 yr.
–Coronary artery disease
–Obstructive lung disease
–Liver disease
–Insulin-dependent diabetes mellitus
–Anticoagulation or history of coagulopathy
–History of mental illness
–Pregnancy

    C. Administer O_2 nasally or by mask.
    D. Insert at least one peripheral intravenous (i.v.) (≥18 gauge).
    E. Perform "stable patient" laboratory studies.
    F. Splint deformed extremities.
    G. Assess for occult injury.
       1. Head, neck, chest, abdomen, pelvis, spine, and extremities.
       2. Selective rectal and pelvic examinations.
    H. Insert nasogastric tube (unnecessary in most stable patients).
    I. Insert urinary catheter (if patient unable to void or pelvic fracture).
    J. Limit i.v. fluid (e.g., 1 L in first 30 minutes).
    K. Select radiologic studies as indicated by mechanism of injury and physical examination.
       1. Chest x-ray (usually routine)
       2. Cervical spine (C-spine)—no x-ray if no symptoms or signs and not intoxicated (see Chapter 30)
       3. Pelvis—no x-ray if no symptoms or signs
       4. Computed tomography (CT) scan of head with any alteration in consciousness, headache, amnesia, or history of anticoagulation
       5. CT scan of abdomen—if tenderness, macroscopic hematuria. or microscopic hematuria with signs and symptoms (see Chapter 31)
       6. Ultrasound (US) of abdomen (selective)—if abdominal tenderness
       7. Spine and extremity films (selective)—if tenderness
  IV. Management of the UNSTABLE adult with blunt trauma
    A. Assess airway (with C-spine immobilization).
       1. Patency, voice, stridor, foreign body, tongue, lacerations, O_2 saturation

2. Treatment **options** (see Chapter 14 for specific indications). **If in doubt, intubate the patient.**
   a. Administration of 100% O_2 (by mask)
   b. Suction
   c. Chin lift
   d. Oral airway (if obtunded)
   e. Nasopharyngeal airway
   f. Laryngeal mask airway (LMA)—very selective
   g. Endotracheal intubation
   h. Surgical airway
B. **Assess breathing**
   1. Facial expression (distress, anguish, flat), depth and quality of respiration (shallow or labored), skin pallor or cyanosis, use of accessory muscles (neck and abdomen)
   2. Trachea (midline, crepitus), neck veins (flat or distended), breath sounds (diminished or absent), chest symmetry (look for anterior or lateral flail, or splinting), respiratory rate, central cyanosis, O_2 saturation (pulse oximetry)
   3. Treatment **options** (see Chapter 26a for specific indications)
      a. Endotracheal tube
      b. Needle decompression of chest, unilateral or bilateral
      c. Chest tube(s), unilateral or bilateral
      d. Ventilator (manual or mechanical)
      e. Thoracotomy
      f. Analgesia (systemic titrated opioids, intercostal block, epidural)
C. **Assess circulation**
   1. Skin color, mentation, palpable pulse
   2. Quality of pulse, blood pressure, capillary refill, peripheral cyanosis, skin temperature, external hemorrhage, agitation, electrocardiographic (ECG) monitoring, O_2 saturation
   3. Treatment **options** (see Chapters 5 and 15 for specific indications)
      a. Two large-bore peripheral i.v., draw "unstable patient" laboratory fluids
      b. Central line if peripheral access unavailable—subclavian or femoral
      c. Warmed Ringer's lactate (1–2 L) i.v. as fast as possible (monitor response)
      d. With profound or persistent hypotension—early blood transfusion
      e. If signs of hypovolemia (e.g., thirst, base deficit, tachycardia, or hypotension), check for occult blood loss in one of six areas
         (1) **External**: (look under dressings), back, buttocks, occiput, axillae
         (2) **Thoracic cavity**: trachea, neck veins, stethoscope, early chest x-ray, chest tube
         (3) **Abdominal cavity**: palpation, diagnostic peritoneal lavage (DPL), US, exploratory laparotomy
         (4) **Pelvis**: physical examination, perineal laceration, unstable pelvic ring, pelvic x-ray, arteriogram, or external fixation
         (5) **Extremities**: fractures, particularly if bilateral or femoral
         (6) **Spine**: extensive fractures with hemorrhage (thoracolumbar)
   4. **If the search for bleeding is unrevealing**, other **causes of hypotension** include the following:
      a. Tension pneumothorax
      b. Cardiac tamponade
      c. Distributive shock (neurogenic, e.g., spinal cord injury)
      d. Severe blunt cardiac injury with acute heart failure (very uncommon)
D. **Neurologic disability**
   1. Perform and document focused neurologic examination (see Chapters 19 and 20) **before** patient is **intubated** and paralyzed: Glasgow Coma Scale (GCS) score, pupils, movement, and gross sensation of **all** extremities.

   2. Palpate head and spine (log roll).
   3. Treatment **options** (see Chapters 19 and 20 for specific indications)
      a. Administration of O_2
      b. Intubation
      c. Mannitol
      d. Consider methylprednisolone (for blunt spinal cord injury with neurologic deficit)
      e. Emergency imaging of brain and spine
      f. Intracranial pressure monitoring
      g. Ventriculostomy
      h. Craniotomy
   E. **Extremities**
      1. Palpate extremities and joints.
      2. Palpate pulses (Doppler).
      3. Perform focused motor and sensory examination.
      4. Treatment **options** (see Chapter 32 for specific indications)
         a. Cover open wounds with sterile dressing.
         b. Apply direct pressure to control hemorrhage.
         c. Realign gross deformities.
         d. Splint
         e. Apply traction (femur fractures).
   F. Place **nasogastric or orogastric tube** and **urinary catheter** at earliest opportunity **if not contraindicated** or **interfering** with assessment or stabilization of airway, breathing, circulation, or neurologic dysfunction.
   G. **Imaging** in the **unstable blunt trauma patient**
      1. **Suggested as time and clinical situation permit (in resuscitation area)**
         a. **Chest x-ray**: cassette under patient preferred rather than under backboard; camera at maximal distance (lower resuscitation litter); inspiratory-hold
         b. **Cervical spine**: lateral (to rule out gross deformity only), delay full C-spine until stable
         c. **Pelvis**: **anteroposterior** (AP)
      2. **Selective** (based on assessment)
         a. Extremities
         b. Thoracic and lumbar spine
      3. In general, **imaging** should be **delayed until airway, breathing, and circulatory dysfunction** have been **stabilized**. Exceptions occur when a chest or pelvic x-ray is needed to identify "occult" blood loss (see above).
      4. **CT scan** (if stabilized hemodynamically). **CT scan done in an unstable patient can be dangerous.** Studies in the trauma patient should be done only in CT scan units with full monitoring capability, easy full patient body viewing, and a nurse-physician team capable of performing any and all life-saving procedures should a crisis arise (e.g., cricothyroidotomy, chest decompression, decision to operate). Newer, rapid helical or spiral scanners can image the head, chest, and abdomen rapidly, allowing studies to be performed in **select transient responders** to fluid challenge when supported by clinical judgment and logistics.
         a. Head: if GCS <15
         b. Chest: if suspected contusion or mediastinal anatomy uncertainty
         c. Abdomen and pelvis: if signs or symptoms or unable to examine
         d. Spine: if suspected by plain films or physical examination
V. **Management of the STABLE adult with penetrating trauma**
   A. Assess patient for airway, breathing, circulatory, and neurologic dysfunction.
   B. Document **number** and **sites** of penetrating wounds.
   C. **Determine trajectory**—this is vital in determining anatomic structures at risk from missiles.
   D. Treatment **options**
      1. Administer O_2

2. Secure at least one peripheral i.v. line
3. Selective placement of nasogastric tube and urinary catheter (e.g., penetrating torso wound)
4. "Stable patient" **laboratory** studies

E. Assess the patient for significant injury, depending on injury sites: physical examination and x-ray studies; both plain film and CT are complementary to accurately determine precise trajectory. Diagnostic **options** include:
   1. **Head**: CT scan without contrast
   2. **Neck**: CT scan with i.v. and oral contrast, AP and lateral x-ray studies, contrast swallow study, endoscopy, arteriogram, neck exploration. (**Caution: check airway repeatedly during diagnostic evaluations with low threshold for intubation.**)
   3. **Chest**: chest x-ray; if transmediastinal, CT with i.v. and oral contrast, or angiography, bronchoscopy, esophageal contrast, cardiac window, echocardiography
   4. **Abdomen, back, or flank**: local wound exploration, DPL, US, CT scan with i.v. and oral contrast (including rectal), laparoscopy, laparotomy
   5. **Extremities**: pulses, motor and sensory examination, ankle brachial index, Duplex US, arteriogram, operative exploration

VI. **Management of the UNSTABLE adult with penetrating trauma**
A. Assess patient for airway, adequate gas exchange, circulatory or neurologic dysfunction.
B. Assess number and sites of penetrating wounds.
C. **Determine trajectory**—this is vital in determining anatomic structures at risk from missiles.
D. **Treatment options** (see Chapter 14 for specific indications)
   1. **Airway**
      a. Administer 100% O_2
      b. Suction
      c. Chin lift
      d. Oral airway (if obtunded)
      e. Nasopharyngeal airway
      f. Endotracheal intubation
      g. Surgical airway (i.e., for shotgun wounds to face)
   2. **Breathing**
      a. Needle decompression of chest, unilateral or bilateral
      b. Chest tube(s), unilateral or bilateral
      c. Ventilator (manual or mechanical)
      d. Thoracotomy or sternotomy
   3. **Circulatory**
      a. Insert two large-bore i.v., draw **unstable** patient **laboratory studies**, consider large-bore central line, warmed Ringer's lactate (1–2 L) i.v., blood transfusion with profound or persistent hypotension
      b. IV **above** and **below** diaphragm in penetrating **torso** trauma
      c. **Avoid i.v.** placement such that the bullet wound is between the i.v. site and the heart.
      d. **If signs of hypovolemia occur (e.g., thirst, base deficit, tachycardia, or hypotension), search for sites of blood loss**.
         (1) **Thoracic cavity**: tracheal deviation, neck veins, bilateral equal breath sounds, chest x-ray study, chest tubes (bilateral if precise trajectory not known).
         (2) **Abdominal cavity**: exploratory laparotomy, US, or DPL (stab wounds).
         (3) If hypotension continues, look for cardiac tamponade, tension pneumothorax.
         (4) Occult spinal cord injury
   4. Place nasogastric or orogastric tube and urinary catheter at earliest convenience.

E. Hemodynamically **unstable patient** with a **penetrating** wound to the **chest** may require chest tube(s) and thoracotomy in emergency department or operating room (OR).

    1. Chest tube may be diagnostic or therapeutic.

    2. If patient is hemodynamically unstable after chest tubes, perform thoracotomy in emergency department or OR.

    3. If stable after chest tubes and mediastinal or transmediastinal trajectory (see Chapter 26a and 26b), then perform the following.

      a. Pericardial window

      b. Echocardiogram (transthoracic or transesophageal)

      c. Aortogram

      d. Bronchoscopy

      e. Esophageal contrast study

      f. CT scan with contrast in selected patients

F. The hemodynamically **unstable** patient with a **penetrating** wound to the **neck, abdomen, or extremity** requires control of hemorrhage in the **operating room**.

VII. Management of the patient in EXTREMIS

  A. The patient *in extremis* presents with anatomic or physiologic findings that will result in **death within minutes** if not immediately corrected. These patients usually have signs of life such as reactive pupils, spontaneous respiratory efforts, spontaneous movement, or a palpable pulse, but otherwise present with profound shock or respiratory failure. This requires a **treat, then diagnose** approach; generally with need for **immediate operation**.

  B. If not intubated, **intubate**.

    1. If unable to intubate, **obtain a surgical airway**.

  C. Penetrating injury, patient in extremis (Fig. 13.2)

    1. Neck

      a. Direct digital pressure if expanding hematoma or active bleeding.

      b. Intravenous fluid and blood

      c. Operating room

    2. Chest

      a. Bilateral chest tubes

      b. Intravenous fluid and blood

      c. Left thoracotomy or bilateral thoracotomy

      d. Operating room

    3. Abdomen

      a. Intravenous fluid and blood, avoid systolic blood pressure >80 mmHg until in the OR.

      b. Move to OR immediately.

        (1) Left thoracotomy for aortic control within the chest if abdomen is expanding and blood pressure remains low despite volume resuscitation. Some prefer control of the aorta through a high midline abdominal incision.

    4. Groin and extremities

      a. Apply pressure if expanding hematoma or active bleeding.

      b. Intravenous fluid and blood

      c. Operating room

    5. Multiple penetrating wounds

      a. Apply pressure to sites of active bleeding.

      b. Bilateral chest tubes

      c. Intravenous fluid and blood

      d. Operating room

      e. Left thoracotomy (see 3. Abdomen, above)

  D. Blunt injury, patient in extremis (Fig. 13.3)

    1. Apply pressure to external hemorrhage

    2. Intravenous fluid and blood

    3. Bilateral chest tubes

      a. If ongoing hemorrhage or >1,500 mL on initial insertion of chest tubes, to OR or resuscitative thoracotomy.

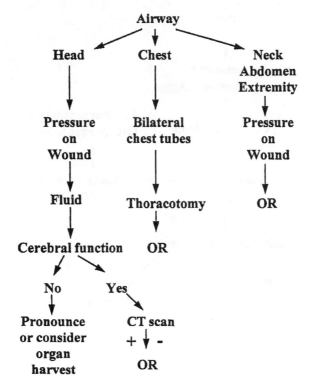

FIG. 13.2. Penetrating trauma patient *in extremis*.

    4. DPL or US of abdomen
       a. If grossly positive, move to OR.
       b. If negative DPL aspirate or US minimal or if no fluid, x-ray study of pelvis.
    5. X-ray of pelvis. The exsanguinating patient with pelvic fracture needs to be identified (A small proportion of patients will have major vascular injury associated with the pelvic fracture and must be taken to the OR).
       a. If positive and no evidence of active bleeding from the chest or abdomen is detected, move to angiography (consider aortography after pelvis).
    6. Priorities with multiple injuries
       a. First →thoracic hemorrhage or tamponade
       b. Second →abdominal hemorrhage
       c. Third →pelvic hemorrhage
       d. Fourth →extremity hemorrhage
       e. Fifth →intracranial injury
       f. Sixth →spinal cord injury
VIII. Laboratory studies
    A. Recent data have suggested a more selective and cost-effective approach to laboratory studies in both blunt and penetrating trauma.
       1. Stable patient
          a. Hemoglobin (Hb) and hematocrit (Hct)
          b. Blood ethanol (ETOH), depending on hospital protocol

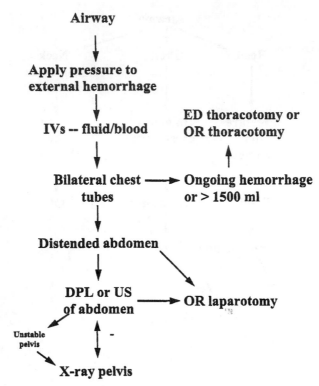

FIG. 13.3. Blunt trauma patient *in extremis*.

    c. Urine dipstick for blood, human chorionic gonadotrophin (HCG) in women of childbearing age (urine or blood)
    d. Blood screening without cross match unless condition changes
    e. Other studies as indicated by disease history
  2. Unstable patient:
    a. Required
      (1) Blood type and cross match
      (2) Arterial blood gas
      (3) Hb/Hct
      (4) Prothrombin time, partial thromboplastin time, platelet count
      (5) Urine dipstick for blood, HCG for women of childbearing age
      (6) ECG
    b. Selective (based on hospital protocol)
      (1) Na, K, CO_2, Cl, blood urea nitrogen (BUN), creatinine, Ca^{++}, Mg^{++}
      (2) Serum amylase or lipase
      (3) Serum ETOH
    c. Point of care testing is available in many trauma centers
IX. Multiple victims
    A. When several trauma victims arrive in the resuscitation area simultaneously, priority should be given to the unstable trauma victims.
    B. Trauma team leader (most senior physician) should assign physicians and nurses to specific areas, and designees should not cover several areas simultaneously.

C. The trauma team leader should rotate from patient to patient to oversee management, prioritize care, and supervise actions of individual trauma teams.

D. The team leader should decide the need for backup assistance or calling a disaster plan when demand outstrips immediate resources. The team leader should err on the side of calling for additional assistance.

Axioms

- The **unstable trauma patient** can be defined by potential requirement for surgery or the ICU as well as cardiopulmonary dysfunction.
- The trauma patient who remains unstable after initial resuscitation usually requires operative intervention.
- The trauma patient **in extremis** may require treatment before diagnosis.

Bibliography

American College of Surgeons Committee on Trauma. *Advanced trauma life support manual.* Chicago: American College of Surgeons, 2001.

Moore FA, Moore EE. Trauma resuscitation. In: *American College of Surgeons Scientific American Surgery.* Section I.2, 2000. New York: Scientific American.

14. AIRWAY MANAGEMENT IN THE TRAUMA PATIENT

Rade B. Vukmir, Kathy J. Rinnert, and Donald M. Yealy

Ensuring adequate oxygenation, ventilation, and protection from aspiration are the cornerstones of airway management and the first priority when treating trauma patients. Appropriate airway management depends on the combination of good judgment, the right equipment, and appropriate skills to perform all necessary procedures. Although airway discussions often focus on the mechanics of intubation, many patients can be treated with basic interventions.

I. **Airway equipment and skills**. A diverse array of equipment and skills are necessary for optimal airway management. These include:
   A. **Basic**
      1. Airway positioning, including chin-lift and jaw-thrust maneuvers, to relieve obstruction caused by the tongue or soft tissues.
      2. Application of supplemental oxygen (100% oxygen by partial or nonrebreather mask).
      3. Use of large-bore suction and oral and nasal airways to maintain or restore patency of the upper airway (each is discussed in Chapter 8).
   B. **Advanced (nonsurgical)**
      1. Bag-valve devices with masks
      2. Availability and knowledge of esophagotracheal airway (Combitube, Sheridan, Argyle, NY) (see Chapter 8)
      3. Direct glottic visualization and oral intubation
      4. Alternatives to direct glottic visualization and oral intubation, including nasal, transillumination (or "lighted stylet"), and tactile (or "digital") intubation and laryngeal mask airway placement
      5. **Cricoid pressure** (or "Sellick's maneuver") to lessen the risk of gastric distention during mask ventilation and aspiration during intubation (see Chapter 8)
   C. **Surgical airway**
      1. **Cricothyroidotomy** (open or percutaneous with dilators)
      2. **Translaryngeal jet insufflation**
      3. **Tracheostomy** (in select cases, e.g., laryngeal fracture)
II. **Indications for intubation**. In spontaneously breathing patients, simple skills (e.g., removal of foreign bodies, airway suctioning, chin-lift or jaw-thrust maneuvers) can establish airway patency and restore adequate respiration. Intubation is reserved for those patients who continue to show signs of inadequate respiration after basic interventions, or patients in whom these interventions alone are not likely to sustain adequate respiration.
   A. **Absolute indications for immediate emergency intubation**
      1. Airway obstruction unrelieved with basic interventions
      2. Apnea or near apnea
      3. Respiratory distress (air hunger, severe tachypnea, cyanosis, hypoxemia, or hypercarbia)
      4. Severe neurologic deficits or depressed consciousness (i.e., focal deficit or Glasgow Coma Scale [GCS] score of ≤8) from head trauma or any other cause
   B. **Urgent (within minutes) indications for intubation**
      1. Penetrating neck injury (with any sign of airway compromise or enlarging hematoma)
      2. Persistent or refractory hypotension, especially if caused by active hemorrhage
      3. Chest wall injury or dysfunction

4. Less severe but prominent altered consciousness, especially after head injury, including both combative and mildly obtunded patients (**Caveat**: reversible causes, including hypoglycemia and opioid or benzodiazepine overdose, should be considered and treated).
C. **Relative indications for nonemergent intubation**
   1. Oromaxillofacial injury.
   2. Pulmonary contusion or impending respiratory failure.
   3. Need for diagnostic or therapeutic procedures in patients at risk for deterioration (e.g., computed tomography or arteriography).
   4. Potential respiratory failure because of intensive systemic analgesic or sedative use.
D. The patient with significant maxillofacial or soft tissue neck injury who is spontaneously breathing, but with some difficulty, is best treated with early intubation, usually orally with direct glottic visualization. This should be performed by the most experienced provider with either topical anesthetics and judicious sedative or analgesic administration. The use of neuromuscular blocking drugs or induction agents to abolish all reflexes and ventilatory drive in these patients can result in an apnea and an inability to intubate or mask ventilate; **this situation can be rapidly fatal**. Other methods to secure the airway, including a surgical airway, must be immediately available in the trauma resuscitation room in this situation. A surgical airway under local anesthesia is another alternative in these situations, and is best performed early (before hypoxemia, hypercarbia, apnea, or extensive tissue deformity occurs).
III. **Approach to intubation**
A. **Oral intubation**. If the patient requires intubation, this is usually performed using direct visualization of the glottis through the mouth while maintaining in-line stabilization of the cervical spine. **No other procedures should be done while intubation is being attempted**; other activities can interfere with this primary intervention. Of all advanced airway-securing techniques, oral intubation is generally associated with the highest success rates (because of familiarity) and a lowest frequency of complications. **Oral intubation requires three people** (Fig. 14.1): one experienced provider to perform laryngoscopy and intubate, another to provide cervical immobilization, and a third to apply cricoid pressure. Large-bore suction must be readily available before any intubation attempt. Pharmacologic agents can be given as part of a systematic approach to those patients who require analgesia, sedation, or muscular relaxation to safely intubate.

To best visualize the glottis, the intubator attempts to align the oropharyngeal and laryngotracheal axes. The "sniffing position" used for nontrauma patients employs neck flexion and head extension to ease alignment. However, this maneuver is **absolutely contraindicated** in the trauma patient suspected of having cervical spine injuries. Aside from those with clear evidence of isolated extremity injuries, all trauma patients are intubated with the head maintained in a midline, neutral position. Care must be taken to ensure that **no** directional forces (distraction or traction) are applied to the cervical spine.
B. **Nasal intubation**, an alternative to oral intubation, is usually performed in a "blind" fashion in patients who are spontaneously breathing (see Chapter 8). **Nasal intubation is contraindicated in apneic patients or those with midface, nasal, or basilar skull fractures**. Nasal intubation is limited by operator inexperience, higher failure rates compared with oral intubation, and frequent development of sinusitis after >48 hours duration. Although possible in many trauma patients, nasal intubation offers little advantage over oral intubation and can be technically more difficult.
C. **Alternatives**. In select cases when oral and nasal intubation are unsuccessful, another intubation method can be an option before a surgical airway is performed. **Tactile, transillumination, and combination** approaches are well described; each requires practice but can establish an airway

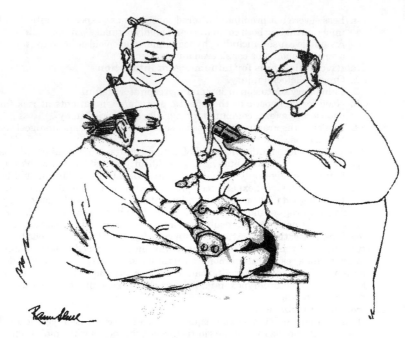

FIG. 14.1. Three-person technique for intubation.

without the need to directly visualize the glottis. Also, use of the **esophago-tracheal Combitube or laryngeal-mask airways** offers an alternative to tracheal intubation. These alternatives are discussed in detail in Chapter 8. Finally, intubation over a flexible bronchoscope is an attractive option that requires special equipment and skill (Fig. 14.2).

D. **Surgical airways** are required when basic interventions and intubation are not likely to succeed (e.g., severe upper airway anatomic distortion from mid or lower facial trauma) or have failed. Cricothyroidotomy and trans-laryngeal jet ventilation are safe and more readily applicable, with the former more familiar to most providers. Appropriate equipment must be ready before any attempt and both procedures must be capable of being completed rapidly. Tracheostomy is generally reserved for nonemergent situations (in favor of cricothyroidotomy), with the exception of patients with laryngeal fractures.

   1. **Percutaneous translaryngeal catheter (jet) insufflation**
      a. **Technique**. The relatively avascular cricothyroid membrane is lo-cated between the shield-shaped thyroid cartilage and the interiorly located, ring-shaped cricoid cartilage. A large-bore (12–14 gauge, preferably designed for this procedure and with side holes) over-the-needle catheter with an attached syringe is directed caudad, pene-trating the skin and cricothyroid membrane until air is aspirated. The catheter is then threaded into the airway and reaspirated to en-sure ongoing intratracheal placement (evidenced by free gas with-drawal or "bubbles" if fluid is in the syringe).

      Then, ventilation occurs via attachment to a jet insufflating de-vice delivering high-flow oxygen at approximately 40 to 50 pounds/square inch (psi) (1 psi = 70 cm H_2O). This device can be a simple high-pressure, one-way valve (to insufflate gas with each manual

Nonemergent

↓

Obtain lateral
cervical spine
film first

↓

Orotracheal intubation
with in-line
stabilization (or
another intubation method)

Urgent and Emergency

↓

Orotracheal intubation
with in-line stabilization

FIG. 14.2. Approach to airway management if potential cervical spine injury.

triggering) or a more elaborate ventilator (with multiple control settings).* The key point is that **the device must be identified and ready for use before the anticipated procedure** rather than "put together on the spot," because the latter frequently fails to deliver adequate volumes or withstand the pressure.

The trachea is used as a passive port for exhalation; because of this, **the only absolute contraindication is complete airway obstruction** (a rare event). By using the aforementioned catheter and oxygen source combination, tidal volumes of 700 to 1,000 mL per 1-second inspiration are achieved. Jet insufflation offers some protection from aspiration (because a portion of the gas insufflated exits cephalad, clearing the upper airway) and an excellent route for alveolar drug delivery, if needed.

A **common mistake** in performing jet ventilation is to ventilate with either a bag-valve or demand-valve device or using another noncompressed oxygen source. A 12- to 14-gauge cannula coupled with these low or nonpressurized oxygen sources will not allow for adequate ventilation, although some (albeit limited) oxygenation can occur. Contrary to popular misconceptions, **correct** jet ventilation using a high-pressure source (40–50 psi—this is **NOT** the same as a 10–15 L/min flow valve) at a rate of 1:3 seconds of inspiration:expiration will allow adequate to supernormal oxygenation and ventilation (with **no** CO_2 accumulation) for unlimited periods of time. The correct gas sources are plentiful, although often overlooked: all oxygen gas cylinders and wall outlets offer 40 to 50 psi oxygen if sampled before the usual "downregulating" devices that offer flow at 1 to 15 L/min.

* See first citation at chapter end for a listing of the many options possible.

b. Complications of jet ventilation include barotrauma, local hemorrhage, hypotension from overventilation and decreased venous return, inadvertent placement with resulting subcutaneous or mediastinal emphysema, hypoxia, hypercarbia, and dysrhythmias from prolonged attempts. The frequency of these complications varies from 5% to 50%, depending on operator skill and preparedness and is similar to that seen with cricothyroidotomy when done by experienced providers.

2. Cricothyroidotomy is preferred to jet insufflation because of familiarity and the ability to provide optimal protection from aspiration and place a large-bore airway for suctioning.

  a. Technique. (Fig. 14.3) The operator **palpates** the thyroid cartilage and the caudad, depressed cricothyroid membrane. A 3-cm midline, longitudinal (if anatomic landmarks are not clearly apparent) or transverse **skin** incision (in the thin neck, with clear landmarks) is performed over the membrane. The skin is spread, and landmarks (thyroid cartilage, cricothyroid membrane) reestablished by palpation. A transverse incision (1.5–2 cm) is made through the **membrane**. The procedure is essentially performed using tactile input; if the membrane cannot be seen, incise where the soft membrane is palpated. A tracheostomy tube or endotracheal tube (at least 5-mm internal diameter, but one size smaller than what would be chosen for oral intubation in an adult) is introduced into the airway and cuff inflated. Adequate oxygenation and ventilation are assured by standard techniques.

  b. Complications include hemorrhage (usually controlled with local pressure and avoided by limiting the size of all incisions), misplacement, hypoxia secondary to prolonged procedure time, esophageal perforation, laryngeal fracture, and subcutaneous emphysema. Stenosis is often a problem if left in place for extended periods because

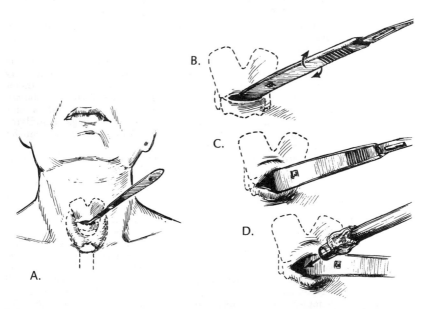

FIG. 14.3. Cricothyroidotomy technique. (From Trunkey DD, Guernsey JM. Cervicothoracic trauma. In: Blaisdell FM, Trunkey DD, eds. *Surgical procedures in trauma management.* New York: Thieme Inc. 1986:303, with permission.)

of the narrow and contained diameter of the cricoid area. **Relative contraindications** include laryngeal trauma or patient age <10 to 12 years.

c. **Percutaneous dilator-based** kits are available that allow for a large-bore cannula to be placed through the cricothyroid membrane. The patient is then ventilated using noncompressed sources (usually a bag-valve device). These kits offer little advantage to formal cricothyroidotomy.

IV. **Pharmacologic assistance during intubation**

A. Some patients can be intubated without drugs (e.g., those deeply comatose or in cardiac arrest), whereas others can be treated with topical or local anesthetics to allow for successful intubation or surgical airway placement. However, most patients must receive systemic sedation, analgesia, and a muscular relaxant to ensure that intubation occurs safely and rapidly. A **never** or **always** approach to the use of pharmacologic adjuncts is strongly discouraged because each approach exposes patients to suboptimal care. For example, mildly obtunded or combative patients can be at greater risk of vomiting and aspiration, prolonged hypoxemia and hypercarbia, and laryngoscopic complications if not given appropriate pharmacologic assistance.

B. Before attenuating or ablating any patient's physiologic responses, the physician must assess the likelihood of ease of intubation and ability to mask ventilate. If laryngoscopy is unlikely to be successful even with systemic induction or muscle relaxant drugs (e.g., severe anatomic distortion or impediments), these agents should not be used to facilitate "a look." In addition, **a plan to deal with failure to intubate and mask ventilate must be discussed**. This includes limiting the number of attempts and providing for rapid surgical airway placement.

C. **Choosing agents**

1. Providers must choose from a variety of sedative, analgesic, hypnotic, and neuromuscular blocking drugs. In the trauma patient, it is best to assume both hypovolemia and a primary central nervous system (CNS) injury exist when choosing a drug regimen. Although these conditions are often not present, this approach allows for a greater margin of safety because either condition can be difficult to exclude in the first minutes after patient arrival.

2. Aside from patients with sedative overdoses, use of a short-acting inductive agent and a neuromuscular blocking agent is preferred. This will optimize intubating conditions, allow for rapid recovery if failure occurs, and limit hemodynamic and intracranial responses, discomfort, and recall.

3. Based on the aforementioned principles, a simple regimen is recommended that meets both effectiveness and safety needs in most trauma patients, recognizing that other regimens, based on local expertise and resources, are possible. We prefer intravenous (i.v.) **etomidate (0.2–0.3 mg/kg) or fentanyl (2–4 µg/kg)** as sedative or inductive agents because of their minimal clinically important side effects at these doses. Hypotension can occur with either of these agents, particularly if severe hypovolemia is present, but is usually less frequent and profound when compared with other regimens. Although barbiturates (especially for isolated head injured patients) and benzodiazepines are used as sedative or inductive agents, their use is to be discouraged because of the more profound and frequent hemodynamic side effects that can occur with their use.

Succinylcholine (1–2 mg/kg i.v.) is our preferred neuromuscular blocking agent because of its long-standing history of rapid reliability and short duration. Pretreatment with a nondepolarizing neuromuscular blocking agent before succinylcholine administration to prevent fasciculations offers little pragmatic benefit and some risk; for these reasons, we do not employ this routinely in emergent situations. For patients with a contraindication to succinylcholine, **vecuronium (0.28 mg/kg i.v. as a single dose or 0.1 mg/kg in a 'priming sequence' where $\frac{1}{10}$ of the total dose is given first followed in 2 minutes by the remainder)** is used, understanding that a more prolonged effect will occur. If paralysis is needed after intubation, either vecuronium or pancuronium (0.05 mg/kg i.v. increments as needed) with further sedation is recommended.

V. **Monitoring during and confirmation after intubation.** Before and during intubation, patients must be monitored to ensure adequate gas exchange is occurring and problems are recognized and treated. In addition, after establishment of an airway, the location of the tube must be confirmed. **No singular method of monitoring or tube confirmation is infallible**; clinicians must use a combination of directed physical examination and adjunct devices to ensure patient safety. Although chest radiography can be used to help confirm tube placement, this is to be avoided. The following methods are easier to perform at the bedside.

   A. **Hemodynamic monitoring**
      1. Observe for signs of poor gas exchange: hypertension and tachycardia (early and sensitive), followed by hypotension and bradycardia (late but specific).

   B. **Directed physical examination**
      1. After intubation, the tube should be examined for condensation and fogging; the epigastrium should be auscultated and quiet; the apices and bases of both lungs should be auscultated and show symmetric breath sounds; and the chest should rise normally. If any uncertainty exists, laryngoscopy should be performed to see the tube passing through the vocal cords. Each of these findings can be misleading or difficult to appreciate.
      2. Although often unrecognized, a declining mental status should prompt an immediate reevaluation of the airway.

   C. **Oxygen saturation and exhaled carbon dioxide measurements**
      1. **Oxygen saturation** is best estimated continuously by pulse oximetry. To maximize O_2 delivery, a saturation of >95% should be sought in all trauma patients. Shock, dyshemoglobinemias (e.g., carbon monoxide related or other substances that bind hemoglobin), dark nail polish, and other physical conditions can limit the accuracy or acquisition of a signal. If pulse oximetry is not possible and any signs of poor oxygen delivery are present, an arterial blood gas analysis should be obtained. **Although arterial oxygen desaturation can indicate incorrect tube placement, this is a late finding**.
      2. **Capnography** is the measurement of expired CO_2 concentrations, with qualitative (waveform), quantitative and semiquantitative (usually colorimetric, with a yellow color indicating CO_2 presence) devices available. In nonintubated patients, capnography accuracy is variable because of mixing with ambient air. However, in intubated patients end-tidal capnography shows excellent correlation with alveolar and arterial CO_2 concentrations.
      Outside of low or no flow states (e.g., massive pulmonary embolus or cardiac arrest), **capnography is the current standard to confirm intratracheal tube placement** and very useful in guiding minute ventilation. In low or no flow states, detectable expired CO_2 for more than four to six breaths confirms that the tube is an upper airway structure, usually the trachea.
      In the rare case where the tracheal tube tip is in the hypopharynx, expired CO_2 will be detected, creating a "false-positive." A capnograph will display an abnormal waveform to help identify this, whereas the commonly used qualitative or semiquantitative (colorimetric) devices will not distinguish this from true tracheal location. The absence of expired CO_2 means either incorrect placement (i.e., esophageal) or little delivery of blood to the pulmonary vascular bed.

D. Other confirmatory devices
   1. Bulb and syringe devices are available to confirm intratracheal tube location; these devices are simple to use and inexpensive, but offer no other information. Rapid and complete reinflation of the deflated bulb (within 5–10 seconds) when attached to the endotracheal tube or unimpeded aspiration of a 30–60 mL syringe similarly attached to the endotracheal tube strongly suggests correct placement.

VI. General intubating procedure
   A. Ensure all equipment—tubes, stylet, blades, handles, suction, bag-valve devices, oxygen, drugs, pulse oximeter, and surgical kits—are available and functioning **before patient arrival**.
   B. Oxygenate with 100% O_2 and assist ventilation for 3 to 4 minutes (if possible) to decrease alveolar nitrogen and arterial CO_2 while maximizing O_2 reserves. This is also the time to asses the ease of intubation and mask ventilation and confirm that a **functioning i.v. catheter is present** for drug administration.
   C. Remove cervical collar and **begin in-line stabilization** by assistant.
   D. Apply **cricoid pressure**.
   E. Optional in nonemergent cases: defasciculate with vecuronium (0.01 mg/kg i.v.) or an equipotent dose of another nondepolarizing agent 2 to 3 minutes before step 5.
   F. Sedation/induction plus relaxation: administer etomidate (0.2–0.3 mg/kg i.v.) or fentanyl (2–4 µg/kg) followed by succinylcholine (1–2 mg/kg) or vecuronium (0.28 mg/kg as a single dose or 0.01 mg/kg followed by 0.1 mg/kg in 2 minutes).
   G. Perform intubation procedure when relaxation optimal (usually 60–90 seconds after last drug dose).
   H. Confirm tube placement and gas exchange using at least three of the following: visualization, physical examination, capnography, oximetry, or bulb or syringe devices.
   I. Release cricoid pressure.
   J. Replace cervical immobilization devices.
   K. Place a nasogastric tube (oral if facial trauma is present) unless contraindicated.

VII. Failed intubation
   A. A clear plan must exist for failed intubation attempts. To ensure preparation, assume all attempts at intubation will fail. The plan must be agreed on between the team leader and airway physician and is best decided in advance. We offer a basic approach, understanding local expertise can alter this plan at each institution.
      1. Reassess, oxygenate, and ventilate followed by second attempt by same or different operator.
      2. If still unsuccessful, an alternative operator can attempt intubation, or skip to step 3 or 4.
      3. If adequate ventilation and oxygenation, attempt alternative technique (e.g., tactile, transillumination, laryngeal mask airway).
      4. If still failed or inadequate gas exchange, immediate surgical airway.
   B. Communication helps avert conflict; however, **the ultimate decision to intubate rests with the trauma team leader**. Each institution should use a multidisciplinary approach to create and practice airway protocols that are clear and well understood by all participants. This include job and task assignments, drug regimens, equipment, and alternatives for each.

Axioms
- All equipment, including oxygen, suction, tubes, stylets, laryngoscopes, and blades, prepared; cricothyroidotomy and jet insufflation trays must be ready before patient arrival.
- A clear plan, agreed on in advance by all physicians involved, detailing the actions and pharmacologic agents to be used must be developed and used in managing the airway of trauma patients.

- Assume all trauma patients have hypovolemia, plus head and cervical spine injuries unless clear evidence exists to refute such; choose drug regimens accordingly.
- The most experienced person should perform any airway procedure, with no competing procedures occurring during intubation or surgical airway attempts.
- Assume all intubation attempts will fail and be prepared to enact alternatives immediately.
- If ablation of airway reflexes is needed to perform intubation, a combination of both a sedative or inductive agent and a neuromuscular blocker should be given together and in the proper dose; trying to limit drugs without one or with smaller doses usually offers more risk of failure than benefit.

Bibliography

Benemouf JL, Scheller MS. The importance of transtracheal jet ventilation in the management of the difficult airway. *Anesthesiology* 1989;71:769–778.

Bivins HG, Ford S, Bezmalinovic Z, et al. The effect of axial traction during orotracheal intubation of the trauma victim with an unstable cervical spine. *Ann Emerg Med* 1988;17:25–30.

Woodard LL, Wolfson AB, Iorg EC, et al. Hemodynamic effects of etomidate for rapid sequence intubation (RSI) in emergency department trauma patients. *Acad Emerg Med* 1995;2:405.

Yealy DM, Paris PM. Recent advances in airway management. *Emerg Med Clin North Am* 1989;7:83–93.

Yealy DM, Plewa MC, Stewart RD. An evaluation of cannulae and oxygen sources for pediatric jet ventilation. *Am J Emerg Med* 1991;9:20–23.

15. VASCULAR ACCESS

Michael D. Pasquale and Michael Rhodes

I. **Venous access**
   A. **Flow through a catheter is determined by Poiseuille's law:**

$$Q = \frac{r^4 \times (\Delta P)}{8 \times \text{viscosity} \times L}$$

   where Q = flow in mL/min, r = radius, (P = pressure gradient, and L = length. The best flow is obtained when dilute, warm (decreased viscosity) fluid is run through a short, wide catheter under pressure. The diameter of the catheter is the most important factor (Table 15.1).
   B. Access to the vascular system should be obtained en route to the hospital or coincident with the primary survey. Choice of the site for an intravenous (i.v.) line depends on location of a potential vascular injury. An i.v. line should not be placed with a vascular injury located between the i.v. access and the heart. For example, if a hypotensive patient has a gunshot wound to the upper right chest, i.v. access in the right arm can exacerbate bleeding from a subclavian vein injury.
   C. Venous access is obtained in all trauma patients for initial blood sampling, fluid resuscitation, and administration of drugs.
   D. **Venous access is usually best obtained peripherally** before consideration is given to placement of a central line.
      1. **Percutaneous**
         a. Preferentially, two large-bore (14- or 16-gauge) i.v. catheters should be placed in large arm veins (e.g., the antecubital fossa). Blood should be drawn before initiation of fluid resuscitation via the catheter, provided the catheter has not been placed proximal to an infusing i.v. line. Sterile technique should always be used. Most peripheral lines placed for resuscitation in the prehospital setting or in the emergency department should be removed within 24 to 48 hours. These catheter sites need to be monitored for complications, particularly cellulitis and phlebitis.
      2. **Cutdown**
         a. Surgical cutdowns are required infrequently in trauma patients, but can be invaluable in instances of difficult i.v. access, particularly in children.
         b. The **correct technique for venous cutdown** is essential for prompt, successful cannulation. Each cutdown site should be selected for its accessibility, vein size, and the urgency for venous access.
         c. Venous cutdowns for trauma have a substantial infection rate; these lines should be removed when alternative access is secured.
         d. **General technical principles**
            (1) The cutdown site should be immobilized, prepared, and draped.
            (2) Appropriate light and instruments should be available.
            (3) Mosquito hemostats and a No. 11 blade are suggested. In the small veins (<2 mm), venous wall elevators and dilators can be useful.
            (4) After anesthetizing the skin with a local anesthetic, a transverse skin incision is made, after which the fat and subcutaneous tissue is spread in a longitudinal direction (i.e., along the course of the vein). A second hemostat or forceps is frequently necessary to secure the vein while it is being mobilized for a distance of approximately 1 to 2 cm.

Table 15.1 Flow rates through commonly used catheters or infusion systems

Level I or rapid infusion system	1500 mL/min (high flow tubing under pressure)
High flow tubing*	250 mL/min
Standard tubing*	165 mL/min
7 F percutaneous sheath*	165 mL/min (high flow tubing)
12-inch, central venous*	65 mL/min (14 gauge)
12-inch, central venous*	35 mL/min (16 gauge)
12-inch, central venous*	20 mL/min (18 gauge)
1.5-inch angiocatheter*	75 mL/min (16 gauge)
1.5-inch angiocatheter*	60 mL/min (18 gauge)

*Standard tubing with gravity flow at 1 M height.

(5) Two silk sutures are then placed under the vein as slings, tying the distal, looping the proximal, and holding each on tension.
(6) With distal retraction, a partial venotomy is made, through which a catheter can be placed.
(7) Special techniques for very small veins
  (a) Consider using magnifying glasses or loupes.
  (b) Place a proximal tourniquet.
  (c) Use a longitudinal rather than a transverse venotomy.
  (d) Small pediatric feeding tubes (size 3F or 5F catheter) have a rounded tip that can bluntly dilate the vein and negotiate proximal venous placement.
(8) The skin incision should be carefully closed and dressed as a surgical wound.
  e. **Cutdown sites.** The saphenous vein is the preferred site for venous cutdown, with the arm veins as the secondary site.
    (1) **Saphenous vein at the ankle**
      (a) **Location**: 1 cm anterior and 1 cm proximal to the medial malleolus (Fig. 15.1)
      (b) **Advantages**
        (i) Performed at a location unencumbered by the rest of the resuscitation team
        (ii) Low morbidity site
        (iii) Safest site for the novice
      (c) **Disadvantages**
        (i) Small veins
        (ii) Distal from the central circulation
        (iii) Frequently inaccessible because of lower leg fractures, casts, splints, or military antishock trousers (MAST)
    (2) **Proximal saphenous vein**
      (a) **Location**: 5 cm inferior to the inguinal ligament and 5 cm medial to the femoral pulse (or 5 cm medial to the midpoint of the inguinal ligament in a pulseless patient) (Fig. 15.2). This is a transverse **medial proximal thigh** incision and **not a groin** incision. The greater saphenous vein is somewhat variable in location because of the amount of fat in this area of the leg.
      (b) **Technique.** After completing a 1- to 2-inch incision in the skin and subcutaneous fat, gentle cephalad and caudal retraction will help to expose the vein. If performing this procedure alone, a small, self-retaining retractor is helpful.
        In an adult, the vein can be identified rapidly by gentle palpation along the medial thigh fascia. The vein can fre-

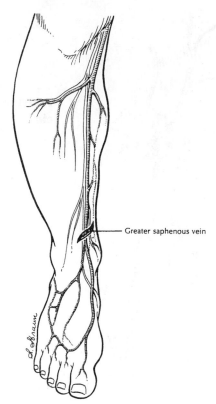

Greater saphenous vein

FIG. 15.1. Saphenous vein cutdown at the ankle. (From Moore EE, Eisman B, van Way CW III. *Critical decisions in trauma.* St Louis: Mosby, 1984, with permission.)

quently be mobilized longitudinally by spreading the hemostat under the vein while the index finger of the other hand is palpating the vein. The vein can then be immobilized over the hemostat, which can be left in place until the catheterization is complete.

Large catheters (8F to 10F) can be placed for rapid flow into the iliac vein. Less commonly, a No. 10 or 12 pediatric nasogastric tube (with its rounded tip) can be introduced into the inferior vena cava via the saphenous vein because the rounded tip can facilitate transversing the saphenofemoral junction. However, flow rate can be reduced by the length of the tube.

  (c) **Advantages**
     (i) Large catheters can be placed quickly into the central circulation
    (ii) Access can be obtained without interfering with resuscitative activities at the head and torso
   (iii) Readily accessed in patients without a pulse
    (iv) Can be obtained intraoperatively
     (v) Useful in experienced hands for infants and small children when no other access is obtainable

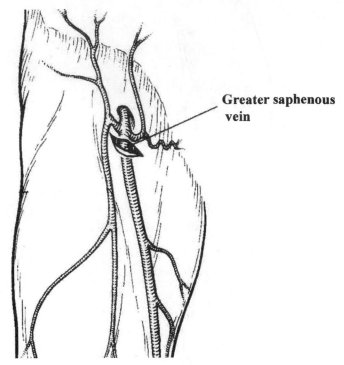

Greater saphenous vein

FIG. 15.2. The greater saphenous vein is accessed at a location one inch inferior to the inguinal ligament and one inch lateral to the pubic tubercle.

    (d) Disadvantages
        (i) Requires experience and familiarity with the anatomy
        (ii) Can be difficult in infants and children because of proximity to the femoral artery and vein
        (iii) An incision in proximity to the groin is required
(3) Antecubital region
    (a) Venous cutdown in the arm is best obtained at a site slightly proximal to the antecubital fossa. Although veins can be identified in the antecubital fossa, this area is frequently inaccessible because (a) of previous attempts to obtain venous access and (b) inadvertent injury to the brachial artery and median nerve can occur. The preferred sites are the basilic vein (located 1 inch proximal and 1 inch medial to the medial epicondyle of the elbow) and the cephalic vein (located 1 inch superior and 1 inch medial to the lateral epicondyle of the humerus) (Fig. 15.3). The technique of venotomy and placement is similar to that described for other sites.
    (b) Advantage
        (i) Easy access, particularly when the patient is draped
    (c) Disadvantage
        (i) More variable in location and somewhat more difficult than saphenous vein at the ankle

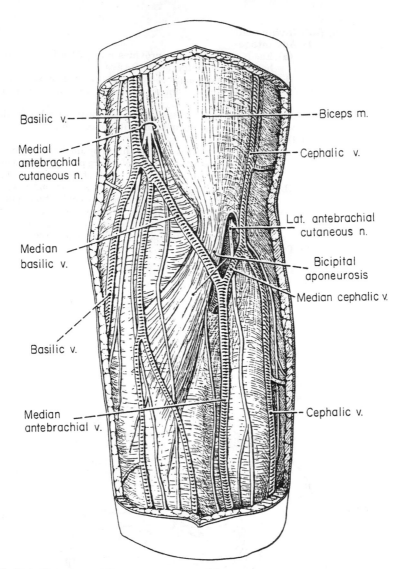

Basilic v.

Medial antebrachial cutaneous n.

Median basilic v.

Basilic v.

Median antebrachial v.

Biceps m.

Cephalic v.

Lat. antebrachial cutaneous n.

Bicipital aponeurosis

Median cephalic v.

Cephalic v.

FIG. 15.3. Upper arm cutdown. (From Woodburne RT. *Essentials of human anatomy.* London: Oxford University Press, 1969:95, with permission.)

E. **Central access.** Although central venous access was initially reserved for postresuscitation stabilization, experience in many trauma centers has led to immediate central access for resuscitation of unstable trauma patients. With the advances of the Seldinger technique (guidewire through needle, followed by catheter over guidewire), central resuscitation catheters (8F to 12F) placed over a dilator sheath have become common practice. These catheters provide very high flow rates because of their large diameters (2.5–4 mm), which are especially useful for rapid-infusion devices.

1. Site

   a. Subclavian vein

      (1) Advantages

         (a) Easily accessible and provides immediate filling of the heart from the superior vena cava

         (b) Allows measurement of the central venous pressure and access for subsequent placement of a pulmonary artery catheter

         (c) The site is easily accessible from the head of the bed for the anesthesia team (supraclavicular approach).

      (2) Disadvantages

         (a) Initial resuscitation does not allow optimal positioning of the patient, such as the Trendelenburg position, placement of a roll between the shoulders, and rotation of the neck.

         (b) Proximity of the pleural space, great vessels, and cervical nerve structures increases the risk of complications; pneumothorax, arterial puncture, hemothorax; and injury to the thoracic duct, phrenic artery, or brachial plexus.

         (c) Radiologic confirmation of proper placement can be delayed.

      (3) Technique (Fig. 15.4)

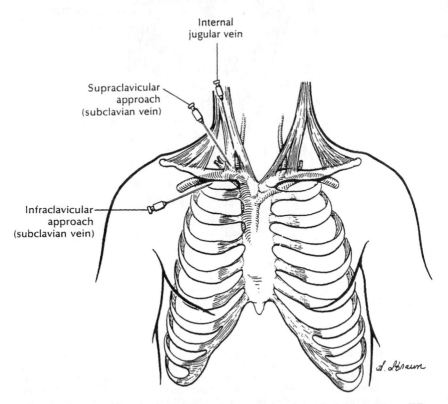

FIG. 15.4. Approach to the subclavian and internal jugular veins. (From Moore EE, Eisman B, van Way CW III. *Critical dimensions in trauma.* St Louis: Mosby, 1984:513, with permission.)

(a) Ideally, the patient is placed in Trendelenburg's position with a roll between the shoulders, although this may not be possible in acute trauma resuscitation.

(b) If a cervical collar is in place, the anterior portion must be removed and the neck immobilized, to allow finger access to palpate the jugular notch. The subclavian area is prepared, and skin and subcutaneous local anesthesia is administered, using the needle to localize the subclavian vein.

(c) The needle is then advanced beneath the clavicle, entering under the junction of the medial third and the middle third of the clavicle and aiming toward the index finger of the other hand, which is placed in the jugular notch of the sternum. The needle is advanced slowly, while hugging the undersurface of the clavicle and withdrawing on the syringe plunger until free blood flow is obtained.

(d) The guidewire should not be advanced unless blood flows freely in the syringe. It is usually helpful to advance the needle approximately 1 mm after obtaining rapid flow in the syringe before advancing the guidewire. The guidewire should be advanced slowly in short intervals, with the index finger and thumb close to the hub of the needle. If the guidewire meets resistance, the needle and guidewire should be removed together to avoid shearing the guidewire.

(e) If the guidewire advances without resistance, the needle is removed, a small skin incision is made with the knife (11 or 15 blade), and the dilator and catheter sheath are advanced firmly but gently over the guidewire. **Some portion of the guidewire is visible and secured at all times**.

(f) It is not necessary to advance the dilator its entire length, because once it is in the vein, the catheter sheath can be advanced over the guidewire, which will help prevent perforation of the superior vena cava during placement.

(g) The ability to freely withdraw blood from the catheter sheath with gentle pressure should be ascertained before initiating i.v. flow. Alternatively, free flow can be assured by connecting the catheter to the i.v. delivery system and lowering the fluid bag toward the floor. If free backflow of blood is seen, i.v. flow can begin. On occasion, the sheath will have to be withdrawn slightly to ascertain blood flow.

(4) **Complications**

(a) **Arterial puncture**. When this occurs, the catheter should be withdrawn and digital pressure applied with the thumb below the clavicle and the index finger above the clavicle for a minimum of 5 minutes.

(b) **Pneumothorax** occurs in up to 5% of patients, even in experienced hands. Withdrawing air in the syringe can occur as a warning sign, but is present in only 20% of the cases in which pneumothorax occurs.

(c) **Catheter malplacement into the internal jugular vein**. As long as free flow occurs, this catheter can still be used for resuscitation but should be repositioned at the first opportunity, which can usually be done without the need for an additional puncture. Hypertonic solutions should not be infused until proper placement of the catheter tip in the superior vena cava is confirmed.

(d) **Exit from the superior vena cava** can result in life-threatening hemorrhage and is usually recognized by signs and symptoms of hemothorax, usually occurring in the opposite side of the chest.

(e) **Dysrhythmia**, particularly if the guidewire is advanced into the heart. In these cases, the guidewire should be slightly withdrawn. If the dysrhythmia does not resolve, the wire should be further withdrawn. **Caution** should be taken in patients with a known **left bundle branch block** because guidewire placement can precipitate a right bundle branch block leading to 3° block requiring pacing.

(5) **Subclavian site selection**

(a) No difference appears to exist in the success or complication rate between right and left subclavian catheter placement. This is more of an issue of judgment, comfort, and experience for the physician placing the catheter. It has been suggested that if a chest injury requiring a chest tube has already been identified, the catheter should be selectively placed on that side to avoid the possibility of an iatrogenic contralateral pneumothorax or injury. This intuitive approach has never been substantiated in the literature. More commonly, selection of the subclavian site is a practical determination based on resuscitative activities in progress on either side of the patient. For example, if a chest tube is being placed on the right side, it is much easier to simultaneously place a subclavian catheter on the left side.

b. **Internal jugular vein.** In blunt trauma, the acute use of an internal jugular catheter is limited by the cervical collar, inability to properly position the neck, or inaccessibility to the head of the patient because of the airway team. However, in **penetrating trauma remote from the neck**, this approach has been found useful.

(1) **Technique**

(a) **The Seldinger technique**, with the precautions noted above for the subclavian vein, is the same. Most clinicians use the anterior approach through the supraclavicular triangle between the heads of the sternocleidomastoid muscle toward the ipsilateral nipple at an angle 45° from the horizontal.

(2) **Advantage**

(a) Better access from the head when the patient is draped or having other resuscitative activity at the chest level

(3) **Disadvantages**

(a) Inability to position the neck and the presence of a cervical collar

(b) Difficult to immobilize and maintain sterile dressing

(4) **Complications**

(a) Same as those for subclavian vein catheter (carotid artery injury rather than subclavian artery)

c. **Femoral vein**

(1) **Technique**

(a) The Seldinger technique described above, with placement of large-bore catheters through the femoral vein, is used frequently in trauma resuscitation. The femoral vein is located approximately 1 cm medial to the femoral artery just at or below the inguinal ligament.

(2) **Advantages**

(a) **Easy access**, particularly when other resuscitative efforts are occurring at the head or torso

(b) **Lower acute morbidity** than the subclavian or internal jugular approach

(3) Disadvantages
  (a) Difficult to locate the vein in a pulseless patient
  (b) Does not guarantee high central flow in patients with intraabdominal or pelvic vascular injury
  (c) Clot can develop at the puncture (frequently nonocclusive)

F. Intraosseous access

1. In children who are aged 6 years or younger, intraosseous access should be established if reliable venous access cannot be established percutaneously after two attempts. It should be used for the initial resuscitation and should be removed when the child has been stabilized and alternative access has been obtained.
2. In general, any i.v. drug or fluid required during the resuscitation of children can be safely administered by the intraosseous route. Fluids generally need to be administered under pressure. Specifically designed needles (modified bone marrow aspiration needles) have been developed for this purpose.
3. **Sites**
   a. The flat anteromedial surface of the proximal tibia, approximately 1 to 3 cm below the tibial tuberosity, is the preferred site for infants and children, because the marrow cavity in this location is very large and the potential for injury to adjacent tissues is minimal (Fig. 15.5).
   b. The anterior surface of the distal tibia, approximately 2 cm above the medial malleolus, is the second preferred site.
   c. The anterior surface of the distal femur has also been used.
4. **Technique**
   a. Identify the insertion site and prepare and drape in a sterile fashion.
   b. Infiltrate skin and subcutaneous with local anesthesia.
   c. Check the needle to ensure that the bevels of the outer needle and internal stylet are properly aligned.
   d. Stabilize the extremity without placing the hand behind the insertion site.

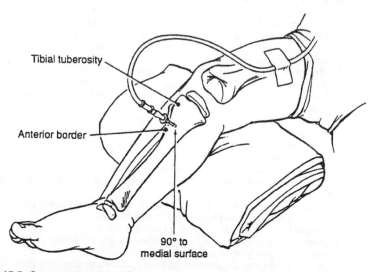

Tibial tuberosity

Anterior border

90° to
medial surface

FIG. 15.5. Intraosseous cannulation.

    e. The needle should be placed through the skin over the identified site, advancing the needle through the bony cortex, directing the needle perpendicular (90° to the long axis of the bone). Use a gentle but firm twisting or drilling motion.

    f. Stop advancing the needle when a sudden decrease in resistance to forward motion of the needle is felt. It is usually possible to aspirate bone marrow at this point. Aspiration of marrow should be followed by irrigation to prevent marrow obstructing the needle.

    g. Unscrew the cap, remove the stylet, and stabilize the needle. A small inverted medicine cup (with the bottom removed) provides protection for the needle when place over the site and taped in place.

    h. Inject 10 mL of normal saline solution through the needle and check for signs of increased resistance to injection, increased circumference of the soft tissues of the calf, or increased firmness of the tissue.

    i. If the test injection is successful, begin infusion.

    j. If the test injection is unsuccessful, remove the needle and attempt the procedure on the other leg.

  5. Complications are rare but include local cellulitis and abscess, osteomyelitis, fracture of the bone, pressure necrosis of the skin, compartment syndrome, epiphyseal plate injury, and hematoma.

II. Arterial access. After the patient has been stabilized or during stabilization, insertion of an arterial catheter allows continuous blood pressure monitoring and frequent blood sampling. In general, the arterial line should be removed when the patient no longer requires continuous pressure monitoring and when frequent blood sampling is unnecessary.

  A. Sites

    1. Radial artery is the preferred site for arterial catheter placement, because the complication rate is lower than other sites. It has been suggested that the Allen test (simultaneous compression of the radial and ulnar arteries, followed by release of the ulnar artery, looking for a flush of perfusion in the hand) be performed before radial artery line puncture. This is not commonly done in most centers because the incidence of distal ischemia is rare, especially in young patients. However, this test should be considered in the elderly, especially under more elective conditions.

    2. Femoral artery is a common line in trauma patients, but requires a somewhat longer catheter. The incidence of infection and distal ischemia is no greater than a radial artery catheter when used in initial resuscitation. However, after stabilization, these lines should be removed because the complication rate increases with time and the location can limit the mobility of the patient.

    3. Dorsalis pedis artery is a more difficult site for percutaneous placement and is difficult to immobilize. This site is more useful in an elective environment, especially in younger patients with limited arterial access.

    4. Axillary artery. Axillary arterial lines have been reported to be very successful in experienced hands in the elective intensive care unit (ICU) environment with low complication rates. They have not been used routinely as part of early resuscitation.

    5. Brachial artery should not be used because it is an end artery with a relatively narrow lumen and a higher incidence of ischemic complications.

  B. Technique

    1. Immobilize the extremity and identify the pulse. Doppler or vascular access ultrasound can be helpful in this regard.

    2. Prepare and drape the area in a sterile fashion.

    3. Anesthetizing the skin with a local anesthetic, even in the unconscious patient, can help reduce vasospasm.

    4. A variety of arterial catheters have been developed and are typically 18 or 20 gauge for the radial artery and 16 or 18 gauge for the femoral artery for an adult. The incidence of thrombosis is related to the diameter of the catheter relative to the size of the artery.

5. Using the catheter-over-the-needle technique, the needle is advanced at a 30° to 45° angle through the skin at the site of maximal pulsation.
6. Two acceptable techniques have been described for the catheter-over-the-needle approach.
    a. The catheter and needle can be passed through both walls of the artery to transfix it, after which the needle is withdrawn, followed by slow withdrawal of the catheter until a pulsatile flow of blood is obtained. The catheter is then advanced slowly through the lumen of the artery. The catheter should not be advanced unless a pulsatile flow extends beyond the hub of the needle.
    b. A second technique is to puncture only the anterior wall of the artery, after which the catheter is slowly advanced until blood appears in the needle. The needle is then lowered to a nearly 10° angle from the horizontal, and the catheter is slowly advanced over the tip of the needle into the lumen of the artery.
    c. Both of these techniques can be facilitated by using a guidewire. The modified Seldinger technique uses a guidewire passed through a needle, followed by catheter placement over a guidewire. Commercial catheters with a self-contained guidewire are also available.
7. The catheter is connected to a **continuous** infusion of heparinized saline solution (the heparin can be withheld in patients with coagulopathy or head injury).
8. The catheter should be sewn into place and a sterile dressing applied.
9. Cutdown for arterial access is sometimes necessary. This is applicable only for the radial and dorsalis pedis areas. In general, a longitudinal skin incision is more useful than the transverse skin incision. The infection rate for an arterial cutdown site is high, and this site should be used only when no alternative exists. Small, curved forceps and vessel dilators (contained in cardiac catheterization kits) facilitate a successful arterial cutdown.

C. The incidence of complications from arterial access are low but can be serious. They include hematoma, cellulitis or abscess, systemic sepsis, ischemia, embolization, malposition, and nerve injury. The incidence of arterial thrombosis is proportional to the size of the catheter and duration of cannulation.

III. Initial fluid resuscitation

A. Details of fluid resuscitation are contained in chapters 5 (*Shock*), 13 (*Adult Trauma Resuscitation*), 40 (*Anesthesia for the Trauma Patient*), and 43 (*Blood Transfusion and Complications*).

B. Injury can result in a decrease in red blood cell mass and intravascular volume, with a reduction in cellular oxygen and nutrient delivery. This can worsen because of the increased metabolic demands of trauma. The goal of initial fluid resuscitation is to **restore effective circulating blood volume** and **avoiding pulmonary and cerebral complications** of fluid overload.

C. **Key points** in initial fluid resuscitation include:
1. Establish access in at least two venous sites. Examine all prehospital lines for catheter size, location, and function. Catheters in the back of the hand wrapped in gauze are commonly dislodged or infiltrated.
2. Calculate the prehospital fluids as part of the initial resuscitation.
3. Infuse warm fluid (40°C). Crystalloids (Ringer's lactate or normal saline solution) are the initial fluid of choice for most trauma patients.
4. In hemodynamically normal patients without obvious injury, limit the initial fluid resuscitation (first hour) to 1 L in adults.
5. In normotensive adults with tachycardia or obvious sources of blood loss, infuse 2 L of crystalloid as rapidly as possible. (Use some caution in this patient category in cases of an associated head injury.)
6. In hypotensive adults who **respond** to initial fluid resuscitation, continue maintenance crystalloids (100–150 mL/h) after the initial 2 L.

7. In hypotensive adults who are **transient** or **nonresponders** to initial fluid resuscitation, infuse **blood** as early as possible to avoid profound hemodilution from excessive crystalloid.

8. Blood component therapy (fresh frozen plasma and platelets) as part of initial fluid resuscitation should be given when clinical or laboratory evidence is seen of coagulopathy or in accord with the institutional massive transfusion protocol. Cryoprecipitate is usually reserved for documented hypofibrinogenemia. **Prophylactic** component therapy as part of initial fluid resuscitation has **not** been shown to be of **value**.

9. **Hypotensive pediatric** patients should have crystalloid infusion using boluses of 20 mL/kg, which can be repeated once. **Transient or nonresponders** should be given blood at **10 mL/kg**.

10. **Rapid infusion devices** provide excellent tools for fluid resuscitation. Warmed fluids, including blood, can be infused at rates of up to 1.5 to 2.0 L/min. Care must be taken to monitor blood pressure, pulse, airway pressures, and arterial oxygen saturation to **avoid inadvertent fluid overload**.

11. Hypertonic saline solution has been shown to improve outcome in selected patients with head or thermal injury. Institutional protocols should be developed for safe and effective use.

Axioms

- Most trauma patients can be resuscitated with peripheral venous access only.
- Short, wide, i.v. catheters and tubing are preferred.
- The technology for central venous access has lowered the threshold for placement of rapid-infusion catheters for resuscitation.
- Placement of large-bore catheters through central access during acute resuscitation should be done by experienced personnel, limiting the advancement of the dilator to avoid mediastinal or intrapleural hemorrhage, which can be fatal.
- Arterial lines can be placed as part of the early resuscitation to afford monitoring and frequent blood sampling. However, this can be delayed until the patient is in the operating room or the ICU, using other noninvasive monitoring and sampling techniques in the resuscitation area.
- A venous line should not be placed at a site such that a penetrating wound is between the line and the heart. If the trajectory of a thoracic wound is not certain, place lines above and below the diaphragm.
- Establishing an i.v. cutdown on a small vein can be difficult. Light, loupes, and appropriate instrumentation and catheters are essential for success.
- Initial fluid resuscitation should be tailored to avoid the pulmonary and cerebral complications of fluid overload.

16. IMAGING OF TRAUMA PATIENTS

Michael P. Federle

I. **Introduction**. The condition of the patient and the specific type of injury that is suspected determine the imaging modality most appropriate (e.g., plain-film tomography versus computed tomographic [CT] scan). In addition, the location of the imaging equipment and the clinical capabilities to support, monitor, and treat the patient during imaging are important in deciding how to image. Regardless of the type of imaging selected, the patient requires constant monitoring and trauma team presence. **The trauma team should plan the sequence of the resuscitation to minimize time loss and avoid radiographs that are likely to be technically impossible or have low diagnostic yield.**

   A. **Plain radiography** remains an essential component of the immediate evaluation of the injured patient, especially the patient with injuries to the chest or skeleton. When hemodynamic stability permits, a seriously injured patient with blunt trauma should have plain radiographs of the cervical spine, chest, and pelvis as part of the initial evaluation. These films should be accomplished without moving the patient from the trauma resuscitation room. The need for further films or studies will be based on the mechanism of injury and findings during the initial and secondary assessments.

   Initial chest x-ray studies are usually performed in the supine position; at a later time, with immobilization or cervical spine clearance, in a sitting, upright position to better assess for aortic injury, pneumothorax, or pleural effusion. Penetrating wounds should have a radiopaque marker placed over each skin penetration site and radiographs obtained to determine trajectory (see Chapters 3 and 13) and retained bullets or fragments.

   B. **Computed tomography** has advanced the diagnosis and management of the injured patient. Management of head, some chest, and many abdominal injuries requires early CT scan. The CT scan, which has become the standard in the early diagnosis of head injury and pelvic fracture, provides a more comprehensive evaluation of chest injuries and maxillofacial fractures and allows specific diagnosis of injury to the organs of the abdomen and retroperitoneum. The accuracy and speed of CT imaging has increased with development of spiral and multislice units.

   C. **Magnetic resonance imaging (MRI)** has several advantages over CT scan, including no need for contrast administration and the ability to obtain images in sagittal, coronal, and oblique planes. MRI can be used to define shear injuries to the brain, injuries to the spinal column and cord, or vascular abnormalities that are not apparent on other radiographs. However, MRI is time-consuming, allows minimal access to the patient during the procedure, and has limited application in the initial evaluation of the trauma patient.

   D. **Ultrasonography** is being used more frequently in the management of trauma patients. The "focused abdominal sonography for trauma" (FAST) is routine in most trauma centers. A rapid diagnosis of hemoperitoneum can be made noninvasively in the trauma patient; sensitivity in this application is approximately 85%. Ultrasound (US) can also be used to assess the hemithoraces and, in experienced hands, peripheral vascular injury.

   E. **Angiography** is used for definitive diagnosis of vascular injuries. Angiography with embolization is the procedure of choice for difficult-to-access injuries (e.g., those to the vertebral artery, pelvic vessels, retroperitoneum) and selected vessels of the chest, abdomen, and large muscle masses.

II. **Skull and brain trauma**
   A. **Plain-film radiography** (i.e., skull x-ray studies) has very limited indications in patients with blunt head injury. Plain films are sometimes indicated

109

for penetrating injuries of the skull to determine the course, location, or number of gunshots or foreign-body fragments, as well as possible depressed skull fragments.

B. Most patients with a significant head injury, history of loss of consciousness (LOC), or postconcussive sequelae require immediate evaluation by CT scan. CT scan of the brain should be the initial screening tool for patients with symptoms indicating moderate to high risk of closed head injury (see Chapter 19). Technically, the CT scan images should be displayed with three windows: brain (shows edema, gray-white interface, ventricles, and cisterns), bone (outlines fractures, bony fragments), and blood (mass lesions, hemorrhage). Contrast enhancement usually is not needed in the initial study.

1. **Common CT findings of brain injury**
   a. **Basilar skull fractures** can occur in 20% of craniofacial injuries, and CT is essential for complete evaluation. However, a negative CT scan does not exclude basilar skull fracture, especially with positive physical findings. Basilar skull fractures have significant associated morbidity, including cerebrospinal fluid (CSF) leak, damage to the internal carotid artery, and facial nerve damage.
   b. **Epidural hematomas** result from the rupture of arteries and large venous sinuses resulting in an accumulation of blood that strips the dura off the inner table of the skull. The temporal region of the skull is commonly injured, resulting in a tear of the middle meningeal artery. The characteristic appearance of an epidural hematoma is a biconvex (lentiform) fluid collection that does not cross the skull suture lines but can cross the midline if venous sinuses are ruptured.
   c. **Subdural hematomas** result from the dissection of blood from ruptured veins that bridge through the subdural space. These hematomas are generally located between the dura and the arachnoid membrane. The typical subdural hematoma is a crescent-shaped fluid collection that conforms to the calvarium and underlying cerebral cortex. Recognition of atypical subdural hematomas is sometimes aided by coronal CT scan or repeat CT scan with enhancement.
   d. **Subarachnoid hemorrhage** is seen commonly in the basilar cisterns of patients following head trauma. Non–contrast-enhanced CT detects about 90% of subarachnoid bleeding within the first 24 hours, regardless of cause, as the higher density of blood replaces the water density of CSF in the cistern and sulci.
   e. **Shear injury or diffuse axonal injury (DAI).** Most brain parenchymal injuries are caused by shear-strain lesions; multiple and bilateral injuries are common. Linear and rotational acceleration-deceleration mechanisms cause shearing along interfaces of tissue of different densities, such as CSF and brain and gray-white junctions with brain and meninges. Unenhanced CT scan may show multiple small focal hemorrhagic lesions with minimal mass effect, but it is an insensitive test. In a patient who is severely depressed neurologically with a relatively normal CT study, the possibility of diffuse brain injury (or cerebrovascular injury) should be considered. MRI is much more accurate in diagnosing diffuse axonal brain injury.
   f. **Cerebral contusions and intraparenchymal hematomas** are relatively common findings on brain CT after injury. Such injuries can coalesce or enlarge and routine followup CT is recommended in these patients in 24 to 48 hours.

III. **Facial trauma.** Facial injuries are seldom life-threatening, but often are associated with more acute problems, such as airway obstruction, head or cervical spine injury, or globe injury. Occasionally, hemorrhage into the nose, nasopharynx, or mouth requires immediate attention.

A. **Plain radiographs** can be helpful for triage and initial management of facial injuries but are less comprehensive and confirmatory than other imaging modalities. Because of this, **CT is preferred to evaluate facial fractures.**

B. **CT scans of the face** can be obtained at the time of CT scan of the brain, but only as patient condition permits. Axial and coronal CT sections are obtained routinely in the stable patient. Computer-aided, three-dimensional (3D) reconstruction from thin axial sections provides optimal delineation of midfacial fractures and the spatial relationship of the fragments.

IV. **Spine injuries.** Every patient with an appropriate mechanism of injury (MOI) must be considered to have a spine injury until such is proved otherwise, either radiographically or clinically.

A. **Cervical spine. An alert, communicative adult trauma victim without distracting injury who denies symptoms, such as neck pain, and has no signs, such as neck tenderness, can be "cleared" on the basis of clinical examination.** Patients with head injury often have accompanying cervical spine (C-spine) injuries, and plain film radiographic evaluation of the C-spine is essential. The unconscious, intoxicated, or non-communicative patient needs radiographic clearance. The cervical collar must not be removed until the C-spine has been evaluated and cleared (see Chapter 20).

   1. **Techniques for obtaining adequate plain film radiographs for C-spine clearance**

      a. The plain-film lateral view of the C-spine is not adequate unless C1 through T1 are visualized. If the shoulders obscure the lower cervical and upper thoracic spine, caudal traction of the arms must be applied during filming, unless contraindicated on clinical grounds. Useful techniques to further define the C-spine include the "swimmer's view" or left and right oblique views. Failure to adequately visualize the cervicothoracic junction or the craniocervical junction will require CT scan or tomography.

      b. **Technically adequate lateral, anteroposterior (AP), and open-mouth odontoid C-spine films are the minimal views necessary to evaluate the C-spine radiographically.** A small percentage of patients with C-spine injury have only ligamentous injury and grossly normal static plain radiographs. Other studies, such as flexion-extension views, left and right oblique views, CT scan, or MRI may be required to delineate these injuries or investigate complex areas or areas not seen on plain films.

         (1) Active flexion-extension views are done voluntarily by the alert and cooperative patient only to the limit of pain tolerance. In the unconscious patient, fluoroscopic examination of passive flexion and extension of the C-spine can be performed. This examination requires a physician familiar with fluoroscopic technique and recognition of the ligamentous instability of the spine.

      c. The purpose of the radiographic evaluation often is to identify possible C-spine bony injury that has not caused a neurologic deficit. In the hemodynamically unstable patient, protect and immobilize the spine, treat the condition causing instability, and clear the spine when the patient's condition permits. **Do not spend time attempting to clear the C-spine in a hemodynamically unstable patient.**

      d. The availability of a CT scan within or near the Emergency Department facilitates emergent evaluation of C-spine trauma. CT scan is the imaging modality of choice for suspected fractures and fracture-dislocations of the spine in which plain films are not diagnostic. These scans are usually performed on an axial plane with thin (1–3 mm) cuts.

      e. MRI is the imaging procedure of choice for evaluation of injuries to the spinal column and cord but is a poor imaging technique for bone.

In patients with myelopathy, MRI can establish the location, extent, and nature of the cord injury, as well as demonstrate the location and nature of nerve root injury in patients with radiculopathy. An MRI should be obtained to evaluate the spinal cord or suspected ligamentous injury, such as disruption of the posterior ligament complex due to anterior subluxation (whiplash).

B. Thoracic and lumbar spine. Plain films of the thoracic and lumbar spine should be taken whenever signs or symptoms suggest a spine injury. In the patient with distracting injuries (e.g., chest or pelvic fractures) or a concomitant C-spine injury, a complete thoracic and lumbar (T&L) spine series is necessary. Certain mechanisms of injury warrant radiographic evaluation of the T&L spine: unprotected victims such as those involved in automobile-pedestrian crashes, rollovers, ejections from a vehicle, thrown about within a vehicle at the time of the crash, motorcycle crashes, or falls from a height.

1. Radiographs must include two views of the area of concern: usually AP and lateral. Oblique views can be helpful, but CT scan directed to the suspected area of injury is preferred. At times, portable studies are not possible because of the patient's large size. In this circumstance, the patient should have these films done in the radiology department, with proper monitoring and trauma team presence.

V. Chest trauma

A. The chest x-ray is the fundamental and primary examination in chest trauma. A frontal AP chest radiograph should be obtained in all major trauma cases. Ideally, an erect chest film is obtained because the anatomic alterations caused by the supine position can simulate disease (e.g., a widened mediastinum or interstitial lung disease) and mask pleural effusions or pneumothorax. However, the sitting upright position is often not possible. To decrease magnification artifacts, the distance from the x-ray tube (camera) to the plate should be maximized to approximately 60 to 72 inches (5–6 ft) in either the supine or reverse Trendelenburg's position.

1. **Acute aortic injury** should be suspected in any patient who suffers a significant deceleration injury. Among those patients who survive, the most common type and site of aortic injury is an incomplete tear through the intima and media of the descending thoracic aorta, just distal to the left subclavian artery. Mediastinal hemorrhage is present in most patients with aortic injury. However, even in retrospect, 7% of patients with thoracic aortic injury have a normal admission chest x-ray study. In addition, only 10% to 20% of patients with plain chest film findings of mediastinal widening prove to have an aortic laceration. In the unstable and multi-injured patient, aortography may not be appropriate; helical CT scan or transesophageal echocardiography can be more expedient. However, the aortogram remains the best test for diagnosis of this injury, in most hospitals.

   a. A patient who has radiographic evidence of mediastinal bleeding may be clinically stable enough to allow definitive imaging evaluation of the aorta. Table 16.1 lists the more common radiographic findings on plain chest film associated with blunt thoracic aortic injury.

2. **CT scan** using spiral and multislice technology preliminarily seems far more accurate than earlier generation CT in the evaluation of the thoracic aorta. With availability of the helical CT scan, recent reports have expanded the role of CT to evaluate the mediastinum and thoracic aorta. CT findings of suspected aortic injury should be considered as representing:

   • Normal (no mediastinal blood, normal aortic contour)
   • Positive (mediastinal hemorrhage plus abnormal aortic contour)
   • Equivocal (mediastinal hemorrhage without an apparent aortic or arterial abnormality)

Table 16.1 Radiographic abnormalities associated with acute thoracic aortic injury

Widened mediastinum (>8 cm)
Aortic knob obliteration
Aortopulmonary window opacification
Left apical pleural cap
Deviation of trachea, endotrachial tube, or nasogastric tube to the right
Depression of left mainstem bronchus
Widened paraspinous "stripe"
Left hemothorax

Depending on other factors, including local experience and expertise and the degree of clinical concern, patients with unequivocally negative or positive studies can often be managed without aortography. Any uncertainty regarding aortic or major vascular injury requires catheter angiography, assuming adequate hemodynamic stability.

3. The diagnosis of diaphragmatic rupture is sometimes difficult to make on plain film. Apparent elevation and distortion of the hemidiaphragm (usually the left) can be evident along with ancillary findings such as pleural effusion or rib fractures. Disruption of the diaphragm, the presence of abdominal contents outside the contour of the diaphragm, nasogastric tube in the chest, and the "pinched" appearance of a herniated bowel are reliable signs. CT scan using sagittal and coronal reformations can be useful in appreciating the altered contour of the diaphragm, but even with CT scan, this diagnosis can be difficult. The optimal imaging procedure for diagnosis of equivocal diaphragmatic rupture is MRI in the sagittal and coronal planes.

4. **Most lung parenchymal and pleural space abnormalities** are adequately evaluated by plain radiograph examinations. CT scan can reveal unsuspected pneumothorax or hemothorax, commonly seen on the upper cuts of an abdominal CT scan.

VI. **Abdominal trauma**

A. **Penetrating trauma** associated with gunshot wounds (GSW) to the abdomen, constitute a special problem in preoperative evaluation. Chest and abdominal plain films are necessary to determine trajectory and localization of opaque foreign bodies and to identify injury in the stable patient. Large radiographs are best used in conjunction with radiographic markers over each skin penetration. This allows determination of trajectory and, therefore, anatomic injury identification. Two films are usually necessary, one under the chest and the second overlapping the chest slightly but covering the abdomen and pelvis.

1. Some authors advocate a single radiograph of the abdomen such as a "one-shot intravenous pyelogram (IVP)," which can assist in evaluating the GSW if the kidney or ureter has been injured. Perhaps, more importantly, it can prove both the presence and the function of the contralateral kidney. The yield is very low in the patient without hematuria. The **technique** for an IVP is

a. Allergy to contrast iodine, shellfish is not present.

b. Large-bore intravenous (i.v.) catheters are used to inject contrast material.

c. Of contrast material, 60% (100 mL) is infused rapidly.

d. A 2-minute postinjection film is obtained to show a bilateral nephrogram.

e. Contrast material should be visualized in the renal collecting system and ureters on a 10-minute film.

2. **Findings include**:
   a. Delayed function and visualization can be seen in renal contusion and minor parenchymal fractures.
   b. Nonvisualization of a portion of the kidney usually indicates injury to that specific area and may require additional studies (i.e., CT scan or angiography).
   c. Nonvisualization on one side is typical of major vascular injury such as renal artery injury, thrombosis, or renal pedicle avulsion. Unilateral nonvisualization prompts immediate arteriography or surgery to establish diagnosis.
      Many centers prefer plain film evaluation and surgical exploration with on-table IVP. This is more expedient if the abdomen requires exploration and avoids unnecessary use of dye and delays in definite surgical evaluation and repair.
3. **Stable** patients with stab wounds to the back or flank can often be evaluated by **triple-contrast-enhanced CT scan.** Gunshot wounds that are thought to be tangential or extraperitoneal also can be evaluated with triple-contrast-enhanced CT scan. Contrast material is administered orally, intravenously, and rectally and has been used to evaluate suspected retroperitoneal structures.

B. **Blunt trauma.** In selecting the various diagnostic methods to evaluate blunt abdominal trauma, many factors are considered: clinical status of the patient, accuracy of the results, experience and expertise of those performing and interpreting the examination, cost, safety, and availability of the procedure.
   1. **Plain radiography is not helpful for identification of significant abdominal injuries following blunt abdominal trauma.**
   2. **CT scan has replaced diagnostic peritoneal lavage (DPL)** as the method for screening blunt abdominal trauma in **stable** patients. (**Focused abdominal sonography for trauma (FAST)** has replaced DPL as the screening tool for abdominal injury in **unstable** patients.) The major time factor in CT evaluation lies in the transport and positioning of the patient. Actual scanning and reconstruction of the images are done quickly. CT is accurate in identifying and quantifying hemoperitoneum, as well as identifying the site and extent of solid-organ injury; CT diagnosis of bowel injury is more challenging. A patient who remains hemodynamically unstable following resuscitation is not a candidate for CT scan or other time-consuming diagnostic imaging studies. Proximity of CT scan to the trauma room will determine safety of transport. In these patients, ultrasonography or DPL is recommended.
      a. CT provides valuable information regarding the depth and extent of abdominal visceral injuries, the extent of hemorrhage, and other criteria that correlate well with the American Association for the Surgery of Trauma (AAST) grade of injury and prognosis. A properly performed and interpreted CT scan reliably demonstrates active bleeding (extravasation), which usually indicates a need for surgery or transcatheter angiographic embolization.
      b. The technique for abdominal CT scan is
         (1) Both i.v. and oral contrast media. No i.v. contrast material should be given until the head scan is completed. The i.v. contrast (100–150 mL of 60% contrast) must be administered at a rate of 2.5 to 3 mL/second.
         (2) The oral contrast material is a dilute solution (2%) of aqueous iodinated contrast medium (e.g., Gastrografin or Gastroview). Alert patients can drink the solution, whereas patients with an altered sensorium have the solution administered through a nasogastric or orogastric tube after evacuation of stomach contents.
         (3) Initial administration of "oral" contrast medium should precede scanning as much as possible to facilitate bowel opacifica-

tion and to minimize delays within the CT scan suite. Delay in obtaining the scan to allow gastrointestinal passage of contrast material is not recommended.

(4) During the scan, i.v. contrast material is administered.

c. Routine scans are done with slices taken at 1-cm intervals from the nipple line (upper heart) to the upper thigh (lesser trochanter). Helical CT scanners allow faster acquisition of higher resolution scans; contiguous 7-mm images are obtained through the abdomen and pelvis.

3. **Ultrasonography** is useful in the diagnosis of hemoperitoneum. US is an alternative to DPL, particularly if personnel with expertise in performance and interpretation are readily available. US is less accurate than CT in the diagnosis of injuries to solid abdominal viscera and does not depict bowel injuries nor the source of hemorrhage. **FAST** examination is used concomitantly with early resuscitation to rapidly determine hemoperitoneum, hemopericardium, or hemothorax.

VII. **Pelvic trauma**

A. **The plain AP pelvic film is key in the early diagnosis of pelvic fracture**. If the alert and communicative patient is asymptomatic, without distracting injuries, this x-ray study is not essential. This radiographic examination requires a frontal pelvic view that includes the iliac crests, both hip joints, and the proximal portion of both femurs. This can be supplemented by angled projections of the pelvis of the caudal ("inlet") and cephalad ("outlet"), because these provide a more accurate delineation of the extent and relationship of pelvic fractures and joint disruptions.

B. **CT scan has a minimal role** in the immediate evaluation of the acutely injured pelvis. However, CT scan is the most accurate method for delineation of the need for operation. Computer-generated 3D images from the axial CT sections of the pelvis assist in preoperative display and reconstruction of complex pelvic fractures. Pelvic CT scan is essential in determining:

1. Pelvic ring disruptions
2. The spatial orientation and relationship of complex or displaced pelvic ring fragments
3. The presence of joint instability
4. Intraarticular fragments
5. Fractures of the articular surface of the acetabulum or femoral head

C. Patients with hemodynamic instability from pelvic fracture should be considered for immediate pelvic angiography. Pelvic angiography assists in the identification of pelvic arterial bleeding sites secondary to fracture that are amenable to percutaneous transcatheter embolization. Between 6% and 18% of patients with unstable pelvic ring disruption have pelvic arterial injuries that warrant embolization. When pelvic arterial bleeding is found at angiography, embolization successfully occludes the bleeding artery in 80% to 90% of cases. Completion arteriography is required to ensure control of hemorrhage after therapeutic embolization. If the patient has a torn venous plexus or cancellous bone fragments are bleeding, these will be unaffected by angiographic embolization and immediate operative intervention is required (see Chapter 33).

D. **Retrograde urethrogram (RUG)** is essential in the evaluation of urethral injuries. Rupture of the bladder or urethral laceration occurs in approximately 20% of patients with significant pelvic ring disruption. Therefore, RUG is the initial diagnostic procedure in patients with pelvic ring disruption and concern for genitourinary injury. It is indicated for any male patient who has blood at the urethral meatus or a scrotal or perineal hematoma. With these findings, a RUG must be performed before insertion of a Foley catheter.

1. **Technique RUG**
   a. An irrigating syringe filled with sterile 30% contrast material (10 mL) is inserted into the urethral meatus.
   b. The penis is stretched slightly to the side.

      c. The urethra is filled with the 10-mL bolus of contrast material.

      d. The film is shot just at the completion of the injection and should be at a 30° oblique angle to demonstrate the prostatic and membranous urethra.

  2. Alternate technique

      a. Pass an 8F Foley catheter into the urethral meatus (approximately 3–4 cm).

      b. Position the balloon of the Foley catheter in the distal urethra with sufficient fluid to maintain a tight fit (usually, 2–4 mL).

      c. Inject the sterile undiluted contrast material (10 mL) in a retrograde fashion, allowing for easy and complete filling of the urethra.

  3. Findings

      a. The most common site of urethral disruption is the prostatomembranous urethral junction.

      b. Extravasation of contrast will be seen at the apex of the prostatic urethra, from the membranous urethra at the triangular ligament.

      c. Partial visualization indicates incomplete disruption.

      d. Complete disruption is indicated by absence of contrast material in the bladder or prostatic urethra.

E. If the urethrogram is negative, a cystogram is performed.

  1. Technique for a cystogram

      a. Pass a 16F Foley catheter into the bladder.

      b. Gravity fill the bladder with 300 to 400 mL of sterile undiluted contrast material.

      c. Frontal and oblique radiographs of the bladder are obtained when the bladder is full.

      d. The bladder is emptied and an AP plain film is obtained to determine if an extraperitoneal bladder rupture is present.

  2. Findings

      a. Severe pelvic and lower abdominal pain, caused by extravasation of the contrast material, is a clinical indication of bladder rupture.

      b. In the unconscious patient, free flow of the diluted contrast fluid can indicate bladder rupture and intraperitoneal extravasation.

      c. These films detect bladder rupture with 98% accuracy.

VIII. Imaging in the intensive care unit (ICU). The imaging techniques discussed in this chapter are applicable to the trauma patient in the ICU. The location of the acute trauma evaluation is not as important as are what questions must be answered with imaging studies. Any trauma patients who are better cared for (monitoring, pharmacologic therapy, and so forth) in the ICU can have their radiographic and other imaging studies performed in the ICU or as their condition permits.

  A. Chest x-rays

    1. A daily chest x-ray may be indicated in any patient who has one or more of the following (can vary with hospital protocol):

      a. Acute respiratory failure

      b. Endotracheal intubation

      c. Positive end-expiratory pressure (PEEP) >5 cm H_2O

      d. FIO_2 >0.5

      e. Chest tube in place

      f. Under treatment for active disease (e.g., pneumonia, atelectasis, etc.)

    2. Selective daily chest x-rays in the ICU for the following patients:

      a. Weaning mode without change in cardiopulmonary status

    3. Chest x-ray is indicated after the following:

      a. Any acute cardiac or pulmonary deterioration

      b. Any invasive chest procedure (e.g., placement of a chest tube, new central venous line, feeding tube, or endoscopy)

    4. Chest x-rays are not necessary when

      a. A central line was changed over a guidewire without difficulty

B. Computed tomography
   1. **CT scan of the head** may be indicated when an unexplained change occurs in neurologic status or as a follow-up for a previous CT scan for head injury. CT scan for encephalopathy of multiple-system organ failure has a low yield.
   2. **CT scan of the chest** can be helpful in delineating the pathology involved in acute pulmonary failure (e.g., consolidated lung, loculated collections, empyema).
   3. **CT scan of the abdomen** without history or physical examination suggesting intraperitoneal pathology is of little benefit. CT scan of the abdomen can be helpful if
      a. Patient has had previous surgery
      b. It is performed to confirm a presumptive clinical diagnosis
      c. Is necessary to direct a percutaneous study or procedure
      d. Missed intraperitoneal injury is suspected
      e. Suspicion of pancreatitis
C. Ultrasound
   1. **Bedside US in the ICU** is helpful to localize fluid collections and to diagnose acalculous cholecystitis.
   2. **Duplex ultrasound** can be useful in detecting venous thrombosis or arterial injury.
   3. **Pericardial tamponade is suspected**.
D. Fluoroscopy
   1. **Fluoroscopy is being used in the ICU** to guide the placement of invasive devices such as pulmonary artery catheters, central lines, inferior vena cava (IVC) filters, or enteral feeding tubes.

Axioms
- The more severely compromised the patient, the less time is available for initial radiographic evaluation.
- Specific images should be obtained to answer the most vital and highest priority questions.
- Do not spend time attempting to clear the C-spine in an unstable patient.
- Axial skeletal and pelvic films may not be indicated in an alert patient without signs or symptoms of these injuries.

Bibliography
Boone DC, Federle MP, Billiar TR, et al. Evolution of management of major hepatic trauma: identification of patterns of injury. *J Trauma* 1995;39:344–350.

DiGiacomo JC, McGonigal MD, Haskal ZJ, et al. Arterial bleeding diagnosed by CT in hemodynamically stable victims of blunt trauma. *J Trauma* 1996;40:249–252.

Dyer DS, Moore EE, Ilke DN, et al. Thoracic aortic injury: how predictive is mechanism and is chest computed tomography a reliable screening tool? *J Trauma* 2000; 48:673–683.

Fabian TC, Davis KA, Gavant ML, et al. Prospective study of blunt aortic injury: helical CT is diagnostic and antihypertensive therapy reduces rupture. *Ann Surg* 1998;227:666–677.

Federle MP, Courcoulas AP, Powell M, et al. Blunt splenic injury in adults: clinical and CT criteria for management, with emphasis on active extravasation. *Radiology* 1998;206:137–142.

Frankel H, Rozycki G, Ochsner M, et al. Indications for obtaining surveillance thoracic and lumbar spine radiographs in injured patients. *J Trauma* 1994;37(4):626–633.

Master SJ, McClean PM, Acarese JS. Skull x-ray examination after head trauma: recommendation by a multidisciplinary panel and validation study. *N Engl J Med* 1987; 316:84–91.

McGonigal MD, Schwab CW, Kauder DK, et al. Supplemental emergent chest computed tomography in the management of blunt torso trauma. *J Trauma* 1990;30: 1431–1435.

Mirvis SE, Shanmuganathan K, Miller BH, et al. Traumatic aortic injury: diagnosis with contrast-enhanced thoracic CT—five-year experience at a major trauma center. *Radiology* 1996;200:413–422.

Shackford SR, Wald SL, Ross SE, et al. The clinical utility of computed tomographic scanning and neurologic examination in the management of patients with minor head injuries. *J Trauma* 1992;33(3):385.

Shanmuganathan K, Mirvis SE, Sherbourne CD, et al. Hemoperitoneum as the sole indicator of abdominal visceral injuries: a potential limitation of screening abdominal US for trauma. *Radiology* 1999;212:423–430.

Shanmuganathan K, Mirvis SE, Sover ER. Value of contrast-enhanced CT in detecting active hemorrhage in patients with blunt abdominal or pelvic trauma. *AJR* 1993;161:65–69.

Shuman WP. CT of blunt abdominal trauma in adults. *Radiology* 1997;205:297–306.

Wechsler RJ, Spettell CM, Kurtz AB, et al. Effects of training and experience in interpretation of emergency body CT. *Radiology* 1996;29:1299–1310.

17. DOCUMENTATION, CODING AND COMPLIANCE, AND EMTALA

Michael Rhodes, C. William Schwab, and Donald M. Yealy

I. **Introduction.** Documentation, coding, and compliance have clinical, legal, reimbursement, and performance improvement implications. These three elements of verification of patient care are defined, interdependent, and require specific efforts.

   A. Scribing the events of trauma care requires attention to detail to avoid coding and subsequent billing errors; the latter can be interpreted as fraud by payors, especially the federal government.

   B. Rules for documentation and billing have evolved and will continue to do so. Failure to properly document or bill for services (**noncompliance**) has legal and financial risks that can cause penalties for physicians and hospitals. These rules, although cumbersome, are the result of governmental and other payer concerns regarding accurate billing; physicians are best equipped to comply when the documentation of care is clear with respect to "who did what and when." Certified coders and compliance officers are now part of many hospital administrative staffs to facilitate interaction between providers and payers or regulators. As electronic medical records emerge, this process will likely become less cumbersome. In the meantime, understanding the requirements allows some techniques to minimize the distractions from patient care.

II. **Documentation.** Documentation should be carried out from prehospital through resuscitation, operating room, intensive care unit, ward, and outpatient care. The requirements for documentation in these areas differ, and tools should be tailored to each phase of trauma care.

   A. In many institutions, the **trauma resuscitation record** is a separate document from the trauma history and physical examination. The trauma resuscitation record is usually a nurse-driven tool, whereas the **trauma history and physical examination** is physician-driven. Frequently, these documents resemble each other and contain much of the same data, but they have distinct purposes. As the electronic medical record emerges, this duplication may not be necessary, because the ideal trauma record would include the history, physical examination, and resuscitation. However, for the purposes of discussion in this chapter, they will be considered separately.

   B. **Trauma resuscitation record.** The trauma resuscitation record is generally two to three pages in length and is a permanent record (see Appendix C). Frequently completed in duplicate by a clerk or nurse recorder, it is designed to minimize writing. Although most are institution-specific, the following elements are usually included:

      1. **Demographic information** should include the patient's name, age, sex, time and mode of arrival, allergies, medications, and significant medical history. This information may not be immediately available, but is generally available as family members arrive.

      2. **Initial assessment**
         a. Initial vital signs, along with information concerning the patient's airway, cervical spine, breathing, and cardiovascular examination
         b. The Revised Trauma Score (RTS) and the Glasgow Coma Score (GCS)
         c. Mechanism of injury
         d. The trauma team members present as well as consultants
         e. A serial record of vital signs, GCS, cardiac rhythm, pulse oximetry, pupil examination, and procedure times
         f. Injury description (anatomic diagram of the body, anterior and posterior, is helpful)

    g. Initial procedures and studies

    h. An accurate account should be made of fluid infused and blood products transfused.

    i. Disposition of the patient and family contacts

C. Trauma history and physical examination (see Appendix C)

    1. The trauma history and physical examination can be written in a standard hospital history and physical examination format, but most trauma centers have developed a preprinted format to minimize writing.

    2. The classic components of a history often cannot be obtained during resuscitation, especially the social history, review of systems, and medical history. Rather than ignoring these (which will not support appropriate coding and billing), identify these items as "unobtainable" with a reason why this is the case (e.g., "Patient was intubated," "Patient was nonverbal," "Patient was critically ill."). To avoid ambiguity, do not use the term "noncontributory."

    3. In many hospitals, a formatted, preprinted checklist or flowchart form is used for the admitting history and physical examination. Although a dictated note is not mandatory, dictation using the flowchart as a reference improves legibility and can enhance reimbursement. The history of the present illness should include the major elements of the resuscitation, including the following information:

        a. Mechanism of injury

        b. Time of the accident

        c. Presence or absence of intrusion, entrapment, restraint, or airbag deployment

        d. Prehospital assessment and evaluation

        e. Initial vital signs

        f. Careful documentation of penetrating wounds

        g. Interpretation of the radiographs and pertinent laboratory studies

    4. A format employing the Advanced Trauma Life Support (ATLS) initial assessment outline is used in many trauma centers:

        a. Primary survey

        b. Resuscitation

        c. Secondary survey

        d. Definitive care

    5. Teaching physician requirements. To generate a bill for services in a teaching setting—whether for evaluation and management (E&M) or for procedures (see more discussion of each in coding section)—the attending physician who supervises housestaff must personally provide service or be present while that service was provided. For the history and examination, the attending physician must either be present for all of this **or** review the resident history and examination and affirm the key aspects independently, noting the latter in his or her teaching physician attestation note. This allows the teaching physician to "link" to the resident documentation, supporting optimal billing. **The phrase "Seen and agree with above" is inadequate to support billing of care delivered together with residents.**

        a. The trauma history and physical examination record should have a separate area for the attending physician to sign with the accompanying statement: "I have evaluated this patient, including a review of the history, physical examination, and laboratory and x-ray studies, and have performed or supervised the procedures outlined in this resuscitation record." However, an additional note (dictated or written) is required that includes the four components of diagnosis (or problem): history and medications, physical examination, studies, and plan.

        b. If billing is planned for any procedures, the attending or supervising physician must either clearly note that he or she performed the procedure or was present "elbow to elbow" (or using another clear statement of bedside presence) with any trainee during the procedure. **Simply stating "I supervised the chest tube insertion" is inadequate**. For those procedures that take 5 minutes or less, the attending physician must be present **and** document his or her presence for the entire procedure. For those requiring more time, the attending physician must note the "key portion(s)" of each and his or her bedside presence plus note immediate availability for remaining portions of the procedure. For example, skin opening and closure is often not a key portion, whereas intraabdominal exploration or repair is a key portion. A supervising physician cannot attest to two key portions occurring simultaneously in different patients (i.e., one cannot "be present or supervising" in two places simultaneously).

   c. Critical care time is that spent by a **teaching physician** in the care on one patient with life- or limb-threatening or impending life- or limb-threatening illness or injury (see later under coding section). It includes bedside care, consultations, laboratory and radiograph interpretations, and discussion with family or other healthcare providers. **Only the attending physician can provide and document billable critical care**, and the time can be summarized. Any note should be specific (e.g., "I spent xx minutes of critical care time providing care, reviewing x-rays"). Similar to procedures, critical care time cannot be billed for two patients at the same time interval, although it can occur sequentially.

   d. All notations must be clearly generated by the attending physician—either handwritten and signed, dictated and signed (some insurers allow electronic signatures), or personally checked off (if a template used) and signed, with clear dates and times included.

  6. The following guidelines should be used to document injuries. Diagnoses should be as specific as possible, because the severity scores assigned are affected by the documentation provided by the physicians.

   a. Central nervous system (CNS) diagnoses
     (1) Document the size of brain lesion, in centimeters.
     (2) Specify type of brain lesion—epidural, subdural, intraparenchymal.
     (3) Indicate duration of loss of consciousness.
     (4) Include neurologic deficits.
     (5) Document cerebrospinal fluid (CSF) leak, hemotympanum, perforated tympanum, Battle's sign, raccoon's eyes.
     (6) Specify cord syndromes as incomplete (anterior, posterior, central, or lateral) or complete, and note their level, if possible.
     (7) Note vertebral body compression fractures.

   b. External injuries
     (1) Document size and location of contusions and abrasions.
     (2) Document length and depth of lacerations.
     (3) Specify involvement of ducts and vessels.
     (4) Document volume of blood loss.
     (5) Specify avulsions and tissue loss >25 cm^2.
     (6) Specify bullet holes by size, location, and presence of soot or powder burns. Do not use the terms **exit wound** or **entrance wound**.

   c. Injuries to internal organs
     (1) Classify length and depth of laceration or perforation of internal organs. Use a grading system if applicable (see Appendix B).
     (2) Specify size and location of hematomas.
     (3) Document involvement of vascular system.
     (4) Specify blood and volume loss (recognizing variability).
     (5) Document any urinary extravasation or fecal contamination associated with injuries to urinary and gastrointestinal (GI) tracts.

> **d. Blood vessel injuries**
>> (1) Specify complete versus incomplete transection of the vessel.
>> (2) Document any segmental loss.
>> (3) Name the specific vessel, if possible.
>
> **e. Orthopedic injuries**
>> (1) Specify fractures as open or closed.
>> (2) Document comminution or displacement, angulation.
>> (3) When making the diagnosis of crush injury, document massive destruction of bone, muscle, nerve, and vascular system of the extremity.
>
> **f. Facial injuries**
>> (1) Use the designation of Le Fort I, II, and III fractures, when applicable.
>> (2) When intraoral lacerations occur with facial fractures, indicate communication with the fracture, and they should be indicated as open injuries.

D. Operating room dictation. The operating room dictation should include efforts at ongoing resuscitation and, if dictated by a resident, should have a notation as to the presence of the attending surgeon during the key portions of the case. A written brief operative note should be placed in the patient's chart to help guide the intensive care unit (ICU) team and other consultants who may be asked to see the patient until the dictated operative report is returned.

E. Intensive Care Unit
> 1. ICU notes should follow a prescribed template outlining the complexities of care. All entries should document the date and time. If written by a resident, a notation should be made that the patient was seen with an attending physician when that occurred.
> 2. The **ICU note** should be structured to include
>> a. Hospital day
>> b. Diagnoses
>> c. Surgical procedures
>> d. Consultants
>> e. Current problems
>> f. System review
>>> (1) CNS
>>> (2) Pulmonary
>>> (3) Hemodynamic
>>> (4) GI
>>> (5) Musculoskeletal
>>> (6) Infectious disease
>>> (7) Skin and wounds
>> g. Laboratory studies and other studies (not covered in the system review)
>> h. Medications
>> i. Plans
> 3. The structured ICU note can be written or typed into a computer template and attached to the chart.
> 4. A notation from the resident that the attending physician was present at rounds is useful, when appropriate. However, a supplemental note by the attending physician may be necessary for reimbursement and should include the following five components:
>> **a. Diagnosis or problem**
>> **b. History**, including medications, major events, and other information relating to the patient's hospital course
>> **c. Physical examination**, with specific mention of the head, chest, abdomen, and extremities and inclusion of laboratory and other diagnostic studies
>> **d. Plan**, which reflects the complexity of the decision making
>> **e. Time spent** is useful except in the resuscitation or emergency area

    f. A sample note:
      Diagnosis or problem: CHI, pulmonary contusion, ICU, ventilator dependent
      History: Fever, leukocytosis, pulmonary infiltrate, continued ventilator dependence, requiring propofol for sedation, on PIP/Tazo
      Physical examination: Tm = 100, pulse = 94, Glasgow Coma Scale (GCS) score = 9, copious pulmonary secretions, culture H. flu, pupils sluggish, no lateralizing signs, abdomen soft, tolerating tube feedings
      Plan: Tracheotomy today, change central line, continue pulmonary toilet, replace magnesium
      Time: 25 minutes

F. Ward. Record date and time of all entries. The ward note also should contain the five components listed above and, when written by the housestaff, should acknowledge the presence of the attending physician, who must, however, include a note detailing his or her specific care or actions. Examples of written or dictated attending notes follow:

    1. Examples:
      Diagnosis: Fx spleen-grade IV, left rib fxs, postsplenectomy
      History: POD 3, minimal complaints, tolerating liquids, OOB in chair, O_2 saturation = 91%, patient-controlled analgesia (PCA) morphine
      Physical examination (PE): Alert, pulse = 94, Tm = 100, chest clear, fair cough, abdomen soft, incision clean
      Plan: Increase mobility, convert PCA to oral (p.o.) Percocet, ultrasound (US) left upper quadrant (LUQ) as baseline, complete blood count (CBC), chest x-ray
      Time: 10 minutes

      Diagnosis: Gunshot wound (GSW) abdomen, small bowel injury, liver injury, exploratory laparotomy, small bowel resection
      History: POD 4, OOB, nasogastric (NG) suction minimal, comfortable, moderate abdominal pain, Amp/sulbactam stopped yesterday
      Physical examination: Tm = 100, pulse = 100, minimal drainage right upper quadrant (RUQ), chest clear, ABD incision clean, positive peristalsis
      Plan: Discontinue NG, advance RUQ drain, mobilize, liquids p.o.
      Time: 15 minutes

      Diagnosis: Multiple contusions and lacerations, advanced age, coronary artery disease (CAD), a fib
      History: Day 3 postfall, confused, painful movement in hip, poor mobility, poor p.o. intake, i.v. fluid therapy, on digitalis and furosemide
      PE: Bewildered, blood pressure = 140/70, pulse = 86 (pacer), multiple ecchymoses, chest and abdomen-normal examination, scalp laceration and facial lacerations clean, neurologic examination—no gross motor or sensory deficit
      Plan: Ice or heat to hip, computed tomography (CT) pelvis, orthopedic consult, check electrolytes, codeine p.o., physical therapy, discuss with home care and family
      Time: 20 minutes

III. Coding
  A. Overview
    1. Basically, two coding systems are used (CPT and ICD-9-CM), both of which are required for billing. **CPT (current procedural terminology)**, published by the American Medical Association (AMA), is widely accepted at the physician component of billing. Three components of the CPT codes: (*a*) procedures, (*b*) E&M (evaluation and management), and (*c*) modifiers. ICD-9-CM (international classification of diseases), developed by the World Health Organization, provides the diagnosis codes necessary to support both physician and hospital billing (ICD9 procedure codes are also used for hospital billing). Lack of understanding by physicians that a **CPT code** (for procedure or evaluation

and management by a physician) **must be accompanied by an ICD9 diagnosis code(s)** is a major obstacle in reimbursement for trauma and critical care.

2. Most CPT procedure codes are straightforward. It is the use of **modifiers** to indicate special situations that is challenging because payors vary considerably in their recognition and acceptance of modifiers. Examples of these special situations include two surgeons, multiple or bilateral procedures, discontinued procedures, surgical team, distinct procedure, repeat procedure, shared procedure, preoperative evaluation only, surgery only, and so forth. However, it is the **E&M coding for trauma** and **critical care** that presents the **greatest challenge** for providers because of the ever-changing and complex rules for documentation. It is the **documentation components, rather than the severity of injury or illness**, that determines the code. With this in mind, what follows are typical patient examples and potential use of E&M codes for trauma and critical care, assuming appropriate documentation (these rules are too lengthy to include).

B. **CPT coding for evaluation and management of the trauma patient**
   1. **(99291)**: Evaluation and management of a critically injured patient, requiring constant attendance (includes peripheral i.v., venous and arterial blood draw, NG and urinary catheters, arterial blood gases, interpretation of hemodynamic or cardiopulmonary monitoring and chest x-ray, and ventilatory management which may in the future become unbundled).
   2. **(99291**: 30–74 min, **99291, 99292**: 75–104 minutes). These codes are used when a critically injured trauma patient requires continued bedside management during initial resuscitation or subsequent critical care. This includes continuous physician attention during transport to CT scan suite, angiography, operating room, or ICU.
      a. This does **not include** the **time** of an **operative procedure** unless the operative procedure is performed by another surgeon while the admitting surgeon is participating in the ongoing resuscitation.
      b. Procedures such as chest tube, central line, diagnostic peritoneal lavage and arterial line are not included in this code and should be billed separately.
      c. These codes are also applicable to subsequent daily critical care management, utilizing the same time parameters.
   3. If initial resuscitation does not rise to the level of critical injury (by the surgeon's judgment and documentation), then the codes for **initial hospital care (99221–23)** should be used, depending on the decision complexity and time spent with the patient.
   4. **(99233): Subsequent hospital care in the ICU (typically 35 minutes)**. This code can be used if the ICU care is for reasons other than specific postoperative care. For example, a patient with a closed head injury, multiple rib fractures, and a femoral fracture who had an exploratory laparotomy and splenectomy can have this code used for ICU care because the ICU care is primarily for reasons other than postoperative splenectomy.
      a. Postoperative care for an isolated splenectomy would be included in the operative code.
      b. Procedures such as chest tube, central line, diagnostic peritoneal lavage (DPL) and arterial line are not included in this code and should be billed separately (modifier required).
      c. The 35 minutes includes time at bedside plus other time in the unit with the patient's chart, images, disposition, and family. **Time** spent **off the unit** in review of patient's data **cannot be reported**, so it is useful to review laboratory studies and images, write or dictate notes, **coordinate patients care** (e.g., discussion with consultants), and conduct family conferences **in or near** the **unit** where the patient is located.

5. **(99232): Subsequent hospital care characteristically performed in the intermediate or step-down unit** when evaluated for reasons other than postoperative care (i.e., a postsplenectomy patient with a head injury, pulmonary contusion, and pelvic injury who has been extubated and is in a step-down unit for cardiac or neurologic monitoring). This code is typically for 25 minutes of total time.

    a. These codes do not apply to care of isolate postoperative injuries because they are included in the operative code.

6. **(99231): Subsequent hospital care, usually rendered on the floor or ward.** This is for follow-up evaluation on the medical surgical floor of the nonoperative or operative trauma patient for reasons other than the postoperative care. Total time is typically 15 minutes.

7. **(99223): Initial hospital care for stable trauma patient with significant injury.** Includes history and physical examination and **complex** decision-making. For example, a 24-year-old man with a fracture-dislocation of the cervical spine, neurologically intact, or a 54-year-old woman with stable vital signs, awake, with multiple contusions and abrasions with a seatbelt sign without peritoneal signs who undergoes an abdominal CT scan. Total time is typically 70 minutes.

8. **(99222): Initial hospital care for a stable trauma patient with a potentially significant injury.** Includes a history and physical examination and moderate decision-making. For example, a 65-year-old man with a cerebral concussion and multiple contusions and abrasions. Total time is typically 50 minutes.

9. **(99221): Initial hospital care for a stable trauma patient who has no apparent significant or potentially significant injury but will require hospitalization.** This includes history and physical examination and **straightforward** decision-making. For example, a 22-year-old man, intoxicated, with multiple contusions and abrasions, triaged to the Trauma Center primarily on the mechanism of injury. Total time is typically 30 minutes.

10. These are just a few of the more common E&M codes used for trauma patients. Consultation codes can also be used. The key issue is to follow the documentation rules for each of these codes, for which you will need a small portable guide, and to provide the appropriate diagnosis for which the E&M codes are being generated. Remember, except for critical care codes (which require continuous bedside attendance), time spent by the physician for each code includes any patient-related activity as long as it occurs in or near the unit on which the patient is located.

C. **Trauma ICD diagnostic coding**

1. **Introduction.** Billing for professional services begins with diagnoses for which care was rendered. Most claim forms accommodate four diagnoses. Since 1988, the Health Care Financing Administration (now called Centers for Medicare and Medicaid Services) has mandated the use of the International Classification of Diseases for diagnosis reporting and most other payors have followed suit. Proper ICD coding can decrease the number of claims sent to manual review, thereby optimizing timely reimbursement. Several principles should be applied whenever possible to ICD coding.

2. **Principles and examples**

    a. ICD coding is contained in two volumes, Volume I (the tabular list) and Volume II (the alphabetical list); use both.

    b. "Unspecified" and "other" codes should be avoided.

        (1) **Example**: You wish to code for blunt hepatic injury. Volume II reveals "Injury, internal, liver 864.00" and "Laceration 864.09." Volume I, however, lists the entire classification scheme for closed hepatic injury with detailed descriptions for each code (e.g., "864.03 Injury to liver, laceration involving parenchyma but without major disruption of parenchyma; i.e., <10 cm long and <3 cm deep"). Using Volume I lets you

choose the best description and avoid "other" (864.09) or "unspecified" (864.00).

c. Diagnoses should reflect information known to you at the time the billed service was rendered. Each CPT code is linked to only those ICD codes related to that CPT code.

   (1) **Example:** You are consulted regarding a patient, AB, who has been assaulted and also stabbed in the abdomen. He was unresponsive in the field but is awake, although incoherent during your evaluation. He has right lower quadrant tenderness. Diagnoses accompanying your Emergency Department consultation claim are (1) "879.2 Open wound, anterior abdominal wall, uncomplicated"; (2) "789.63 Abdominal tenderness, right lower quadrant"; and (3) "850.1 Concussion with brief loss of consciousness." You perform DPL. For this procedure, your diagnoses are 1 and 2. DPL is positive, and at laparotomy you repair two distal ileal holes and one ascending colon hole. For the operation, you list (1) "863.39 Open injury, small intestine, other or multiple for CPT 44603 (repair multiple small bowel)" and (2) "863.51 Open injury, ascending colon for 44604 (repair colon)."

d. ICD diagnoses must contain fourth or fifth digits where required. Failure to use required digits often leads to manual review.

   (1) **Example:** 789.63 Abdominal tenderness, right lower quadrant compared with 789 Abdominal pain and tenderness. 863.51 Open injury, ascending colon compared with 863.50 Open wound, colon.

e. Thorough ICD coding supports CPT coding for critical care services and for complex evaluation and management services. Not all ICU patients require critical care services daily, and auditors are likely to visit physicians with apparent excess critical care or complex visit charges.

   (1) **Example:** You admit EF to the ICU after a motor vehicle crash in which he sustained a liver laceration and a cardiac contusion. He presented with hypotension, and developed a supraventricular tachycardia soon after arrival in the ICU. The use of diagnoses (1) "864.04 Injury to liver, closed, major laceration"; (2) "958.4 Traumatic shock"; (3) "861.01 Cardiac contusion"; and (4) "427.0 Paroxysmal supraventricular tachycardia" better supports a critical care service CPT code than any of these codes used alone.

f. Initial diagnostic code selection can have an impact on reimbursement for services provided later in the patient's course.

   (1) **Example:** Critical care services performed by the operating surgeon are normally not reimbursed during a postoperative global period. However, if the diagnostic codes for the operation are for injury, fracture, burns, open wounds, or other trauma, that surgeon also can charge and collect for critical care services (although not other evaluation and management services). Patient AB (see Example 3) remains somewhat obtunded; he aspirates and develops pneumonia and then septic shock. You perform endotracheal intubation, initiate and manage mechanical ventilation, and institute and manage vasopressors and antibiotics. Because your CPT codes for AB's operation were linked to diagnostic codes for small bowel and colon injuries, you can now bill for critical care services. You list "482.89 Bacterial pneumonia" and "518.5 Pulmonary insufficiency following trauma and surgery" for CPT "31500 Endotracheal intubation, emergency." You list "482.89, 518.5, and 785.59 Shock" without mention of trauma for the critical care services.

    g. Use of E or V codes as primary diagnoses often leads to manual review or to automatic denial. E or V codes can be appropriately used in addition to other ICD codes, although they should not replace non-E, non-V codes. V codes can be appropriate as primary diagnoses for "no charge" visits.

      (1) Example: AB (see Example 3) returns to your office for followup 6 weeks after laparotomy. You link diagnosis "V67.09 Postoperative follow-up" with a "no charge" office visit code. This documents that you provided the postoperative outpatient care required in the global surgical package.

IV. EMTALA. Beginning in the mid 1980s, federal legislation had evolved to protect patients seeking emergency care. Initially referred to as "antidumping" laws, these actions have evolved into the "Emergency Medical Treatment and Active Labor Act." All hospitals and providers that offer emergency services are bound by EMTALA.

    A. EMTALA states that any person seeking emergency care (including trauma) must receive a screening examination and stabilization, irrespective of the ability to pay. The providers and hospitals must provide and document that care, or document refusal by a patient who has the capacity to do so and with the knowledge that care will be provided without financial concerns. All life- and limb-threatening injuries must be sought and initial care given. Hospitals must have policies that ensure physician availability (including functional on-call lists of providers across specialties) to provide this initial emergency care.

      1. The screening examination and stabilizing actions were not defined in the statute. Based on interpretations and case law, however, these should be similar to those provided to any patient presenting with the same symptoms or findings. This means the same or similar tests by the same or similar providers (e.g., a nurse screening examination would not suffice unless this was the only examination done routinely for all patients with that complaint). Definitive care is not mandated. The only exception to the stabilization requirement is when attempts to do so would jeopardize the patient's health or outcome.

      2. Transfer to a more appropriate facility can occur after this screening and stabilization has occurred if the receiving facility offers services not available at the original site. Trauma centers often receive patients for this reason from nontrauma centers or lower level centers. The transfer must be accompanied by notification and acceptance between providers, documented agreement by the patient (if capable), and all pertinent medical records. Local policy and practice must assure these steps and documentation.

      3. EMTALA covers all hospital property—including clinics and other care sites—and the obligation begins with patient arrival to the facility. That includes patients who reach the hospital driveway or sidewalks (if for the purpose of seeking care). Also, patients in an ambulance requesting transport to a hospital are covered, irrespective of which entity owns or operates the ambulance. This has profound and uncertain implications for ambulance diversion practices. Finally, it can extend to the hospital floor, especially if early discharge before identification of injuries occurs or an acute decompensation happens without care.

      4. The possible penalties for failure to comply with EMTALA include imprisonment, fines (with multiple violations possible in a given case), and potential exclusion from Medicare for up to 5 years. The fines can be tripled in selected circumstances where egregious behavior exists. These penalties are separate and unrelated to civil actions (i.e., malpractice).

      5. The best emergency department and trauma bay policies are to evaluate and treat all patients the same, and ask insurance information only after the initial care and plan is complete.

Axioms

- Notes should be factual. Avoid the temptation to express disappointment (e.g., "sequential compression boots found at foot of bed" or "patient not taken for scan because of inadequate number of staff on floor").
- Do not use **noncontributory** or **not applicable** for absent data. Use the word "unobtainable," and state the reason why.
- Dating and timing of notes are essential for medical-legal and reimbursement reasons.
- Teaching physicians must personally provide care to bill professional fees in a training setting. Thus, they must clearly review housestaff care and independently confirm findings to bill for care and procedures **or** do a complete examination alone (the latter being rare).
- Teaching physician notes need not be lengthy, and should link to any resident documentation. Do not write "Seen and agree with above" alone if billing is planned. Simply put, to generate a professional bill for care, the teaching physician must have "been there, done it, and wrote it down."
- To avoid EMTALA problems, care for all patients first, leaving insurance questions until after the resuscitation and emergent care is complete.

Bibliography

American College of Surgeons Committee on Trauma. *Resources for optimal care of the injured patient*. Chicago: American College of Surgeons, 1998.

American Medical Association. *International classification of diseases*, 9th revision, clinical modification (ICD-9-CM). Chicago: American Medical Association, 1999.

American Medical Association. *Physicians' current procedural terminology (CPT) 2000*. Chicago: American Medical Association, 1999.

American Medical Association and US Health Care Financing Administration. Washington, DC. *Documentation guidelines for evaluation and management services*, May 1997.

18. OPERATING ROOM PRACTICE

Michael Rhodes and Michael Russell

I. **Conducting a trauma operation**
   A. The ideal location for a trauma operating room (OR) is adjacent to the resuscitation area. This, however, depends on hospital-specific geography and resources. In general, it is more practical to have the trauma operating room within the main OR suite for more flexibility of equipment and personnel. It is **better** to **take** the **patient** and the **resuscitation team** to an **OR** than to attempt to bring the OR to the patient. A protocol for elevator standby and priority transport must be in place. When possible, obtain an operative consent from the patient or family. With a hemodynamically unstable patient or patient with closed head injury, obtaining consent may not be possible. A lifesaving operation should not be delayed to complete a formal operative consent.
   B. A trauma OR should have a minimum space of 400 to 450 ft^2. The following equipment should be available:
      1. A large, high-quality OR light with two peripheral satellite lights for patients requiring multiple, simultaneous procedures
      2. Dedicated x-ray equipment (built-in, if possible) to move in and out of the operative field
      3. An OR table capable of plain radiography and fluoroscopy
      4. A minimum of four suction connections
      5. A minimum of eight electrical outlets
      6. Warm intravenous (i.v.) fluids
      7. A rapid-infusion device
      8. A blood salvage device
      9. A multipurpose anesthesia machine capable of high minute ventilation (up to 30 L/min), 20 cm H_2O of positive end-expiratory pressure (PEEP), and pressure-support or inverse-ratio ventilation
      10. Multichannel pressure monitoring with a remote slave monitor
      11. Multiple x-ray view boxes (minimum eight)
      12. Patient heating devices
      13. Electrocautery with argon beam capability
      14. A general trauma tray that should include aortic compressor, rib spreader, sternal retractor, and a variety of vascular clamps
      15. Headlight, face shields or goggles, boots, and impervious gowns for the operating team
   C. **The resuscitation team should accompany the critically injured patient to the OR.** Adequate assistance should be available to move the patient from the resuscitation litter to the OR table; this movement should be directed by the trauma team. In general, the patient should be removed from the backboard and military antishock trousers (MAST) before start of the operation.
   D. For urgent exploratory laparotomy, the patient should have both arms available for adequate access during the operative procedure. Access to the central veins should be in place for most critically injured patients. A **cervical collar** can be removed after the patient is anesthetized and **replaced with two 5-pound sandbags** on each side of the head with large **tape** across the forehead. This allows exposure of the lower neck and clavicular area for central access or subsequent thoracic incisions.
   E. Pulse oximetry, capnometry, pressure monitoring, and electrocardiographic (ECG) monitoring should be applied. The ECG pads should be strategically placed to avoid interference with subsequent operative intervention. Warming devices should be placed over those areas not in the surgical field. The patient should be **prepared** from **midthighs to midneck** and **laterally to the table** (Fig. 18.1). In agonal patients, even a 15-second painting or

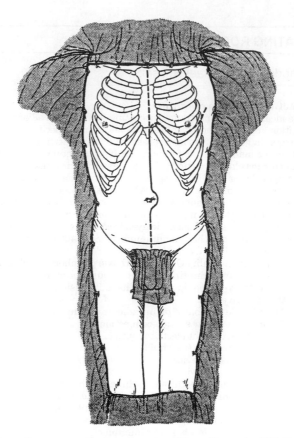

FIG. 18.1. Operating room patient preparation. (From Champion HR, Robbs JV, Trunkey DD. Trauma surgery, parts 1 and 2. In: Dudley H, Carter D, Russell RCG, eds. *Rob and Smith's operative surgery.* Boston: Butterworth, 1989:540, with permission.)

spray with antiseptic is superior to no skin preparation. Draping should be wide and secured in place with staples or sutures.

F. In a **hypotensive** patient with an obtainable blood pressure, the **abdomen** should **not** be **opened until** blood is available in the room, adequate i.v. is in place, and the **anesthesia team is prepared** to deal with possible sudden cardiovascular collapse.

G. A number of techniques are used in the OR to care for the injured patient, depending on the body region and stability of the patient. In general, the following are useful guidelines:

1. Ensure adequate help, light, and suction.
2. The incision should be large enough for rapid and thorough exploration. **The operation should not be compromised by inadequate exposure**.
3. Blood salvage capability should be ready before opening a body cavity suspected of massive hemorrhage.
4. Hemorrhage in most areas can be controlled by precise packing before attempting definitive repair.

   5. In an unstable patient, it is valuable to frequently monitor hematocrit, arterial blood gases, ionized calcium, and potassium. A tableside point-of-service analyzer can be useful.
   6. Conduct of specific OR procedures is presented in Chapters 19 through 37.
 II. **Operating room team**
   A. A physician team includes the trauma surgeon, the resident or assistant surgeons, and the anesthesiologist. Continuous communication between the physician members of the team is essential. In a **persistently unstable** patient with complex anatomic injuries, a **second trauma surgeon** can be invaluable in the resuscitative and technical aspects of the patient's care.
   B. An OR scrub nurse, a circulating nurse, a nurse anesthetist, an emergency department nurse, and a critical care nurse can all be participants in a major operating room resuscitation. Operating room technicians, perfusionists, laboratory technicians, and respiratory therapists can be assigned vital responsibilities as part of the OR resuscitation.
III. **Operating room communication**
   A. The OR should be notified of all level I trauma patients arriving at the hospital. This occurs whether or not the need for immediate operative intervention is known. **OR personnel** should be notified and placed on **standby** when the trauma team is activated. The OR personnel should communicate with the trauma team to determine the need for operative intervention.
   B. A system should be in place for the operating team to provide periodic updates to family members.
   C. Direct communication between the OR and the blood bank or laboratory should be available.
 IV. **Priorities for multiple procedures**
   A. The decisions in prioritization of operative procedures can be challenging. Following are some general guidelines:
      1. After airway and ventilatory control, major hemorrhage, either external or body cavity, takes priority.
      2. External hemorrhage from the face, scalp, and extremities can be controlled by pressure, packing, or temporary suture closure until major body cavity hemorrhage is controlled.
      3. In general, uncontrolled thoracic hemorrhage or cardiac tamponade takes priority over uncontrolled abdominal hemorrhage.
      4. Damage control techniques with hemorrhage control, stapling of intestine, and packing should be seriously considered in the massively injured patient who is coagulopathic, acidotic, and cold (see Chapter 29).
      5. Craniotomy without a preceding imaging study is rarely required in the OR, especially in the absence of lateralizing signs.
      6. Body cavity hemorrhage (chest, abdomen, pelvis) takes priority over head injury.
      7. A patient with a wide mediastinum and active intraabdominal hemorrhage should have exploratory laparotomy and simultaneous evaluation of the mediastinum with transesophageal echocardiography.

Axioms
• The resuscitation initiated in the emergency department should be continued in the OR.
• Identify early the patient requiring a damage control approach.
• Actively bleeding patients should be resuscitated in the OR; control of the hemorrhage and resuscitation should occur simultaneously.
• Severely injured trauma patients may require a specially designed OR with a team of physicians and nurses trained to respond in a flexible fashion to a variety of operative and logistic challenges.

Bibliography
Rhodes M, Brader A, Lucke J, Gillott A. Direct transport to the operating room for resuscitation of trauma patients. *J Trauma* 1989;29:907–915.

19. HEAD INJURY

Donald W. Marion

Traumatic Brain Injury

Central nervous system (CNS) injury is the most common cause of death from injury. Two million people per year suffer traumatic brain injuries, many as the result of motor vehicle crashes. Most of these victims are between the ages of 16 and 30 years. The increasing use of seatbelts and airbags has resulted in an estimated 20% to 25% reduction in these traffic fatalities. However, the incidence of penetrating injury to the brain and spinal cord is increasing.

I. **Anatomy and physiology**
   A. The skull is particularly thin in the temporal region. The floor of the cranial cavity is divided into three regions: anterior (frontal lobes), middle (temporal lobes), and posterior (lower brainstem and cerebellum).
   B. The **meninges** cover the brain in three layers: dura mater (fibrous membrane that adheres to the internal surface of the skull), arachnoid membrane, and pia mater (attached to the surface of the brain). Cerebrospinal fluid (CSF) circulates between the arachnoid and pia mater in the subarachnoid space.
   C. The brain is composed of the cerebrum, cerebellum, and the brainstem. The brainstem consists of the midbrain, pons, and medulla. The reticular activating system (responsible for state of alertness) is within the midbrain and upper pons. The cardiorespiratory centers reside in the medulla. Small lesions in the brainstem can cause profound neurologic deficit.
   D. The Monro-Kellie Doctrine states that the total volume of intracranial contents must remain constant because of the rigid bony cranium. With an expanding mass lesion, the intracranial pressure (ICP) is generally within normal limits until the point of decompensation on the pressure-volume curve is reached; ICP then dramatically increases.
   E. **Cerebral perfusion pressure (CPP)** = Mean arterial pressure − ICP. Maintenance of cerebral perfusion is essential in the management of patients with severe closed head injury. Normal **cerebral blood flow (CBF)** is approximately 50 mL/100 g brain/minute. CBF <20 mL/100 g brain/minute represents cerebral ischemia and cell death occurs at approximately 5 mL/100 g brain/minute. In addition to cerebral ischemia in response to injury, the injured brain loses its ability to autoregulate blood flow, increasing susceptibility of the injured brain to further ischemia.
II. **Traumatic brain injuries (TBI)** are categorized as mild (80%), moderate (10%), or severe (10%), depending on the level of neurologic dysfunction at the time of initial evaluation. **Determination of the Glasgow Coma Scale (GCS) score as early as possible and then serially is essential. Loss of consciousness (LOC)** is an important indicator of traumatic brain injury. Classification of traumatic brain injury is based on the GCS.
   A. **Mild head injury**
      1. GCS score of 13 to 15
      2. Brief period of LOC
      3. Prognosis is excellent
      4. Mortality rate <1%
   B. **Moderate head injury**
      1. GCS score of 9 to 12
      2. Typically, confused and may have focal neurologic deficits; able to follow simple commands
      3. Prognosis is good
      4. Mortality rate <5%

C. Severe head injury
  1. GCS of ≤8—generally, the accepted definition of coma
  2. Unable to follow commands
  3. Until recently, mortality >40%
  4. Most survivors have significant disabilities
  5. Elevated ICP is a common cause of death and neurologic disability

III. Initial evaluation and treatment of head injury
  A. General
  1. Patients suspected of having suffered a head injury, particularly if confused or unresponsive, require emergency evaluation and treatment at a center with capabilities for immediate neurosurgical intervention. General objectives are rapid diagnosis and evacuation of intracranial mass lesions, expedient treatment of extracranial injuries, and avoidance of secondary brain injury.
  2. Severe brain injury is associated with cerebral ischemia. Therefore, a principal therapeutic goal is to enhance cerebral perfusion and oxygenation and avoid further ischemic injury to the brain.

  B. Initial management of the unresponsive patient with head injury
  1. **Intubation** with controlled ventilation (avoid routine hyperventilation). If possible, a focused neurologic examination, including assessment of GCS, pupillary response, and extremity movement, is critical before intubation and pharmacologic paralysis.
  2. **Venous access**
    a. Restore intravascular volume, blood pressure, and perfusion.
    b. Avoid hypotonic or dextrose-containing solutions.
  3. **Immobilize the patient with rigid backboard and cervical spine (C-spine) collar.** Assume that all patients with TBI have a spine injury until proved otherwise.
  4. **Pharmacologic paralysis** and sedation, if agitated or combative
    a. Short-acting agents are recommended.
      (1) Vecuronium bromide, cisatracurium, or succinylcholine
      (2) Opioid sedation: fentanyl or morphine
      (3) Avoid benzodiazepines
  5. **Monitor blood pressure and O₂** saturation continuously.
  6. Check arterial blood gases (ABG), blood glucose, electrolytes, prothrombin time (PT), partial thromboplastin time (PTT), hematocrit, and platelet count.
  7. **Initiate medical management of the head injury.** Proceed with rapid acquisition of a computed tomographic (CT) scan of the head, if promptly available. Based on time, distance, and local capabilities, transfer may be necessary. **Rapid referral** to a center capable of immediate neurosurgical intervention may be required. **Do not delay transport to obtain a CT scan of the head. Early diagnosis and evacuation of cranial mass lesions are critical.**
  8. **Repeated neurologic examination and assessment of GCS.** Documentation of the GCS in patients who are intubated should be noted by a T (i.e., 11[T]; patients who are pharmacologically paralyzed are noted by a P (i.e., 3[P]); and patients who are intubated and pharmacologically paralyzed are noted by a TP (i.e., 3[TP]). This is needed for meaningful interpretation of the GCS values.
  9. Hyperventilation causes cerebral vasoconstriction and can worsen cerebral ischemia. Hyperventilation, however, can be indicated in the setting of abrupt neurologic deterioration.

  C. Secondary management
  1. **The avoidance of secondary brain injury is essential. A single episode of hypotension (systolic blood pressure <90 mmHg) in the adult will increase mortality 50%.**
  2. The GCS obtained in the emergency department can be a more reliable assessment of the severity of brain injury than the GCS obtained in the field.

3. The GCS cannot be assessed by simple observation and requires stimulation of the patient. In cases of asymmetry in either eye opening or motor scores, the best score is used.

4. If time permits, a lateral cervical spine x-ray study usually can be obtained during secondary survey of the patient, which may detect gross injury or malalignment of the cervical spine (Fig.19.1).

D. **Indications for ICP monitoring.** As a general approach, liberal use of ICP monitoring in patients with severe TBI (GCS ≤8) is recommended. ICP monitoring is not routinely indicated for patients with moderate or mild closed head injury. **ICP monitoring is indicated for**:

1. Severe closed head injury (GCS ≤8) and abnormal CT of head
   a. **Definition of abnormal CT**:
      (1) Hematoma
      (2) Contusion
      (3) Edema
      (4) Compressed basal cisterns

2. Severe closed head injury (GCS ≤8) and normal CT of head, but two or more of the following exist:
   a. Age >40 years
   b. Unilateral or bilateral flexor or extensor posturing
   c. Systolic blood pressure <90 mmHg (rapid correction of hypotension is essential)

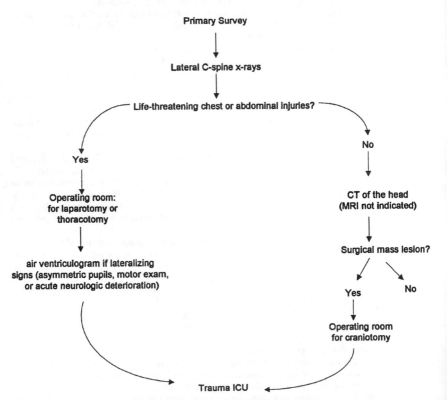

FIG. 19.1. Emergency department triage of severe brain injury.

E. Intensive care management of patients with severe TBI (GCS ≤8).
The goal is to prevent secondary brain injury by limiting focal cerebral ischemia and enhancing cerebral perfusion. This can best be accomplished by the continuous monitoring of several physiologic parameters and the judicious use of therapies to lower elevated ICP.

1. **Recommendations for physiologic monitoring of the patient with severe TBI**
   a. Arterial blood pressure. Noninvasive monitoring can be used, but an arterial catheter is preferred
   b. Heart rate, electrocardiogram (ECG), temperature, and pulse oximetry
   c. Central venous pressure or pulmonary artery catheter monitoring if the patient's volume status is in question
   d. ICP monitoring
   e. Fluid balance (intake and output)
   f. Arterial blood gases every 4 to 6 hours initially; electrolytes and serum osmolality (if receiving mannitol) every 6 hours; hematocrit, PT, PTT, platelets every 12 hours
   g. Jugular venous O_2 saturation or O_2 content by local protocol

2. **Goals of therapy**
   a. Mean arterial blood pressure of 90 to 110 mmHg in the adult
   b. O_2 saturation (arterial) 100%
   c. ICP <20 mmHg
   d. CPP >60–70 mmHg
   Note: CPP = mean arterial pressure (MAP) – ICP
   e. $Paco_2$ = 35 ± 2 mmHg
   f. Hematocrit = 32 ± 2%
   g. Central venous pressure = 8 to 14 cm H_2O
   h. Avoid dextrose-containing intravenous solutions for first 24 hours
   i. Maintain jugular venous O_2 saturation >50% or O_2 content of 4 to 6 vol%
   j. Ensure normal PT, PTT, and platelet count
   k. Maintain a normal temperature

3. **Management of elevated ICP**
   a. Improved outcomes can be expected if ICP is kept below 20 mmHg. The preferred ICP monitoring device is a ventriculostomy catheter coupled with a strain gauge. This system is relatively inexpensive, accurate, and allows CSF drainage when needed to control ICP.
   b. Fiberoptic white matter catheters are also accurate. They can be easier to insert, but they are more expensive and do not allow for CSF drainage (Fig. 19.2).
   c. Continuous CSF drainage is not recommended because the ventricular walls can collapse around the catheter tip and occlude its ports.
   d. A repeat CT scan of the head should be obtained within 24 hours after the initial scan to detect delayed posttraumatic hematomas, and a scan should be obtained with any abrupt increase in ICP or worsening of the neurologic examination.
   e. When using barbiturates, the depression of myocardial contractility can be minimized by maintenance of a high-normal intravascular volume. All patients receiving barbiturate therapy (for elevated ICP) should have frequent measurements of cardiac output and preload.
   f. Avoid hypovolemia and hyperosmolality if mannitol is used. Osmolality should be maintained at <310 to 320 mOsm.

4. **Anticonvulsant prophylaxis.** Prolonged use of anticonvulsant therapy is not indicated for patients with TBI. Current recommendations are for the use of phenytoin during the first 7 days following injury in patients at high risk for early posttraumatic seizures. These risk factors include cortical contusion, subdural hematoma, penetrating head wound,

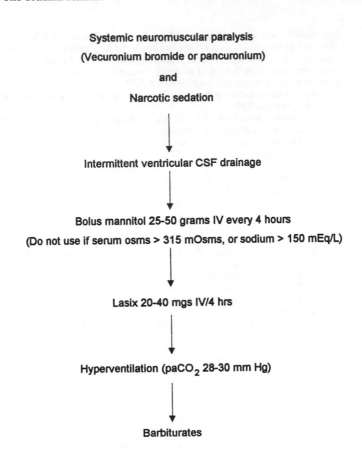

Systemic neuromuscular paralysis

(Vecuronium bromide or pancuronium)

and

Narcotic sedation

Intermittent ventricular CSF drainage

Bolus mannitol 25-50 grams IV every 4 hours

(Do not use if serum osms > 315 mOsms, or sodium > 150 mEq/L)

Lasix 20-40 mgs IV/4 hrs

Hyperventilation (paCO$_2$ 28-30 mm Hg)

Barbiturates

(Pentobarbital 400-1000 mg IV over 1 hr, then 40-100 mg/hr)

- titrate to maintain normal cardiac output

FIG. 19.2. Steps for the management of elevated intracranial pressure (ICP).

epidural hematoma, depressed skull fracture, intracerebral hematoma, and seizure within 24 hours of injury.

5. **Begin nutritional supplementation within 48 hours of the injury.** Aim for approximately 25 to 30 kcal/kg/day with either enteral (preferred) or parenteral supplementation. Most of these patients will tolerate jejunostomy feeding.

6. **Prognosis**
   a. The outcome following severe TBI is strongly correlated with initial GCS score, pupil reactivity and size, age, ICP (pressures >20 mmHg or inability to reduce elevated ICP), surgical intracranial mass lesions, hypotension (systolic blood pressure <90 mmHg), and jugular venous O$_2$ saturation <50%.
   b. The establishment and availability of dedicated head injury rehabilitation facilities have greatly improved long-term outcome for these patients. Every effort should be made to transfer these patients to such a rehabilitation facility for aggressive inpatient therapy once they are medically and neurologically stable.

IV. Mild to moderate head injuries

A. The distinction between mild and moderate head injuries is based on the initial Glasgow Coma Scale score and appearance of the initial CT scan of the head. Patients who have an initial GCS score of 13 to 15 are considered to have a mild brain injury. Those patients with a GCS score of 9 to 12 are classified as having a moderate brain injury. Some recommend that any patient who has a posttraumatic abnormality such as contusion or subdural or epidural hematoma on initial CT scan should be classified categorically as either a moderate or severe head injury patient regardless of initial GCS score. As many as 10% to 35% of those patients with GCS scores of 13 to 15 will have posttraumatic abnormalities on CT scan, and 2% to 9% ultimately will require a craniotomy for these lesions. Except for these empiric classification systems, the distinction between mild and moderate head injury is merely one of degree of severity of parenchymal injury. Thus, these two categories will be considered together in this section.

B. Most patients with **mild head injury** can be observed safely in the emergency department and discharged, although a few are at risk for delayed posttraumatic intracerebral hematomas or brain swelling. Identification of these patients requires careful neurologic assessment and liberal use of the CT scan.

   1. Clinical characteristics associated with an increased risk for subsequent brain swelling or hemorrhage are loss of consciousness associated with posttraumatic or retrograde amnesia. These patients should have a CT scan of the head.

   2. Patients with an abnormal CT scan or those who have a focal neurologic deficit on evaluation in the emergency department should be admitted for observation.

C. Decision on return to play after **sports-related head injuries** is determined by loss of consciousness or amnesia. The following guidelines are recommended:

   1. No loss of consciousness and no amnesia following a minor head injury: The patient can return 5 to 15 minutes after becoming completely lucid and asymptomatic.

   2. Posttraumatic amnesia but no loss of consciousness or retrograde amnesia: No return to play that day.

   3. Posttraumatic and retrograde amnesia with loss of consciousness: No return to play for 1 week after becoming completely lucid and asymptomatic and only after a detailed neurologic examination and CT scan.

   4. Posttraumatic and retrograde amnesia and prolonged loss of consciousness: No return to play for 1 month and only after detailed neurologic evaluation and CT scan.

D. The likelihood of sustaining one or more head injuries after an initial minor head injury is increased, and subsequent head injuries have an additive, deleterious effect on complex processing abilities and reaction times.

V. Penetrating brain injuries

A. Penetrating injuries can be subcategorized into gunshot wounds and lower-velocity injuries; the prognosis between the two is very different.

   1. Gunshot wounds to the brain carry a very high mortality rate. As the bullet traverses the brain tissue, it causes a cylinder of tissue destruction extending perpendicular from the bullet tract to a distance of as much as ten times the diameter of the bullet.

   2. General management of gunshot wounds to the brain follows the same principles of cerebral resuscitation as other brain injuries. The incidence of elevated ICP is high.

   3. Superficial debridement of the entrance and exit wounds is generally recommended, although it is usually not necessary to retrieve all deep-seated bullet and bone fragments.

   4. Broad-spectrum intravenous antibiotics and prophylactic anticonvulsant therapy are recommended.

    5. Prognosis depends largely on the trajectory of the bullet through the brain. If the bullet traverses deep brain structures (e.g., the basal ganglia or brainstem) or traverses the posterior fossa, the mortality rate is extremely high. If the bullet avoids these structures, the outcome can be more optimistic.

    6. Patients with an initial GCS score of 3 to 4 will have a high mortality rate (>80%). Conversely, 80% of patients who are able to follow commands on admission to the hospital (GCS >8) will have mild or no disability.

  B. Lower-velocity missile wounds. The most important factor determining outcome from lower-velocity missile wounds (e.g., stab or arrow wounds) to the head is the location of brain injury. If the missile damages the motor cortex, for example, contralateral motor weakness should be confined to the area of cortex that was damaged.

    1. The missile may be tamponading a major intracranial artery, so it is best to remove protruding knives or other objects **only in the operating room and only when the surgeon is prepared to deal with the consequences of major arterial bleeding.**

    2. A 7- to 14-day course of broad-spectrum antibiotics and prophylactic anticonvulsants (7 days) is indicated.

VI. Skull fractures

  A. Linear skull fractures are most common and typically occur over the lateral convexities of the skull. The squamous portion of the temporal bone in this region is thin and closely associated with the middle meningeal artery. Fractures in this area can tear the artery, which is the most common cause for epidural hematoma. For most skull fractures, it is not the fracture but rather the underlying blood clot or brain contusion that raises concern. Because these associated lesions are best detected with CT and are not recognized with plain skull x-rays, **a CT of the head is the diagnostic study of choice for patients suspected of having a skull fracture.**

  B. Depressed skull fractures. The surgical elevation and repair of these fractures will not lead to a change in any associated neurologic deficit or a decrease in the risk for subsequent seizures. These fractures may be open (associated with an overlying scalp laceration) or closed. Indications for surgical repair of depressed skull fractures are evidence of CSF leak, cosmetic deformity, or contaminated bone or scalp fragments pushed into the brain. Treatment includes:

    1. Broad-spectrum antibiotics for 7 to 14 days

    2. Prophylactic anticonvulsant therapy for 7 days

  C. Basilar skull fractures, which occur most commonly through the floor of the anterior cranial fossa, can disrupt the ethmoid bones and lead to leak of CSF through the nose (rhinorrhea). Fractures also can occur through the petrous bones posteriorly, leading to CSF drainage through the ear (otorrhea). Cranial nerve injuries are commonly associated with posterior basilar skull fractures, and findings should be sought on clinical examination.

    1. The primary concern with basilar skull fractures is associated CSF leak and risk of meningitis.

    2. Prophylactic antibiotic treatment is not recommended. Several investigations have found that morbidity is actually increased with prophylactic antibiotics because of selection of more virulent organisms.

    3. Attempts to stop the leak should begin with elevation of the head of the bed to 60°. If the leak does not stop within 6 to 8 hours, a lumbar CSF drainage catheter should be placed, and 50 to 100 mL of CSF should be drained every 8 hours. If this fails to stop the leak within 24 hours, the patient should be taken to surgery for repair of the dural laceration.

VII. Postconcussion syndrome

  A. Postconcussion syndrome can result from relatively minor head injuries.

  B. Most commonly involves headaches, tinnitus, vertigo, gait unsteadiness, emotional lability, sleep disturbances, intermittent blurring of vision, and irritability.

C. Symptoms can continue for weeks, months, or several years, but are rarely permanent.

D. Of patients who suffer postconcussion syndrome, 90% have spontaneous resolution of their symptoms within 2 weeks of injury. Beta-blocking agents, tricyclic antidepressants, or nonsteroidal anti-inflammatory agents can be beneficial, as well as psychotherapy and physical therapy.

Axioms

• Loss of consciousness is an important indicator of brain injury.
• Determine the GCS score as early as possible.
• A principal therapeutic goal is to enhance cerebral perfusion and avoid further ischemic injury.
• Early diagnosis and evacuation of mass lesions are critical.
• CT scan is the diagnostic test of choice for patients with skull fractures.

Bibliography

American College of Surgeons. *Advanced trauma life support.* Chicago: American College of Surgeons, 1998.

Bouma GJ, Muizelaar JP, Choi SC, et al. Cerebral circulation and metabolism after severe traumatic brain injury: the elusive role of ischemia. *J Neurosurg* 1991;685–693.

Chesnut RM, Marshall LF, Klauber MR, et al. The role of secondary brain injury in determining outcome from severe head injury. *J Trauma* 1993;34:216–222.

Chesnut RM, Marshall SB, Piek J, et al. Early and late systemic hypotension as a frequent and fundamental source of cerebral ischemia following severe brain injury in the traumatic coma data bank. *Acta Neurochir Suppl (Wien)* 1993;59:121–125.

Clifton GL, Kreutzer JS, Choi SC, et al. Relationship between Glasgow outcome scale and neuropsychological measures after brain injury. *Neurosurgery* 1994;33:34–39.

Fletcher JM, Ewing-Cobbs L, Miner ME, et al. Behavioral changes after closed head injury in children. *J Consult Clin Psychol* 1990;58:93–98.

Joint Section on Neurotrauma and Critical Care. *Guidelines for the management of severe head injury.* New York, New York. Brain Trauma Foundation, 1996.

Levin HS, Grossman RG, Rose JE, et al. Long-term neuropsychological outcome of closed head injury. *J Neurosurg* 1979;50:412–422.

Levin HS, Williams DH, Eisenberg HM, et al. Serial MRI and neurobehavioral findings after mild to moderate closed head injury. *J Neurol Neurosurg Psychiatry* 1992;55:255–262.

Marion DW, ed. *Traumatic brain injury.* New York: Thieme Medical Publishers, Inc., 1999.

Marion DW, Carlier PM. Problems with initial Glasgow Coma score assessment caused by the prehospital treatment of head-injured patients: results of a national survey. *J Trauma* 1994;36:89–95.

Marion DW, Darby J, Yonas H. Acute regional cerebral blood flow changes caused by severe head injuries. *J Neurosurg* 1991;74:407–414.

Muizelaar JP, Marmarou A, Ward JD, et al. Adverse effects of prolonged hyperventilation in patients with severe head injury: a randomized clinical trial. *J Neurosurg* 1991;75:731–739.

Vollmer DG, Torner JC, Jane JA, et al. Age and outcome following traumatic coma: why do older patients fare worse. *J Neurosurg* 1991;75:S37–S49.

20. INJURIES TO THE SPINAL CORD AND SPINAL COLUMN

William C. Welch, William F. Donaldson, III and Donald W. Marion

I. **Introduction.** Each year, approximately 10,000 new spinal cord injuries result in paralysis, with an estimated societal cost of $10 billion. The average age of the injured is about 30 years and 82% of victims are male. Motor vehicle accidents account for about 50% of the spinal cord injuries, sports 14%, falls 21%, and violence 15%. Of patients with spinal cord injuries, 44% also suffer from other significant trauma, with 14% having head and facial trauma. About half of all spinal cord injuries involve the cervical spine, most occurring between C4 and C7. The most commonly missed injuries are C1-C2 and C7–T1. Half of the spinal injuries involve complete quadriplegia.

II. **Anatomy and biomechanical definitions**

    A. The spinal cord is a continuation of the brainstem (medulla). This area is the cervicomedullary junction, which is located at the foramen magnum of the skull. The spinal cord continues through the vertebral canal of the cervical, thoracic, and upper lumbar vertebra, generally ending at the L1-L2 space. The spinal cord contains the **upper motor neurons (UMN)** that synapse with **lower motor neurons (LMN)** to form the nerve roots (Table 20.1) and cauda equina. The nerve roots in the cervical and lumbar regions fuse as the cervical and lumbar plexuses before separating again as specific nerves. Generally speaking, UMN lesions carry a worse prognosis than LMN lesions, as nerve roots have better capacity for repair than does the spinal cord.

    B. The spinal column is composed of seven cervical, twelve thoracic, five lumbar, and five fused sacral vertebrae. With the exception of the sacral vertebra, the vertebral bodies articulate with each other across the intervertebral disc and facet joints, forming a functional spinal unit. The facet joints, associated ligamentous structures, and other bone articulations (e.g., the rib cage) determine the motion across two vertebral bodies. The motions are considered in the sagittal plane (flexion and extension), coronal plane (lateral flexion), and in the transverse plane (rotation). In the cervical spine, about 50% of flexion and extension occurs between the occiput and C1, whereas 50% of rotation occurs between C1 and C2. The remainder of cervical movement takes place in the subaxial region. The thoracic spine has very little motion because of the facet joint orientation and added stabilization of the rib cage. The facet joints of the lumbar spine have a more sagittal orientation and allow moderate motion in the sagittal plane while resisting rotation. This accounts for the high number of injuries at the thoracolumbar junction where it goes from a stiff thoracic area to a mobile lumbar area.

    C. Injuries to the spinal column occur as a result of excessive forces applied to the spine. These forces can cause axial loading, hyperflexion, hyperextension, distraction, rotation, or a combination of forces. Injury to the spinal column can cause spinal instability, which can be defined on radiographic or clinical grounds. In the acute setting, radiographic features are most commonly used to determine spinal stability. This is reviewed below.

    D. The conceptualization of the spine as a series of support columns increases our biomechanical understanding of stability. **Three columns of the spine** have been described for the lower thoracic and lumbar spine. The **anterior column** (anterior longitudinal ligament and the anterior two thirds of the vertebral body and disc), the **middle column** (posterior third of the vertebral body and disc, the posterior longitudinal ligament), and the **posterior column** (the facet joints, capsule, ligamentum flavum, and posterior ligaments) describe the main columns of overall biomechanical support of the spine well, especially with regard to the thoracic and lumbar spine (Fig. 20.1). The three-column theory may not be completely applicable to the cervical

Table 20.1 Chart of muscle groups and nerve and nerve root supply

Muscle	Nerve root	Nerve
Cervical flexors	C1–C4	
Cervical extensors	C1–C4	
Trapezius		Cranial nerve XI
Sternocleidomastoid		Cranial nerve XI
Arm abduction		
–0 to 15°, supraspinatus	C4–C6	Suprascapular
–15 to 90°, deltoid	C5–C6	Axillary
–>90°, trapezius and serratus anterior	C5–C7	Long thoracic
Biceps	C5–C6	Musculocutaneous
Forearm supination	C5–C6	Musculocutaneous
Forearm pronation	C6–C7	Median
Wrist flexors	C7–C8, T1	Median
Wrist extensors	C6–C8	Radial
Hand intrinsics	C7–T1	Median and ulnar
Hip flexion	L1–L3	Femoral
Hip extension	L4–S1	Sciatic
Thigh abduction	L4–S2	Superior gluteal
Thigh adduction	L2–L4	Obturator
Leg flexion	L4–S2	Sciatic
Leg extension	L2–L4	Femoral
Foot plantar flexion	L5–S1	Superficial peroneal and tibial
Foot dorsiflexion	L4–L5	Deep peroneal
Great toe extension	L4–L5, S1	Deep peroneal
Foot inversion	L4–L5	Deep peroneal
Foot eversion	L5–S1	Superficial peroneal
Rectal sphincters	S2–S4	Pudendal

spine, but it is still generally used. **Injuries or deficits of two of three columns can denote biomechanical instability** and the patient may require surgical stabilization.

    E. Spinal cord injuries can be separate and distinct from spinal column injuries. **The diagnosis of a spinal cord injury is made on clinical grounds and** supplemented with diagnostic tests such as magnetic resonance imaging (MRI), myelography or electrodiagnostic studies. The level of spinal cord injury frequently correlates with the level of spinal column injury. Spinal cord injury can occur without spinal column injury. For example, patients with severe cervical canal stenosis are at risk of spinal cord injury if they experience hyperextension injuries.

    F. **Spinal column injuries** are bone or ligamentous disruptions that result in bone fractures or ligamentous instability. The loss of these stabilizing and supporting elements can result in compression and injury of neural elements. The diagnosis of spinal column injury is based on clinical and radiographic criteria, such as pain and ecchymosis at the level of fracture and plain film evidence of fracture. Spinal column injuries can occur without spinal cord injury.

III. Neurologic evaluation

    A. A standard neurologic examination is performed on each patient. This includes evaluation of mental status, cranial nerves, motor testing, sensory testing, and reflex assessment. Further specialized neurologic testing, such as determination of cerebellar functions, straight leg raise testing, and other tests can be deferred.

Posterior   **Middle**   **Anterior**
Element   **Element**   **Element**

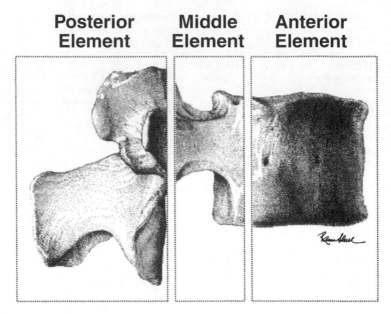

FIG. 20.1. Drawing showing the three columns of support in the spine.

B. The Glasgow Coma Score (GCS) is determined and recorded. The mental status is established as to person, place, date, and events surrounding the events. Cranial nerve evaluation is done as best as possible, with special attention directed to the third nerve and pupillary size and symmetry. Acute changes in the pupillary diameter can indicate a brain herniation syndrome and may require emergent surgery, hyperventilation, or diuresis.

C. Motor evaluation is performed for the GCS and spinal cord injury (SCI) evaluation. The patient is asked to move all extremities individually and strength is assessed according to the American Spinal Injury Association/ International Medical Society of Paraplegia (ASIA/IMSOP) protocol. Normal strength is graded 5/5, the ability to fully overcome gravity through a full range of motion is graded 3/5. No movement is graded 0/5, flicker movement 1/5, movement throughout a range of motion but unable to overcome gravity is graded 2/5, and mild weakness is graded 4/5. Tenodesis, the substitution of muscle groups, is also recorded.

D. When performing the GCS and SCI evaluations, be cognizant that patients with C5 levels of spinal cord function will only be able to flex their arms. This is not necessarily a posturing motion, but reflects the level of the cord injury.

E. **Sensory testing** is performed with regard to light touch and position sense (Fig. 20.2).

F. Impairment to pain sensation and temperature is useful when confirming central cord and Brown-Sequard syndrome.

G. **Reflex testing** is performed at the biceps, triceps, brachioradialis, knee, and ankle areas. Special reflex testing including jaw jerk, deltoid, pectoral, superficial abdominal, bulbo- or cliterocavernositis, and Babinski reflexes are tested and recorded as appropriate. The extremity reflexes are graded on a scale of 0–4, with 0 being absent, 1 being decreased, 2 representing the normal range, 3 representing increased reflex activity, and 4 is grossly exaggerated activity with sustained clonus. Babinski responses are recorded as present or absent. The presence of upper motor neuron findings (hyperreflexia, loss of superficial abdominal reflexes, Babinski responses) indicates spinal cord or conus medullaris injury. Decreased reflexes imply lower motor neuron (cauda equina and nerve root) injury. Weakness, sensory loss, and bladder, bowel, and sexual dysfunction can be seen with either upper or lower motor neuron injuries.

H. Determination of SCI is made following the neurologic examination. **The neurologic level(s) are determined and recorded based on the most caudal sensory and motor function**. SCI are initially defined as complete or incomplete. **Complete injury** is seen in the patient without sensory or motor function below the level of neurologic injury, as well as perianal sensation and sphincteric function. The patient with **incomplete injury** has partial preservation of sensory or motor function below the level of neurologic injury, with preservation of perianal sensation and motor function.

I. In the acute setting, the use of specific terms denoting neurologic level is preferable to more general terms (e.g., paraparesis, paraplegia, quadriparesis, quadriplegia). The **ASIA impairment scale** used to grade impairment is as follows:

1. Complete loss of sensory and motor function (including the sacral area) below the neurologic level
2. Incomplete injury, whereby sensory function is preserved below the level of neurologic injury including the sacral area
3. Incomplete injury with motor function preserved below the neurologic level and most preserved groups exhibiting strength of ≤3
4. Incomplete injury with motor function preserved below the neurologic level and most preserved groups exhibiting ≤3 strength
5. **Normal sensory and motor examination**. Even patients with ASIA 1 scores can improve neurologically, although few of these patients will achieve functional motor recovery

J. Another useful descriptor of spinal cord injuries involves pathologic criteria. The injuries can be described as central cord, posterior cord, anterior cord, and Brown-Sequard types.

1. **Posterior cord injuries** with loss of position sense (posterior columns) are rarely traumatic. This injury is usually related to vitamin deficiencies and infections (e.g., syphilis). The patients will develop a loss of position and vibratory sense.
2. **Central cord injuries** are very common in patients who experience excessive motion in the sagittal plane (e.g., hyperflexion and hyperextension). These injuries represent a centripetal force applied to the spinal cord with central necrosis of the spinal cord. The hallmark features are hand weakness, more so than leg weakness, and loss of pain and temperature sensation.
3. **Anterior cord injury** suggests anterior spinal artery occlusion and results in loss of all motor and sensory function other than position sense.
4. **Brown-Sequard (cord hemisection) syndrome** is identified by loss of ipsilateral motor function, ipsilateral position sense and contralateral loss of pain and temperature sensation two to three segments below the level of injury.
5. It is possible to have mixed cord syndromes as well. The findings in these cases are described by the neurologic deficits and are not assigned to a specific cord-type syndrome.

K. **Conus medullaris and cauda equina syndromes** must be considered. Both of these occur at the thoracolumbar level and result in varying degrees of weakness, sensory loss, and bladder, bowel, and sexual dysfunction. Conus injuries affect upper motor neurons and Babinski responses are identified.

IV. **Acute treatment**

A. Treatment in the field of patients with spinal column and spinal cord injuries follows the basic prehospital protocols (Chapter 8). Treatment is directed to establishment of an adequate airway, ventilation of the lungs, and maintenance of circulatory support to prevent secondary neurologic injuries. Once

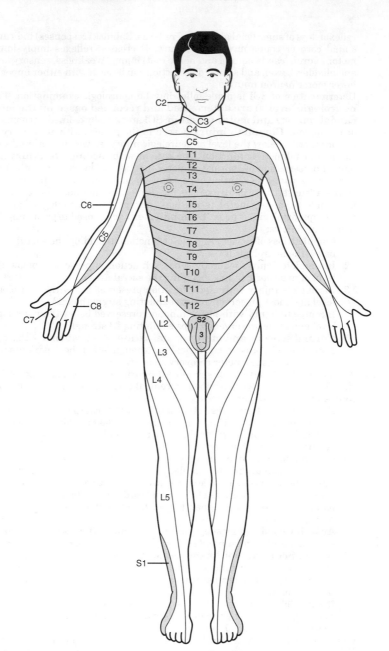

FIG. 20.2. Anterior (**A**) and posterior

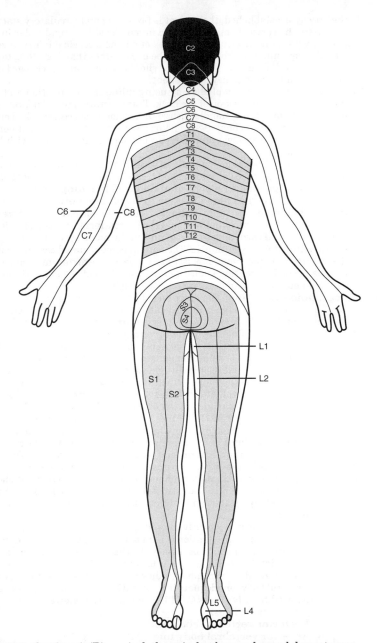

FIG. 20.2. *Continued.* (**B**) cervical, thoracic, lumbar, and sacral dermatomes.
(From McDonald JV, Welch WC. Patient history and neurologic examination.
In: Welch WC, Jacobs GB, Jackson RP, eds. *Operative spinal surgery*. Stamford,
CT: Appleton & Lange, 1999;3:15, with permission.)

the airway is established, the patient is breathing and circulatory status is adequate, the cervical spine should be immobilized in a rigid collar in any patient who is unconscious or suspected of having a cervical injury. A scoop stretcher or similar backboard should be used, rather than logrolling to prevent uncontrolled motion. The patient should remain on a backboard until evaluated in the emergency department.

B. Intubation is best accomplished by using inline immobilization and oral intubation, avoiding flexion of the neck. Transportation to the nearest hospital that is equipped to handle such injuries should be accomplished either on ground or in air. The patient's neurologic status as well as pulmonary function should be assessed and recorded, especially patients with high quadriplegia.

C. Hypovolemic and neurogenic shock can occur in the setting of SCI. The cause of hypotension must be determined and treated immediately. **Hypotension should be regarded as a sign of abdominal bleeding, aortic or cardiac injury, external blood loss, or to result from other sources before considering neurogenic shock.** Neurogenic shock should be treated to prevent further injury to the spinal cord. Treatment consists of fluid administration and cardiopressors to maintain the mean systemic blood pressure at approximately 90 mmHg. The patient is reevaluated continuously in the emergency department. Resuscitative measures are continued and modified as needed. Attention is directed to evaluation of the spine through a detailed neurologic examination and radiographs.

V. Radiographic evaluation. The diagnosis of spinal cord or spinal column injury is of paramount importance in the acute trauma setting. The diagnosis is reached by obtaining a history of the events, performing a neurologic evaluation of the patient, and obtaining the appropriate radiographic evaluation. The initial studies should cover the area of suspected injury. Patients with persistent complaints of pain along the spine should be assumed to have a spinal column injury until proved otherwise. Generally, patients with normal x-ray study and severe neck pain should receive follow-up flexion or extension films about 3 days after injury to rule out instability that was masked by muscle spasm. Keep in mind that **10% to 15% of patients with one spine fracture will have another fracture elsewhere in the spine.** Patients who have suffered neurologic injury rendering them comatose or who have other conditions that prevent them from fully cooperating with the examining physician should have complete spine radiographic evaluation. Approximately 1% of patients who are obtunded will have ligamentous instability that is missed when x-ray studies are normal. Dynamic studies (flexion and extension films) as well as the static films should be considered in these patients. The "skeletal level" is used to denote the area of greatest vertebral injury and can be different from the neurologic level(s).

A. Cervical spine

1. Because the most commonly missed fractures are at the C1-C2 and C7–T1 levels, special attention is paid to these areas and more detailed studies are performed, if necessary. In the cervical spine, the lateral view provides 90% of the needed information.

2. The basic lateral radiographic studies must include the skull base and T1 vertebral body for adequate interpretation. A "swimmer's view" may be required to fully assess C7–T1. The films are reviewed with careful attention to three lines:

   a. Posterior vertebral body line
   b. Anterior vertebral body line
   c. Spinolaminar line (Fig. 20.3)
   These lines should be uninterrupted and smooth. The appearance of a straight spine (loss of the normal cervical lordosis) indicates extensor muscular spasm and can suggest spinal injury.

3. Next, **the soft tissues** are examined. The trachea contains air and provides a line of contrast against the vertebral bodies. Prevertebral swelling indicates a hematoma consistent with spinal column injury. The

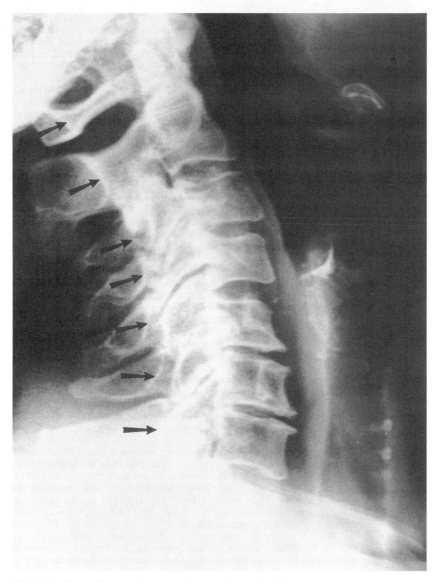

FIG. 20.3. Normal cervical spine lateral radiograph with demonstration of spinolaminar line (*arrows*).

hematoma can also compromise the patient's airway, leading to respiratory collapse. The soft tissue space should be no greater than 5 mm measured at the inferior aspect of the C2 vertebral body and no greater than 20 mm at the level of C6. Another important distance is the atlantodens interval. This is the space between the anterior aspect of the odontoid (dens) and the ring of C1. This space should not exceed 3.5 mm in the adult and 5 mm in the child. Distances greater than those indicate disruption of the transverse ligament, with resultant instability.

4. **Vertebral height** is examined next, including vertebral body morphology. The vertebral bodies should be similar in appearance, without evidence of compression or fracture. The distance between the posterior spinous process should be examined and this distance should be similar at each level. In summary, the lateral cervical spine film yields a tremendous amount of information when interpreted carefully.

5. Other radiographs obtained of the cervical spine include the open mouth view of C1-C2. This study shows the base of the odontoid and helps to determine whether a type I, II, or III odontoid fracture (discussed below) is present. The lateral masses of C1 are examined with regard to their relationship to C2. Little or no overhang of the lateral masses should be seen and overhang ≥6.5 mm indicates a fracture of the ring of C1, with probable disruption of the transverse ligament. The odontoid bone should be symmetrically located between the lateral masses of C2.

6. The **Anteroposterior (AP) view of the spine** is examined for the distance between spinous processes, alignment and rotation. Facet anatomy is more closely observed with oblique views of the cervical spine. Areas suspected of having fracture can be further assessed with fine-cut CT. MRI is indicated in patients with neurologic deficits or significant fractures that will require reduction. The MRI yields information as to ligamentous integrity, subtle compression fractures, traumatic disc rupture, and SCI. Patients with neurologic deficits should be evaluated in consultation with the spine surgery service.

7. If a conscious patient has no neck pain to palpation and can voluntarily flex, extend and rotate without pain, and initial x-rays are normal, the collar may be removed. Should a patient have neck pain and yet have normal preliminary x-rays, further studies should be undertaken. At a minimum, flexion and extension films should be performed to rule-out ligamentous instability. Further radiographs, including oblique studies, focused or "cone-down" views of suspicious areas, computed tomography (CT) with sagittal and coronal reconstruction, magnetic resonance imaging (MRI), and even bone scan, can be appropriate to rule out possible bone or ligamentous injury. The collar should remain in place until the neck is cleared clinically and radiographically.

B. **Thoracolumbar spine**
1. The thoracolumbar spine is commonly injured at the T12–L1 levels. This occurs because of the large lever arm created by the inflexible thoracic spine as it joins the lumbar spine. This area of the spine is well examined with lateral and AP views. Three lines are observed along the anterior and posterior aspects of the vertebral bodies, and along the posterior aspect of the spinous processes. The distance between these processes should also remain equal.

2. On the AP view, the distance between pedicles is determined as is the distance between the posterior spinous processes. The transverse processes and ribs are evaluated for fractures and the soft tissues are examined for swelling.

3. More specialized imaging studies are obtained as necessary. CT is useful for a closer examination of bone anatomy. These studies can be ordered with 1- to 3-mm cuts, and sagittal and coronal reconstruction to better define bony anatomy. MRI provides excellent visualization of the spinal cord and nerve roots and helps to define spinal cord and ligamentous injury.

4. AP and lateral films are indicated in those patients with symptoms referable to the thoracic area or those who have a mechanism that is consistent with such an injury. This would include patients involved in motorcycle accidents, falls from height, ejection from vehicle, or pedestrian–automobile collisions. Flexion and extension films are not as helpful in this area as compared with the cervical spine. CT is indi-

cated for those patients with fractures noted on x-ray film or when the anatomy is not well seen on plain films. MRI is indicated for all patients with neurologic findings.

C. Lumbar spine
1. The lumbar spine is subjected to injurious forces in falls, motor vehicle crashes, and by other means. Because the spinal cord ends at the L1-L2 level, true SCI from lumbar fractures is infrequent. Injuries to the conus medullaris and cauda equina can occur if the spinal canal is compromised. Commonly, no neurologic injury is noted with lumbar spine fractures.
2. The lumbar spine is evaluated similar to the thoracolumbar spine. AP and lateral spine films are the initial studies.
3. CT can be useful to determine the amount of canal compromise in cases of burst fracture. MRI and myelography are also helpful in cases of traumatic nerve root injury, canal compression, and conus medullaris and cauda equina syndromes.

VI. Medical management of SCI. Once the patient has arrived in the trauma resuscitation area, more sophisticated medical management can begin. These management protocols include definitive treatment of other injuries; maintenance of adequate blood pressure; detailed radiographic studies, as described above; high-dose steroids, if appropriate; determination of the need for surgical intervention; and postoperative rehabilitation. Treatment of shock is discussed above. The potential negative effects of definitive treatment of other injuries must be discussed with the consulting neurosurgeon or orthopedic spine surgeon before intervention.

A. Methylprednisolone. A number of studies have suggested that neurologic improvement can occur following the administration of high-dose steroids after closed, nonpenetrating injury to the spinal cord. The NASCIS 2 study showed that methylprednisolone given in a dose of 30 mg/kg intravenously (i.v.) over 45 minutes within 8 hours after injury in those with incomplete or suspected incomplete SCI can improve neurologic outcome. The initial dose is followed by 5.4 mg/kg/h i.v. given over the next 23 hours by continuous drip. No increase was seen in infection rate, duodenal perforation, or other complications associated with short-term steroid use.

B. Other medical issues to be considered in patients with SCI include prevention and treatment of **pulmonary complications.** Aggressive pulmonary toilet, specialized rotating beds, and antibiotics are often appropriate. **Urinary tract infections** are common in paralyzed patients because of repeated catheterization. **Decubitus ulcers** can occur rapidly in insensate patients. Aggressive nursing care is the mainstay of treatment. **Stress gastric and duodenal ulcers** are common and prophylaxis is recommended. **Joint contractures and heterotopic ossification** are common in paralyzed patients. These complications can be reduced by physical therapy. Spinal cord injured patients are more sensitive to acetylcholine and the use of succinylcholine can precipitate a hyperkalemic crisis.

VII. Surgical management of cervical spinal column injuries
A. Occiput C1-C2 injuries
1. Occipital C1 injuries, which are rare, are usually not associated with patient survival. These injuries typically cause a dislocation between the occipital and C1 condyles. Subarachnoid blood seen on brain CT can provide an early clue to the diagnosis. Treatment is surgical if patient survival is expected.
2. C1-C2 injuries, which are common, are frequently missed because of the relatively complex anatomy of the C1-C2 junction and the difficulty in obtaining a full set of films in the multiply injured patient. The bony odontoid fractures can be divided into types I, II, and III (Fig. 20.4).
   a. Type I is simply a chip off of the odontoid bone. This is a stable fracture.
   b. Type II fractures are those that occur at the base of the dens. These fractures are considered to be unstable in the acute setting. They require external stabilization (rigid cervical collar or halo-vest

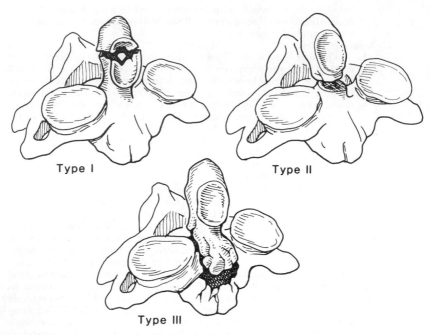

Type I

Type II

Type III

FIG. 20.4. Drawing of type I, II, and III odontoid fractures.

device) or internal fixation (odontoid screw or C1-C2 posterior fixation using a Gallie or Brooks-type construct, potentially with the use of screws placed across the articulating surfaces of C1-C2). Airway management is critical in these patients as upper airway swelling and subsequent respiratory compromise can occur.

   c. **Type III fractures** involve the vertebral body of C2. These fractures are treated in the same fashion as type II fractures. They generally have a better healing rate than type II fractures.

3. **Jefferson fractures** occur when an axial load is placed on the head. The C1 bone, which is circular in nature, is forced apart. Fractures occur anteriorly and posteriorly. This fracture can be stable in nature and can heal with external mobilization.

4. It is important to consider that the main ligament stabilizing the dens within the ring of C1 is the transverse ligament. This ligament keeps the dens in close approximation to the ring of C1. The space between the posterior aspect of the ring of C1 and the anterior border of the dens is called the "atlantodens" interval. This space should not exceed 3.5 mm in the adult (Fig. 20.5).

   a. The ligament can be torn whenever the ring of C1 is fractured. The amount of medial-lateral displacement of the ring of C1 can be measured on AP radiographs or CT reconstructions. Normally, the C1 lateral masses do not overlap the C2 vertebral body. Should the combined amount of lateral mass overlap of C1 on C2 exceed 6.5 mm, consider the transverse ligament to be torn and the C1-C2 area unstable (Fig. 20.6).

5. **"Hangman's fracture"** or spondylolisthesis of the C2 pedicles occurs in the C1-C2 area. This type of fracture is also unstable and requires external, or rarely, internal fixation.

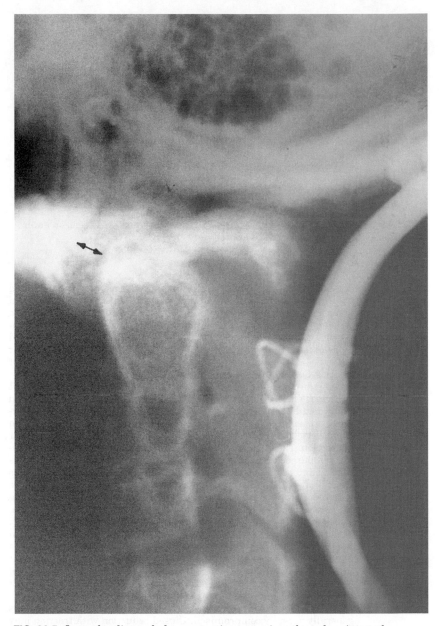

FIG. 20.5. Lateral radiograph demonstrating excessive atlantodens interval.

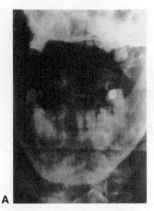 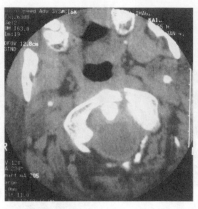

A   **B**

FIG. 20.6. C1 fracture with overhanging of the C1 lateral masses as seen on antero-posterior plain film (**A**) and axial computed tomography scan (**B**).

B. C3–C7 Injuries

1. Most of the C3–C7 injuries can be diagnosed from a lateral film using the three lines to determine alignment and stability. Also on flexion and extension views, no >3.5 mm of listhesis should be seen between two vertebrae and no >11° of angulation between vertebral bodies, as measured at the adjoining endplates. The spinous process distances should be symmetric. CT will define the bone anatomy and MRI will better show the ligamentous injury, cord anatomy, and disc pathology. In most injuries, both studies should be obtained.

2. A common type of injury involves **unilateral and bilateral facet injuries**. These injuries include both fractures of the facet joints and injury to the capsules with resultant "perched" facets. Both types of injuries are noted on plain films and CT. The presence of 25% subluxation of one vertebra on another can represent a unilateral facet fracture or dislocation. The CT scan appearance of this fracture looks like "opposing hamburger buns" (Fig. 20.7). Subluxation of 50% generally means that a bilateral facet injury has occurred. Patients with these injuries should have MRI to diagnose any disc herniation that could interfere with reduction of the two vertebral bodies, potentially causing a neurologic catastrophe if the disc compromises the cord during reduction. Those patients will need anterior discectomy before reduction.

3. Generally, unilateral and bilateral facet dislocations are reduced in tong or halo traction under close supervision by the spine surgeon or the reduction can be performed intraoperatively. Although unilateral facet fractures can be stable, surgical fusion is often the preferred method of treatment. Occasionally, pure bony injuries can be handled by halo-vest immobilization, once the fracture has been reduced.

4. **Bilateral facet injuries are unstable** because the spinal canal is generally severely compromised. Closed reduction with traction may be unsuccessful. Intraoperative reduction and stabilization with neurophysiologic monitoring is the treatment method of choice if traction fails.

C. Burst fractures generally occur as a result of flexion or axial loading. The columns may appear well aligned at first glance on the lateral radiograph. Generally noted is an expansion of the prevertebral space and loss of vertebral height. The CT scan will show the vertebral comminution involving all three columns and generally has neural canal compromise and subsequent neuro-

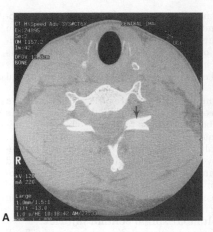

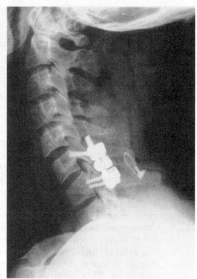

C

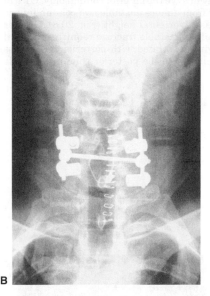

B

FIG. 20.7. Preoperative axial computed tomography scan demonstrating a unilateral jumped and locked facet fracture and dislocation (**A**). The left jumped facet has the appearance of two opposing hamburger buns (*arrow*). Anteroposterior (**B**) and lateral (**C**) radiographs demonstrating the instrumented fusion using lateral mass screws and rods with interspinous wiring and bone grafting.

logic deficit. These will require surgical stabilization but should have gentle traction or collar immobilization during studies and before surgery.

   D. Teardrop fractures must be differentiated from the less ominous extension injury with a small chip off of the anterior cortex of the vertebral body to the true teardrop that is highly unstable. CT will show the sagittal split in the vertebral body in a true teardrop-type injury. MRI will often demonstrate an early spinal cord contusion. Most of these patients are neurologically impaired and will need surgery to stabilize the neck and decompress the spinal cord.

   E. Spinal cord injuries without radiographic abnormality (SCIWORA). A number of patients will appear to be neurologically impaired without fractures or ligamentous injuries noted on initial radiographic studies. Generally, patients in this group are at the ends of the age spectrum. Young patients are susceptible to this type of injury because of the elasticity of their ligaments. In the older patient, generally is found underlying cervical stenosis, either degenerative or congenital. Mild hyperflexion or hyperextension injuries will cause spinal cord compression without bony fracture. Early spinal cord changes are often noted on the MRI. A central cord-type injury is often the result in these types of injuries. Although some of these patients will slowly recover, a number will need to have decompressions of the spinal cord to promote recovery.

   F. **Ankylosing spondylitis** is a condition that creates the appearance of a "bamboo spine." Despite the osteoporotic quality of the bone, the spine is fused at multiple segments. The bone also has a tendency to bleed and epidural spinal hematomas are common and associated with neurologic injury. The exact fracture can be difficult to identify on plain radiographs. Frequently, the underlying deformity is not known, positioning is difficult and dangerous for imaging studies, and these patients can deteriorate neurologically because of malposition of the neck and their propensity to develop epidural hematomas. A spine specialist should manage x-ray and imaging studies to prevent the neck going into further flexion or extension.

VIII. **Surgical management of thoracolumbar spinal column injuries**
   A. **Compression fractures** typically involve the anterior column only. CT will differentiate a one-column injury from a more unstable two-column injury. The lateral film will show the loss of vertebral height (Fig. 20.8). Greater than 40% loss of height can signal an unstable fracture requiring surgical treatment. This amount of wedging associated with posterior tenderness generally signals a ligamentous injury to the posterior column. Multiple

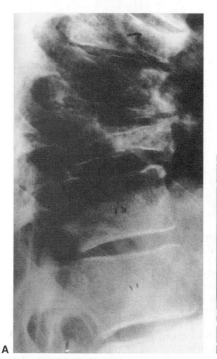
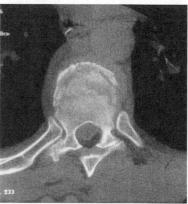

A   B

FIG. 20.8. T9 compression fracture as seen on lateral radiograph (**A**) and axial computed tomography scan (**B**).

compression fractures can be unstable and should be watched closely. Higher fractures (T1–T9) require much more energy to fracture because of rib cage stability and are associated with more serious injury. Multiple rib fractures and sternal fractures are associated with instability. Most T10–L5 compression fractures with <40% loss of height and no posterior tenderness can be managed in a brace.

    1. Imaging (CT, MRI) is indicated for any compression fracture associated with neurologic injury, >30% loss of height of vertebral body, and any patient with posterior tenderness or widening of the pedicles on an AP view. These patients should be evaluated by a spine surgeon.

B. Burst fractures involve two of the three columns and are generally considered unstable. X-ray findings are positive when the lateral view shows loss of vertebral height, widening of the spinous processes, or interruption of the posterior vertebral body line. The AP view shows widening of the pedicles, widening between the spinous processes, and loss of vertebral height. Many of these patients have neurologic injury. All of these fractures should have detailed imaging studies and the patients should receive spine service consultation.

C. Flexion or distraction (seat belt or Chance) fractures. This axially oriented fracture is caused by a flexion injury around an anterior fulcrum (lap belt without shoulder harness). The fracture can split the pedicles in half, tear open the disc space, or spare bone elements and be ligamentous in nature. The excessive flexion motion places the spine in kyphosis. This injury is associated with a 30% to 45% incidence of abdominal injury and 13% paralysis. Some of the pure bony injuries can be managed nonoperatively by placing the patients in an extension brace to bring the fractured bony elements into apposition, but ligamentous injuries require surgery. These injuries require detailed imaging studies.

D. Fracture-dislocations are highly unstable and require imaging studies on all patients. Most occur at the thoracolumbar junction. The more cephalad the injury, the more likely paraplegia will result (90% above T10 and 60% below T10). The AP and lateral views will show translation of the spine as well as fractures in the facets, dislocations, or comminution fraction. These injuries require detailed radiographic studies, followed by surgical intervention.

E. Sacral fractures are difficult to see on x-ray film and will require CT for delineation. Fractures lateral to the sacral foramen have a 6% incidence of neurologic injury (L5 root) and fractures through the foramen have a 28% incidence. Fractures medial to the foramen through the canal have an associated neurologic injury in 57%, most involving bowel and bladder function. Displaced fractures can require surgery.

IX. Gunshot wounds to the spine

A. Penetrating injuries to the spine should be treated as elsewhere in the body. The standard surgical principles of debridement and closure can be applied. The caveat is that patients with cerebrospinal fluid (CSF) leaks are at risk of meningitis and paravertebral abscess formation, unless CSF egress is controlled.

B. In general, large exit wounds require exploration and debridement. Wound cultures are taken and all potentially contaminating material (e.g., clothing fragments or shotgun wadding) is removed. Passage through the esophagus, pharynx, or colon before traversing the spine has the potential to cause spinal sepsis. Radical debridement of the spine is no longer advocated in this situation. Minimal debridement of bullet tract and 1 to 2 weeks of broad-spectrum antibiotics is sufficient to decrease the chance of spinal infection to about 10% of cases when the bullet traverses the colon, esophagus, or pharynx.

C. Removing bullet fragments may necessarily be delayed if an abnormal lead level develops. Removal of a bullet from the spinal canal is recommended with a worsening neurologic picture or evidence of neurologic compression on radiographic studies. These procedures can be facilitated if performed in a delayed fashion to allow easier dural repair. CSF diversion (e.g., lumbar,

cervical or ventricular drainage) may be required for persistent leakage. Neurologic deterioration mandates a more urgent approach to debridement.
D. Surprisingly, few spinal injuries caused by the bullet striking the spinal column are unstable enough to require surgical stabilization. The three-column theory can be used to dictate treatment. If two of three columns are involved, a rigid orthosis is necessary. Flexion or extension films may be necessary to determine stability.

Axioms

* The most important factors when treating injuries to the spine are attention to the mechanism of injury, understanding the level of neurologic function at the time of injury compared to later presentation, maintaining a continual awareness of other injuries to the spine, confounding injuries, and patient variables.
* The most commonly missed fractures occur at the C1-C2 and C7 levels.
* The general assumption is that all patients have an unstable spine until proved otherwise.
* Patients with continued complaints of spine-related pain must be thoroughly evaluated and this evaluation must be repeated if the symptoms persist.
* Should any doubt about the injury persist, evaluation by a spine surgeon is necessary.

Bibliography

American College of Surgeons Committee on Trauma. *Advanced trauma life support instructor manual.* Chicago: American College of Surgeons, 1997.
Bracken MB, Holford TR. Effects of timing of methylprednisolone or naloxone administration on recovery of segmental and long-tract neurological function in NASCIS 2. *J Neurosurg* 1993;79:500–507.
Carlson GD, Gorden C. Invited Review. Spinal cord injury research: current status and clinical implications. *SpineLine* 2000;1:7–18.
International standards for neurological and functional classification of spinal cord injury, 4th ed. Chicago: American Spinal Injury Association, International Medical Society of Paraplegia (ASIA/IMSOP) American Spinal Injury Association, 1992.
Przybylski G, Welch WC, Jacobs GB. Spinal instability and biomechanics. In: Welch WC, Jacobs GB, Jackson RP, eds. *Operative spinal surgery.* Stamford, CT: Appleton & Lange, 1999;7:104–112.

21. SOFT TISSUE WOUNDS OF THE FACE

James M. Russavage and Gary T. Patterson

I. **General**
   A. Careful examination and evaluation of the wound should be made before any treatment. Lacerations or contusions should be considered evidence of underlying bone injury and alert the clinician to inspect the radiographs of the bone in that area. Fractures of the underlying bone should be detected and, in many cases, treated before definitive soft tissue management. Treatment of the fracture after the soft tissue management often disrupts the soft tissue closure and further damages the soft tissue. If the fractures are exposed through soft tissue lacerations, perform fracture fixation through the open wound rather than use the standard incisions for facial fracture treatment.
   B. Injuries to associated nerves, ducts, glands, and sinuses require assessment, and a thorough investigation of the structural functions in the vicinity of the laceration is important.
   C. Tissue that is contaminated and damaged by crush and contusion presents a hazard for infection if primary repair is undertaken. The probability of contamination increases rapidly and is directly proportional to the length of time that has elapsed since injury. The history and circumstances of the injury provide evidence signaling the possibility of deeply imbedded foreign material.
   D. **Delayed primary wound closure**
      1. **Indications**
         a. Patient seen late after injury
         b. Extensive tissue edema
         c. Subcutaneous hematoma
         d. Crush injury
         e. Wound edges are badly contused
         f. Tissue is devitalized
      2. **Treatment**
         a. Limited debridement to remove devitalized tissue
         b. Wet dressings
         c. Antibiotic therapy
      3. **Treatment continued** until resolution of edema and acute inflammation and a cleaner appearance of the wound; delayed primary closure is likely to be successful.
   E. Primary closure under unsatisfactory conditions can contribute to increased soft tissue loss, with tension, infection, and tissue necrosis. If the wound edges cannot be approximated because of contracture after open treatment, the wound can be covered with a skin graft, which can be secondarily excised.
II. **Photography** should be done for the following reasons
   A. Accurate record keeping
   B. Insurance and legal purposes
   C. Supplement the written evaluations
   D. Assess the effectiveness of the therapy
III. **Anesthesia.** An attitude of reassurance and sympathy, together with adequate premedication, permits extensive operation under local anesthesia.
   A. Nerve blocks can be used to establish regional anesthesia in a wide field, with reduced dosage of medication and less discomfort. Less complicated wounds (e.g., small cuts, bruises, lacerations) and some uncomplicated fractures of the facial bones (e.g., the nose) can be treated under local anesthesia, either in the operating room or in an outpatient treatment area.
   B. More extensive injuries may require general anesthesia
IV. **Debridement and care.** Thorough cleansing of soft tissue wounds is imperative before any definitive treatment is attempted. All blood and debris should be carefully washed from the tissues with copious amounts of water and mild

detergents. Remove any foreign materials, such as glass, hair, clothing, tooth structures, pieces of artificial dentures, paint, grease, gravel, and dirt.

A. Except for the removal of obviously devitalized portions of tissue, extensive debridement of soft tissue has little place in the management of facial injuries. All tissue that can participate in a satisfactory repair should be retained.

    1. Err on the side of retaining tissues that may not survive rather than to debride or destroy any tissues that might be important in a final result. The excellent blood supply of the face usually makes extensive debridement unnecessary.

V. **Cleaning of the wound**. All wounds should be carefully inspected for foreign material. Its removal is imperative to prevent separation, infection, delayed healing, and subsequent pigmentation of skin. The presence of foreign material and hematoma reduces the bacterial inoculum necessary for infection to develop.

A. The tissue edges can be cleansed with antiseptics, detergent soaps, and water.

B. In rare cases, solvents (e.g., ether, benzene, or alcohol) are necessary to remove materials not soluble in water or removable by scrubbing or debridement. Scrubbing with a brush under adequate anesthesia is required to remove foreign material and prevent the development of infection and "traumatic tattoo." The material can be removed initially with scrubbing, the point of a No. 11 blade, or a small dermatologic curette.

VI. **Wound type**

A. **Abrasion**

    1. Clean with mild, nonirritating soap or Hibiclens (Zeneca, Wilmington, DE), Betadine (Purdue Frederick, Norwalk, CT), or pHisoHex (Sanofi Winthrop, New York, NY).

    2. Dirt, grease, carbon, and other pigments should be carefully scrubbed out of the wound.

    3. Apply light lubricating dressing.

    4. Moist compresses (wet to wet) or the application of an antibacterial ointment (Neosporin or Bacitracin; Warner Wellcome, Morris Plains, NJ) will prevent drying and desiccation of the exposed wound surfaces.

B. **Contused wounds**

    1. Generally subside without active treatment.

    2. Most hematomas are diffuse and absorb gradually.

    3. Eyelid, cheek, or forehead hematoma may require drainage.

    4. Nasal septal hematoma needs to be evacuated through a small incision in the septal mucosa or through a large-bore needle.

C. **Simple laceration**

    1. Repair should be undertaken after underlying structures have been assessed and foreign bodies removed.

    2. Time lapse between injury and repair is important relative to risk of infection and the choice of repair technique.

    3. With the exception of animal bites and traumatic tattoo, most soft tissue wounds of the face, properly cleansed and dressed, can await primary repair up to 24 hours, without serious risk of infection.

    4. Tissue that is devitalized must be excised, regardless of its location or of how important it was.

        a. Although debridement should be conservative, it must be adequate. Ragged, severely contused wound edges should be conservatively excised to provide perpendicular skin edges that will heal primarily with minimal scarring.

    5. Closely parallel lacerations can be converted to a single wound by excising the intervening skin bridge, facilitating repair and reducing scar formation.

    6. Displaced tissue should be returned to its original position.

    7. Occasionally, immediately changing the direction of a wound by Z-plasty or making tissue allowance for scar contracture at the time of primary wound repair is appropriate.

    8. If the contused marginal tissues are of anatomic importance, it is best to avoid debridement and consider secondary reconstructive surgery.

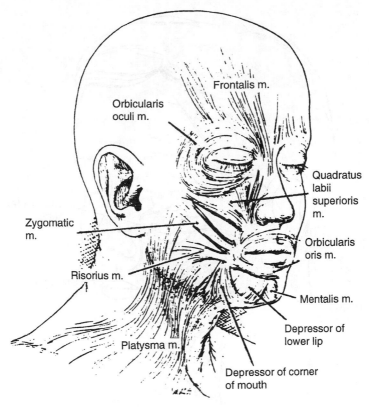

FIG. 21.1. Muscles of facial expression.

D. **Deep lacerations**. The muscles of facial expression (Fig. 21.1) are so closely associated with the skin that careful closure of the wound in layers gives adequate approximation of the muscle.
    1. If possible, facial muscle layers should be identified and closed separately with fine absorbable sutures.
    2. Closure of the muscle and fascia in layers, including the subcutaneous tissue, restores adequate function and prevents adherence of cheek skin to the muscle.
VII. **Anatomic considerations in repairing soft tissue**
    A. **Facial nerve**. It is often impractical and unnecessary to identify and suture the terminal branches of the facial nerve. The plexus of nerve fibers makes regeneration of activity a common occurrence, despite the absence of direct facial nerve suturing. Reasonably accurate approximation of the tissues usually allows some element of nerve regeneration by neurotization of muscle.
        1. Nerve repair need not be performed anterior to a line drawn at the lateral canthus of the eyelids.
        2. Suture of named branches of the facial nerve should be performed and the branches should be sought (Fig. 21.2). Primary repair at the time of initial treatment is recommended.
    B. **Trigeminal nerve**. The sensory branches of the trigeminal (Fig. 21.3) nerve in the region of the skin are small, and approximation is impractical and unnecessary. Partial or complete recovery of sensation usually occurs within a

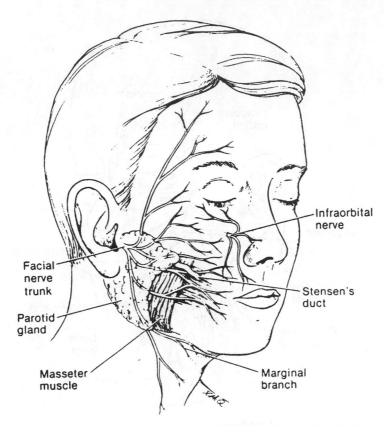

FIG. 21.2. Deep anatomy of the cheek showing facial nerve, parotid gland, Stensen's duct, and masseter muscle.

few months to a year, with slight hypesthesia often present. Contusion of trigeminal nerve branches also occurs as a result of fractures.

C. **Parotid duct lacerations.** Lacerations of the parotid duct should be repaired at the time of wound closure to prevent fistula to the skin or to the mucous membrane of the mouth.

1. To identify the course of the parotid duct, a line is drawn from the tragus of the ear to the midportion of the upper lip. The duct traverses the middle third of the line.

2. The parotid duct travels adjacent to the buccal branch of the facial nerve. Buccal branch paralysis with an overlying laceration should suggest the possibility of a parotid duct injury.

3. The parotid duct empties into the mouth opposite the maxillary second molar.

   a. A Silastic tube or silver probe can be inserted into the opening of the duct and the course of the duct followed. The duct can be irrigated with saline using a No. 22 Angiocath sleeve. The appearance of saline in the wound indicates that the duct is injured. The proximal end of the duct can be identified in the wound expressing secretion of saliva.

   b. A Silastic catheter is placed in the duct and the wound repaired with fine sutures. The tube is left in for a 2-week period, as tolerated (Fig. 21.4).

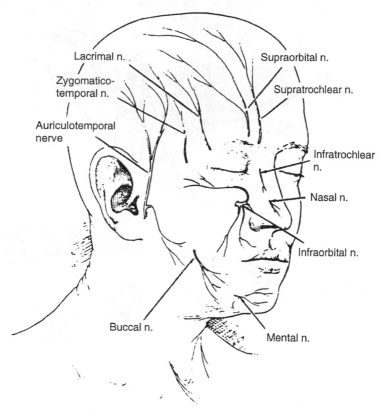

FIG. 21.3. Trigeminal sensory nerve distribution to the face.

VIII. **Regional considerations in repairing soft tissue**
  A. **Forehead and brow**
    1. Preserve the eyebrow
    2. Do not shave eyebrow
    3. Repair muscle layer
  B. **Ears.** Assess adjacent wounds and the middle and inner ear. The presence of hearing loss, hemorrhagic otorrhea, cerebrospinal fluid (CSF) leak, or facial nerve injury suggest middle- or inner-ear injury.
    1. Ecchymosis over the mastoid area is known as **Battle's sign**, a finding associated with basilar skull fracture.
    2. The ear may be involved in abrasions, contusions, lacerations, and hematomas.
      a. Abrasions heal with the continued application of light dressing and ointment. A well-designed dressing, suitably padded (with mineral oil-soaked cotton), minimizes edema and hemorrhage. Care must be taken that this does not exert inordinate pressure that prevents circulation to the auricle.
      b. Lacerations of the auricle are usually associated with lacerations of the cartilage. The ear can be totally or incompletely avulsed, but is often viable when even a small pedicle remains. Appropriate debridement and cleansing of the wound minimizes the likelihood of subsequent chondritis or deformity.

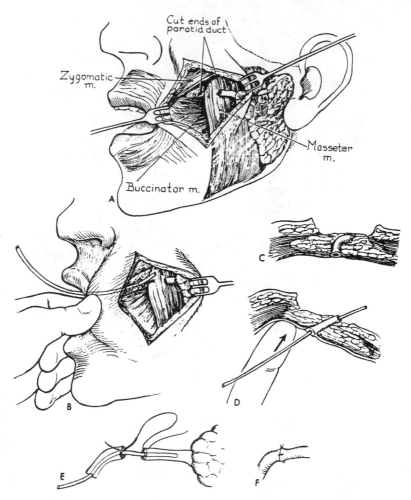

FIG. 21.4. Repair of a severed parotid duct (**A**), severed duct (**B**), Silastic tube in duct (**C**), angulation of Stensen's duct in cheek (**D**), stretching of mucosa facilitates stent placement (**E**), suturing of duct under magnification (**F**), stent remains in 10 to 14 days.

(1) The ear should be carefully sutured into place and adequately supported with dressings.

(2) The ear canal can be stented with Xeroform (Sherwood-Davis & Geck, St. Louis) gauze.

(3) The cartilage should be trimmed accurately to the skin margin.

(4) The auricle has numerous landmarks that allow accurate placement of skin sutures, providing excellent realignment and minimal deformity.

3. **Repair**

   a. Conservative debridement.

   b. Return tissues to point of origin.

   c. Repair cartilage with 5-0 **clear** monofilament nonabsorbable suture.

   d. Repair skin with 6-0 monofilament nonabsorbable suture.

C. Nose. Lacerations of the nose can involve the skin, the lining in the vestibule of the nose, or the mucous membrane of the nasal cavity, most commonly at the junction of the bone and the cartilages.

1. Wounds must be **approximated with anatomic** accuracy, aligning the nostril borders precisely.
2. Septal hematoma can be diagnosed easily with a nasal speculum examination. Immediately evacuate the septal hematoma through a small mucosal incision or by needle aspiration. An untreated septal hematoma will typically resorb and destroy the septal cartilage, especially when becoming infected; a "saddle nose" deformity results.
3. When treating injuries penetrating all soft tissue layers of the nose, it is easiest to repair the mucous membrane lining first, with 4-0 plain catgut or another absorbable suture.
4. Torn septal, upper lateral, alar, and columellar cartilages can usually be reapproximated under direct vision through the wound and held in good position simply by accurate repair of the underlying mucoperichondrium and the overlying skin. Interrupted sutures with 6-0 monofilament polypropylene are ideal for such skin closure.
   a. The nose is sometimes packed with a petroleum-impregnated gauze to maintain position of cartilaginous or bony fragments.

D. Lips

1. Lacerations of the lips can involve only the superficial skin and subcutaneous tissues or extend into the orbicularis oris muscle. Full-thickness lacerations can also be encountered.
2. Bleeding can be profuse if the labial artery is severed. Local pressure or ligation of the vessel controls the bleeding.
3. The vermilion-cutaneous margin and the vermilion-mucosal margin provide accurate landmarks that must be precisely approximated.
   a. Lip musculature should be closed first, using 3-0 or 4-0 chromic gut sutures.

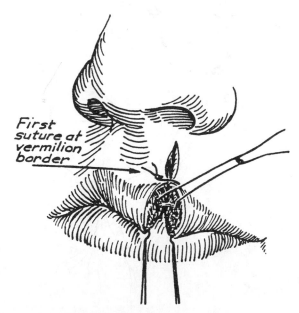

FIG. 21.5. Repair of vertical laceration of lip.

    b. Blood should then be completely cleansed from the vermilion border
    and an accurate approximation made.

    c. The mucous membrane should be closed with 4-0 or 5-0 chromic
    suture.

    d. Close skin with 6-0 polypropylene (Fig. 21.5).

IX. Nonsuture technique of wound closure. Some superficial wounds, especially in children, respond well to approximation with commercially available sterile adhesive strips. Benzoin can be placed on the wound edges to assist tape adherence. The tape is reinforced and provides strong resistance to traction in the lateral direction.

    A. Adhesive strips can provide uniform approximation of tissue margins and eliminate trauma from sutures.

    B. The disadvantage is the potential for uneven alignment of the wound edges. Adhesive strips can be left in place for 2 to 3 weeks, if indicated, and the wound, thus reinforced, prevents lateral pull on the incision.

X. Suturing. The most satisfactory scars after repair of facial lacerations are seen in cases in which the laceration parallels the relaxed lines skin tension (Fig. 21.6). The basic techniques are illustrated in Figure 21.7. Choice of suture materials and surgical needles is wide.

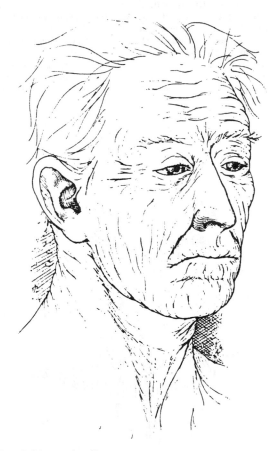

FIG. 21.6. Relaxed skin tension lines.

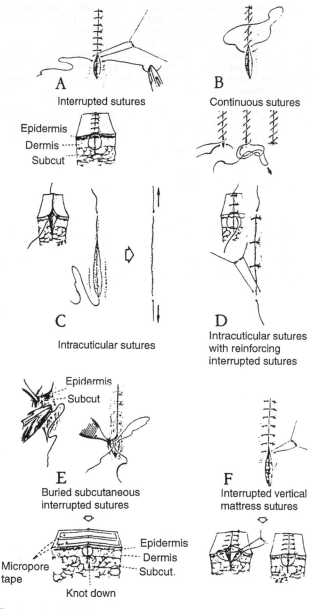

A Interrupted sutures

Epidermis
Dermis
Subcut

B Continuous sutures

C Intracuticular sutures

D Intracuticular sutures
with reinforcing
interrupted sutures

Epidermis
Subcut

E Buried subcutaneous
interrupted sutures

Micropore
tape

Epidermis
Dermis
Subcut.

Knot down

F Interrupted vertical
mattress sutures

FIG. 21.7. Basic suture techniques.

    A. If proper closure of the subcutaneous and dermal tissues has been achieved, minimal tension in the skin closure should result. Skin sutures, therefore, can be removed to prevent residual suture-hole scars.

XI. Removal of sutures. Facial wounds have the advantage of a rich vascular supply, which contributes to early healing. Where skin is thin, as in the eyelids, sutures can be removed in 3 days. Elsewhere on the face, sutures can be left 4 to 6 days. Sutures in the ears can remain 10 to 14 days when associated with injury to underlying cartilage.

XII. Animal bites

    A. The surgical creation of a clean wound is an essential precaution before primary suture. Irrigate the wound with large amounts of saline.

    B. Alternatively, surgical debridement and excision of the wound edges can convert the wound into a clean injury.

    C. Broad-spectrum antibiotic coverage is mandatory.

    D. Because the risk of infection from human bites is significant, some surgeons perform only secondary closures in such injuries.

Axioms

- Careful assessment of a facial wound is required before treatment.
- Extensive debridement of soft tissues is rarely required for facial injuries; preserve as much tissue as possible.
- Scars from facial wounds are determined less by suture materials and needles than by the character of the wound, appropriate debridement, and the skill of the surgeon.

22. BONY ORAL-MAXILLOFACIAL INJURIES

Mark W. Ochs

I. **Evaluation of the patient with suspected facial trauma**
   A. Initial evaluation
   1. Relieve airway obstruction.
   2. Control hemorrhage.
   3. Search for more immediately life-threatening injuries (thoracic, abdominal, head, extremity).
   4. Assume cervical spine (C-spine) injury and stabilize until it is cleared.
   5. Neurologic assessment.
   B. **Secondary evaluation**
   1. Complete head, eye, ear, nose, throat (HEENT) examination.
      a. Scalp and skull evaluation (palpate)
      b. Cranial nerve evaluation
      c. Otologic evaluation (external ear, otoscopic examination)
      d. Ophthalmologic evaluation (pupil symmetry, reactivity, visual acuity, and ocular movement)

II. **Dentoalveolar trauma**
   A. **Anatomy**
   1. Adult dentition is composed of 32 teeth, including bilateral maxillary and mandibular central and lateral incisors, canines, first and second premolars, and three molars. Typically, the third molars are either absent or impacted.
   2. The pediatric dentition consists of 20 total deciduous teeth, including bilateral maxillary and mandibular central and lateral incisors, canines, and two molars (Fig. 22.1). Exfoliation of the deciduous teeth begins at approximately 6 years of age and the mixed dentition stage continues until 12 to 14 years of age. The teeth are attached to the alveolar processes of the maxilla and mandible by periodontal ligaments. Alveolar bone in younger age groups undergoes plastic deformation when subjected to trauma.
   B. **Evaluation**
   1. Clinical
      a. Account for all teeth. Count the teeth; attempt to locate any missing teeth at the location of the injury. With unaccounted for missing teeth, consider traumatic impaction into the local bone or surrounding soft tissues; also, dislodged teeth can be aspirated or swallowed. Appropriate radiographs should be obtained to locate missing teeth.
      b. Evaluate the occlusion. Ask the patient if the bite feels normal? This is a very simple yet sensitive screening tool to detect dentoalveolar and facial fractures. Occlusion should be evaluated for stability and symmetry. Occlusal discrepancies, traumatic gaps in the dental arches, and tears of the pink, firm attached gingiva should raise the suspicion of maxillary and mandibular fractures.
      c. Evaluate damaged or displaced teeth. Fractured teeth can be classified to the depth and location of fracture (Fig. 22.2). Dislocated teeth can be totally avulsed or subluxed or an associated alveolar fracture may be present.
   2. Radiographs. A Panorex is a good screening radiograph for most dentoalveolar trauma. If not available, plain radiographs of the maxillofacial complex often suffice (posteroanterior, lateral, or oblique views). Isolated tooth fractures are best evaluated with intraoral dental radiographs. If these are not available, early dental referral should be sought.

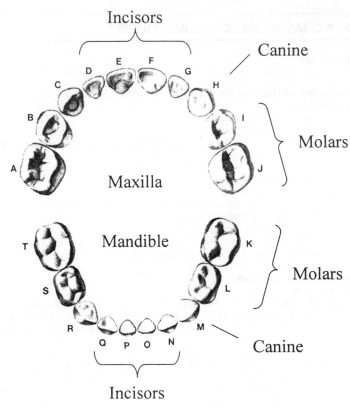

FIG. 22.1. Pediatric dental arches (**A**)

C. Management

1. Age of the patient, type of tooth (deciduous or permanent), status of tooth development, condition of tooth before trauma, patient motivation, time elapsed since injury, and associated injuries must be considered when deciding on management of dentoalveolar trauma.
2. Intraoral soft-tissue lacerations are usually best treated by conservative debridement, irrigation, and primary repair with absorbable sutures after stabilization or definitive treatment of the dentoalveolar fracture.
3. In general, isolated tooth crown fractures need emergent referral if the dental pulp (dark pink or red appearance) is exposed or if teeth are sensitive.

    a. Dislocated or subluxed teeth and dentoalveolar fractures need to be emergently reduced and stabilized with wire and composite resin bonding. Composite resins are opaque white filling material that is either chemically or UV light activated.

    b. Avulsed deciduous teeth should not be reimplanted because of low success rate and possibility of damage to the underlying developing permanent dentition.

    c. Avulsed permanent teeth should be replaced into the tooth socket as soon as possible after the trauma. Immediate reimplantation is ideal. If this is not possible, the tooth should be stored in appropriate storage medium (avulsed tooth storage system → buccal vestibule → milk → saline → moist towel) and replaced as soon as

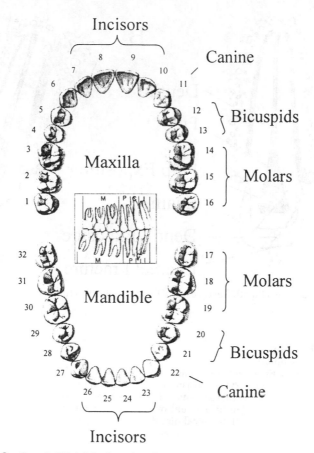

FIG. 22.1. *Continued.* (**B**) Adult dental arches.

possible. A delay of >2 hours or desiccation of the tooth root significantly affects the overall prognosis of the tooth. Once reimplanted, the tooth still requires composite resin splinting to the adjacent stable teeth and should not be in heavy contact with the opposing dentition during chewing motions.

III. Mandibular fractures. Aside from nasal fractures, mandibular fractures account for approximately two thirds of all bony maxillofacial trauma. The mechanism of injury is usually blunt trauma sustained from assault or motor vehicle accident.

   A. Anatomy and location of injury. Fractures tend to occur at the local site of impact, areas of weakness, and are often multiple. The anatomic regions and associated incidence of fracture are shown in Figure 22.3. In edentulous patients, the incidence of subcondylar fractures accounts for 37% of all mandible fractures and is often paired with a contralateral body fracture. The inferior alveolar neurovascular bundle enters the mandible on the medial aspect of the mid ramus through the mandibular foramen and traverses an intrabony canal, exiting through the mental foramen located just inferior to the mandibular premolar root tips. It is strictly a sensory nerve (V_3) supplying the ipsilateral lower lip, teeth, and gingiva.

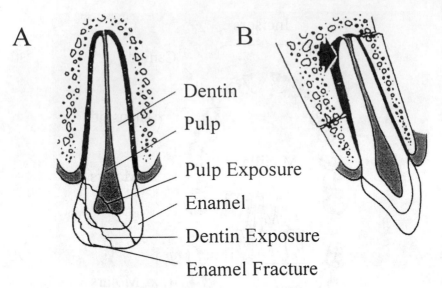

FIG. 22.2. A. Level of tooth fractures. **B.** Dentoalveolar fracture.

B. Evaluation
    1. Clinical
        a. Emergent situations
            (1) Airway obstruction. Foreign bodies (e.g., dentures, avulsed teeth) can cause airway obstruction; remove them at the time of initial evaluation. In addition, airway obstruction can occur with bilateral mandibular parasymphyseal or body fractures.

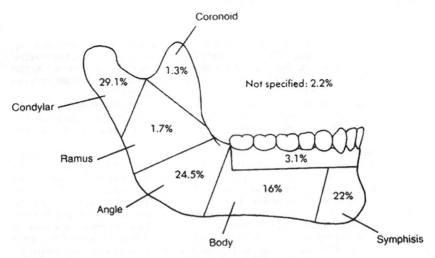

FIG. 22.3. Mandibular anatomy and fracture zones.

Manual anterior distraction of the flail anterior mandibular segment, allowing the patient to be semisupine or to sit up, and oral suctioning can provide temporary relief, but a definitive airway should be secured urgently.

(2) Hemorrhage is rarely a significant problem with mandibular fractures.

(a) The inferior alveolar artery traveling in the mandibular canal can be lacerated during the initial injury, but simple fracture reduction, direct pressure, or infiltration with epinephrine containing anesthetic solutions is usually adequate for hemostasis.

(b) Persistent or profuse bleeding is often associated with penetrating injuries and a secure airway should be the primary concern. Hemorrhage control should then be performed by direct surgical exploration or, rarely, by interventional radiologic means. With mandibular bleeding, fracture reduction and temporary stabilization are preferable to local packing, which usually distracts and destabilizes the bony segments, allowing continued hemorrhage.

b. Occlusion. Malocclusion is one of the first clinical signs detected in patients with mandibular fractures. If the fracture is in the tooth-bearing segment of the mandible, a noticeable step deformity or interdental gap may be detected. Floor of mouth ecchymosis is pathognomonic for a mandibular parasymphyseal or body fracture. If the fracture is located in the subcondylar region, a shift of the chin toward the affected side or an anterior or lateral open bite may be present (Fig. 22.4).

c. Soft-tissue signs, such as ecchymosis, edema, pain, and gingival or mucosal lacerations, may be present at the fracture site.

d. Sensation. Lower lip and chin paraesthesia or anesthesia is common in patients with mandible fractures located between the mid ramus and canine region. Greater bony displacement increases the risk for inferior alveolar nerve injury or transection.

2. Radiographs. Plain radiographs usually suffice for evaluation of mandibular fractures. At least two views at 90° should be used to evaluate most injuries. This is especially important in the subcondylar region, where superimposition of other structures can mimic or obscure a fracture. The best initial radiograph is the Panorex, accompanied by an open mouth Towne's view. Other radiographs that can be used to evaluate mandibular fractures are the posteroanterior (PA) and lateral oblique views. Computed tomography (CT) can be helpful for the evaluation of patients with condylar or subcondylar fractures. This is particularly true in children because their condyles are developing and incompletely ossified, making plain radiology detection difficult. Any patient (especially children) with a chin laceration and preauricular pain or swelling should be evaluated for a condylar or subcondylar fracture. Coronoid fractures account for <1% of all mandible fractures and are almost always associated with an overlying zygomatic complex fracture that was displaced medially, creating the injury.

C. Management

1. Cervical immobilization

a. Cervical immobilization should be maintained until C-spine injury can be definitively ruled out.

2. Management of emergent problems

a. Initial management should be to control airway and bleeding. Control of the airway is performed with distraction of flail bony segments, if possible. In the event of a compromised airway, endotracheal intubation or surgical airway should be established before surgical repair and stabilization of the mandibular fracture.

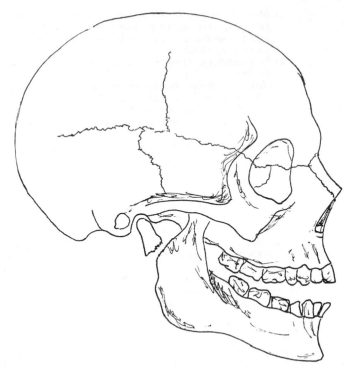

FIG. 22.4. Anterior open bite caused by a condyle fracture with posterior vertical collapse.

   3. Temporary immobilization
      a. Temporary partial reduction and stabilization of the fracture segments can provide symptomatic relief, help control bleeding, and minimize damage to the inferior alveolar neurovascular bundle. This can be performed with a modified Barton's bandage or by placing a stainless steel bridal wire (24–26 gauge) around the necks of two teeth on either side of the line of fracture (Fig. 22.5).
   4. Definitive treatment. Fractures should be reduced adequately, fixated, and immobilized for adequate healing to occur. This is typically accomplished via open reduction, with internal plate and screw fixation. Without immobilization, fracture segments usually become displaced by the attached muscle pull, leading to a malunion or nonunion. Isolated non- or minimally displaced fractures, particularly condylar and subcondylar, can be suitably treated by wiring the teeth together (maxillomandibular fixation [MMF]). The period of MMF is usually for 6 to 8 weeks, except for condylar fractures where, because of the risk of temporomandibular joint fibro-osseous ankylosis, 2 weeks is the standard.
   5. Prophylactic antibiotics. Mandibular fractures that include tooth-bearing segments are considered compound fractures because of the egress of saliva, bacteria, and other contaminants through the periodontal ligament or fracture site. Prophylactic antibiotics that cover most oral microorganisms (e.g., penicillin) or a first-generation cephalosporin are recommended, along with oral saline or antimicrobial rinses. In the penicillin-allergic patient, clindamycin is a good alternative.

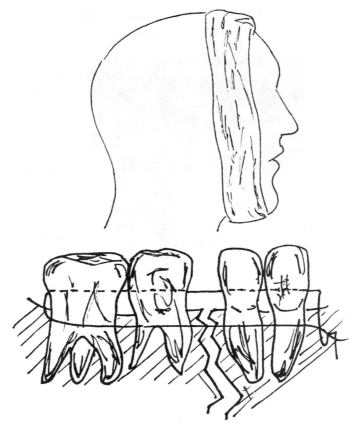

FIG. 22.5. Bridal wiring to stabilize an anterior mandibular fracture site.

IV. **Midface fractures** can be defined as any fracture of the orbital-zygomatic-maxillary complex. The mechanism of injury is usually blunt from assault or motor vehicle accident.

A. **General midfacial fracture management**

1. **Anatomy and location of injury**. The midface is divided into the maxilla, the zygomatic complexes, and the nasal-orbital-ethmoid (NOE) complex (Fig. 22.6). Fractures tend to occur at the site of impact and inherently weak regions of the midfacial complex, including bony sutures, foramina, and apertures.

a. The infraorbital neurovascular bundle enters the midfacial complex via the orbital region through the inferior orbital fissure and then traversing partially through a bony canal along the floor of the orbit to exit through the infraorbital foramen on the anterior surface of the maxilla. The infraorbital nerve (V_2) supplies general sensation to the ipsilateral lower eyelid, lateral nose, upper lip, and anterior maxilla.

2. **Evaluation**

a. Clinical

(1) Emergent situations

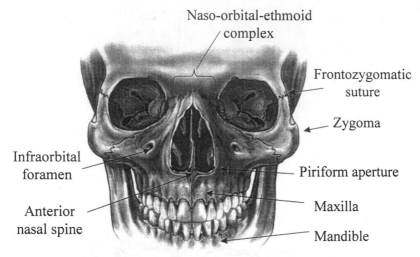

FIG. 22.6. Midfacial anatomy.

     (a) Airway obstruction. Foreign bodies (e.g., dentures, avulsed teeth) can cause airway obstruction and should be removed at the initial evaluation. In most clinical situations, airway obstruction occurs in patients with panfacial trauma, including significant mandibular fractures.

     (b) Hemorrhage. Significant hemorrhage is more common with midfacial fractures than with mandibular fractures. The descending palatine arteries, which travel in a bony canal along the posterolateral surface of the nasal cavity within the palatine bone, can cause profuse posterior nasal hemorrhage. Other vessels that may be injured include nasal septal, sphenopalatine, and pterygoid plexus.

   (2) Occlusion. Occlusal discrepancies are one of the first clinical signs detected in patients with certain midfacial fractures. Mobility of the maxillary dentition relative to other midfacial structures is indicative of a maxillary fracture. A posteriorly directed force of significant magnitude can cause a posteriorly impacted maxilla. Either an anterior or posterior open bite, or relative protrusion of the lower teeth, is indicative of a maxillary or midfacial fracture.

   (3) Soft-tissue signs include ecchymosis, edema, pain, and mucosal lacerations.

   (4) Palpation. Palpate all bones of the midface, including maxilla, orbital rims, zygomas, and nose; often, the patient is too sensitive to allow a complete examination. However, grasping the anterior maxillary teeth with the thumb and forefinger and attempting upward and side-to-side movement while stabilizing the entire forehead with the opposite hand is crucial to detecting a midfacial fracture.

   (5) Sensation. Upper lateral lip, nose, and cheek paraesthesia or anesthesia is common in patients with a fracture extending

through the infraorbital foramen. Complete transection of the infraorbital nerve is uncommon in blunt trauma.

(6) Ophthalmologic examination. Any fracture involving the bony orbit or zygomatic complex can cause injuries to the globe or other orbital contents. Complete examination includes pupils, visual acuity, range of motion of the globe, globe position, and the globe itself, including a funduscopic examination. Extraocular movements in multiple fields of gaze are often diminished in patients with significant orbital edema, but tend to be mild without a firm fixed sudden stop. Blowout fracture of one of the orbital walls (most commonly the medial orbital floor) can cause entrapment of the extraocular muscles (inferior rectus muscles or inferior oblique). A firm, fixed and reproducible point of limitation in upgaze or, more likely, downgaze should alert the practitioner to this possibility. An urgent specialist consultation is appropriate because prolonged muscle ischemia can lead to long-term impairment of movement.

(7) Nasal examination. Significant nasal trauma can be associated with nasal airway obstruction and significant epistaxis.

   (a) Epistaxis from anterior vessels can be controlled with upright positioning, cold compresses, topical nasal vasoconstrictor sprays, local direct pressure, or, infrequently, anterior nasal packing.

   (b) Posterior epistaxis may require compression tamponade.

   (c) The nasal septum must be evaluated for the presence of a septal hematoma, which can lead to localized loss of septal support of the nasal dorsum and a "saddle nose" deformity.

(8) Examination for cerebrospinal fluid (CSF) leak. CSF leaks most commonly occur with midfacial, frontal sinus, or basilar skull fractures.

   (a) Fractures involving the NOE complex occasionally involve the cribriform plate in the superior aspect of the nasal cavity and floor of the anterior cranial fossa.

   (b) Basilar skull fractures can involve the petrous temporal bone, resulting in leakage of CSF.

   (c) Various tests, including the ring test and chloride or glucose sampling, have been described to establish a diagnosis of CSF leak, but contemporary testing for potential CSF leakage is with a beta$_2$-transferrin determination (positive with CSF leak) on the collected drainage sample.

(9) Radiographs

   (a) CT is the diagnostic modality of choice for the complete evaluation of midfacial trauma with thin sections (3 mm) in axial planes through the midface and the orbits. Direct coronal views are particularly helpful with orbital fractures but the patient's C-spine status may preclude obtaining them.

   (b) Plain radiographs sometimes can be used as an initial screening tool, but soft-tissue swelling and superimposition of other anatomic structures usually obscure some fracture lines. The best plain radiographic series includes the Water's view, the submental vertex view, and the lateral facial view.

   (c) The panoramic radiograph is of little use in the evaluation of midfacial trauma, except in determining if a concomitant mandibular fracture exists.

3. Management

  a. Cervical immobilization is maintained until C-spine injury can be definitively excluded.

b. Management of emergent problems

(1) Initial management should consist of control of the airway and bleeding.

(2) Significant posterior nasal hemorrhage can be controlled with posterior nasopharynx occlusion with a Foley catheter that has been inserted transnasally into the nasopharynx, inflated with water or saline, then gentle anterior traction applied with anterior nasal packing.

(3) Persistent deep hemorrhage can be problematic, and control may require surgical ligation of branches of the external carotid artery in the neck or, preferably, with interventional radiology.

(4) Because of risk of inadvertent intracranial placement, blind (nonfiberoptic) nasal intubation with endotracheal tubes or nasogastric tubes are contraindicated in patients with suspected midfacial trauma involving the NOE complex.

c. Treatment of ophthalmologic problems. Obtain ophthalmologic consultation for individuals with potential globe injuries. Fat herniation through an upper eyelid laceration or an irregular (not round) pointing pupil suggests a penetrating globe injury (see Chapter 23).

d. Decongestants. Spray decongestants should be used in patients with significant midfacial trauma to provide symptomatic relief for nasal airway obstruction and to minimize epistaxis.

(1) Phenylephrine

(2) Oxymetazoline

Edema prevention. Open surgical treatment of midfacial trauma can be difficult in an operative field with significant edema. Operative repair is usually delayed until edema has significantly resolved. Prevention of facial edema can provide symptomatic relief for the patient as well as expedite definitive treatment.

(3) Steroids. Pharmacologic administration of glucocorticoids can hasten the resolution of facial edema in patients with maxillofacial trauma. Dexamethasone (4–8 mg) administered intravenously (i.v.) every 6 hours or methylprednisolone (125 mg) i.v. every 6 hours for 24 to 48 hours may be used. Administration of steroids is of questionable benefit after the edema is present. Caution should be used when administering steroids in insulin-dependent diabetic patients.

(4) The head of bed. Elevate to at least 30° for the first several days after sustaining facial trauma.

(5) Intermittent application of cold compresses for the first 24 hours may be beneficial for the prevention of facial edema (20 minutes on and 20 minutes off).

e. Definitive treatment of midfacial trauma fractures should be deferred until after a full clinical and radiographic evaluation and the patient is stabilized. The beginning of osseous healing can occur as early as 7 days after the injury. Reduction and repair can be exceedingly difficult if surgery is delayed for more than 2 weeks. Contemporary treatment of midfacial fractures involves open reduction and internal fixation using titanium miniplates and screws. Minimally or nondisplaced nasal, orbital, zygomatic complex (tripod), and zygomatic arch fractures may not require surgical treatment. Nonunion of these isolated fractures is exceedingly rare.

B. LeFort fractures are those of the midface that involve the maxillary dentoalveolar segment. The mechanism and location of impact usually determine the type of fracture sustained. Fractures tend to occur in certain patterns of the midface and are traditionally classified by the highest level of fracture (Fig. 22.7). Most LeFort fractures are not pure and can have comminution, additional levels or lines of fracture, and other associated facial fractures.

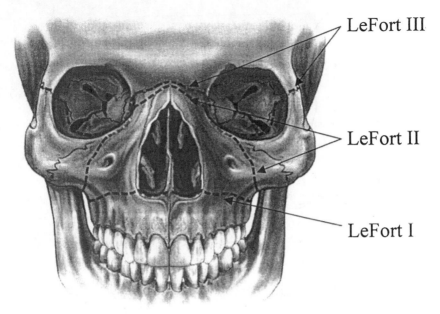

LeFort III

LeFort II

LeFort I

FIG. 22.7. LeFort levels of fracture.

C. **Zygomaticomaxillary complex fractures**. Zygomaticomaxillary complex (ZMC, tripod or malar) fractures usually are sustained with direct blunt trauma to the zygomatic buttress of the face. The zygoma has four major stability points, with connections as follows: (a) the frontal bone at the frontozygomatic suture; (b) the maxilla at the medial inferior orbital rim; (c) at the zygomaticomaxillary buttress; and (d) the temporal bone at the zygomatic arch. A complete fracture of the complex usually involves all four of these major stability points (Fig. 22.8). Anteriorly, the fracture usually occurs in the maxilla obliquely through the infraorbital foramen because of the relatively weak nature of this bone (high incidence of V_2 sensory division paraesthesia). Other significant physical findings associated with ZMC fractures are depression of the zygomatic eminence, lateral subconjunctival hemorrhage, ocular dystopia (uneven pupillary levels), lateral canthal ptosis, enophthalmos, and palpable fractures at the inferior and lateral orbital rims. With extreme medial and posterior displacement, the patient can exhibit limited mouth opening because of impingement of the fractured complex against the coronoid process of the mandible. For oral access or intubation, initial deviation of the mandible toward the uninjured side can sufficiently clear this mechanical obstruction.

D. **Zygomatic arch fractures**. Isolated zygomatic arch fractures usually are sustained by focal direct blunt trauma to the zygomatic arch, creating three breakpoints with a "classic W-pattern" (Fig. 22.9). Common physical findings are a depression at the location of trauma and pain on mandibular opening caused by masseteric muscle pull. Limited mandibular opening can also exist because of mechanical obstruction of the coronoid process. A submental vertex or "jug-handle" view is usually sufficient to identify this fracture. Early (24–72 hours) surgical reduction without internal fixation via a lateral brow, temporal hairline (Gille's), or maxillary vestibular incision is desirable. Stability of the fracture reduction decreases beyond this time and

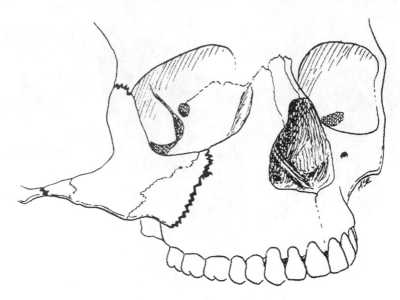

FIG. 22.8. Right zygomaticomaxillary complex (ZMC) fracture.

tends to sag back inward, thus requiring a much more extensive exposure (e.g., a hemicoronal incision) for direct access and plating.

E. Orbital blowout fractures occur from direct impact to the orbit or globe (Fig. 22.10). The floor of the orbit and the medial orbital wall are the thinnest walls and most commonly involved with this type of fracture. The surrounding maxillary sinus and ethmoid air cells act as "airbags of the orbit," cushioning the blow and absorbing the force, thus, protecting to some degree against globe rupture. The prolapse of some of the orbital contents into these spaces can produce enophthalmos or orbital dystopia because of a relative increase in the orbital volume. Additionally, suspensory fascia (Tenon's capsule) or extraocular muscles can be entrapped in the fracture line, leading to restricted eye movement and diplopia in certain fields of gaze. Coronal CT scans are invaluable when evaluating this injury and should be correlated with clinical findings. Indications for surgical correction include a significant cosmetic or functional deformity. A relative indication is >25% to 50% of the surface area of an orbital wall being involved in the fracture. If edema allows, optimal time for repair is within 24 hours. If significant edema exists, reevaluation and repair within 5 to 7 days is desirable. Systemic corticosteroids have limited usefulness in hastening resolution of this edema. Patients should be cautioned not to blow the nose, which can cause significant orbital emphysema. Repair usually entails open reduction or removal of the fractured segments, then reducing the orbital contents with possible autogenous or alloplastic implant reconstruction.

F. Nasal fracture is the most common fracture to the face. Complete examination should include evaluation for a septal hematoma. Epistaxis should be controlled. The diagnosis of a nasal fracture is primarily a clinical one. Nasal deformity, deviation, and bony crepitus with movement are the usual findings. Occasionally, radiographs can aid in the diagnosis. If edema allows, early reduction (within 24–48 hours) of isolated nasal and septal fractures affords the greatest stability. If not, repair should be performed within

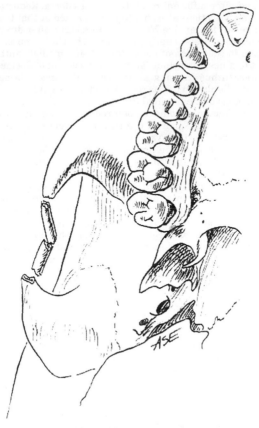

FIG. 22.9. Right zygomatic arch fracture viewed from below.

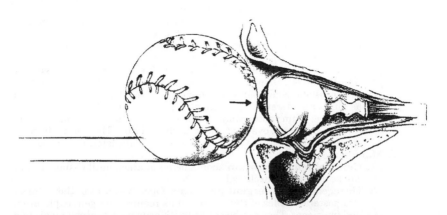

FIG. 22.10. Orbital floor blowout fracture.

5 to 7 days after sufficient resolution of the edema. Reduction of septal fractures and dislocations also should be performed at that time.

G. **Fractures of the entire NOE complex** occur after direct high impact to the region. Diagnosis usually can be made by clinical observation and direct palpation in the region of nasal dorsum and medial canthal tendons. Significant findings can include lateral displacement of the medial canthal tendons (telecanthus) causing an increased distance (normally 30–34 mm). Significant disruption in this region can lead to epiphora secondary to swelling or damage of the lacrimal drainage system. Primary surgical repair of significant fractures includes open reduction and plating of the bony segments, with direct repair of the canthal tendons. Repair should be done within the first 7 to 10 days, because secondary repair is exceedingly difficult and often leads to compromised results. Globe injuries and CSF leaks should be sought when a NOE injury is being evaluated.

V. **Frontal sinus fractures**

A. **Anatomy and location of injury**. The frontal sinus is usually divided into left and right halves by a midline septum; both sides drain into the middle meatus of the nose through their respective nasofrontal ducts or foramina. Of adults, 5% have no frontal sinus and 5% have only a unilateral sinus. Trauma to the forehead region can fracture the anterior or posterior walls of the frontal sinus or damage the nasofrontal ducts. With fracture of the posterior wall of the frontal sinus, consider the potential for a dural laceration or cerebral injury.

B. **Evaluation**

1. **Clinical**

a. Emergent situations

(1) Open fracture of the anterior and posterior table of the frontal sinus are considered emergencies because of the high risk of meningitis from direct cerebral exposure. Emergent surgical intervention is indicated.

(2) Cerebral contusions are common, with injuries to the frontal sinus.

b. Local signs include ecchymosis, edema, pain, and cutaneous lacerations at the location of fracture, and fractures and deformity of the forehead and superior orbital rims.

c. Sensation. Forehead and scalp paraesthesia or anesthesia. The supraorbital and supratrochlear nerves (V_1) supply this region.

d. Nasal examination and CSF leaks. NOE complex trauma can be associated with frontal sinus fractures. CSF leaks can occur in patients with frontal sinus fractures. Questionable nasal discharge should be submitted for a β_2-transferrin level.

2. **Radiographs**. CT is the diagnostic modality of choice for the complete evaluation of frontal sinus trauma. Thin sections (2–3 mm) in the axial plane through the paranasal sinuses are usually adequate for most purposes. Both the anterior and posterior tables of the frontal sinus should be categorized as **fractured or noninvolved** and **displaced versus nondisplaced**. Displacement is defined as overlap by the amount of thickness of the adjacent cortical bone. Intermediate distinctions such as mild or moderate displacement are confusing and have no clinical relevance. Plain radiographs can be used as initial screening for bony injury but will not evaluate the underlying brain. The best plain radiographic series includes the Caldwell view and the lateral cephalogram.

C. **Management**

1. **Cervical immobilization** should be maintained until C-spine injury can be definitively excluded.

2. Management of **emergent problems**. Open fractures of the anterior and posterior tables of the frontal sinus require emergent exploration and treatment. They can be treated with primary cutaneous repair and delayed treatment of the frontal sinus injury, as indicated.

3. **Prophylactic antibiotics**. Most frontal sinus fractures fill with blood and mucus early after trauma. Prophylactic antibiotics that cover most sinus microorganisms (e.g., ampicillin with clavulanate) or a first-generation cephalosporin usually are recommended in these situations. Posterior table involvement often is covered with a broader spectrum antibiotic that can cross the blood–brain barrier.
4. **Decongestants**. Because of mucosal edema and the potential for compromised frontal sinus drainage, decongestants should be used in patients with significant frontal sinus trauma.
5. Definitive treatment of frontal sinus fractures depends on the extent of the fracture. If the drainage system of the sinuses is significantly compromised, obliteration is usually recommended. If only the anterior table is involved and nondisplaced, no surgical treatment is generally necessary. A displaced frontal sinus that is either extensive or creates a cosmetic deformity can be accessed directly through the fracture or via a liberal sinusotomy. The mucosal lining is then completely removed with curettage and drilling to deter formation of a mucocele at a usually much later date—such as years later. The nasofrontal ducts can then be obliterated with fascia or bone grafts and the frontal sinus can be obliterated with autologous fat, bone, pericranium, or alloplastic materials. If only the anterior table is displaced without involvement of the nasofrontal ducts, primary repair without obliteration can be performed. Significant involvement or displacement of the posterior table usually requires direct exploration, with repair or cranialization depending on the degree of damage. Smaller frontal sinuses in young patients can be cranialized by simply removing the posterior sinus wall, smoothing the edges, removing the mucosal lining, and obliterating the frontonasal ducts. This treatment in older patients and those with large frontal sinuses may predispose them to developing chronic subdural fluid accumulations. With displaced posterior table fractures, associated dural tears requiring neurosurgical repair is the rule rather than the exception.

Axioms

• Control of both the airway and hemorrhage is the immediate goal in the management of bony injuries to the face.
• Assume that all patients with facial fractures have concomitant cervical spine injury.
• Malocclusion is an important clinical sign of mandibular or maxillary fractures.
• A nasal septal hematoma must be identified and evacuated to avoid saddle nose deformity.

23. OPHTHALMIC INJURIES

Randall L. Beatty

I. **Introduction**
    A. Eye injuries are common and require prompt evaluation and treatment to minimize the risk of loss of sight. These injuries may be obvious (as with penetrating trauma), but also can be more difficult to detect, especially in the unresponsive, multiply injured patient. All injured patients require physical and visual examinations as part of their early management.
    B. Prompt consultation with an ophthalmologist is strongly recommended in all cases of periorbital or ocular trauma.
    C. Following is a brief overview of how to conduct appropriate physical and visual examinations and document them in the medical record, and a description of several of the more common injuries.

II. **History**
    A. Obtain a history of preexisting ocular disease. Does the patient wear glasses? Is there a history of glaucoma?
    B. Circumstances surrounding the injury.
    C. Patient complaints: photophobia or pain, change in vision (double vision or decreased vision).

III. **Physical examination and visual acuity**. Irrespective of how minor an injury may appear, documentation of visual acuity is the first step in evaluating any patient with possible ocular trauma. **Visual acuity is the single most sensitive test to alert the treating physician to the presence of an eye injury**. In general, the ultimate visual outcome is directly related to the presenting visual acuity.
    A. Test for vision in each eye separately by covering the opposite eye with either the palm of the patient's hand or some occluding device such as an eye patch or bandage. Any means of documenting the vision can be used.
        1. In the emergency setting, patients are often supine. A description of the ability to see letters on a card, a pen, or name tag is sufficient. In the case of a patient with reduced vision, the distance at which the patient can count fingers, see a hand wave, tell the direction of a light (light projection), or detect the presence of a light (light perception) provides an adequate preliminary assessment.
        2. If the patient has eyeglasses, check visual acuity with their use. For older patients with bifocal glasses, test near vision with the patient looking through the bifocal portion at the bottom of the glasses.
            a. If the glasses have been lost or are not with the patient, have the patient look through a small pinhole (in a piece of paper or cardboard or a commercial device) to approximate the eyeglass correction.
        3. Obtain visual field evaluation by confrontation testing and document whether the patient is cooperative enough to undergo the test.
        4. **Documentation in the medical record of "vision intact," "vision okay," "fine," or "the same" is inadequate**. The first test in any ophthalmic workup is adequate documentation of visual acuity (Fig. 23.1).
        5. If the patient is unconscious or uncooperative, it may not be possible to assess vision by having the patient read. However, it may still be possible to assess the visual status by measuring pupillary responses. These are direct responses to light, consensual responses in the opposite eye, and testing for an afferent pupillary defect (which, if present, would indicate optic nerve damage) (Table 23.1.)
    B. **Eyelids**. Assess for edema, laceration, ptosis, or other evidence of injury.
    C. **Palpate the orbital rim** for deformity or crepitation.
    D. **Examine the globe without applying pressure**. Assess the globe for possible displacement or entrapment, ocular movement, and diplopia.

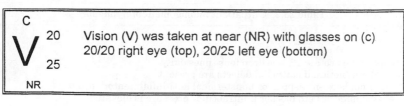

FIG. 23.1. Documentation of visual acuity.

E. **Pupils**. Evaluate for shape, equality, and response to light. An irregular peaked pupil may indicate an open globe with the peaked pupil pointing to the area of the laceration.

F. **Cornea**. Assess for opacity, abrasions, foreign bodies, or contact lenses. Contacts should be removed from trauma patients. If unsure whether a patient has a contact lens, a small amount of fluorescein will make the presence obvious. An unconscious patient can develop a perforating bacterial corneal ulcer from a contact lens left in the eye for several days.

G. **Conjunctivae**. Evaluate for subconjunctival hemorrhage, chemosis (swelling), or foreign bodies.

H. **Anterior chamber**. Assess for blood (hyphema) or abnormal depth. A shallow anterior chamber can result from an anterior penetrating wound, and a deep anterior chamber from injury to the posterior portion of the globe.

I. **Iris** should be reactive and of regular shape.

J. **Lens** should be in the normal location and transparent.

K. **Vitreous** should be transparent. Blood in the vitreous will produce a black rather than a red reflex. Assess for foreign bodies.

L. **Retina**. Assess for hemorrhage or detachment.

IV. **Common injuries**

  A. **Traumatic hyphema**. Blood in the anterior chamber of the eye behind the cornea can obscure the detail of the iris or lens. A hyphema can be associated with a more serious injury (e.g., a ruptured globe).

    1. **Microhyphema** has red blood cells floating in the anterior chamber and is best seen with a slit-lamp examination. A **gross hyphema** can be detected with a penlight examination, and a total hyphema represents an anterior chamber that is packed with a blood clot. **"Eight-ball hyphema"** refers to a dark-colored clot, usually indicating a nonacute injury. An acute injury usually has bright red blood within the anterior chamber.

    2. **Evaluation of the hyphema**

      a. **Visual acuity**

      b. **Slit-lamp examination** with intraocular pressure testing

      c. **Imaging studies** may be indicated to rule out orbital fractures, intraocular foreign bodies, or open globe. A B-mode ultrasound can show details of the posterior eye and help detect a retinal detachment.

    3. **Management of hyphema** remains controversial to whether patients with traumatic hyphema are treated as inpatients or outpatients. Most patients with microhyphemas and small hyphemas are treated as outpatients. Patients with larger hyphemas, other periocular trauma, and sickle cell disease usually are treated as inpatients.

Table 23.1. Documentation of pupillary responses

PERRL - APD (normal pupil responses to light, negative afferent pupillary defect)

Table 23.2. Outpatient management of hyphema

Medications
−Atropine 1% three times daily
−Prednisolone acetate 1% one drop four times daily
−Topical antibiotics, if epithelial defects are present
−Acetaminophen—no aspirin or nonsteroidal anti-inflammatory drugs
−Acetazolamide or beta blocker if intraocular pressure is elevated

Activities
−Bedrest with head elevated
−Limited activity—no bending, lifting (straining)
−Shield over injured eye

Follow-up
−Seen daily for 4–5 days

---

     a. Corneal staining or glaucoma can result from hyphema. Increase in pain after hyphema suggests rebleeding or glaucoma (Tables 23.2 and 23.3).

B. Eyelid lacerations. Perform a complete ophthalmic examination on every patient with eyelid or periorbital lacerations. Soft-tissue injuries are repaired only after globe injuries are excluded and imaging studies performed. Even the most complex eyelid laceration repairs can be delayed for 24 to 48 hours with excellent surgical results.

    1. Specific eyelid complications include canthal tendon disinsertion, lacrimal drainage system canalicular lacerations, levator aponeurosis disinsertion or laceration, and lacrimal sac lacerations. These and transmarginal eyelid lacerations require special attention.

    2. Any laceration in the medial aspect of the eyelid is likely to cause a canalicular laceration. Careful inspection and probing and irrigation of the lacrimal apparatus are required to detect this injury. Irrigate and examine all wounds for the presence of foreign bodies.

    3. Complicated injuries are best repaired in the operating room under monitored sedation or general anesthesia. Most superficial lacerations can be repaired with local eyelid blocks in the emergency department. In severe eyelid disruptions, the medial canthus should be addressed

Table 23.3. Inpatient acute management of hyphema

Medications
−Atropine 1% three times daily
−Prednisolone acetate 1% four times daily
−Antiglaucoma medication: timolol maleate 0.5% twice daily acetazolamide 500 mg twice daily
−Acetaminophen for pain: as needed
−Aminocaproic acid (50 mg/kg liquid every 4 hours; maximum dose 30 g/24 hours)

Activities
−Bedrest with bathroom privileges and decreased activity
−Shield full time to injured eye

Indications for surgery
−Bloodstaining of the cornea
−Elevated intraocular pressure of 50 mmHg for 5 days, 35 mmHg for 7 days, or, eight ball hyphema. In patients with, sickle cell surgery recommended with intraocular pressure over 24 mmHg for 24 hours on maximal medications.

first with repair of the canalicular injury, silicone tube intubation of the nasal lacrimal system, and repair of the deep head of the medial canthal tendon before closure of any other eyelid lacerations.

a. Close lid defects before lateral fixation because a rotational flap or canthotomy may be necessary to achieve closure without producing pressure on the transmarginal lacerations.

b. Eyelid laceration repair requires at least a two-layered closure with 5-0 absorbable sutures in the deep tissue and nonabsorbable sutures in the eyelid margins (6-0 silk).

c. Superficial skin closure is best accomplished with 6-0 or 7-0 monofilament or 6-0 fast-absorbing plain gut sutures.

d. Take care when closing deep eyelid tissue—**never place sutures in contact with the surface of the eyeball**.

4. Ptosis secondary to the trauma is best observed for 6 to 12 months and then treated by a levator resection or advancement. Mechanical ptosis from hematoma or tissue edema usually improves slowly.

a. Topical antibiotic ointments give good bacterial prophylaxis and also provide corneal protection in circumstances of poor eyelid closure. Corticosteroids are helpful in the postoperative period to reduce tissue edema. Ice packs and nondependent head positioning are important posttreatment maneuvers.

b. Avoid occluding the eye with pressure patching because of the risk of orbital hemorrhage. Check vision and pupils at regular intervals. The skin sutures usually are removed in 4 to 5 days; however, leave lid margin sutures in place 10 to 12 days.

C. **Open globe**. An open globe is the most serious sight-threatening ocular injury occurring in blunt maxillofacial trauma; this is a laceration with extrusion of intraocular contents. **With a suspected globe laceration, never place pressure on the globe. Even slight pressure can cause extrusion of intraocular contents and reduce the chance of restoring useful vision or avoiding enucleation**. This includes the pressure exerted by the eyelids in a forced squeeze, local anesthesia injection into the periocular region, or inadvertent pressure while closing lacerations on the face.

1. **An immediate ophthalmology consult is required for patients suspected of having an open globe**.

2. Prehospital care of a suspected open globe involves protecting the eye with a plastic or metal shield taped from the forehead to the cheekbone.

a. Additional maneuvers that may help save an eye include administration of pain medication so that the grimacing and Valsalva movements of the patient are avoided.

b. Administer antiemetics to prevent vomiting (which also can further extrude intraocular contents).

3. Perform ocular explorations under general anesthesia without local anesthetics.

4. The most common site for an open globe is at the limbus, the junction between the cornea and sclera. The second most common site for a scleral laceration is just posterior to the insertion of the four recti muscles.

5. Signs that suggest a ruptured globe include:

a. Any distortion of the front of the eye

b. Loss of vision

c. Displaced lens

d. Traumatic hyphema

e. Hemorrhagic chemosis

f. Shallow or deep anterior chamber

6. After the initial evaluation, obtain a computed tomographic (CT) scan of the orbit.

7. Attempt primary repair of all ruptured globes.

8. In the emergency department, prophylactic intravenous (i.v.) antibiotics, usually a cephalosporin, are usually started. Wounds contaminated with

Table 23.4. Open globe evaluation

Vision
"Gentle examination"
Shield
Intravenous or intramuscular medications
Operating room

---

soil or dirt require clindamycin to prevent *Bacillus cereus* endophthalmitis. **Never place topical eyedrops, particularly topical antibiotic ointments, on a lacerated globe because they are toxic to the intraocular contents.**

9. Once an open globe is suspected, further examination of the eye is aborted in the emergency setting and is continued only after the patient is anesthetized in the operating room (OR). This minimizes manipulation of the globe. A shield placed on the eye remains in place until the surgical preparation is done in the OR (Table 23.4).

D. **Intraocular foreign bodies** (IOFB) can be present despite excellent visual acuity. Small metallic fragments can enter the eye without the patient experiencing much discomfort. These metallic pieces are often <1 mm in diameter and can be multiple.

1. Suspect an IOFB in any eye injury, especially in a patient with a history of metal-on-metal hammering. The most useful imaging test is a high-resolution, thin-cut CT scan through the globe. Obtain axial and coronal views. Small IOFB can indicate that other ocular injuries are present, and a detailed ophthalmologic examination must be performed (surgical removal is usually done by vitrectomy) (Table 23.5).

E. **Corneal abrasions** cause pain, the sensation that a foreign body is in the eye, photophobia, chemosis, and decreased visual acuity. Fluorescein will stain the corneal abrasion. Superficial corneal foreign bodies can be removed with irrigation. If the foreign bodies are embedded in the cornea, refer the patient to an ophthalmologist.

F. **Hemorrhage and orbital bone fractures**

1. Orbital fractures can lead to acute, compressive orbital hemorrhage, one of the most urgent ophthalmologic emergencies. The increasing intraorbital pressure and intraocular pressure resulting from an expanding hemorrhage can quickly lead to vascular compromise of the retina and optic nerve and result in permanent vision loss. Timely orbital decompression with a lateral canthotomy may be required to save vision in an eye with an expanding hemorrhage.

2. Of orbital fractures, 40% are associated with serious ocular injuries, including retinal tears and detachments, retinal hemorrhage, vitreous hemorrhage, dislocation of the lens, hyphema, glaucoma, and traumatic cataract. Ocular injuries occur with midface, supraorbital, and frontal fractures. An open globe, retinal detachment, or traumatic optic neuropathy, along with orbital fractures, presents a contraindication to early

Table 23.5. Intraocular foreign bodies evaluation

Visual acuity
Dilated fundus examination
Shield
Computed tomography scan
Operating room

---

bony repair. As a general guideline, fix the globe first. The bone can then be repaired in approximately 2 weeks.

3. Elevated intraocular pressure suggests increased orbital pressure, whereas lower intraocular pressure suggests a penetrating or perforating injury with globe disruption. Recognition of these ocular injuries is essential. Repair of isolated orbital fractures is never an operative emergency, and a complete ocular evaluation should be done before any orbital bone surgery (Table 23.6).

G. **Traumatic optic neuropathies.** Traumatic vision loss with complete blindness occurs in approximately 3% of patients suffering blunt maxillofacial injuries. Of midface, supraorbital, or frontal sinus fractures, 4% are associated with severe optic nerve injuries. Early diagnosis and treatment of optic nerve injuries may avoid irreversible vision loss.

1. With a greater number of patients with closed head trauma surviving, more surviving patients have permanent loss of vision. Decreased visual acuity or visual fields with an afferent pupillary defect in the involved eye points to traumatic optic nerve injury. It is sometimes difficult for the nonophthalmologist to make this determination because multiply injured trauma patients are often uncooperative or even unconscious and, on ophthalmoscopy, the optic disc appears normal. The eyelids may be swollen, and it is technically difficult to evaluate ocular status. It is necessary to examine the pupils to make the diagnosis of an afferent pupillary defect. This can be done, even in an unconscious patient, and also in a patient who has a traumatically dilated pupil.

2. Obtain thin-section CT scans through the orbit and optic canal to exclude the possibility of a bone fracture compromising the optic nerve.

3. High-dose steroids are given intravenously. The loading dose is methylprednisolone (30 mg/kg) i.v., followed by 15 mg/kg 2 hours later, with a maintenance dose (15 mg/kg) i.v. every 6 hours.

4. With improvement in vision over the next 48 to 72 hours, the dosage is continued for 5 days and then tapered rapidly. A surgical optic nerve decompression may be required if vision deteriorates when tapering begins. If, after 24 to 48 hours, no improvement in visual acuity has occurred, discontinue medication (Table 23.7).

H. **Lens.** A blunt injury to the eye can result in clouding (cataract) or displacement of the lens. A sharp injury to the lens capsule can also cause a cataract, but lens particles can also leak into the anterior chamber, resulting in severe uveitis, lens-induced glaucoma, and sometimes lens anaphylaxis (similar to sympathetic ophthalmia). A leaking lens must be removed.

I. **Retina**

1. **Retinal detachment.** Blunt trauma can cause retinal detachment, especially in patients who are nearsighted, have had previous ocular injury, or have had cataract surgery.

   a. Most retinal detachments caused by trauma do not occur at the time of injury, but do occur weeks to months later. Although the risk never drops to zero, most detachments occur within 6 months of injury.

   b. Slow, progressive peeling away of the retina from the underlying choroid from the accumulation of fluid under the retina through a small hole, tear, or disinsertion of the retina causes the detachment.

Table 23.6. General approach to orbital bone fractures

Treat ocular injury
Follow vision
Pupil examinations

Table 23.7. Management of traumatic optic neuropathy

Workup	Medications	Further treatment, based on response
	Methylprednisolone	
Visual acuity	Loading dose 30 mg/kg i.v. followed by 2 hours later with 15 mg/kg i.v.	No visual recovery by 48 hours→ discontinue steroids
Visual field	Maintenance dose: methylprednisolone, 15 mg/kg i.v. every 6 hours	Vision improved→ continue and taper steroids over 5 days
Pupil examination		
Rule out other cause for decreased visual acuity		Optic canal decompression may be required for worsening vision

i.v., intravenous

    c. The diagnosis is suspected when a patient presents with complaints of flashing lights and a curtain or shade interfering with some portion of the visual field. Confrontation visual fields may detect the field loss. The diagnosis is made by indirect ophthalmoscopy through a dilated pupil.
    2. Retina commotion. A finger or other object directly hitting the eye or orbit can cause retinal damage that appears like edema on ophthalmoscopy, but is really damage to the photoreceptors that causes vision decrease and visual field defects. Blood may also appear under the retina. Recovery can be complete or very limited.
  J. Sympathetic ophthalmia. A penetrating injury to one globe can cause the development of sympathetic ophthalmia in the uninjured eye. Sympathetic ophthalmia is a bilateral inflammation (thought to be autoimmune) of the uveal tract (iris, ciliary body, choroid).
    1. Can result in loss of vision in both eyes
    2. Very rare (i.e., 10 to 20 cases annually in the United States)
    3. The risk of sympathetic ophthalmia is thought to be low if enucleation of the injured eye is completed within 10 to 14 days of injury. Only when loss of vision is clearly nonreversible in the injured eye should enucleation be performed.
    4. Corticosteroids can be of benefit in preventing sympathetic ophthalmia.

Axioms
- Determination of visual acuity is essential for early detection of serious eye injury.
- Sutures are never placed in direct contact with the globe.
- If an open globe is suspected, put no pressure on the eye.

Bibliography
Catalano R, Belin M. *Ocular emergencies*. Philadelphia: WB Saunders, 1992.
Cullom RD, Chang B. *The Wills eye manual: office and emergency room diagnosis and treatment of eye disease*. Philadelphia: JB Lippincott, 1990.
Eagling E, Roper-Hall M. *Eye injuries: an illustrated guide*. Philadelphia: JB Lippincott, 1986.
Linberg J. *Oculoplastic and orbital emergencies*. Norwalk, CT: Appleton & Lange, 1990.
Ocular trauma. In: *Advanced trauma life support manual*. Philadelphia: American College of Surgeons, 1993:385–390.
Spoor T, Nesi F. *Management of ocular, orbital and adnexal trauma*. New York: Raven Press, 1988.

24. PENETRATING NECK INJURY

Robert A. Maxwell

I. **Introduction.** Management of penetrating cervical injury has undergone major change during the last decade. Stable patients without obvious evidence of vascular or aerodigestive injury and penetration of the platysma can now be managed nonoperatively, with appropriate diagnostic evaluation, whereas patients with obvious major wounds or airway injury should have traditional operative exploration. Patients **without** violation of the platysma are unlikely to have significant injury and can simply be treated with local wound management. Inappropriate evaluation or management resulting in missed injury can result in mortality rates of 15%. The high density of vascular, neurologic, and visceral structures warrants suspicion of injury and thorough appreciation of cervical anatomy (Fig. 24.1). Stable patients with positive findings on their diagnostic workup should proceed with appropriate intervention.

II. **Initial assessment and management**
   A. Patients with signs of penetrating neck injury or who are unstable; explore promptly once rapid initial assessment is completed and the airway is secured (Table 24.1). **The major initial concern in any patient with a penetrating neck wound is early control of the airway.** Intubation in these patients is complicated by the possibility of associated cervical spine injury, laryngeal injury, and large hematomas in the neck. **The key is to intubate early.** Cervical spine injury may be present and appropriate protective measures must be implemented. **If at all possible, Glasgow Coma Scale and neurologic deficit should be documented before sedation or chemical paralysis** because neurologic status can influence future operative management.

III. **Operative versus nonoperative management.** The initial assessment will generally determine which path of the operative or nonoperative algorithm to take (Fig 24.2). The main factors are **stability**, presence of **hard signs**, and **location of injury**.
   A. **Signs mandating exploration.** Older literature has discussed "hard signs" and "soft signs" for neck exploration; this terminology is confusing. Here, however, indications have been separated into those requiring immediate neck exploration and signs that mandate further workup. Physical findings such as **bleeding, expanding hematoma**, and **stridor** are indicative of major or life-threatening injury that will require surgical intervention (Table 24.1.) Signs that mandate further evaluation in the stable patient include hoarseness, dysphonia or change in voice, hemoptysis, dysphagia or odynophagia, or hematemesis.
   B. **Injury location.** The neck is divided into three **anatomic** zones that dictate the type of operative approach and the structures at risk for injury (Fig. 24.3). For zone II injuries with hard signs, proceed immediately with exploration; the operative approach is generally the same regardless of the structures injured. "Stable" patients with zone I or III injuries should have appropriate workup to identify the anatomy of injury and allow planning of the appropriate operative approach.
      1. **Zone I** extends from the clavicles and thoracic outlet to the cricoid cartilage. The trachea, great vessels, esophagus, thoracic duct, upper mediastinum, and lung apices reside in this area.
      2. **Zone II** extends from the cricoid cartilage to the angle of the mandible. The carotid and vertebral arteries, jugular veins, esophagus, pharynx, trachea, and larynx reside in this area.
      3. **Zone III** extends from the angle of the mandible to the base of the skull; it contains the distal extracranial carotid arteries, vertebral arteries, and jugular veins.

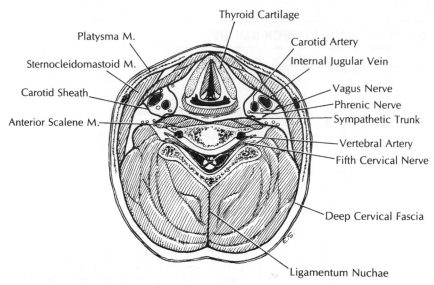

Thyroid Cartilage

Platysma M.

Sternocleidomastoid M.

Carotid Sheath

Anterior Scalene M.

Carotid Artery

Internal Jugular Vein

Vagus Nerve

Phrenic Nerve

Sympathetic Trunk

Vertebral Artery

Fifth Cervical Nerve

Deep Cervical Fascia

Ligamentum Nuchae

FIG. 24.1. Neck anatomy. (From Goodnight JE Jr. Cervical injury. In: Blaisdell FW, Trunkey DD, eds. *Trauma management: cervicothoracic trauma*. New York: Thieme, 1986:96, with permission.)

 C. Mechanism. As in other anatomic locations, **gunshot wounds** are generally more destructive than **stab injuries** and more likely to be associated with a significant injury (~50% of patients with low-velocity gunshot wounds vs 10% to 20% knife stab wounds have injuries requiring operative intervention). High-velocity gunshot wounds require mandatory exploration and debridement.

 D. Frequency of injury. The carotid artery, internal jugular vein, larynx, and esophagus are injured in approximately 5% to 10% of patients requiring exploratory surgery. The vertebral artery is injured in about 1% to 1.5%.

IV. Nonoperative evaluation. For stable patients presenting with zone I or III injuries or zone II injuries without hard signs proceed with appropriate diagnostic workup. This will generally entail arteriography, pharyngoesophagoscopy and tracheobronchoscopy for zones I and II. Injuries that transverse more than one zone require the appropriate combination of diagnostic modalities.

 A. Arteriography. An arteriographic road map is invaluable in excluding injury or planning the operative approach for zone I or III injuries, time permitting. An adequate arteriogram should visualize the innominate, carotid,

Table 24.1. Signs warranting immediate surgical exploration for zone II injuries

Ongoing hemorrhage
Large-sized or expanding hematoma
Bruit
Massive blood loss at scene
Hemiparesis or hemiplegia (presumed carotid injury)
Extensive subcutaneous emphysema
Stridor

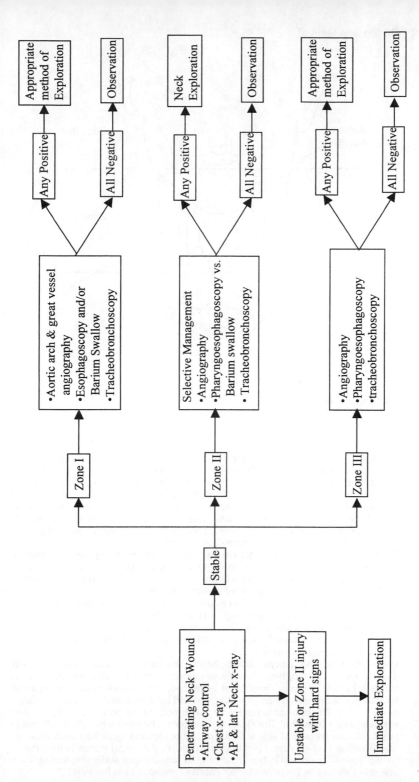

FIG. 24.2. Penetrating neck injury management algorithm.

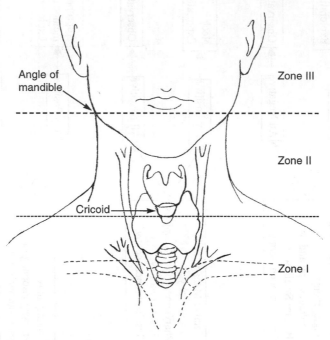

FIG. 24.3. Zones of the neck.

subclavian, and vertebral arteries for zone I and carotids and vertebral arteries for zones II and III. "Four-vessel" arteriography is essential to exclude arterial injury in zone II injuries with signs such as proximity, stable hematoma, or history of significant bleeding. A complete arteriogram for zone II injuries should also include visualization of the inferior thyroid artery via the thyrocervical trunk. The role of magnetic resonance angiography (MRA) and computed tomographic angiography (CTA) are not yet defined in evaluation of cerebrovascular injury.

   B. Endoscopy and esophagography. Alone, either modality has a sensitivity of approximately 60% for detecting esophageal injury. Combining modalities increases sensitivity to approximately 90%, and such should be considered based on trajectory and index of suspicion when a single modality has failed to reveal an injury. Direct pharyngoscopy is essential in evaluating all zone II and III injuries. Laryngoscopy and tracheobronchoscopy are recommended to evaluate zone I and II injuries managed selectively.

   C. Duplex ultrasound for the evaluation of the carotid arteries may be useful in experienced hands.

V. General operative preparation. Active bleeding should be controlled with digital pressure throughout the skin preparation and until direct vascular control is achieved. Wounds should **not** be probed, cannulated, or locally explored because these maneuvers can dislodge clot and lead to uncontrolled hemorrhage or embolism. The patient is generally positioned supine on the operating table with the arms tucked at the sides. Extension of the neck with 15° to 20° rotation to the contralateral side is desirable if the cervical spine has been cleared. Stabilization in the neutral position is necessary if cervical status is uncertain. Skin preparation should extend from the ear to the upper abdomen, and at least one groin should be prepared for potential saphenous vein harvest.

VI. Operative approach. Zone I injuries are usually the most challenging and require the most preoperative planning based on diagnostic workup. In **every operation, exposure is the key to technical success**. Appreciation of the anatomy is essential and care must be taken to avoid injury to the phrenic, vagus, or recurrent laryngeal nerves or thoracic duct whenever operating in the neck. Heparinization can be used to manage carotid injuries, if not precluded by other findings.

   A. Zone I. Life-threatening injuries usually result from zone I injuries and aggressive management is required. A median sternotomy with supraclavicular extension is the most versatile approach when time does not permit preoperative evaluation. Control of the proximal third of the left subclavian artery is initially best achieved through an anterolateral thoracotomy in the third intercostal space (Fig. 24.4). A supraclavicular counter incision is then made for distal control. Extension into a trapdoor sternotomy may then be necessary for definitive repair (Fig. 24.5). Exposure of innominate and zone I common carotid injuries is best achieved through a median sternotomy. Control of the proximal right subclavian and distal two thirds of the left subclavian injuries is best achieved through a supraclavicular incision, with resection of the clavicular head (Fig. 24.6).

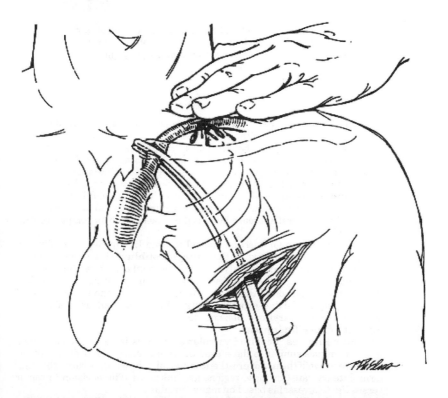

FIG. 24.4. Control of the proximal left subclavian artery can be achieved rapidly through an anterolateral thoracotomy in the third intercostal space. (From Feliciano DV, Graham JM. Major thoracic vascular injury. In: *Rob & Smith's operative surgery: trauma surgery*, part 1. Boston: Butterworth, 1989:289, with permission.)

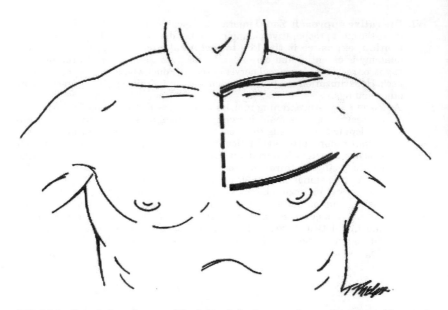

FIG. 24.5. Complete exposure of the left subclavian vessels can be obtained by creating a trapdoor type incision. (From Feliciano DV, Graham JM. Major thoracic vascular injury. In: *Rob & Smith's operative surgery: trauma surgery*, part 1. Boston: Butterworth, 1989:286, with permission.)

    B. Zone II exposure is generally best facilitated by a standard cervical incision along the anterior border of the sternocleidomastoid muscle from the angle of the mandible to the sternal notch (Fig. 24.7). Proximal control is obtained by starting low in the neck and dissecting out the common carotid, followed by distal control above the injury before proceeding directly into the wound tract. This approach then allows adequate visualization of the carotid sheath, trachea, and esophagus as well as other structures in this area. Bilateral injuries or transcervical wounds can be exposed by bilateral cervical incisions or conversion of a unilateral approach into a collar type incision for complex central neck repairs.

    C. Zone III. Exposure for vascular control in zone III injuries generally proceeds similarly to zone II except that **anterior subluxation** of the mandible may be necessary preoperatively to afford maximal exposure. Care must be taken not to damage the hypoglossal nerve when operating in this region. Intracranial extension of the injury will likely require the participation of neurosurgery for further exposure. Notify this team in advance of the possibility that these services will be needed.

VII. Treatment of specific injuries

    A. Vascular injuries. Repair of vascular structures is generally performed with techniques similar to those used in other areas of the body. However, take care to avoid the use of prosthetic material, if possible, because the long-term patency rates in these regions are unknown. The decision to repair versus ligate a vessel is based on many variables.

        a. If a patient is neurologically intact preoperatively, all carotid injuries should be repaired. **The one exception** may be if complete obstruction of flow is found and the clot cannot be adequately back-flushed from the vessel with retrograde flow. Repair can cause embolization.

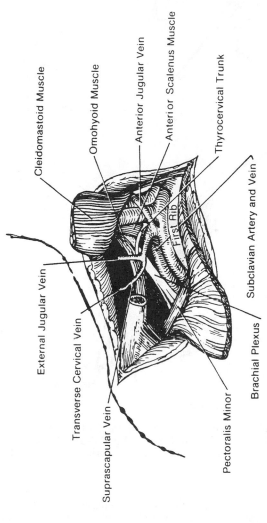

External Jugular Vein

Cleidomastoid Muscle

Transverse Cervical Vein

Omohyoid Muscle

Anterior Jugular Vein

Anterior Scalenus Muscle

Thyrocervical Trunk

First Rib

Suprascapular Vein

Pectoralis Minor

Brachial Plexus

Subclavian Artery and Vein

FIG. 24.6. Proximal exposure of the right subclavian vessels via resection of the clavicular head. (From Flint LM, Snyder WH, Perry MO, et al. Management of major vascular injuries in the base of the neck. *Arch Surg* 1975;106:407–413, with permission.)

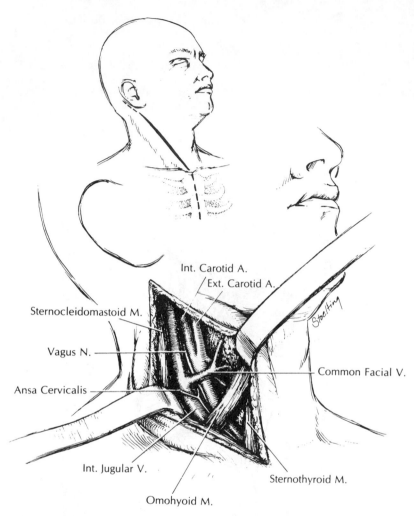

FIG. 24.7. Exposure of zone II injuries through a standard cervical incision. (From Ward RE. Injury to the cervical cerebral vessels. In: Blaisdell FW, Trunkey DD, eds. *Trauma management: cervicothoracic trauma*. New York: Thieme, 1986:273, with permission.)

    b. Controversy arises over preoperative management of patients with neurologic deficits. Patients with mild to moderate deficits should generally have repair, whereas patients with dense hemiplegias or Glasgow Coma Scale scores <8 can have repair if the injury is less than **3 hours** old. In older injuries, repair should generally be avoided to prevent converting an ischemic infarct to a hemorrhagic lesion.

    c. Occasionally, high zone III carotid injuries are not amenable to repair and hemorrhage must be controlled by leaving an inflated Fogarty catheter in place until complete thrombosis of the vessel occurs.

    d. Vertebral artery injuries are difficult to expose operatively and should generally be managed by radiographic embolization if the contralateral

side is patent. Injuries discovered operatively should be packed and taken for radiographic embolization postoperatively.
  e. Injuries to the jugular vein should be repaired primarily, if possible. Extensive injuries requiring an interposition graft should be ligated rather than repaired.
B. **Tracheal injury.** Simple tracheal lacerations can be repaired in a single layer with an absorbable polyglactin suture. Complex injuries can require **tracheostomy**, and extensive injuries can require delayed reconstruction with cartilage graft and fascial flaps. Patients with tracheal injury should remain **intubated** postoperatively until it is certain that they will not develop significant airway edema.
C. **Pharyngeal/esophageal injuries.** Meticulous preoperative pharyngoscopy and operative dissection must be employed to avoid missed injuries. These injuries should be adequately debrided and repaired in two layers. **Rotation of the sternohyoid** muscle over the cervical esophageal repairs will decrease the incidence of fistula formation and obviate the need for drainage. Extensive esophageal injury may require the creation of a cervical esophagostomy.

Axioms

- Patients with obvious major penetrating cervical injuries need early control of the airway.
- Presence of hard signs, radiologic or endoscopic diagnosis, and zone of injury dictate operative management.
- Appropriate choice of surgical approach in zone I injuries is essential in obtaining adequate exposure.

Bibliography

Biffl WL, Moore EE, Rehse DH, et al. Selective management of penetrating neck trauma based on cervical level of injury. *Am J Surg* 1997;174:678–682.

Thal ER, Meyer DM. Penetrating neck trauma. *Curr Probl Surg* 1992;29(1):1–56.

Velmahos GC, Souter I, Degiannis E, et al. Selective surgical management in penetrating neck injuries. *Can J Surg* 1994;37:487 491.

25. BLUNT NECK INJURY

Tiffany K. Bee, Martin A. Croce, and Juan B. Ochoa

I. **Introduction.** Compared with other sites of the body (e.g., head, thorax, abdomen), significant blunt neck trauma is infrequent, with the exception of cervical spine injuries (see Chapter 20). Despite this, awareness of the occurrence of blunt neck injuries is essential for any trauma practitioner because (a) injuries can be devastating, producing high morbidity and mortality; (b) signs of direct injury are often subtle or absent; and (c) once clinical manifestations make the diagnosis obvious, it is often too late for adequate treatment. This chapter discusses the multiplicity of injuries that can occur with blunt neck trauma and to help the reader determine basic principles of diagnosis and treatment.

Three broad types of blunt forces can cause neck injury:

   A. Direct impact to the neck, which can be observed as part of the shoulder restraint of the seatbelt, and also in all-terrain vehicles (ATV) or snowmobile accidents where the driver receives a direct impact to the neck by a clothesline or a wire.

   B. Injuries secondary to excessive extension, flexion, or rotation, which may leave **no** external signs of injury.

   C. Compression injuries (e.g., as that observed with hanging or garroting), in which central nervous system (CNS) manifestations secondary to asphyxiation may be prominent.

II. **Anatomy.** A significant portion of the experience reported in the literature refers to penetrating neck injuries. Clinicians have applied similar principles in the management of blunt trauma. A common and practical approach to neck injuries is to classify them according to the anatomic location of the injury itself. Location determines the structures more susceptible to injury and also helps in designing a diagnostic and therapeutic strategy.

   A. Zones

     1. Zone I: clavicle to cricoid

     2. Zone II: cricoid to angle of mandible

     3. Zone III: angle of mandible to skull base

     As a general principle, injuries to zones I and III are more difficult to approach surgically. Therefore, in physiologically stable patients, most benefit derives from the use of diagnostic maneuvers.

III. **Initial evaluation**

   A. All trauma patients should be systematically evaluated according to the Advanced Trauma Life Support protocols. A high index of suspicion of an occult injury cannot be overemphasized. Most patients will come already immobilized from the scene. Remove the anterior portion of the collar and perform a complete examination while the patient is being provided with adequate inline immobilization (see below).

     1. Airway. Loss of the airway is a life-threatening emergency. Airway loss from blunt neck trauma can occur secondary to (a) expanding hematoma (i.e., retropharyngeal, deep cervical fascia); (b) thyroid fracture or trachea rupture; (c) neurologic injury that produces sensory or motor loss in the aerodigestive tract; and (d) accumulation of secretions and blood. The airway in most conscious patients can be evaluated by assessing the presence of stridor and evaluating the quality of the patient's voice. Obtain control of the airway when abnormalities of oxygenation, ventilation, or sensorium are detected. Oral endotracheal intubation is the route of choice in most patients, unless injuries to the cricothyroid or trachea are suspected, when a tracheostomy is preferred. Be aware that abnormal or obscured anatomic landmarks can make endotracheal intubation a difficult challenge. Obtain the best expertise available and, ideally, have both an anesthesiologist and an experienced surgeon present in the room. **Discuss alternative strategies for securing the airway if your first strategy fails**.

2. **Breathing**
   a. Pneumothorax can occur when laryngeotracheal or esophageal trauma results in tension pneumothorax. Lower neck injuries (zone 1) are also associated with violation of the pleura and the presence of pneumothorax. If a tension pneumothorax is present, needle decompression followed by tube thoracostomy is indicated. Pneumomediastinum can be present, but it usually does not compromise breathing.

3. **Circulation**
   a. Two large-bore peripheral intravenous (i.v.) lines should be placed. Remember, lower neck trauma can be associated with subclavian vein injuries. Therefore, i.v. lines placed in the upper extremities of these patients may not be appropriate.
   b. Careful monitoring of peripheral pulses is necessary, evaluating for signs of deficit. Check for carotid and temporal arterial pulses.
   c. Direct pressure should be applied to bleeding areas in the neck without probing or blind clamp placement. Occult bleeding can occur in the neck, especially in zone I. Expanding hematomas are especially dangerous, with the possibility of loss of airway patency. Bleeding can also be associated with loss of blood flow to the brain, neurologic dysfunction, and loss of airway protection.

B. **Physical examination**
1. **Inspection**
   a. Evaluate the neck for lacerations, abrasions, contusions, crepitation, jugular venous distension, or other gross deformities. Stridor, hoarseness, odynophagia, or dysphagia is suggestive of laryngotracheal or aerodigestive injury. Signs can be subtle, and appear as simple discoloration or minimal abrasions, as observed in seatbelt and "clothesline" injuries.

2. **Auscultation**
   a. A bruit over carotid vessels—an uncommon finding—requires further investigation.

3. **Palpation**
   a. A pulse deficit or thrill is suggestive of vascular injury.
   b. Loss of the normal anatomic contours of the anterior neck, thyroid cartilage, and cricoid cartilage is suggestive of laryngeal fracture.
   c. A defect in the tracheal wall ("step-off") is indicative of a tracheal disruption.
   d. Subcutaneous emphysema is suggestive of pneumothorax or airway injury. It is unlikely that an esophageal injury will cause significant subcutaneous emphysema, but retropharyngeal air will likely be present.

4. **Systemic manifestations**. Fever, tachycardia, and generalized sepsis are signs of missed esophagus or upper aerodigestive tract injuries. Missed injuries of this nature can be especially devastating and must be aggressively approached.

C. **Radiographic evaluation**
1. Lateral cervical spine radiograph
   a. Pretracheal soft tissue thickness >5.0 mm is suggestive of cervical spine fracture.
   b. Signs of subcutaneous emphysema or retropharyngeal air are suggestive of laryngotracheal or esophageal injury.
   c. Cervical immobilization should continue until radiographically and clinically cleared.

2. Chest radiograph
   a. Pneumothorax, subcutaneous emphysema, pneumomediastinum, and pneumopericardium can occur with upper airway injuries.

   b. Tube thoracostomy may be indicated, especially with positive pressure ventilation.
IV. Diagnostic modalities. Patients with expanding hematomas or active hemorrhage should be taken immediately to the operating room. For hemodynamically stable patients, however, further diagnostic evaluation is necessary. Lateral cervical spine and chest radiographs should be obtained in the resuscitation area for all patients with blunt injury. Several modalities used to diagnose specific injuries may be available at a given institution or at different times during the day or night. Therefore, be aware of the advantages and limitations of the diagnostic modalities used. At times, complementary tests need to be done to overcome the limitations of a given test or procedure. For example, the use of a barium swallow along with flexible esophagoscopy can be used to exclude a high esophageal injury. Other tests may depend on the availability of qualified technicians or radiologists. Carefully evaluate the limitations in resources when dealing with a patient suspected of having a blunt neck injury.
   A. Computed tomography (CT) scan
      1. Strengths
         a. Excellent for identifying injuries to the larynx and vertebral column; may identify small collections of extraluminal air in the unusual case of blunt esophageal injury.
      2. Weaknesses
         a. Not sensitive enough for blunt vascular injuries.
         b. Requires time and a physiologically stable patient. Do NOT take the patient for a CT scan if the patient is at a risk of losing his or her airway or of becoming hemodynamically stable.
         c. Requires the use of intravenous contrast.
   B. Laryngoscopy and bronchoscopy
      1. Strengths
         a. Direct visualization of larynx and trachea
      2. Weaknesses
         a. Injury to larynx or trachea can be obscured by the endotracheal tube.
         b. Requires patient cooperation and, frequently, sedation. Perform the procedure where an airway can be easily secured, if airway loss occurs.
   C. Duplex ultrasound
      1. Strengths
         a. Noninvasive test for occlusive carotid disease
      2. Weaknesses
         a. Operator dependent
         b. Difficult with hematoma or subcutaneous emphysema
         c. Unreliable for identification of blunt internal carotid artery dissection
         d. Inadequate examination with cervical immobilization
   D. Angiography
      1. Strengths
         a. Remains the standard for diagnosis of carotid or vertebral artery injuries
      2. Weaknesses
         a. Invasive
   E. Contrast esophagram
      1. Strengths
         a. Barium adequately distends the esophagus for easier identification of injury; water-soluble contrast is inadequate
      2. Weaknesses
         a. Technically difficult in the intubated patient
   F. Flexible esophagoscopy
      1. Strengths
         a. Good visualization of esophagus
         b. Can safely be performed in patient with cervical immobilization (unlike rigid esophagoscopy)
      2. Weaknesses

      a. May be difficult to adequately distend esophagus to identify small injuries

      b. May lack sensitivity for the detection of all injuries

V. Specific injuries

  A. Carotid artery

    1. Common carotid artery

      a. Usually caused by a direct blow to neck, with surrounding soft tissue hematoma or contusion

      b. Can present with hemiparesis that is unexplained by brain CT findings. **Abnormal neurologic clinical findings in the presence of a normal CT scan of the brain demands a full vascular workup.**

      c. Associated facial and cervical fractures are signs of severe trauma and should increase suspicion of vascular injury.

      d. Angiography. A complete four vessel angiogram is necessary to evaluate the presence or lack of cross-filling via the circle of Willis.

    2. Internal carotid artery

      a. Injury usually caused by rapid deceleration with neck rotation and hyperextension, causing the internal carotid to stretch, usually over the second to third cervical transverse process, resulting in an intimal injury. Typically, dissection extends up to the skull base; can be associated pseudoaneurysm. However, external signs of injury can be completely absent when hyperextension or neck rotation occurs.

      b. Delayed diagnosis in 50% of cases. May present with hemiparesis or other neurologic deficit that is unexplained by brain CT findings. Horner's syndrome may be present because of associated injury to the sympathetic fibers, which are in close proximity to the distal internal carotid artery. Although the complete Horner's syndrome is not usually present, miosis typically is.

      c. Complete four-vessel angiography is the standard for diagnosis.

  B. Vertebral artery

    1. Associated with flexion and rotation of the neck, also cervical spine fractures or subluxation. Fractures of the foramen transversarium are likewise associated with vascular injuries.

    2. With associated cervical injuries, angiography is indicated. Again, a four-vessel study is indicated.

  C. Larynx and trachea

    1. Usually caused by a direct blow to the neck.

    2. Generally associated with subcutaneous emphysema and loss of the normal contour of the thyroid cartilage. A palpable defect may be felt in the tracheal wall.

    3. Awake patients with laryngotracheal injuries will assume a position in which they have a patent airway.

    4. The airway must be secured. The best option is a surgical airway using local anesthesia in the operating room.

  D. Esophagus

    1. Usually caused by a direct blow to neck; however, these injuries are rare. Injuries tend to occur at the level of the hypopharyngeal–esophageal junction.

    2. Diagnosis is by barium swallow and endoscopy. The combination of both techniques improves diagnostic accuracy and minimizes the risk of false-negative findings.

VI. Treatment

  A. Carotid artery

    1. Operative management should be reserved for injuries to the common carotid or the proximal internal carotid. Blunt injuries, which are usually dissections (with or without associated pseudoaneurysm), typically extend distally, making primary repair impractical. Interposition grafting is usually necessary, and a long segment may be required. Because controversy exists whether carotid injuries associated with a neurologic deficit should be repaired, seek expertise to manage these patients.

2. Nonoperative therapy, consisting of anticoagulation to prevent clot propagation or embolization, is the primary treatment for blunt, traumatic internal carotid artery dissections. Although continuous heparin is the preferred treatment, use it with extreme caution in patients with associated injuries; it can be relatively contraindicated in patients with cerebral intraparenchymal hemorrhage or contusion. Partial thromboplastin time (PTT) should be closely monitored, and the goal is 40 to 45 seconds. Perform follow-up angiography in approximately 7 days to assess for progression of injury. Therapy can be converted to warfarin and should continue for approximately 6 months. Follow-up studies may include magnetic resonance angiography because it is less invasive than conventional angiography. In the future, treatment may involve stent grafts.

B. **Vertebral artery**
1. Operative management is usually not necessary. Surgical approach is difficult and can be associated with significant bleeding.
2. Nonoperative management is similar to the anticoagulation for internal carotid injuries. Antiplatelet therapy can be substituted in cases of occluded vessels.
3. Radiologic embolization should be reserved for arteriovenous fistula or active extravasation.

C. **Larynx and Trachea**
1. The first priority is to secure the airway, which may require emergent incision and intubation of the disrupted distal trachea.
2. For destructive injuries, tracheal reconstruction may be necessary. Mathison and Grillo have established basic management principles.
   a. Avoid searching for recurrent laryngeal nerves.
   b. Separate tracheal and esophageal suture lines.
   c. Conserve viable trachea.
   d. Avoid tracheostomy through the repair.
   e. Flex the neck to avoid tension on the repair.
3. Manage less destructive injuries (usually to the larynx) with tracheostomy distal to the injury and primary repair of the injury.
4. Treat mild injuries with minimal swelling or nondisplaced cartilage with observation, voice rest, and humidified air.

D. **Esophagus**
1. Operative repair should be undertaken promptly when the diagnosis is made. The esophagus should be repaired in two layers (inner mucosal, outer muscularis). The repair can be buttressed by surrounding strap muscles. Drainage is not necessary for simple repairs. However, if a drain is deemed necessary, it should be a closed suction drain.

Axioms
- The first priority is to obtain a secure airway, as with all trauma patients. This can be difficult in a patient with severe neck trauma.
- Significant injuries to the larynx, trachea, carotid, or esophagus are not common, but are associated with relatively high morbidity and mortality.
- Neurologic deficit associated with a normal CT of the brain mandates four-vessel angiography.

26A. THORACIC INJURY

John P. Pryor, C. William Schwab, and Andrew B. Peitzman

I. **Introduction.** Thoracic injuries account for approximately 25% of all trauma deaths and contribute to an additional 25% of deaths annually in the United States. Death can be immediate (within seconds to minutes), early (minutes to hours), or late (days to weeks) after injury. Immediate deaths usually involve disruption of the heart or great vessel injury. Early deaths are frequently caused by airway obstruction, tension pneumothorax, pulmonary contusion, or cardiac tamponade. Pulmonary complications, sepsis, and missed injuries account for the late deaths.

Most patients with thoracic injury are managed nonoperatively. Treatment options include analgesia, pulmonary hygiene, endotracheal intubation, and tube thoracostomy. Only 10% to 15% of patients with chest trauma will require thoracotomy or sternotomy.

II. **Immediate evaluation**
   A. **Physical examination** includes evaluation of upper airway, chest wall symmetry and stability, breath sounds, and heart tones. Findings of subcutaneous emphysema, jugular venous distention (JVD), and tracheal deviation are specifically sought early in the evaluation.
   B. **Begin resuscitation** while performing concurrent diagnostic procedures. **Administer oxygen** by high flow, non-rebreathing mask. If the patient does not respond adequately to volume resuscitation (persistent hypotension, acidosis, and base deficit), consider ongoing blood loss, and reevaluate for cardiac tamponade, tension pneumothorax, and acute cardiogenic shock (rare from blunt trauma).
   C. Monitor pulse oximetry and electrocardiogram (ECG) continuously.
   D. Obtain a **chest x-ray (CXR)** early in the evaluation of patients with thoracic injury. Sites of missile entry or penetration should be identified with radiopaque markers (e.g., metallic markers, paper clips).
   E. Obtain medical history, arterial blood gas (ABG), ECG.
   F. Identify **indications for immediate operation**.
      1. Massive hemothorax (>1,500 mL blood returned on insertion of chest tube)
      2. Ongoing bleeding from chest (>200 mL/hour for ≥4 hours)
      3. Cardiac tamponade
      4. Acute deterioration from penetrating transmediastinal chest wounds
      5. Chest wall disruption
      6. Massive air leak from the chest tube or major tracheobronchial injury
      7. Vascular injury at the thoracic outlet with hemodynamic instability
      8. Esophageal injury
      9. Radiographic evidence of great vessel injury
      10. Suspected air embolism
      11. Impalement wounds to the chest

III. Immediate management of **penetrating chest wounds**
   A. Avoid probing the wound to determine depth or angle, which can produce pneumothorax or hemothorax.
   B. Obtain a **CXR** with metallic markers placed on all penetrating wounds.
      1. Attempt to **determine trajectory to delineate anatomic injury**.
      2. Perform tube thoracostomy for pneumothorax or hemothorax.
      3. If negative, repeat film in 6 hours; 7% to 10% of this population will develop delayed pneumothorax.
   C. Administer tetanus prophylaxis.
   D. Antibiotics **are not** used for routine penetrating wounds treated without an operation or procedure.

IV. Immediate evaluation of **transmediastinal penetrating wounds** (Fig. 26a.1)

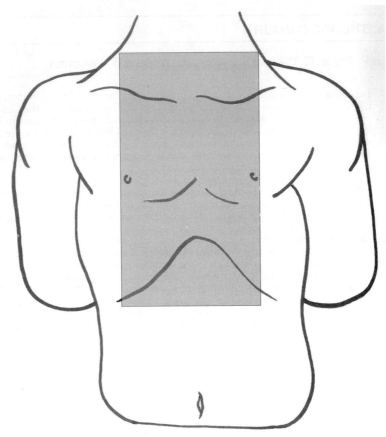

FIG. 26A.1. The box of death. *Shaded area* represents the danger zone for transmediastinal injury.

A. Diagnosis of transmediastinal penetration is based on clinical suspicion, trajectory of the bullet, or CXR findings. Perform a rapid assessment of patient to evaluate airway, hemodynamic status, and the need for hemorrhage control.
B. Classify the patient, based on hemodynamics, as **in extremis, unstable, or stable** (Fig. 26a.2).
C. The patient **in extremis** has agonal respirations without measurable blood pressure.
  1. Intubate, oxygenate, and start volume resuscitation.
  2. Perform immediate left anterolateral thoracotomy to control hemorrhage or relieve cardiac tamponade. If needed, extend across sternum to a right thoracotomy ("clamshell thoracotomy").
D. The **unstable patient** has a measurable blood pressure but is hypotensive, with a systolic blood pressure <100 mmHg. These patients, with associated transmediastinal trajectory, often have injuries to the following organs (in descending frequency): lung, heart, chest wall vessel, great vessels, esophagus, trachea or bronchi, and pulmonary artery or vein.
  1. Assess the need for intubation, oxygenate, and start volume resuscitation.
  2. Obtain a CXR.

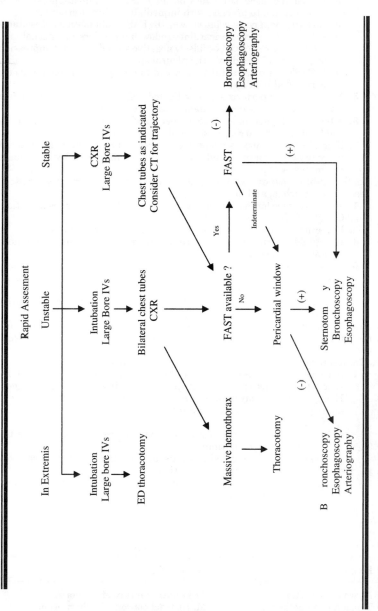

FIG. 26A.2. Diagnostic algorithm for transmediastinal penetrating trauma. Focused assessment sonography for trauma (FAST); chest x-ray (CXR); emergency department (ED), computed tomography (CT).

3. Perform tube thoracostomy for pneumothorax or hemothorax.
4. If available, perform a **focused abdominal sonography for trauma (FAST) ultrasound examination** to diagnose pericardial effusion.
   a. A **positive** pericardial view on the FAST in an unstable patient is an indication to proceed with immediate median sternotomy.
   b. An **equivocal** pericardial view on the FAST examination necessitates either an operative pericardial window or an exploratory sternotomy.
   c. A **negative** FAST can be falsely negative secondary to decompression of pericardial blood into the pleural space.
   d. If FAST is **not available**, proceed to the operating room (OR) for pericardial window.
5. Thoracotomy is performed, as indicated, based on the volume of chest tube return and the hemodynamic stability (see II.F.)
6. After major hemorrhage is controlled, perform flexible esophagoscopy and bronchoscopy to diagnose aerodigestive tract injury.
7. If great vessel injury is suspected by trajectory and the patient is not taken to the OR for other indications, perform **angiography** to evaluate potential vascular injury.

E. In the **stable patient**, evaluate possible injury to the heart, great vessels, esophagus, trachea, and bronchi.
   1. Assess the need for intubation, oxygenate, and start volume resuscitation.
   2. Obtain a CXR.
   3. Perform tube thoracostomy for pneumothorax or hemothorax.
   4. If available, perform a **FAST ultrasound examination** to diagnose pericardial effusion.
   5. If FAST is not available, proceed to the OR for pericardial window, where esophagoscopy and bronchoscopy can be performed at this time or completed postoperatively.
   6. If great vessel injury is suspected by trajectory, perform **angiography** to evaluate potential vascular injury.

V. **Major thoracic injuries** can be divided into those that are immediately life threatening ("lethal six") and those that can be difficult to diagnose ("hidden six") (Table 26a.1).
   A. **Immediately life-threatening injuries** ("lethal six")
      1. **Airway obstruction**. Control of the airway is foremost in trauma resuscitation. Protect the cervical spine as the airway is being managed. However, do not delay definitive airway management because of concern about possible cervical spine injury.
         a. **Causes**
            (1) The tongue most commonly causes airway obstruction in the unconscious patient.
            (2) Dentures, avulsed teeth, tissue, secretions, and blood can contribute to airway obstruction.
            (3) Bilateral mandibular fracture can allow the tongue to collapse into the hypopharynx.

Table 26a.1. Major thoracic injury

Lethal six	Hidden six
Airway obstruction	Traumatic rupture of the aorta
Tension pneumothorax	Major tracheobronchial disruption
Cardiac tamponade	Blunt cardiac injury
Open pneumothorax	Diaphragmatic tear
Massive hemothorax	Esophageal perforation
Flail chest	Pulmonary contusion

      (4) Expanding neck hematomas produce deviation of the larynx and mechanical compression of the trachea.

      (5) Laryngeal trauma (e.g., thyroid cartilage or cricoid fractures) produce submucosal hemorrhage and edema, leading to obstruction.

      (6) Tracheal tear or transection

   b. **Physical findings** include stridor, hoarseness, subcutaneous emphysema, altered mental status, accessory muscle use, air hunger, apnea, and cyanosis (sign of preterminal hypoxemia).

   c. Any suspicion of airway obstruction or inability to exchange air adequately mandates early intubation.

   d. Management (see Chapter 14)

      (1) **When in doubt, intubate** using a controlled rapid sequence.

      (2) Provide inline cervical spine immobilization during intubation.

      (3) Intubate early, especially in cases of neck hematoma or possible airway edema; airway edema can be insidious and progressive and can make delayed intubation more difficult.

      (4) Have equipment for emergency cricothyroidotomy readily available if endotracheal intubation fails.

2. **Tension pneumothorax** occurs when air enters the pleural space from lung injury or through the chest wall without a means of exit. The affected lung collapses, with subsequent mediastinal shift, kinking of the superior and inferior vena cava, impaired venous return, and decreased cardiac output. Ventilation of the contralateral lung is also decreased by the mediastinal shift.

   a. **Most common causes**

      (1) Penetrating injury to the chest

      (2) Blunt trauma with parenchymal lung injury

      (3) Mechanical ventilation with high airway pressure

      (4) Spontaneous pneumothorax with blebs that failed to seal

   b. **Clinical diagnosis—not a radiographic diagnosis**

      (1) Severe respiratory distress

      (2) Hypotension

      (3) Unilateral absence of breath sounds

      (4) Hyperresonance to percussion over affected hemithorax

      (5) Neck vein distention (can be absent in hypovolemic patients)

      (6) Tracheal deviation (late finding—not necessary to confirm clinical diagnosis)

      (7) Cyanosis (preterminal)

      (8) Rapid onset can occur after intubation and positive pressure ventilation

   c. **Treatment**

      (1) Immediately decompress by inserting a 12- or 14-gauge i.v. catheter into the second intercostal space in the midclavicular line or the fifth intercostal space in the anterior axillary line; this converts the tension pneumothorax into a simple pneumothorax.

      (2) Follow immediately with tube thoracostomy.

3. **Pericardial tamponade** is commonly the result of penetrating trauma, but it can also be seen in blunt chest trauma. The pericardial sac does not acutely distend; 75 to 100 mL of blood can produce tamponade physiology in the adult.

   a. **Diagnosis** (Fig. 26a.3)

      (1) If awake, these patients are extremely anxious; they will state that they sense "impending doom," and may appear "deathlike."

      (2) Suspect tamponade in those with persistent hypotension, acidosis, and base deficit, despite adequate blood and fluid resuscitation, especially if ongoing blood loss is not evident.

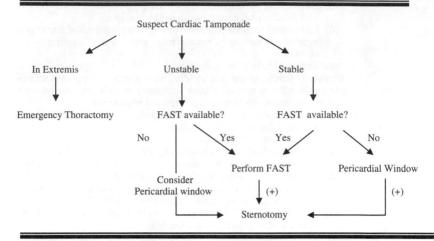

FIG. 26A.3. Diagnostic algorithm for suspected cardiac tamponade. Focused assessment sonography for trauma (FAST).

(3) **Classic signs**: JVD, hypotension, and muffled heart tones (**Beck's triad**) are present in only 33% of patients with confirmed tamponade. JVD may not be present secondary to hypovolemia. **Pulsus paradoxus** is a decrease in systolic pressure of >10 mmHg during inspiration and suggests tamponade. **Kussmaul's sign** is a hard and true sign of tamponade; inspiration in a spontaneously breathing patient results in a rise in central venous pressure. The classic signs of cardiac tamponade are uncommon—**shock or ongoing hypotension without blood loss is the usual trigger to suggest this injury**.

(4) If a pulmonary artery catheter is present, right- and left-side heart pressures will appear to equalize. Central venous pressure approaches the pulmonary arterial wedge pressure, and both will be elevated.

(5) If available, a **FAST ultrasound examination** should be performed to identify pericardial fluid.

  (a) A **positive** pericardial view on the FAST in an **unstable** patient is an indication to proceed with median sternotomy or left anterolateral thoracotomy.

  (b) An **equivocal** pericardial view on the FAST examination or a positive examination in a **stable** patient necessitates an operative pericardial window.

  (c) A **negative** FAST in penetrating injury can be falsely negative secondary to decompression of pericardial fluid into the pleural space.

b. **Treatment**. Generally, the multiple interventions mentioned below occur simultaneously. These can be performed in either the emergency department (ED) or the OR, based on the clinical condition of the patient.

  (1) Assess the need for intubation, oxygenate, and start volume resuscitation.

  (2) Pericardiocentesis can be used as a temporizing maneuver to relieve tamponade until definitive repair is possible. This is often difficult to successfully perform because of the "blind" nature of the procedure and relatively small blood volume in the sac.

(3) If the patient is **in extremis**, an emergent left anterolateral thoracotomy should be performed to relieve the tamponade.

    (a) If the patient is **unstable**, urgent sternotomy should be performed in the OR.

    (b) If the patient is **stable**, a diagnostic pericardial window can be performed in the OR to confirm the diagnosis. If this reveals blood in the sac, extend the incision to a sternotomy.

4. **Open pneumothorax** (sucking chest wound)

    a. Usually caused by impalement injury or destructive penetrating wound (shotgun).

    b. Large open defect in chest wall (>3 cm diameter) with equilibration between intrathoracic and atmospheric pressure

        (1) If the opening is greater than two thirds the diameter of the trachea, then air follows the path of least resistance through the chest wall with each inspiration, leading to profound hypoventilation and hypoxia. Signs and symptoms are usually proportional to the size of the defect.

    c. **Management**

        (1) Intubate, if patient is unstable or in any respiratory distress.

        (2) Close the chest wall defect with a sterile occlusive dressing taped on three sides to act as a flutter-type valve. Avoid securing the dressing on all four sides in the absence of a chest tube, which can produce a tension pneumothorax.

        (3) Perform tube thoracostomy on the affected side. Avoid placing the tube near or through the traumatic wound.

        (4) Perform urgent thoracotomy to evacuate blood clot and treat associated intrathoracic injuries.

           (a) Irrigate, debride, and close the chest wall defect in the OR.

           (b) Large defects may require flap closure.

5. **Massive hemothorax**

    a. Common in penetrating trauma with hilar or systemic vessel disruption

        (1) Intercostal and internal mammary vessels are most commonly injured.

        (2) Each hemithorax can hold up to 3 L of blood.

        (3) Neck veins can be flat secondary to hypovolemia or distended because of the mechanical effects of intrathoracic blood.

        (4) Hilar or great vessel disruption will present with severe shock.

    b. **Diagnosis**

        (1) Hemorrhagic shock

        (2) Unilateral absence or diminution of breath sounds

        (3) Unilateral dullness to percussion

        (4) Flat neck veins

        (5) CXR will show unilateral "white out" (opacification)

    c. **Treatment**

        (1) Intubate a patient in shock or with any respiratory difficulty.

        (2) Establish large-bore i.v. access and have blood available for infusion before decompression.

        (3) If available, have an autotransfusion setup for the chest tube collection system.

        (4) Perform tube thoracostomy with a large tube catheter (36F or 40F) in fifth intercostal space.

           (a) A second chest tube is occasionally necessary to adequately drain the hemothorax.

        (5) Thoracotomy is indicated for:

           (a) Hemodynamic decompensation or ongoing instability because of chest bleeding

           (b) ≥1,500 mL blood evacuated initially

           (c) Ongoing bleeding of >200 mL/hour for ≥4 hours

        (d) Failure to completely drain hemothorax, despite at least two functioning and appropriately positioned chest tubes

    (6) Consider early thoracoscopy for incompletely drained or clotted hemothorax.

6. Flail chest usually results from direct high energy impact. The flail segment classically involves anterior (costochondral cartilage) or lateral rib fractures. Posterior rib fractures usually do not produce a flail segment because the heavy musculature provides stability.

  a. Diagnosis

    (1) Diagnosis is made when two or more ribs are fractured in two or more locations, which often leads to paradoxical motion of that chest wall segment. Patients on positive pressure ventilation may not show this paradoxical motion.

    (2) Diagnosis is clinical, not radiographic.

    (3) Chest wall must be observed for several respiratory cycles and during coughing.

    (4) Blunt force of injury typically produces an underlying pulmonary contusion. Morbidity and mortality are generally related to the lung parenchymal injury rather than the chest wall injury.

    (5) The patient is at high risk for pneumothorax or hemothorax, as both an immediate and a delayed presentation.

    (6) The flail segment, underlying pulmonary contusion, and splinting caused by pain all exacerbate hypoxemia.

    (7) Abdominal injuries occur in approximately 15% of patients.

  b. Management

    (1) Immediately intubate for shock or signs of respiratory distress, such as:

      (a) Labored breathing requiring accessory muscle use

      (b) Respiratory rate >35/minute or <8/minute

      (c) Oxygen saturation <90%, PaO_2 <60 mmHg

      (d) $PaCO_2$ >55 mmHg

    (2) Consider intubation for patients with a history of hemodynamic instability, the need for surgical repair of another problem, chronic obstructive pulmonary disease, cardiac disease, or advanced age.

    (3) Admit patient to the intensive care unit (ICU). The natural progression of the injury is worsening hypoxemia and respiratory insufficiency.

    (4) Control pain (see Chapter 41). Regional analgesia in the form of an epidural block is the most effective way to deliver pain relief for patients with chest wall trauma. Alternatives include:

      (a) Systemic opioids by continuous infusion or patient-controlled anesthesia (PCA)

      (b) Intercostal nerve blocks

      (c) Intrapleural local anesthesia via the chest tube

    (5) Avoid steroids or prophylactic antibiotics.

    (6) Monitor pulse oximetry.

    (7) Provide aggressive pulmonary hygiene, including incentive spirometry and cough-deep breathing. Adequate pain control and CPAP may preclude intubation.

B. Potentially life-threatening injuries ("hidden six")

  1. Traumatic rupture of the aorta is defined as a tear in the wall of the aorta that is contained by the adventitia of artery and the parietal pleura.

    a. The mechanism of injury is rapid deceleration, such as falls from significant height, high-speed motor vehicle crashes, and ejected occupants. Thoracic aortic injury can also occur with lateral crashes or rear-end crashes. Of these victims, 80% die at the scene. The remaining patients are at risk for delayed free rupture into the mediastinum or pleural space.

b. Usually, survivors are initially hypotensive but respond to fluid resuscitation. Because free rupture of the transected aorta is rapidly fatal, persistent or recurring hypotension usually results from a secondary bleeding source, not the aortic injury.

c. Laceration is usually located near the ligamentum arteriosum (85%). Less often, injury is situated in the ascending aorta, at the diaphragm, or in the mid descending thoracic aorta. Survivors usually have a contained hematoma held only by an intact adventitial layer.

d. Diagnosis (Fig. 26a.4)

(1) Clinical signs

    (a) Asymmetry in upper extremity blood pressures and upper extremity hypertension

    (b) Widened pulse pressure

    (c) Chest wall contusion

    (d) Posterior scapular pain, intrascapular murmur

    (e) One half of patients with great vessel injury from blunt trauma have no external signs of blunt chest injury.

(2) Signs on **CXR**

    (a) Widened mediastinum (>8 cm); this is the most consistent finding

    (b) Fracture of first three ribs, scapula, or sternum

    (c) Obliteration of aortic knob

    (d) Deviation of trachea to right

    (e) Presence of pleural cap, usually on the left but occasionally bilaterally

    (f) Elevation and rightward shift of the right mainstem bronchus

    (g) Depression of the left mainstem bronchus >40° from horizontal

    (h) Obliteration of aortopulmonary window

    (i) Deviation of esophagus (nasogastric tube) to right

    (j) Left pleural effusion

    (k) No single sign reliably confirms or excludes aortic injury. However, a widened mediastinum is the most consistent finding on CXR and should prompt further evaluation.

(3) Historically, **aortography** was the gold standard for diagnosis. Approximately 10% of all angiograms are positive when liberal indications are used, and only 2% to 3% are falsely negative.

(4) Chest computed tomography (CT) has recently become a valuable diagnostic tool for aortic injury. Standard CT scanners can characterize mediastinal hematomas that are suggestive of aortic injury. Helical and new high-speed, high-resolution scanners can provide definitive diagnosis of the aortic injury, rivaling angiography with respect to overall accuracy.

    (a) Mediastinal hematomas found on chest CT mandate aortogram for definitive diagnosis.

    (b) Definitive diagnostic aortic injuries found on helical scanners may also require aortography, depending on the practices of the surgeon who will perform the repair.

    (c) Negative scans rule out aortic injury with a 92% sensitivity. Small intimal tears and dissections may be missed on CT scan.

(5) Transesophageal echocardiogram (TEE) may not be as reliable as angiogram in the diagnosis of aortic injury (sensitivity of 63% and specificity of 84%). A positive TEE will confirm the location of the injury and expedite management. If the TEE is negative, an aortogram will be required to reliably exclude the injury. TEE is an excellent alternative for unstable patients who:

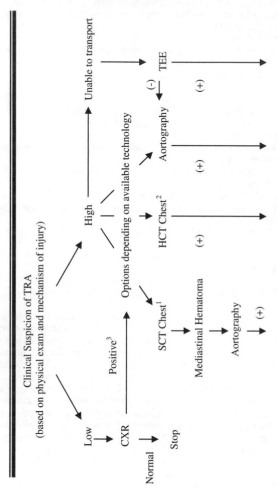

FIG. 26A.4. Diagnostic algorithm for suspected traumatic rupture of the aorta (TRA). [1]Standard computed tomography; [2]helical computed tomography; [3]positive findings are those listed in IV.B.1.d.(2).

[1]Standard conventional computed tomography; [2]Helical computed tomography; [3]Positive = findings listed in (IV.B.1.d.(2)). TEE = Tranesophageal echocardiogram

(a) Must be transported directly to the OR for other cavitary bleeding
(b) Have a very wide mediastinum and a high suspicion of thoracic aortic injury exists
(c) Patients in the ICU who are high risk for transport to radiology.

  e. **Management**
   (1) Establish airway, as needed.
   (2) Control and prevent hypertension. Maneuvers to decrease wall tension in the aorta preoperatively may decrease risk of rupture. Beta blockade should be instituted only after significant hemorrhage from other injuries has been ruled out. The goal for systolic blood pressure should be approximately 100 mm/Hg.
      (a) **Esmolol** is a short-acting beta-blocker that can be easily titrated to desired blood pressure. The loading dose is **500 µg/kg** followed by a continuous infusion of **50 µg/kg/min** titrated to a systolic blood pressure of 100 mmHg and a heart rate <100 beats/minute.
      (b) **Labetolol** is a longer acting beta- and alpha-blocker that can decrease wall tension. An initial i.v. dose of **20 mg** is given. Additional doses can be given to obtain parameters as above, up to **300 mg total**.
      (c) **Nitroprusside** can be added as a second agent if blood pressure is not controlled with beta blockade. It is administered as a continuous infusion at **0.1 µg/kg/min** titrated to effect up to a dose of 10 µg/kg/min.
   (3) If the patient has a stable mediastinal hematoma and concomitant abdominal injury, perform a truncated laparotomy first. Take care not to pack the abdomen tightly or clamp the aorta, causing increased proximal aortic pressure. An intraoperative TEE can be used to evaluate the thoracic aorta.

2. **Tracheobronchial injuries**
  a. Most patients with major airway injuries die at the scene as a result of asphyxia. Those who survive to reach the hospital are usually *in extremis*. An incomplete injury can lead to granuloma formation with late stenosis, persistent atelectasis, and recurring pneumonia.
  b. Location
   (1) **Cervical tracheal injuries**
      (a) Usually present with upper airway obstruction and cyanosis unrelieved with O_2
      (b) Symptoms include local pain, dysphagia, cough, and hemoptysis
      (c) Subcutaneous emphysema
      (d) Blunt transection is uncommon and tends to occur at the cricotracheal junction
   (2) Thoracic tracheal or bronchial injuries
      (a) Of major bronchial injuries, 80% occur within 2 cm of carina.
      (b) Intrapleural laceration. The patient develops persistent dyspnea, massive air leak, and massive pneumothorax that does not reexpand with chest tube drainage. Intraparenchymal injuries usually seal spontaneously if the lung is adequately expanded.
      (c) Extrapleural rupture into the mediastinum. The patient will have pneumomediastinum and subcutaneous emphysema. Respiratory distress may be minimal, especially with partial bronchial transections. Of partial bronchial disruptions, 25% will go undetected for 2 to 4 weeks, but persistent atelectasis, recurrent pneumonia, and suppuration should prompt further investigation.

(d) **Radiographic signs on CXR**
  (i) An abnormal admission CXR will be seen in 90% of cases; findings include pneumothorax, pleural effusion, subcutaneous emphysema, fractures of ipsilateral ribs 1 through 5, and mediastinal hematoma.
  (ii) Specific findings
  • Peribronchial air
  • Deep cervical emphysema; radiolucent line along prevertebral fascia (early and reliable sign)
  • "Fallen lung" refers to a pattern of lung collapse sometimes seen with these injuries. The lung collapses laterally with a medial pneumothorax.
(f) **Management**
  (i) Administer 100% O_2.
  (ii) Perform immediate bronchoscopy if the patient is stable.
  (iii) Place endotracheal tube into mainstem bronchus of uninjured side to improve ventilation of uninjured lung and protect it from spillover bleeding. Consider dual-lumen tube or Univent tube if possible. (Vitaid, Ltd., Lewiston, NY)
  (iv) Definitive treatment includes primary repair with mucosa-to-mucosa closure using nonabsorbable, interrupted polypropylene sutures.
  (v) Exposure for injuries
  • Median sternotomy provides access to the anterior or left lateral portion of the mediastinal trachea.
  • Right posterolateral thoracotomy provides exposure of the right lateral or posterior aspect of the trachea or right lung bronchi or parenchymal injury.
  • Left posterolateral thoracotomy provides access to the left lung bronchi or parenchymal laceration.
3. **Blunt cardiac injury (BCI)**
  a. **Definition**. BCI is a phrase used to describe a spectrum of injury to the heart. It can range from asymptomatic myocardial muscle contusion to clinically significant dysrhythmia, acute heart failure, valvular injury, or cardiac rupture. Critical blunt cardiac injury, particularly that which causes hemodynamic instability, is rare.
    (1) The most common complication of blunt injury to the myocardial is dysrhythmia. The most common dysrhythmia is sinus tachycardia, although other dysrhythmias, including premature atrial contractions, atrial fibrillation, and premature ventricular contractions, are possible. Other ECG changes that may be seen are right bundle branch block or acute current of injury with ST elevation and T-wave flattening. Myocardial injuries that produce significant dysrhythmias usually have ECG abnormalities on admission, although these ECG findings are generally not specific.
  b. **Diagnosis**. Debate is seen in the literature regarding the criteria for the diagnosis and significance of blunt cardiac injury. (Fig. 26a.5).
    (1) An admission 12-lead ECG should be performed as a screening test for all patients suspected of having BCI. An ECG is considered positive if it demonstrates dysrhythmia, atrial or ventricular ectopy, S-T changes, bundle branch block, or hemifascicular blocks.
    (2) If the ECG is positive, an echocardiogram should be considered to assess wall motion and valvular competency. An echocardiogram may be the most sensitive test for the diagnosis of

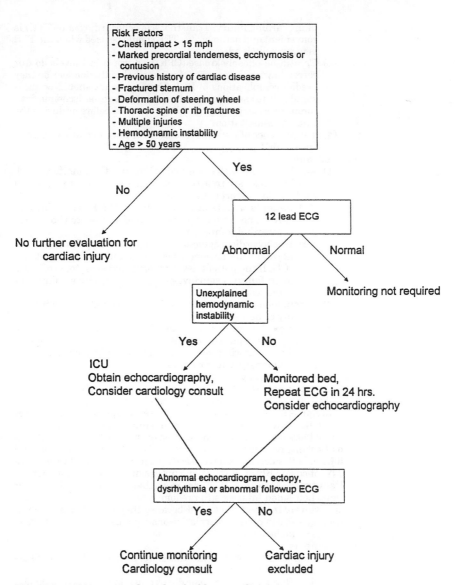

FIG. 26A.5. Diagnostic algorithm for blunt cardiac injury.

blunt cardiac injury. Transthoracic echocardiogram (TTE) is convenient and noninvasive. TEE should be used when the TTE is technically inadequate.

   (3) Creatinine phosphokinase (CPK) and troponin-I levels do **not** correlate with the severity of myocardial contusion; nor do they predict complications of BCI. These enzymes should be measured only to assess potential concomitant cardiac ischemia from coronary occlusion that may have occurred before or during the trauma resuscitation.

   (4) The presence of a sternal fracture does not correlate with presence of BCI.

  c. Treatment

   (1) Admit patients with suspected BCI to an ECG-monitored bed. Dysrhythmias are treated as necessary according to advanced cardiac life support (ACLS) protocol.

    (a) Patients with ischemic changes on the ECG or elevated cardiac enzyme levels are treated similar to those with myocardial infarction.

    (b) If echocardiographic-proved contusion (hypokinesis or abnormal wall movement) is seen, admit the patient to an ICU. If the patient develops signs and symptoms of acute heart failure, begin invasive monitoring with a pulmonary artery catheter.

   (3) Obtain follow-up ECG only for those with an abnormal tracing initially or new signs.

   (4) Blunt cardiac injury is not an absolute contraindication to surgery. If the patient with BCI requires noncardiac surgery, invasive monitoring perioperatively is usually needed (arterial line, pulmonary artery catheter).

4. Diaphragmatic injury

  a. Blunt trauma. Diaphragmatic injury from blunt forces is classically large, radial, and located posterolaterally. The left hemidiaphragm is involved in 65% to 80% of cases. Diaphragmatic ruptures are markers for severe intraabdominal injuries. Central diaphragmatic tears can occur with herniation of the heart. Right diaphragmatic ruptures are markers for severe associated intraabdominal injury. Left-sided tears have associated intraabdominal injuries in 77% of cases. Blunt diaphragm rupture mandates exploration.

  b. Penetrating trauma. Wounds are smaller but tend to enlarge over time. Left-sided injuries still predominate. These injuries need operative repair when diagnosed because they do not heal spontaneously and can produce herniation or strangulation of the intestine as late sequelae.

  c. Diagnosis

   (1) Diagnosis can be difficult, therefore, have a high index of suspicion based on mechanism.

    (a) Rapid deceleration or direct crush to the upper abdomen

    (b) Severe chest trauma, lower rib fractures

    (c) Penetrating injuries to the chest and upper abdomen

   (2) CXR is diagnostic in only 25% to 50% of cases of blunt trauma. Possible findings include:

    (a) Hemidiaphragmatic elevation or lower lobe atelectasis

    (b) Nasogastric tube in left hemithorax

    (c) Stomach, colon, or small bowel in chest

    (d) In penetrating trauma and small defects, the diaphragm appears normal.

    (e) Positive pressure can tamponade viscera herniation and make the CXR appear normal. After extubation, herniation may become apparent on CXR.

(3) Right hemidiaphragm tears are less likely to be diagnosed by CXR because of the presence of the liver in the defect.

(4) CT scan may miss diaphragmatic injury in the absence of gross hollow visceral herniation.

(5) Diagnostic peritoneal lavage (DPL) yields false-negative results in 25% to 34% of diaphragmatic injuries. If an ipsilateral chest tube is present, DPL fluid may be observed exiting the chest tube.

(6) Direct visualization of the injury by laparotomy, laparoscopy, or thoracoscopy remains the gold standard for diagnosis.

d. **Treatment**

(1) Most diaphragmatic tears require repair.

(2) Viscera tend to herniate as a result of changes in intrathoracic pressure during respiration, with strangulation as a possible late complication.

(3) Acute repair is accomplished via laparotomy, in most cases, with nonabsorbable, interrupted horizontal mattress sutures.

(4) Thoracotomy may be needed to reduce large defects in chronic herniation.

(5) Prosthetic material or flaps are rarely needed to close the defect.

(6) The mortality rate is 25% to 40% because of the severity of associated injuries.

5. **Esophageal injury**

a. Most injuries result from penetrating trauma. Blunt injury is rare (<0.1% incidence). Presentation varies according to location of injury:

(1) **Cervical esophagus**: subcutaneous emphysema, hematemesis (see Chapters 24 and 25)

(2) **Thoracic esophagus**: mediastinal emphysema, subcutaneous emphysema, pleural effusion, retroesophageal air, unexplained fever within 24 hours of injury

(3) **Intraabdominal esophagus**: commonly asymptomatic initially; may have pneumoperitoneum, hemoperitoneum

b. **Diagnosis**

(1) Penetrating trajectories involving the mediastinum or neck mandate diagnostic workup to exclude injury to the esophagus.

(2) Many penetrating injuries are detected at the time of emergency thoracotomy or laparotomy.

(3) **Esophagoscopy** and **esophagogram** are used with equal sensitivity (60%). Combining both studies will detect almost all esophageal injuries.

(4) CT scan may have a role in determining trajectory in stable patients.

c. **Management**

(1) **Operative exposure**

(a) **Cervical**: unilateral neck incision along the sternocleidomastoid muscle

(b) **Proximal thoracic**: right posterolateral thoracotomy in fifth intercostal space

(c) **Distal thoracic**: left posterolateral thoracotomy in sixth intercostal space

(2) **Definitive repair**

(a) **Injury <6 hours old**: close primarily in two layers with absorbable suture and cover with pleural or intercostal muscle flap. Distal esophageal repair can also be reinforced with Nissen wrap. Drain.

(b) **Complex injury or >12 hours old**: repair wound as above. Diverting cervical esophagostomy and oversewing of the distal esophagus should be considered with signs of mediastinitis. Wide drainage with chest tubes and feeding gastrostomy are both indicated.

(c) **Injury 6 to 12 hours old**: controversial, however if there is shock with multiple injuries divert as above.

6. **Pulmonary contusion**
   a. The most common potentially lethal chest injury
   b. Caused by hemorrhage into lung parenchyma
   c. Commonly, this accompanies a flail segment or multiple fractured ribs. Pulmonary contusion can also accompany a penetrating injury.
   d. Children may have a pulmonary contusion in the absence of rib fractures because of the resilience of the chest wall.
   e. The natural progression is worsening hypoxemia for the first 24 to 48 hours.
      (1) **Diagnosis**. CXR findings are typically delayed in appearance and nonsegmental. If abnormalities are seen on the admission CXR, the pulmonary contusion is severe. Hemoptysis or blood in the endotracheal tube is a sign of pulmonary contusion.
      (2) **Treatment**
         (a) Although excessive lung water can exacerbate pulmonary contusions, adequate volume resuscitation should not be withheld in patients with other injuries.
         (b) If the fluid status is in question, a pulmonary artery catheter may help facilitate fluid management.
         (c) Prophylactic antibiotics or steroids are **not** indicated.
         (d) **Mild contusion**: give supplemental oxygen, monitor oxygen saturations, perform aggressive pulmonary toilet, and administer analgesia.
         (e) **Moderate to severe contusion**: In addition to above, intubate and mechanically ventilate with positive end-expiratory pressure.
         (f) **Catastrophic contusion**: if the patient is not responsive to conventional ventilation, consider pressure-limiting ventilatory modes, such as pressure controlled or inverse ratio ventilation or high frequency jet ventilation. Extracorporeal membrane oxygenation (ECMO) is an option in centers with this expertise. For severe unilateral contusions, consider independent lung ventilation through a double lumen tube.

VI. **Other thoracic injuries**
   A. **Traumatic asphyxia**
      1. **Definition**
         a. Occurs with a severe crushing injury to the chest or upper abdomen. Intrathoracic and superior vena cava pressures increase and, together with reflux closure of the glottis, produce reversal of flow in the valveless veins of the head and neck with subsequent capillary disruption.
         b. Chest wall, intrathoracic, and intraabdominal injuries (heart, lung, liver) are frequently associated injuries.
         c. Increased intracranial pressure, cerebral edema, and hypoxic brain injury are rare sequelae.
      2. **Diagnosis**
         a. Craniocervical cyanosis, followed by craniocervical rubor
         b. Facial edema
         c. Petechiae
         d. Subconjunctival hemorrhage
         e. Neurologic symptoms (e.g., loss of consciousness, seizures, confusion, and temporary or permanent blindness) occur occasionally.
         f. Hematuria, hematotympanum, or epistaxis occur rarely.
      3. **Treatment**
         a. Elevate head of bed 30°.
         b. Administer oxygen.

    c. Treat any underlying injuries.

    d. Perform adequate pulmonary hygiene.

B. Chest wall injury

    1. Fractures of the scapula or first or second rib result from significant force. The risk of associated intrathoracic injury is >50%.

    2. Sternal fractures. Of these, 40% will have associated rib fractures and 25% will have associated long bone injury.

    3. Fractures of ribs 3 through 8

        a. The main clinical issues are pain and restriction of ventilation.

        b. Search for pulmonary contusion and blunt cardiac injury.

        c. Provide adequate pain relief by epidural anesthesia, PCA, or intercostal nerve blocks.

    4. Fractures of ribs 9 through 12. A 25% risk exists of associated liver (right-sided fractures), spleen (left-sided fractures), or kidney injury.

VII. Emergency thoracic procedures

  A. Tube thoracostomy (Fig. 26a.6)

    1. The usual insertion site is the fourth or fifth intercostal space just anterior to the midaxillary line. Identify the space between the pectoralis major anteriorly and the latissimus dorsi posteriorly (Fig. 26a.6A). Do not insert tubes through traumatic wounds. Use a large caliber tube (≥32F) to ensure adequate drainage of the pleural space.

    2. Prepare and drape the chest.

    3. Anesthetize the site locally with 1% lidocaine (10–20 mL), including the skin, periosteum, subpleural space, and pleura. Except under the most life-threatening circumstances, proper local anesthesia must be used to minimize patient discomfort.

    4. Make a 3- to 4-cm horizontal skin incision below the selected interspace and insert a large, curved hemostat through the subcutaneous tissue and muscle to the upper edge of the rib (Fig. 26a.6B). Separate the intercostal muscles as you pass over the rib.

    5. Puncture the parietal pleura just above the rib, avoiding the neurovascular bundle running along the inferior border. Spread the intercostal muscles.

    6. Remove the clamp and place a finger into the pleural space to confirm appropriate position and to clear any adhesions that may be present (Fig. 26a.6C).

    7. Use the clamp or a finger as a guide to advance the tube into the pleural space. Guide the tube posteriorly and toward the apex of the pleural space (Fig. 26a.6D–F).

    8. If correctly placed, the tube should "fog" with expiration. After placement, run a finger along the tube to confirm proper placement. Confirm that all of the holes are within the pleural space. Rotating the tube 360° ensures that it is not kinked in the chest.

    9. Connect the tube to an underwater-seal apparatus and place at 20 cm of water suction. For known hemothoraces, use an autotransfusion reservoir.

    10. Secure tube with a heavy Prolene or silk suture. Tape all tube connections to prevent separation.

    11. Obtain a CXR.

  B. Chest tube removal

    1. The tube should be removed when:

        a. It has ceased to function (the water level no longer fluctuates with inspiration), **or**

        b. No air leak **and** the drainage of blood or fluid is <100 mL in 24 hours.

    2. After the dressings and sutures have been removed, the tube should be quickly extracted as the patient holds a full inspiration.

        a. Cooperative patients should practice taking a full inspiration and holding this before the actual removal of the tube.

        b. For the patient who cannot cooperate, the tube should be pulled at the end of observed inspiration.

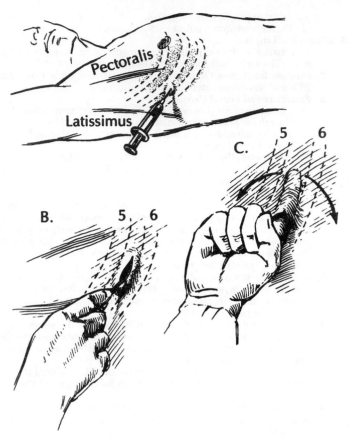

FIG. 26A.6. Steps for chest tube insertion. (From Trunkey DD, Guernsey JM. Surgical procedures. In: Blaisdell FW, Trunkey DD, eds. *Trauma management-cervicothoracic trauma.* New York: Thieme, 1986:310, with permission.)

      c. An occlusive gauze dressing should be secured over the exit site to provide an airtight seal. A dry gauze dressing is placed over this.

      d. A horizontal mattress suture can also be used to close the skin hole.

   3. Repeat CXR. A small pneumothorax after tube removal does not mandate immediate replacement of the chest tube.

C. Pericardiocentesis (Fig. 26a.7)

   1. Indications

      a. Acute distention of the pericardial sac with as little as 75 to 100 mL of blood can produce tamponade physiology. Withdrawal of this fluid is lifesaving. However, it is difficult to tap this small pocket of fluid, especially if it accumulates posteriorly.

      b. When used for diagnosis, pericardiocentesis can produce false-negative results in 50% to 60% of cases because of pericardial blood clotting or needle misplacement.

      c. In acute cardiac tamponade, pericardiocentesis can be used as a temporizing maneuver until definitive pericardiotomy is possible.

      d. Pericardiocentesis is rarely indicated in a level I trauma center.

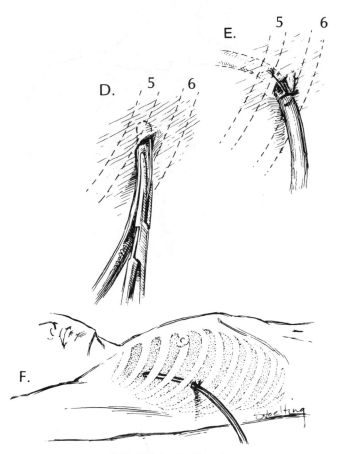

FIG. 26A.6. *Continued.*

2. Technique

    a. A 16- or 18-gauge long (6") needle is connected to a 30-mL syringe. The needle is introduced under the xiphoid and directed toward the left shoulder and at a 45° angle to the skin. Back pressure is placed on the plunger of the syringe as the needle is advanced.

    b. Blood (30 mL) is withdrawn and the clinical situation is reassessed. If no improvement is noted, aspiration is repeated.

3. Complications

    a. Iatrogenic coronary artery injury, myocardial laceration, pneumothorax, hemothorax, and mediastinal hematoma can occur.

    b. False-positive return can occur when the ventricle or a hemothorax is inadvertently tapped.

D. Pericardial window (Fig. 26a.8)

    1. Pericardial window should be considered in the patient who is at risk of having cardiac injury but who has maintained adequate vital signs. As mentioned, pericardial tamponade is rapidly fatal. If the patient is *in extremis* or hypotensive, prompt left thoracotomy is indicated. However, in a more stable patient with a parasternal penetrating wound suggestive

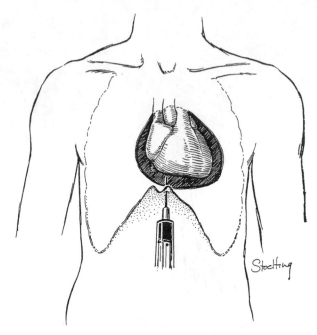

FIG. 26A.7. Pericardiocentesis. (From Rich NM, Spencer FC. *Vascular trauma.* Philadelphia: WB Saunders, 1978:409, with permission.)

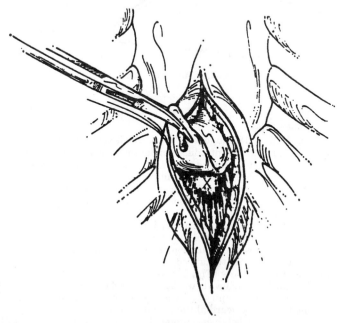

FIG. 26A.8. Pericardial window.

of possible cardiac injury, a pericardial window using a subxiphoid approach is safer and more definitive than pericardiocentesis.
2. **Technique**
   a. Pericardial window is performed in the OR under general anesthesia.
   b. Prepare the patient from chin to mid thighs before the induction of general anesthesia in anticipation of acute hemodynamic decompensation.
   c. An incision is made over the xiphoid process and in the upper midline of the abdomen.
   d. Excision of the xiphoid process may facilitate the procedure. The diaphragmatic attachments immediately deep to the sternum should be freed with finger dissection. The diaphragm can then be retracted toward the patient's feet with Kocher clamps. Reverse Trendelenburg's position helps to expose the pericardium. A sponge stick can be used to mobilize the pericardial fat off the anterior surface of the pericardium. The white pericardium is then identified.
   e. An incision is made with scissors on the anterior surface of the pericardium using forceps to lift the pericardium away from the heart, and the incision is extended 1 to 2 cm.
   f. If blood is found in the pericardial sac, the procedure should be quickly converted to median sternotomy and the cardiac wound definitively repaired. The sternal saw should always be in the OR during pericardial window for the possibility of need for prompt median sternotomy.

Bibliography

Biffl WL, Moore FA, Moore EE, et al. Cardiac enzymes are irrelevant in the patient with suspected myocardial contusion. *Am J Surg* 1994;169:523–528.

Fabian TC, Davis KA, Gavant ML, et al. Prospective study of blunt aortic injury: helical CT is diagnostic and anti-hypertensive therapy reduces rupture. *Ann Surg* 1998;227:666–670.

Ferjani M, Droc G, Dreus S, et al. Circulating cardiac troponin T in myocardial contusion. *Chest* 1997;111:427–433.

Flowers JL, Graham SM, Ugarte MA, et al. Flexible endoscopy for the diagnosis of esophageal trauma. *J Trauma* 1996;40:261–265.

Gammie JS, Pham AS, Hattler BG, et al. Traumatic aortic rupture: diagnosis and management. *Ann Thorac Surg* 1998;66:1295–300.

Guth A, Pachter HL, Kim U. Pitfalls in the diagnosis of blunt diaphragmatic injury. *Am J Surg* 1995;170:5–9.

Heniford BT, Carillo EH, Spain DA, et al. The role of thoracoscopy in the management of retained thoracic collections after trauma. *Ann Thorac Surg* 1997;63:940–943.

Maenza RL, Seaberg D, DiAmico F. A meta-analysis of blunt cardiac trauma: ending myocardial confusion. *Am J Emerg Med* 1996;14:237.

Meyers BF, McCabe CJ. Traumatic diaphragmatic hernia: occult marker of serious injury. *Ann Surg* 1993;218:783–790.

Moon RM, Luchette FA, Gibson SW, et al. Prospective, randomized comparison between epidural versus parenteral opioid analgesia in thoracic trauma. *Ann Surg* 1999;229:684–692.

Reber PU, Schmeid B, Seiler CA, et al. Missed diaphragmatic injuries and their long term sequelae. *J Trauma* 1998;44:183–188.

Richardson JD, Miller FB. Injury to the lung and pleura. In: Feliciano DV, Moore EE, Mattox KL, eds. *Trauma*. Stamford, CT: Appleton & Lange, 1996:387–407.

Richardson JD, Miller FB, Carillo EH, et al. Complex thoracic injuries. *Surg Clin North Am* 1996;76:725–748.

Richardson JD, Flint LM, Snow NJ, et al. Management of transmediastinal gunshot wounds. *Surgery* 1981;90:671–676.

Roszycki GS, Feliciano DV, Oschner MG, et al. The role of ultrasound in patients with possible penetrating cardiac wounds: a prospective multicenter study. *J Trauma* 1999;46:543–552.

Wolfman NT, Myers WS, Glauser SJ, et al. Validity of CT classification on management of occult pneumothorax: a prospective study. *AJR* 1998;171:1317–1320.

26B. THORACIC VASCULAR INJURY

John P. Pryor, C. William Schwab, and Andrew B. Peitzman

I. **Introduction**
   A. Clinical features dictate the initial care of patients with chest injuries. Hemodynamic instability from a chest wound indicates a major vascular or cardiac injury that mandates prompt control of bleeding. Ideally, emergency operations on the chest should be performed in the operating room (OR) after a brief resuscitation. However, cardiac tamponade or exsanguination requires definitive procedures in the trauma resuscitation area. Otherwise, use a structured evaluation with ongoing resuscitation, with operation on those patients with specific injuries (see later) or deterioration.
   B. The chest cavity is more compartmentalized than the abdomen. The bony chest wall, clavicles, and shoulders make operative exposure of injured viscera difficult. Large, relatively fixed structures limit exposure of the posterior mediastinum. The choice of chest incision is determined by the expected anatomic injury, the urgency with which surgical access is required, and the patient's stability. **Control of hemorrhage is the priority and the approach selected must not compromise adequate exposure.**
   C. Patients with severe chest trauma are often initially evaluated by general surgeons and emergency physicians. All surgeons must be proficient in thoracic exposure and control of exsanguinating hemorrhage. After control of major bleeding, intraoperative consultation with a cardiothoracic surgeon is advised. This is especially important with complex injuries to the hilum, coronary arteries or internal structures of the heart. The repair of these complex injuries is beyond the scope of this chapter.

II. **Mechanism of injury**
   A. Blunt thoracic injury is frequently associated with abdominal injuries. In those patients requiring emergency operative control of a thoracic vascular injury, perform either concurrent exploration of the abdomen or diagnostic peritoneal lavage to evaluate for injuries below the diaphragm.
   B. In penetrating injury, the trajectory of the weapon or bullet is the key to determining the anatomic structures at risk.

III. **Presentation and diagnosis**
   A. **Presentation**. Major thoracic or cardiac injuries will frequently present with hemodynamic instability. The goal is to quickly determine that a major injury exists and to prepare for emergent exploration and repair. Patients who arrive unresponsive without a measurable blood pressure are *in extremis* and should have immediate emergency thoracotomy (see section VI).
   B. **Clinical signs of thoracic vascular or cardiac injury**
      1. Hemodynamic instability (hypotension, altered sensorium, or other signs of shock) with a penetrating chest wound
      2. Massive hemothorax (>1,500 mL on insertion of a chest tube, persistent hemothorax on chest x-ray (CXR), or >200 mL/hour for 4 hours)
      3. Cardiac tamponade
      4. Large mediastinal hematoma
   C. **Diagnosis**
      1. Use **CXR** to diagnose a hemothorax or mediastinal hematoma. Penetrating wound sites should be marked with metallic clips to help determine trajectories. Anteroposterior and lateral views can help to determine trajectory. The cardiac silhouette does not change appreciably in acute tamponade.
      2. **Ultrasound**. Focused abdominal sonography for trauma (FAST) examination, with special attention to the pericardial view, can determine the presence of fluid in the pericardium or abdomen.

3. **Tube thoracostomy can be both diagnostic and therapeutic**. Pneumothorax or hemothorax can be confirmed by tube thoracostomy. For patients *in extremis*, thoracostomy should be used as the initial diagnostic and therapeutic intervention, rather than CXR.

D. **Injury complexes**. Certain thoracic vascular injuries can be predicted by the injury mechanism, trajectory, and findings on the initial CXR:

1. **Massive hemothorax** involves injury to pulmonary hilum, proximal subclavian artery on the left, proximal innominate artery on the right, heart with a communication through the pericardium, intercostal artery, internal mammary artery, and azygous vein. For unstable patients who do not respond to chest tube drainage, choice of incision is a **thoracotomy** on side of hemothorax.

2. **Superior mediastinal hematoma** involves injury to innominate artery and vein, subclavian and carotid arteries bilaterally, superior vena cava, and heart. The best approach is through a median sternotomy with extensions into the neck as needed.

3. **Middle mediastinal hematoma** includes heart wound with intact pericardium, aortic arch, proximal innominate, and left proximal carotid and subclavian arteries. Best approached through a sternotomy or posterolateral thoracotomy.

IV. **Initial evaluation and resuscitation**. When a major thoracic vascular injury is suspected, initiate prompt resuscitation while searching for the cause.

A. Perform immediate endotracheal intubation.

B. Place two large-bore intravenous (i.v.) lines for volume infusion, ideally one above and one below the diaphragm.

C. Infuse pre-warmed crystalloids.

1. Transfuse warmed blood immediately, using other blood products as needed (see Chapter 43).

D. Have rapid infusion and cell saver devices immediately available.

E. Administer tetanus prophylaxis and preoperative antibiotics.

V. **Thoracic operations** (Table 26b.1). Position the patient to allow maximal exposure to the chest; including the neck, abdomen, and groins in the operative field. If a median sternotomy is planned, the prepared area must include both lateral chest walls to the bed posteriorly. It also helps to have a beanbag in position under the patient for a thoracotomy incision. If concurrent access to the abdomen is necessary, a modified "taxi hailing" position can be used (Fig. 26b.1). Other preparations include:

A. Double-lumen endotracheal tube, if time permits

B. Large-bore central i.v. access

C. Foley catheter

D. Nasogastric tube

E. Tube thoracostomy of the contralateral hemithorax, if any potential exists for contralateral injury

F. Appropriate padding of potential pressure areas and careful positioning to prevent nerve injury. The surgical team must actively participate in this process.

G. Internal defibrillation paddles

H. Vascular clamps to control pulmonary hilum and atrial appendage bleeding

I. Staplers for lung parenchymal and hilar injury

VI. **Thoracic surgery approaches**

A. **Emergency department thoracotomy (EDT)**. Enthusiasm for EDT has waned over the past several years. The overall mortality of patients receiving EDT is >95%, a marker of the severity of illness rather than technique-related issues. Young patients with an isolated penetrating thoracic injury are the most likely to survive. Other salvageable situations include a patient with a penetrating thoracic wound who has acute deterioration in the hospital, patient with uncontrollable hemorrhage, an unstable patient suspected of having a major thoracic vascular injury, and a patient with clinical evidence of an air embolism because of lung parenchymal or hilar injuries.

Table 26b.1. Conduct of operations for thoracic vascular injury

---

Preparation
–Allow early notice to operating room staff to prepare for thoracic procedures
–Maintain operating room temperature >80° F (27° C)
–Have cell saver and rapid transfuser unit available
–Notify cardiopulmonary bypass (CPB) technicians of possible need for CPB
–Have blood products immediately available
Position
–Median sternotomy—supine with arms out at 90°
　—Prepare from chin to midthighs, laterally to bed
–Emergency department thoracotomy—supine with left arm raised
　—Preparation is deferred
–Urgent left thoracotomy—taxi-hailing position with bump under left back
　—Prepare from chin to pubis and laterally to bed
　—Prepare out left arm
–Right thoracotomy—lateral decubitus position with bean bag
Anesthesia
–Place double lumen tube, if indicated
–Place arterial line in uninjured side
–Chest tubes in cavities not being explored should be put to suction
–Ensure access to peripheral and central intravenous lines
–Place urometer at patient's head to monitor urinary output
–Monitor central temperature via esophagus or bladder
–Warm the patient
　—Surface warming, where possible
　—Fluid warmer
　—Turn humidified heat on ventilator to maximum
Scrub Staff
–Open thoracotomy, sternotomy, and laparotomy sets
–Have long instruments available
–Have aortic clamp immediately available
–Assemble equipment for CPB in room for possible use
–Have GIA, endovascular GIA and TA staplers available

GIA = gastrointestinal anastomasis; TA = thoracoabdominal

1. **Indications (Table 26b.2)**
    a. EDT should be considered in patients who are *in extremis* or in trauma arrest without **vitals signs**, which is defined as a measurable blood pressure or pulse. Patients should then be evaluated for when signs of life (SOL) were present and lost. SOL include:
        (1) Spontaneous movements
        (2) Pupillary response, eye movement
        (3) Spontaneous respirations
        (4) Electrical complexes >40/minute on electrocardiogram (ECG)
    b. In **blunt trauma arrest**, EDT is indicated only if the patient has SOL **on arrival to the hospital**. Patients who have SOL in the field and lose them in route are considered dead on arrival (DOA).
    c. In **penetrating trauma arrest**, EDT is indicated if the patient had SOL in the field. Patients with penetrating injury should receive EDT even if SOL are lost en route. This expanded indication (compared with blunt trauma arrest) is specific because of the higher frequency of reparable lesions being present.
    d. Patients **without SOL in the field**, regardless of mechanism are DOA.
2. **Technique**
    a. Perform a left thoracotomy below the left nipple at the fourth intercostal space. The incision should be made from the edge of the

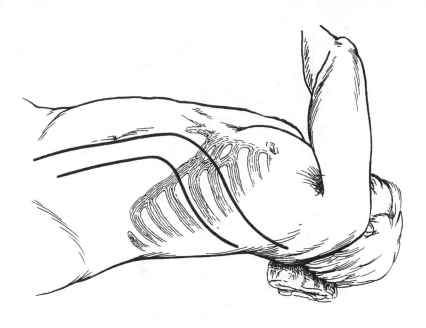

FIG. 26B.1. The "taxi-hailing" position that allows for access to the abdomen and left chest. (Adapted from Rutherford RB. *Atlas of vascular surgery: basic techniques and exposures*, 1st ed. Philadelphia: WB Saunders, 1993:223, with permission.)

sternum to the latissimus dorsi posteriorly (Fig. 26b.2). In a woman, make the skin incision in the inframammary crease. Incise the intercostal muscle with scissors and insert a large rib spreader. Take care to insert the rib spreader with the "T" bar posteriorly near the bed; this will allow free access to extend the thoracotomy across the sternum to the right side if necessary (Fig. 26b.3).

b. Open the pericardium. This relieves tamponade and allows more effective internal compressions. This should be done in the anterior

Table 26b.2. Indications for Emergency Department thoracotomy

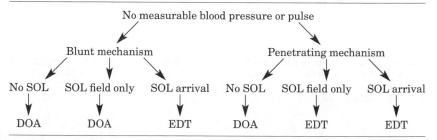

SOL, signs of life = eye movement, pupillary response, spontaneous respiration, electrical activity (>40 complexes per minute) on electrogram. DOA, dead on arrival; EDT, Emergency Department thoracotomy.

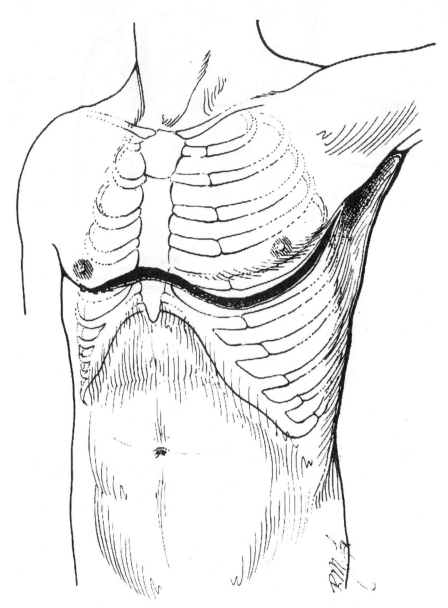

FIG. 26B.2. Emergency department thoracotomy. Extend the incision to the right side below the right nipple for easy access to the right chest. (Adapted from Moore EE, Eiseman B, Van Way CW. *Critical decisions in trauma*, 1st ed. St. Louis: Mosby, 1984:524, with permission.)

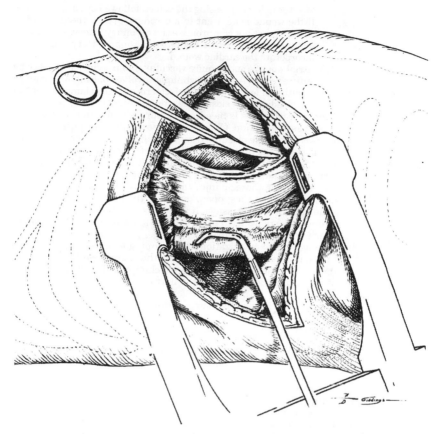

FIG. 26B.3. A view into the left chest during emergency department thoracotomy. A clamp is shown on the descending aorta and a sharp pericardiotomy is shown proceeding cephalad anterior to the phrenic vessels. (Adapted from Moore EE, Eiseman B, Van Way CW. *Critical decisions in trauma*, 1st ed. St. Louis: Mosby, 1984:529, with permission.)

portion of the pericardium in a caudal to cephalad plane, avoiding injury to the phrenic nerve. The opening should extend from the cardiac apex to the root of the aorta.

c. If the heart is not beating, perform internal massage. If the heart is fibrillating, attempt internal cardioversion at 20 J followed by 30 J. If cardioversion fails, temporarily tamponade the ascending aorta and perform gentle internal compression to perfuse the coronaries and reattempt cardioversion.

d. If the myocardium is ruptured or injured, compress the wound together gently or place a finger over the hole. Repair anterior wounds with a 2-0 pledgeted suture. Approximate but do not strangulate the myocardium as the suture is tied.

(1) Do not insert a balloon catheter into the hole, or attempt to place a clamp on a ventricular wound. These maneuvers will often enlarge the hole in the myocardium and block ventricular outflow. If a ventricular wound is found, control bleeding with a finger

over the hole compressing the defect, followed by suture closure. If the wound is adjacent to a coronary artery, the myocardial closure must not compromise the coronary artery. Pass a horizontal mattress suture under the coronary artery and tie it to incorporate the cardiac wound.

    (2) Atrial wounds may require vascular clamp occlusion followed by suture repair. Another technique involves placing Allis clamps on either side of the atrial defect, crossing the clamps to control the bleeding, and closing the wound with 2.0 pledgeted suture.

  e. If the thoracic aorta is bleeding, compress and clamp with a side-biting vascular clamp. Check for the possibility of a posterior hole.

  f. In cases of massive bleeding from the pulmonary parenchyma or the hilum, clamp the hilum. This is best performed by releasing the inferior pulmonary ligament, passing a hand around the vascular structures, and safely guiding a vascular clamp on the hilum.

  g. If no reparable thoracic injury is found, the patient is unlikely to survive. With the chest open, compress the thoracic aorta and continue open cardiac massage. If this successfully restores a palpable carotid pulse in a short period of time, move to the OR for repair of injuries below the diaphragm.

  h. Although aortic mobilization and clamping is useful in experienced hands, it is safer to simply compress the thoracic aorta against the spine without formal mobilization or clamping. This helps avoid the risk of injury to the esophagus or aorta.

B. Median sternotomy

  1. Advantage. Provides excellent exposure of the heart and proximal great vessels, but not the posterior mediastinal structures. The incision can be extended into the neck or supraclavicular for more distal vascular control and repair (Fig. 26b.4).

  2. Disadvantages. Requires a sternal saw or Lipski knife and usually takes more time than left anterolateral thoracotomy; because of this, it is not recommended for EDT. Also, access is limited to the esophagus and descending aorta.

  3. Technique

    a. The patient is supine on the OR table with both arms abducted to 90°.

    b. The skin and subcutaneous tissues are divided from the sternal notch to inferior to the xiphoid onto the upper midline of the abdomen.

    c. A plane on the posterior surface of the sternum is developed bluntly from above and below before division of the sternum with the oscillating saw or Lipski knife. Begin this at the caudal edge of the sternum, and lift the saw or knife and sternum as you proceed in the cephalad direction. Stay in the center of the sternum to avoid injury to the costal cartilages and entry into either hemithorax.

    d. Bone wax may be required for cancellous bone bleeding.

    e. To facilitate exposure of the great vessels, the incision can be extended laterally into the neck, dividing sternocleidomastoid, platysma, strap, and anterior scalene muscles (protecting the phrenic nerve).

    f. Further exposure of the second and third portions of the subclavian vessels can be enhanced by resection or division of the clavicle.

    g. Extension into the abdomen with a midline incision is easily accomplished.

C. Left anterolateral thoracotomy

  1. Advantage. Permits rapid access to the chest, especially for decompression of pericardial tamponade and for repair of the heart, left lung and hilum, and aorta. This can be extended across the sternum (bilateral or clamshell thoracotomy) to access the right chest. Left anterolateral thoracotomy is the best initial operative approach for unstable patients or when the location of the intrathoracic injury is unclear.

  2. Disadvantage. Poor access to the posterior mediastinum, distal subclavian vessels, and right chest.

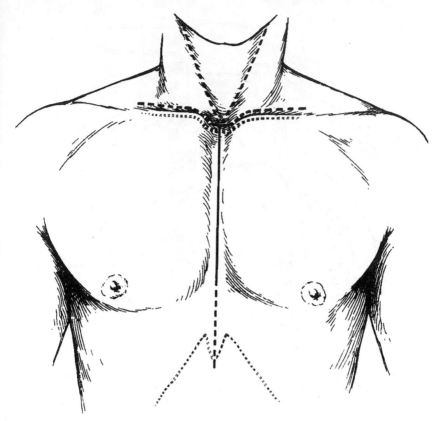

FIG. 26B.4. Extensions of the median sternotomy. Superclavicular and neck extensions are shown (*dotted lines*). (Adapted from Rutherford RB. *Atlas of vascular surgery: basic techniques and exposures*, 1st ed. Philadelphia: WB Saunders, 1993:235, with permission.)

    3. Technique
        a. The patient should have a sandbag under the left chest to tilt the torso 30°. The left arm should be fully extended over the patient's head to provide extension of the incision on the posterior chest wall.
        b. An incision is made in the fourth or fifth intercostal space, from the sternal edge to the scapula.
        c. The muscles are divided with electrocautery and the intercostal muscles are divided or stripped from the rib below to avoid injury to the neurovascular bundle.
        d. A rib spreader is inserted with the "T" bar toward the back and opened widely.
        e. A thoracoabdominal incision can be accomplished by dividing the costal margin with heavy scissors or bone cutters and extending the incision into the abdomen.
D. Bilateral thoracotomy (clamshell thoracotomy) (Fig. 26b.5)
    1. Advantage. Permits wide exposure to all structures in the chest. Best incision for patients with multiple gunshot wounds that violate pleural spaces, bilateral hemothoraces, and superior mediastinal hematomas.

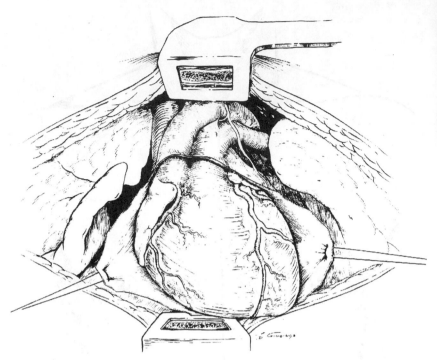

FIG. 26B.5. A view into the chest during a bilateral "clamshell" thoracotomy. Note the excellent exposure of the heart and great vessels. (Adapted from Moore EE, Eiseman B, Van Way CW. *Critical decisions in trauma*, 1st ed. St. Louis: Mosby, 1984:528, with permission.)

2. **Disadvantage**. Large incision, extensive heat loss from wound, both internal mammary arteries are ligated.
3. **Technique**. After the anterolateral thoracotomy, the sternum is divided transversely with heavy scissors, Gigli saw, or sternal saw. The sternal incision is opened with the rib spreader. The incision is extended through the fourth interspace as far into the contralateral chest as possible.

E. **Left or right posterolateral thoracotomy**
1. **Advantages**. Provides excellent access to the hemithorax. The left posterolateral thoracotomy permits access to the aorta and proximal left subclavian artery, the left lung, the left chest wall, and the distal esophagus. The right posterolateral thoracotomy provides access to the trachea, the right lung, the right chest wall, and the proximal esophagus.
2. **Disadvantages**. The decubitus position for the posterior approach leaves little flexibility in gaining access to opposite chest or abdominal structures. Injuries elsewhere cannot be accessed.
3. **Technique**
   a. Use the standard incision for elective thoracic surgery. By varying the interspace used, all regions of the thoracic cavity can be exposed.
   b. The patient is placed in full lateral decubitus position with the upper arm supported over the head, the lower arm extended and padded with an axillary roll, the lower leg is flexed, and the upper leg extended with padding between the knees. The pelvis should be secured with tape and a sandbag (Fig. 26b.6).

     c. Using the tip of the scapula as a landmark, the muscles of the lateral chest wall are divided down to and including the intercostal muscles. In more stable patients requiring less exposure, sparing of the latissimus dorsi muscle is possible.

F. Other approaches include:

    1. Right thoracotomy can be useful for isolated right hemothorax. It is also the incision of choice with high esophageal wounds and wounds to the carina.

    2. Thoracoabdominal incision is useful to expose the inferior thoracic and supraceliac aorta on the left side. It is also indicated to gain control of the proximal thoracic inferior vena cava on the right side.

VII. Specific injuries

    A. Pulmonary hilum

      1. Presentation. Massive hemothorax on side of injury.

      2. Exposure. Anterolateral thoracotomy on the side of injury. Control can also be gained initially through a median sternotomy.

      3. Technique. Control of hilar bleeding can be accomplished initially by manual compression. Quick dissection of the inferior pulmonary ligament

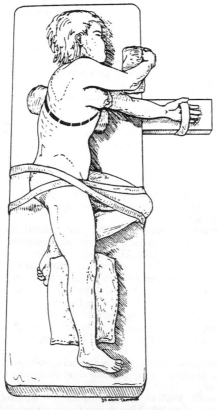

FIG. 26 B.6. Position for an urgent right posterolateral thoracotomy. (From Champion HR, Robbs JV, Trunkey DD. Trauma surgery, parts 1 and 2. In: *Rob and Smith's operative surgery*. London: Butterworth, 1989:273, with permission.)

aids in the isolation and identification of the bleeding site. Exsanguinating hemorrhage can then be definitively stopped with a clamp across the entire hilum. Intrapericardial control of hilar vessels is used for proximal injuries to the pulmonary artery or vein, if necessary. Primary repair is desirable; however, lobectomy should be considered early if bleeding is not easily controlled. Pneumonectomy is rarely required to stop hilar bleeding and carries a high postoperative morbidity and mortality.

B. Aorta and innominate artery
   1. **Presentation**. Superior or middle mediastinal hematoma, but can also present with massive hemothorax if there is a communication with a pleural space.
   2. **Exposure**. The proximal innominate artery and aortic arch are best approached by a median sternotomy. Early ligation of the innominate vein and associated thymic tissue in the anterior mediastinum will aid in exposing the aortic arch. The proximal descending aorta is approached by a posterolateral thoracotomy. Traumatic blunt ruptures of the aorta are typically found in this location just distal to the ligamentum arteriosum.
   3. **Technique**
      a. Control of the aorta at the arch is difficult. Small injuries can be controlled initially with finger occlusion and at times with a side-biting Statinski clamp. Primary repair can be accomplished using nonabsorbable suture with pledgets. Treat proximal innominate artery injuries by ligating proximally and performing a bypass from the aorta to the distal innominate.
      b. Blunt, traumatic rupture of the aorta is repaired either primarily or with a short interposition graft. Options include direct repair without distal shunting, repair with passive shunting of blood distally using a Gott shunt, or repair after active bypass.

C. Carotid artery
   1. **Presentation**. Superior mediastinal hematoma or neck hematoma. Hemiplegia on physical examination is suggestive of a carotid injury.
   2. **Exposure**. Median sternotomy with either a right or left cervical extension along the medial boarder of the sternocleidomastoid muscle (with proximal carotid artery injury).
   3. **Technique**. Primary repair or interposition graft with vein or polytetrafluoroethylene (PTFE). Proximal internal carotid artery injuries can be treated by ligation and reconstitution by performing an end-to-end external to internal carotid artery bypass. Consider simple ligation without bypass for injuries that show no prograde flow preoperatively.

D. Subclavian artery
   1. **Presentation**. Superior mediastinal hematoma or neck hematoma. Proximal injuries on the left can present with massive left hemothorax.
   2. **Exposure**. The proximal right subclavian artery is accessed by a median sternotomy. An infra- or supraclavicular extension is used to gain distal control. The proximal left subclavian artery is best approached through a left lateral thoracotomy through the third intercostal space. Distal control on the left can be accomplished with an infraclavicular incision, with or without removal of the clavicle.
   3. **Technique**. Primary repair or interposition graft with PTFE. Treat proximal injuries by ligation and end-to-side carotid-subclavian bypass.

E. Heart
   1. **Presentation**. Pericardial tamponade, mediastinal hematoma, or massive hemothorax with wounds that communicate through the pericardium.
   2. **Exposure**. Median sternotomy or left anterolateral thoracotomy. Extension of the left thoracotomy across to the right (clamshell) provides excellent exposure to the entire middle mediastinum.
   3. **Technique**. Wounds of the atria and auricles can be controlled with a side-biting Statinski clamp and repaired primarily with 3-0 or 4-0 non-

absorbable suture. Wounds in the ventricle are repaired with individual mattress pledgeted sutures of 3-0 or 4-0 Prolene. Take care not to obstruct coronary vessels in repairs.

F. Intercostal arteries
   1. **Presentation**. Hemothorax or subcutaneous hematoma.
   2. **Exposure**. Thoracotomy on side of injury.
   3. **Technique**. Simple ligation proximal and distal to the injury.

G. Internal mammary artery
   1. **Presentation**. Hemothorax, superior or middle mediastinal hematoma.
   2. **Exposure**. Median sternotomy or anterior thoracotomy.
   3. **Technique**. Simple ligation proximal and distal to the injury. Bilateral internal mammary artery ligation can be performed safely in most patients.

H. Azygous and hemiazygous veins
   1. **Presentation**. Hemothorax
   2. **Exposure**. Thoracotomy on side of hemothorax
   3. **Technique**. Suture ligation proximal and distal to injury. Take care to avoid inadvertent injury to the thoracic duct on the left.

Bibliography

Blostein PA, Hodgman CG. Computed tomography of the chest in blunt thoracic trauma: results of a prospective trial. *J Trauma* 1997;43:13–18.

Eisenberg HM, Middleton JD, Narayan RK. *Resources for the optimal care of the injured patient: 1993*. Committee on Trauma, American College of Surgeons, 1993.

Mitchell ME, Muakkassan FF, Poole GV, et al. Surgical approach of choice for penetrating cardiac wounds. *J Trauma* 1993;34:17–20.

Pate JW. Tracheobronchial and esophageal injuries. *Surg Clin North Am* 1989;69:111.

Richardson JD, Miller FB, Carrillo EH, et al. Complex thoracic injuries. *Surg Clin North Am* 1999;76:725–748.

Richardson JD, Flint LM, Snow NJ. Management of transmediastinal gunshot wounds. *Surgery* 1981;90:671.

Rozycki GS, Feliciano DV, Ochsner G, et al. The role of ultrasound in patients with possible penetrating cardiac wounds; a prospective multicenter study. *J Trauma* 1999;46:543–552.

Schwab CW, Adcock OT, Max MH. Emergency department thoracotomy (EDT): a 26-month experience using an "agonal" protocol. *Am Surg* 1986;52:20–29.

Wall MJ, Granchi T, Liscum K, et al. Penetrating thoracic vascular injuries. *Surg Clin North Am* 1999;76:749–762.

27. ABDOMINAL INJURY

Heidi L. Frankel, Darrell C. Boone, and Andrew B. Peitzman

I. **Overview**. Abdominal injuries are divided into two broad categories, based on the mechanism of injury: **blunt** and **penetrating** abdominal trauma. Abdominal injury is a significant cause of morbidity and mortality; expedient diagnosis and treatment of intraabdominal injuries are essential to avoid preventable morbidity and death. Because management guidelines are different for blunt and penetrating abdominal trauma, they will be discussed separately.

II. **Blunt abdominal trauma**. Motor vehicle crashes account for 75% of blunt abdominal injuries. Other mechanisms include falls, motorcycle or bicycle crashes, sporting mishaps, and assaults.

   A. **Intraabdominal injuries result from:**
   1. Compression causing a crush injury
   2. An abrupt shearing force causing tears of organs or vascular pedicles
   3. A sudden rise in intraabdominal pressure causing rupture of an intraabdominal viscus

   B. **Evaluation**
   1. **Clinical**. Information regarding the mechanism of injury is essential in determining the likelihood of an intraabdominal injury (see Chapter 2). Abdominal examination after blunt trauma is often unreliable. Nearly one half of patients without obvious findings on physical examination will have positive findings at laparotomy. Altered level of consciousness, spinal cord or other distracting injury, and medication or substance effects can further confound the physical examination. Although adjunctive tests are important in the evaluation of blunt abdominal trauma, **careful, repeated physical examination of the patient remains essential in the early diagnosis of abdominal injury**. The choice of adjunctive diagnostic tests depends, in part, on the hemodynamic stability of the patient, the associated injuries and the patient volume at the treating institution (i.e., extremely busy centers may not have the personnel to perform serial physical examinations reliably) (Fig. 27.1).

   In **hemodynamically unstable patients or patients with ongoing fluid requirements**, rapid evaluation of the abdomen while the patient is in the trauma resuscitation area is mandatory. Ultrasound (focused abdominal sonography for trauma [**FAST**]) and diagnostic peritoneal lavage (**DPL**) are appropriate diagnostic tools to determine the presence of hemoperitoneum. In **the stable patient without immediate need for the operating room (OR)**, computed tomography (CT) is the investigation of choice.
   a. **Physical examination**. Evaluation of the patient will often uncover signs of hypoperfusion (e.g., obtundation, cool skin temperature, and delayed capillary refill), which should initiate a search for a source of blood loss. Factors that have been associated with abdominal injury requiring laparotomy include chest injury, base deficit, pelvic fracture, and hypotension in the field or trauma resuscitation area.
      (1) Evaluation of the abdomen may indicate distension or signs of peritoneal irritation (usually associated with injury to a hollow viscus). However, blood in the peritoneum often does not produce peritoneal signs.
      (2) Commonly injured abdominal organs include the liver, spleen, bowel mesentery, and kidney. If the patient is a restrained victim in a motor vehicle crash, particularly with a visible contusion on the abdomen from a lap belt, suspect hollow viscus injury, an injury commonly missed.

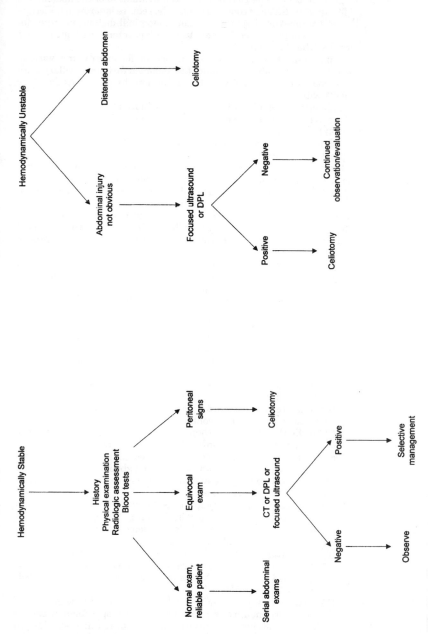

FIG. 27.1. Algorithm for the management of blunt abdominal trauma.

2. **Diagnostic tests**. The goal of the initial evaluation of the abdomen is to identify expeditiously those patients who require laparotomy. Victims of blunt trauma with hypotension and abdominal distension or peritoneal signs should proceed immediately to laparotomy without further workup of the abdomen.

For patients without an obvious indication for laparotomy, various modalities are available to evaluate the abdomen further. Ancillary evaluation above and beyond physical examination should be considered for patients with:

- An abnormal or equivocal abdominal evaluation
- Concurrent injury to the chest or pelvic ring
- Gross hematuria
- A diminished level of consciousness
- Spinal cord injury
- Other injuries requiring a long general anesthetic for management, so that repeat abdominal examination is not feasible
- Diminished capacity to tolerate a delay in diagnosis of abdominal injury (e.g., extremes of age)

The diagnostic test used depends on the mechanism of injury, associated injuries and hemodynamic stability. **Remember that control of cavitary bleeding takes precedence over further diagnostic testing**.

a. **Plain radiographs**. The chest radiograph may reveal a ruptured hemidiaphragm or pneumoperitoneum. Plain abdominal films are rarely productive, but may show retroperitoneal gas or findings associated with abdominal injuries (e.g., fractures of the lumbar spine or lower rib cage).

b. **Laboratory evaluation**. Individual serum tests may not provide evidence of blunt abdominal injury. Patients with blunt injury received promptly from the scene may not be anemic or acidotic on presentation. Similarly, amylase levels can be normal, even with significant pancreatic or intestinal injury.

c. **Focused assessment by sonography in trauma (FAST)** is primarily a rapid, noninvasive means of identifying hemoperitoneum in the trauma resuscitation area and, as such, has replaced diagnostic peritoneal lavage in many centers (Fig. 27.2).

   (1) **Indications** include a hemodynamically unstable patient without obvious indication for laparotomy; any patient requiring prompt transfer to the OR for nonabdominal cause; or use as a screening test for all others requiring abdominal evaluation.

   (2) **Contraindications** include obvious need for laparotomy or lack of FAST expertise.

   (3) **Accuracy**. Sensitivity and specificity (70% to 95%) are generally less than those of CT in detecting hemoperitoneum. It is much less accurate than CT for the detection and anatomic characterization of solid organ injury.

   (4) **Advantages**. Ultrasound is rapid and noninvasive; no need to transfer the patient to the radiology suite; can be performed by a trained member of the trauma team; can be repeated; is less expensive than CT.

   (5) **Disadvantages**. Can miss solid organ injury in the absence of hemoperitoneum or small amounts of hemoperitoneum; cannot distinguish between ascites and blood; requires specialized training and competency; and is difficult to interpret in the obese and in patients with extensive subcutaneous emphysema.

   (6) **Technique of FAST**. A 3 to 5.0 MHz transducer is placed in the subxiphoid region in the sagittal plane to set the machine gain. Sagittal views of Morison's pouch and the splenorenal recess are performed, followed by a pelvic transverse view. Free

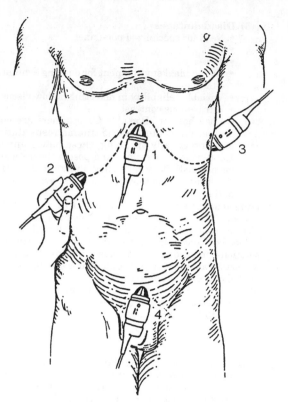

FIG. 27.2. Ultrasound. (From Rozycki GS, Ochsner MG, Schmidt JA, et al. A prospective study of surgeon performed ultrasound as the primary adjuvant modality for injured patient assessment. *J Trauma* 1995;39:493, with permission.)

fluid appears anechoic (black) compared with the surrounding structures.

d. CT can evaluate solid organ injury; intraabdominal fluid, blood, air; and retroperitoneal organ injury in hemodynamically stable patients suspected of having intraabdominal injuries. CT scans should be obtained of the abdomen and pelvis (upper abdominal cuts will show caudad pulmonary parenchyma and may reveal occult pneumothorax; pelvic cuts may reveal dependent hemoperitoneum), using both oral and intravenous (i.v.) contrast.

   (1) Indications. Hemodynamically stable patients requiring abdominal evaluation

   (2) Contraindications. Hemodynamically unstable patients or those with an obvious need for laparotomy

   (3) Accuracy. Recent experience with modern high-resolution scanners shows accuracy rates of 92% to 98%. Hollow viscus and pancreatic injuries are those most likely to be missed by CT.

   (4) Advantages
- Noninvasive
- Reveals solid organ injury with anatomic characterization
- Estimates free fluid volume
- Provides assessment of retroperitoneal injuries

(5) Disadvantages
- Need for specialized personnel
- Cost
- Time
- Not an ideal environment for ongoing evaluation and resuscitation
- Variable reliability in detecting hollow viscus injuries
- Intravenous contrast

(6) On the horizon. Portable CT scanners are currently being used at few centers in the trauma resuscitation area. However, practically speaking, these new scanners still weigh 1,300 pounds, are slow, and pose a theoretical radiation exposure risk. New technology may increase the reliance on CT scanning for thoracoabdominal evaluation in less stable patients.

e. **Diagnostic peritoneal lavage (DPL)** is a rapid and accurate modality for the diagnosis of intraabdominal injury in blunt trauma victims. A catheter is placed into the peritoneal cavity for aspiration of blood or fluid. If this is negative, a liter of warmed normal saline solution is infused (or 10 mL/kg in children) into the abdomen and allowed to drain by gravity. The effluent is sent for laboratory analysis.

(1) Criteria for positive DPL
- 10 mL gross blood on aspiration
- >100,000 red blood cells/mm^3
- >500 white blood cells/mm^3
- Bacteria
- Bile
- Food particles

(2) Indications are as for FAST.

(3) Contraindications are obvious need for laparotomy, previous abdominal operations (relative), pregnancy, or pelvic ring fracture (relative, may be performed supraumbilically).

(4) Accuracy. The sensitivity and specificity of DPL approach 95%. The false-negative rate is 4%.

(5) Advantages. DPL is quick, accurate, sensitive, and low cost.

(6) Disadvantages. DPL is invasive and has a nontherapeutic rate of 15% to 27% (i.e., injuries that have bled into the peritoneal cavity but do not require repair). DPL can fail to detect diaphragmatic and retroperitoneal injuries.

(7) Technique. DPL can be performed in an open, semiopen, or closed technique. In the open technique, skin, subcutaneous tissue fascia, and peritoneum are incised under direct vision for catheter insertion. In the semiopen technique, the catheter is blindly inserted through preperitoneal fat and peritoneum into the peritoneal space. Seldinger technique is used for the closed method.

III. Penetrating abdominal trauma is usually caused by a gunshot wound (GSW) or stab wound. The likelihood of injury requiring operative repair is higher for abdominal GSW (80% to 95%) than for stab wounds (25% to 33%) and the management algorithms differ. Abdominal organs commonly injured with penetrating wounds include the small bowel, liver, stomach, colon, and vascular structures. Any penetrating wound from the nipple line anteriorly or scapular tip posteriorly to the buttocks inferiorly can produce an intraperitoneal injury (Fig. 27.3).

A. **Gunshot injuries.** In most instances, patients sustaining gunshot wounds to the abdomen require laparotomy as their diagnostic and therapeutic modality.

1. **Physical examination.** Carefully inspect the patient so as not to miss wounds. Bullets that do not strike bone or other solid objects generally travel in a straight line. **Trajectory determination is the key to in-**

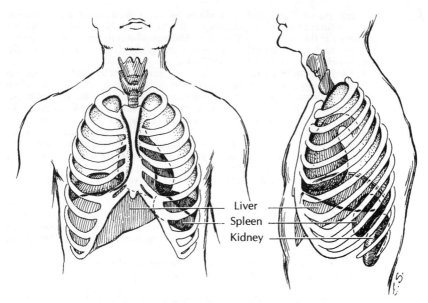

FIG. 27.3. The intrathoracic abdomen. (From Blaisdell FW. Initial assessment. In: Blaisdell FW, Trunkey DD, eds. *Trauma management—cervicothoracic trauma.* New York: Thieme, 1989:6, with permission.)

jury identification. Nonetheless, hemodynamically unstable patients with abdominal GSW should not have extensive evaluation before celiotomy. Carefully examine the patient paying special attention to the body creases, perineum, and rectum. Bullet wounds should be counted and assessed. An odd number of wounds suggests a retained bullet; elongated wounds without penetration typify graze injuries. Palpate the abdomen for signs of tenderness. A neurologic examination should be performed to exclude spinal cord injury.

2. **Plain radiographs** assist in determining trajectory. This is facilitated by marking cutaneous bullet wounds with radiopaque markers. In addition, the presence of pneumoperitoneum, spinal fractures, pneumo-, or hemothorax can be appreciated.

3. **CT scan** has a limited role in the evaluation of patients with abdominal GSW. However, in hemodynamically stable patients in whom it is questioned, peritoneal penetration can be excluded. If any doubt exists, laparotomy is mandatory. In addition, selected patients with right upper quadrant GSW isolated to the liver can be candidates for nonoperative management.

4. **FAST**, similarly, has a limited role in evaluating those with abdominal GSW. It can be useful to assist in operative planning in hypotensive patients with multiple cavitary wounds.

5. **Laparoscopy can be useful** in assessing hemodynamically stable patients with tangential GSW. Its use may prevent unnecessary laparotomy and shorten the hospital stay.

B. **Stab wounds**. Indications for immediate exploration include hypotension, peritoneal signs, and evisceration. If these are not present, a selective management approach is justified. Anterior stab wounds refer to those in front of the anterior axillary line. One third are extraperitoneal, one third are intraperitoneal requiring repair, and one third are intraperitoneal not requiring visceral repair. Flank stab wounds lie between the anterior and posterior axillary lines from the scapular tip to the iliac crest. Back stab wounds are posterior to the posterior axillary line. Abdominal organs are at risk with thoracic wounds inferior to the nipple line anteriorly (ICS 4) and scapular tip posteriorly (ICS 7) (Figs. 27.3 and 27.4).

1. **Serial examination** (selective management) can be used to detect the development of peritoneal signs in a hemodynamically stable patient. The same surgeon should repeat abdominal examinations noting and documenting temperature, pulse rate, and white blood count. With this evaluation method, the delayed laparotomy rate is 40% with <3% mortality.

2. **Local wound exploration** can be performed in the trauma resuscitation area on patients without indications for operation after anterior abdominal stab. The skin is prepared and anesthetized and the original wound is enlarged. Exploration is considered positive if posterior fascial penetration is observed. Patients with positive local wound explorations progress to laparoscopy or laparotomy.

3. **CT scan with triple contrast** (oral, i.v., and rectal) can be used to evaluate back and flank SW with a sensitivity of 89%, specificity of 98% and accuracy of 97%. CT is not helpful in the evaluation of anterior abdominal stab wounds, especially in thin patients with slight abdominal musculature.

4. **FAST** is minimally useful in the workup of stable patients with abdominal stab wounds. If positive, visceral injury can be inferred.

5. **DPL** can be performed to evaluate abdominal stab wounds. The criteria for red blood cell (RBC) counts is generally lower than that for patients with blunt injury (i.e., 1,000 vs 100,000/mm^3). Lower threshold values will improve the sensitivity of the modality, but increase the negative or nontherapeutic laparotomy rate.

C. **Shotgun wounds**. Close-range shotgun wounds are high-velocity injuries. As such, they can result in blast and penetrating abdominal wounds. Shotgun wounds with peritoneal penetration mandate laparotomy. Those delivered from a distance can be evaluated with CT scan to determine peritoneal penetration by pellets.

D. **Impalement injuries**. The impaled object is secured in place and removed in the OR under direct visualization with the abdomen open.

IV. **Conducting an exploratory laparotomy**. Refinements in diagnostic capabilities have allowed a more selective application of laparotomy, reducing the number of nontherapeutic laparotomies without increasing morbidity and mortality.

A. **Indications for exploratory laparotomy**. Laparotomy for trauma can be performed on the basis of physical examination findings alone or on the basis of results of further diagnostic tests.

1. **Clinical**
   - Obvious peritoneal signs on physical examination
   - Hypotension with a distended abdomen on physical examination
   - Abdominal GSW with peritoneal penetration
   - Abdominal stab wound with evisceration, hypotension, or peritonitis

2. **Diagnostic tests**
   - Positive DPL
   - Findings with any other diagnostic intervention (e.g., chest x-ray [ruptured diaphragm, pneumoperitoneum], abdominal ultrasound, abdominal CT, or laparoscopy suggestive of an intraabdominal injury requiring repair)

B. **General setup**
1. **Availability of the OR**. An OR appropriately stocked with appropriate anesthetics and nursing and support staff should be immediately available 24 hours a day.

2. **Rapid transport**. Once the decision is made to operate, the patient must be rapidly transported directly to the OR with appropriate airway support personnel, trauma team surgeons, and trauma team nursing staff in attendance.

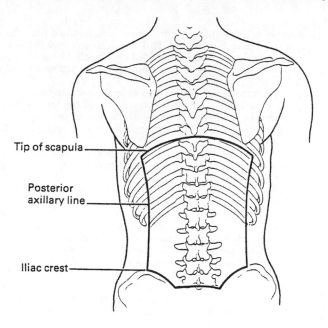

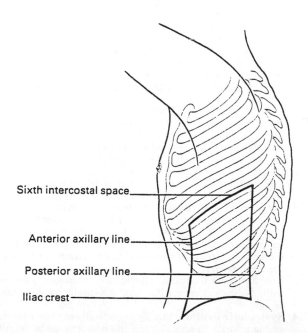

FIG. 27.4. Posterior and flank zones of the abdomen. (From Champion HR, Robbs JV, Trunkey DD, eds. Trauma surgery, parts 1 and 2. In: *Rob and Smith's operative surgery*. London: Butterworth 1989:102, with permission.)

3. **Consent**. If possible, informed consent is obtained from the patient or relative before laparotomy. This is not always possible or practicable, depending on the injuries involved and the clinical state of the patient; in such cases, the operation should proceed without life-threatening delays to obtain consent.

4. **Intravenous lines, tubes, and spinal precautions**
   a. The patient should already have at least two large-bore i.v. placed; other i.v. and arterial access can be placed as necessary in the OR. Control of cavitary bleeding should not be delayed by fluid resuscitation.
   b. Administer broad-spectrum, gram-negative and anaerobic antibiotic coverage (e.g., an extended spectrum penicillin or a third-generation cephalosporin).
   c. Place chest tubes to underwater seal, **not clamped**, during transport and immediately to suction drainage on arrival in the OR.
   d. Place nasogastric or orogastric tubes and a Foley catheter before laparotomy. No procedure should be performed in such a way as to delay control of bleeding and contamination.
   e. Move the patient onto the operating table with appropriate cervical spine and thoracolumbar spine precautions; in many cases, spinal injury will not have been excluded before arrival in the OR. If the patient is still immobilized on a backboard, he or she should be log rolled and the board removed before beginning surgery. **Occult penetrating wounds must be sought before beginning laparotomy**.
   f. Sequential compression devices can be used for hemodynamically stable patients, if readily available.

5. **Rapid infusion system**. Prime the infusion system to infuse blood products and "cell-saved blood" quickly via large-bore lines before the incision releases the tamponade. Ascertain that packed RBC are in the OR and plasma and platelets are available for the patient with active hemorrhage.

6. **Preparation of the patient**. The patient is shaved, and then the entire anterolateral neck (remove anterior portion of cervical collar and then sandbag to maintain cervical spine immobilization), chest to the table bilaterally, abdomen, groin, and thigh region (to the knees bilaterally) are prepared and draped in sterile fashion (see Fig. 18.1).

C. **Initial goals. Stop bleeding and control gastrointestinal contamination**. The exploratory laparotomy for trauma is a sequential, consistently conducted, operative procedure.

1. **Incision**. For urgent laparotomy, a generous midline incision is preferred. Alternative abdominal incisions can be useful for known injuries in stable patients. Adequate exposure is critical. Self-retaining retractor systems and headlights are useful.

2. **Bleeding control**. Scoop free blood and rapidly pack all four quadrants to control bleeding as a first step. **With blunt injuries**, the likely sources of bleeding are the liver, spleen, and mesentery. Pack the liver and spleen, and quickly clamp the mesenteric bleeders. **With penetrating injuries**, the likely sources of significant bleeding are the liver, retroperitoneal vascular structures, and mesentery. Pack the liver and retroperitoneum, and quickly clamp mesenteric bleeding vessels. **If packing does not control a bleeding site, this source of hemorrhage must be controlled as the first priority**.

3. **Contamination control**. Quickly control bowel content contamination using Babcock clamps, Allis clamps, a stapler, rapid temporary sutures, or ligatures.

4. **Systematic exploration**. Systematically explore the entire abdomen, giving priority to areas of ongoing hemorrhage to definitively control bleeding:
   • Liver
   • Spleen

- Stomach
- Right colon, transverse colon, descending colon, sigmoid colon, rectum, and small bowel, from ligament of Treitz to terminal ileum, looking at the entire bowel wall and the mesentery
- Pancreas, by opening lesser sac (visualize and palpate)
- Kocher maneuver to visualize the duodenum, with evidence of possible injury
- Left and right hemidiaphragms and retroperitoneum
- Pelvic structures, including the bladder
    a. **With penetrating injuries**, exploration should focus on following the track of the weapon or missile.
5. Injury repair (section V.A–H)
6. **Closure**
    a. Running nonabsorbable or absorbable monofilament suture (e.g., No. 1 nylon or No. 1 looped absorbable suture)
    b. Leave skin open with delayed secondary closure if there is contamination
    c. If gross edema of abdominal contents precludes closure, absorbable mesh, sterile i.v. bags, or intestinal bags can be used with moist gauze and an impermeable dressing (e.g., Op-Site) to prevent possible abdominal compartment syndrome (see Chapters 28, 29, and 30). Recognize the combination of complex injuries and physiologic signs (generally, hypothermia, acidosis, and coagulopathy) that dictate abbreviated laparotomy (damage control).
V. **Specific organ injuries.** Treatment of organ injuries is similar whether the injury mechanism is penetrating or blunt. An exception to the rule is a retroperitoneal hematoma. Explore all retroperitoneal hematomas caused by penetrating injuries.
    A. **Diaphragm**
        1. **Incidence**
            a. Injuries to the diaphragm account for 1% to 8% of blunt injuries; up to two thirds of ruptures occur on the left; 5% are central; and the heart will be seen through the defect.
            b. High-speed motor vehicle crashes account for 90% of injuries. Injuries from penetrating trauma are generally small.
            c. High incidence of associated intraabdominal injury (60% to 80%); the stomach has usually herniated through the defect, which may not be appreciated in the patient on positive pressure ventilation.
        2. **Anatomy.** The anterior portion of the diaphragm attaches to the inferior portion of the sternum and the costal margin. Posteriorly, the diaphragm is attached to the 11th and 12th ribs. The central portion of the diaphragm is attached to the pericardium. Innervation is via the phrenic nerve (C3–C5).
        3. **Diagnosis.** Clinical diagnosis of diaphragmatic injury is difficult.
            a. Findings can include diminished breath sounds on the affected side, bowel sounds audible in the hemithorax, or a scaphoid abdomen. The patient may complain of respiratory distress, chest pain, or abdominal pain.
            b. A chest radiograph may show hemopneumothorax and an elevated or indistinct hemidiaphragm with a stomach bubble or bowel gas pattern in the hemithorax. Of diaphragmatic ruptures, 40% present as an obvious finding on chest x-ray (CXR); in 40% the CXR is abnormal but not diagnostic; and in 20% the CXR is normal. Placement of a nasogastric tube with a follow-up chest radiograph may confirm displacement of the stomach through a torn diaphragm.
            c. DPL is not sensitive.
            d. Injuries to the diaphragm are easily missed on CT.
            e. Real-time ultrasound, laparoscopy, thoracoscopy, or laparotomy can be useful in equivocal cases.

4. **Treatment**
   a. Approach is via laparotomy with repair for acute injuries.
   b. Perform primary repair with a horizontal mattress suture of non-absorbable material.
   c. Irrigate the thoracic cavity; generally, leave a chest tube in place.
   d. Perform repair via thoracotomy for delayed diagnosis (i.e., injuries presenting after many years); this facilitates lysis of adhesions between lung and abdominal contents.
   e. Selected isolated injuries to the right diaphragm from penetrating mechanisms can be managed expectantly.
5. **Outcome**
   a. The mortality rate is 40% and the morbidity rate is 80%, mostly because of associated injuries.
   b. If diaphragmatic injury is recognized and repaired early, the morbidity related to the diaphragm injury is rare. If a diaphragmatic injury (whether from blunt or penetrating injury) is missed, morbidity is significant.
6. **Organ injury scale (see Appendix A)**

B. **Stomach**
1. **Incidence**
   a. Blunt gastric injuries are rare, with an incidence of 0.9% to 1.8%. Gastric injury occurs in 10% to 15% of penetrating trauma.
2. **Anatomy**. The gastric wall has mucosal, submucosal, serosal, and three smooth muscle layers. The stomach has an extensive blood supply that includes the right gastric, left gastric, right gastroepiploic artery, and the left gastroepiploic and the short gastric arteries. The normal stomach contains few bacteria because of its high acid content.
3. **Diagnosis**
   a. Signs of chemical peritonitis (acid pH) on physical examination
   b. Blood in nasogastric aspirate (present in one third of patients with penetrating gastric wounds)
   c. Free subdiaphragmatic air on CXR in <50% of blunt gastric ruptures
   d. DPL or CT findings
4. **Treatment is operative**
   a. Administer preoperative antibiotics.
   b. Perform laparotomy through a long midline incision. Because other intraperitoneal injuries are generally more immediately life-threatening, address them first. Carefully visualize the gastric wall, including the posterior wall via the lesser sac, the gastroesophageal junction, and the greater and lesser curvatures (where injury may be obscured by the greater or lesser omentum).
   c. Debride and repair the stomach in two layers—the inner layer with running absorbable suture and the outer layer with nonabsorbable suture. Gastric resection is rarely required. Irrigate and remove gastric contents from the peritoneal cavity.
   d. Pyloroplasty may be required to avoid stenosis, or, rarely resection and esophagogastrostomy are necessary for gastroesophageal junction injuries.
5. **The outcome** is generally good. Morbidity and mortality are usually caused by associated injuries, which are common. On the other hand, recent papers have reported a high risk of abdominal infection with gastric injury.
6. **Organ injury scale (see Appendix A)**

C. **Small bowel**
1. **Incidence**
   a. The small bowel is the most commonly injured intraabdominal organ in penetrating trauma; a blunt mechanism of injury is less common, but not rare (5% to 15%).
   b. Small isolated perforations probably result from blowouts of pseudo-closed loops (lap belt injuries).

    c. Larger perforations, complete disruptions, and injuries associated with large mesenteric hematoma or lacerations are caused by direct blows or shearing injury.

    d. Perforation from blunt injury is most common at the ligament of Treitz, ileocecal valve, mid-jejunum, or in areas of adhesions.

2. Anatomy. The adult small bowel averages 6.5 m in length; the proximal 40% is jejunum. The proximal small bowel has few bacteria and is pH neutral; the bacterial content increases toward the distal small bowel. The blood supply is primarily from the superior mesenteric artery (SMA), with drainage via the superior mesenteric vein (SMV).

3. Diagnosis

    a. Suspect small-bowel injury with evidence of an abdominal wall lap belt contusion; also, 30% to 60% risk of bowel injury with a Chance fracture of the lumbar spine.

    b. Small-bowel injury is often not diagnosed on initial presentation. This delay contributes significantly to morbidity and mortality. Small-bowel contents have a neutral pH, so the patient is less likely to have peritonitis on initial examination.

    c. DPL findings generally reveal blood. Positive DPL on the basis of only elevated white blood cell (WBC) count with a negative RBC count is unusual. False-negative DPL findings can occur with small-bowel injury.

    d. CT has a significant false-negative rate in the diagnosis of small-bowel injury. Findings suggestive of small-bowel injury include:

        (1) Fluid collections without solid viscus injury

        (2) Bowel wall thickening

        (3) Mesenteric infiltration

        (4) Free intraperitoneal air

4. Treatment is operative

    a. Perform laparotomy and repair, and administer preoperative antibiotics.

    b. Imbricate antimesenteric wall hematomas with serosal injuries with Lembert stitches to reduce the risk of delayed perforation.

    c. Debride simple lacerations and close transversely to avoid stenosis.

    d. Similarly connect and close adjacent small lacerations (Fig. 27.5).

    e. Resect larger injuries and perform an end-to-end anastomosis.

    f. Injuries to the mesentery of the small bowel, which can bleed massively, must be rapidly controlled, with definitive repair of the small bowel delayed until later in the operation. Injury to the proximal SMA may require a saphenous vein interposition graft or shunting in a damage control scenario.

5. Outcome

    a. The outcome is generally good if the diagnosis is made quickly and the operation is promptly performed. The anastomotic leak rate is 1% to 2%, which can manifest as enterocutaneous fistula, peritonitis, or intraabdominal abscess.

    b. The incidence of subsequent bowel obstruction is 1% to 2%.

6. Organ injury scale (see Appendix A)

D. Colon and rectum

1. Incidence. The colon is injured in 25% of GSW and 5% of stab wounds. Colonic injury occurs in 2% to 5% of blunt injuries. Rectal injuries represent up to 5% of all colon injuries. Blunt rectal perforation can be associated with pelvic fractures or concussion injuries (e.g., injuries from underwater explosions), or with devascularization from mesenteric injury. The morbidity and mortality rates are 5% to 10% with colonic injury and associated injuries.

2. Anatomy. The colon is 1.5 m in length. Its major function is the absorption of water. The predominant organisms are anaerobes, gram-negative

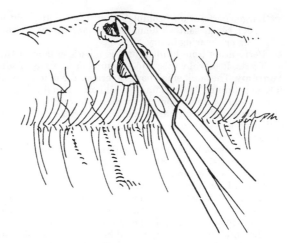

FIG. 27.5. Adjacent small bowel lacerations are connected and closed. (From Champion HR, Robbs JV, Trunkey DD, eds. Trauma surgery, parts 1 and 2. In: *Rob and Smith's operative surgery*. London: Butterworth, 1989:406, with permission.)

enteric organisms, and enterococci. The extraperitoneal rectum is 12 cm in length. The splenic flexure is the "watershed area" in terms of blood supply.

3. **Diagnosis**
   a. Peritoneal signs on examination or free intraperitoneal air. At laparotomy, small injuries in the wall of the colon can be missed. Carefully explore all blood staining or hematomas of the colonic wall.
   b. Gross blood on rectal examination in the presence of a pelvic fracture should prompt proctoscopy in an effort to identify a rectal injury. Consider proctoscopy for any patient with a major pelvic fracture; devascularization of the sigmoid colon may result.
   c. Gross blood on rectal examination with a penetrating abdominal, buttock, or pelvic wound is pathognomonic of colorectal injury. If the patient is hemodynamically stable, perform proctoscopy in the OR to visualize the injury. The location of the injury can be important in planning the operation. **Even if the hole cannot be visualized on proctoscopy, assume the patient has a colorectal injury.** In hemodynamically unstable patients, proceed with laparotomy first.

4. **Treatment is operative**
   a. **Colon**. The conventional treatment for colonic injury involves exteriorization or repair with a proximal diverting colostomy. (This was based on an extremely high pre-World War I (WWI) mortality with nonoperative treatment, a mortality >60% associated with suture closure of colon wounds during WWI, and a 35% mortality during World War II (WWII) when a policy of exteriorization or repair with proximal colostomy was adopted.)
      (1) Current operative options include primary repair of the injury, resection and anastomosis, and colostomy. Recent data have indicated that primary repair (including resection and anastomosis, although this is more controversial) of selected injuries can be applied in most colonic injuries; anatomic location of the injury is not an absolute contraindication to this approach.
         (a) The guidelines for primary repair or resection include minimal fecal spillage, no shock (defined as systolic blood

pressure <90 mmHg), minimal associated intraabdominal injuries, <8-hour delay in diagnosis and treatment, and <1-L blood loss.

   (b) Traditional contraindications to primary repair include extensive intraperitoneal spillage of feces, extensive colonic injury requiring resection, and major loss of the abdominal wall or mesh repair of the abdominal wall; these contraindications have been challenged in recent papers.

   (c) If a primary repair cannot be performed safely, a colostomy or resection and anastomosis are options.

   b. Rectum. Injuries to the rectum should be defined as intraperitoneal rectum or extraperitoneal rectal injuries. Often, intraperitoneal rectal injuries can be primarily repaired. Treat extraperitoneal rectal tears by diverting sigmoid colostomy. Acceptable options include Hartmann resection with end colostomy, end colostomy with a mucus fistula, or loop colostomy with a stapled distal end. If the defect is not readily identified on proctoscopy, do not extensively mobilize the rectum in attempting to identify the hole. Presacral drainage (closed suction or Penrose drains) and irrigation of the distal rectal stump have been recommended, but no consensus exists on these issues.

   c. If a colostomy is necessary in a patient with a pelvic fracture requiring fixation, place the colostomy in the left upper quadrant to facilitate the orthopedic procedure. This procedure can be delayed until the hemodynamically unstable patient is resuscitated.

   d. Perioperative broad-spectrum antibiotics should be administered for colon and rectal wounds.

5. Outcome

   a. Morbidity occurs in proportion to the magnitude of the original injury.

   (1) 1% to 2% incidence of fecal fistula.

   (2) 5% incidence of intraabdominal abscess with primary repair.

   (3) 17% incidence of abscess formation in those requiring colostomy.

   (4) Most postoperative abscesses can be percutaneously drained.

   (5) The mortality rate for pelvic fracture with rectal perforation is 20%.

   (6) Morbidity for the initial trauma laparotomy and subsequent colostomy takedown when colostomy was performed is higher than primary repair in a single procedure. The current approach is to avoid colostomy whenever possible. In the setting of colostomy, return to the OR within the first 10 days for colostomy reversal can be applied.

6. Organ injury scale (see Appendix A)

E. Duodenum and pancreas. Pancreatic and duodenal injuries are listed together because of their shared blood supply and incidence of concomitant injury (Fig. 27.6). Preoperative diagnosis of these injuries is often difficult; operative solutions can be complex.

1. Pancreatic injuries

   a. Incidence

   (1) Relatively uncommon; most are caused by penetrating injury (70% to 75%); constitute <10% of abdominal trauma but represent a major diagnostic challenge, especially in blunt trauma cases. Blunt injury is more common in children. Blunt pancreatic injury generally occurs from a crushing injury of the pancreas between the spine and another object (e.g., steering wheel, handlebar, or blunt weapon).

   (2) Associated intraabdominal injury is found in >90% of pancreatic injuries, with vascular injury responsible for more than half of the morbidity and most of the immediate deaths. Major vascular injury (aorta, portal vein, or inferior vena cava [IVC]) is associated with 50% to 75% of penetrating pancreatic injuries and 12% of blunt pancreatic injuries. Intraabdominal

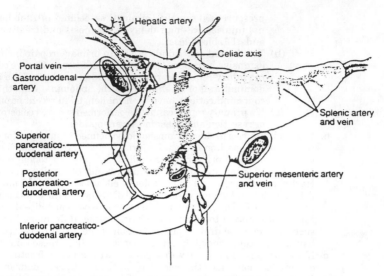

FIG. 27.6. Anatomy of the pancreas. (From Frey W. Abdominal arterial trauma. In: Blaisdell FW, Trunkey DD, eds. *Abdominal trauma*, 2nd ed. New York: Thieme, 1993:346, with permission.)

organs most commonly injured in conjunction with pancreatic injury (whether blunt or penetrating) include the liver, spleen, duodenum, and small intestine. Early deaths are from hemorrhage and late deaths are from infection.

b. Anatomy. The pancreas is retroperitoneal. The head of the pancreas lies to the right of the midline originating at the level of L-2. The body crosses the midline with the pancreatic tail ending in the hilum of the spleen at the level of L-1. The SMA and SMV lie posteriorly in a groove in the neck of the pancreas.

 (1) The main pancreatic duct of Wirsung usually runs the length of the pancreas. The accessory duct of Santorini usually branches from the pancreatic duct in the pancreas and empties separately into the duodenum; in 20%, the accessory duct drains into the main pancreatic duct and in 8% it is the sole drainage of the pancreas.

c. Diagnosis

 (1) Pancreatic injury should be suspected, based on the mechanism of injury and the high incidence of associated intraabdominal injury. Physical examination, FAST, DPL, and CT findings consistent with other injuries may indicate the need for laparotomy in patients with preoperatively unrecognized pancreatic injuries. Isolated pancreatic injury is uncommon.

 (2) Generally, laparotomy is indicated for patients with pancreatic injury because of concomitant abdominal injuries. If not, the initial complaints with pancreatic injury may be vague and nonspecific; 6 to 24 hours after the injury, the patient will complain of mid-epigastric or back pain. Physical findings include nonspecific or mid-epigastric abdominal tenderness. Eventually, the patient will develop peritoneal signs.

 (3) Serum hyperamylasemia is neither sensitive nor specific.

 (4) DPL is not reliable in the diagnosis of retroperitoneal injuries but will frequently identify intraperitoneal blood or the presence of associated injuries.

(5) CT may identify peripancreatic hematomas but may not identify pancreatic lacerations or even complete transections early in the postinjury period.

(6) Endoscopic retrograde cholangiopancreatography (ERCP) or magnetic resonance cholangiopancreatogram (MRCP) can be used to diagnose pancreatic ductal injury in hemodynamically stable patients.

(7) Intraoperative diagnosis depends on visual inspection and bimanual palpation of the pancreas by opening the gastrocolic ligament and entering the lesser sac, and by performing a Kocher maneuver. Mobilization of the spleen along with the tail of the pancreas and opening of the retroperitoneum to facilitate palpation of the substance of the gland may be necessary to determine transection versus contusion. **Identification of injury to the major duct is the critical issue in intraoperative management of pancreatic injury**.

   (a) Intraoperative pancreatography may be useful for suspected pancreatic head ductal injuries but is rarely needed with careful inspection and palpation of the pancreas.

d. Treatment. Suspected pancreatic injuries should be surgically explored. Treatment principles include

(1) Control hemorrhage

(2) Debride devitalized pancreas, which can require resection

(3) Preserve maximal amount of viable pancreatic tissue

(4) Wide drainage of pancreatic secretions with closed-suction drains

(5) Feeding jejunostomy for postoperative care with significant lesions

e. Treatment options

(1) **Pancreatic contusion or capsular laceration without ductal injury → wide drainage**. Do not repair capsular lacerations; this can produce a pseudocyst. The operative goal is to develop a controlled pancreatic fistula postoperatively, which will generally close spontaneously.

(2) **Pancreatic transection distal to the SMA → distal pancreatectomy**. Attempt splenic conservation in the stable patient. Control the resection line by stapling the pancreatic stump or closing with horizontal mattress sutures made with nonabsorbable materials. Attempt to visualize and directly oversew the pancreatic duct. Place closed suction drains.

(3) **Pancreatic transection to the right of the SMA (not involving the ampulla) → no optimal operation**. The options include wide drainage of the area of injury to develop a controlled pancreatic fistula; ligation of both ends of the distal duct and wide drainage; and oversewing the proximal pancreas and performing a Roux-en-Y jejunostomy to the distal pancreas (indicated uncommonly).

(4) Severe injury to both the head of the pancreas and the duodenum may require pancreaticoduodenectomy; however, this is rarely indicated. It can be performed in staged, damage control fashion.

f. Outcome

(1) 70% to 35% incidence of pancreatic fistula; most spontaneously resolve.

(2) Intraabdominal abscess or wound infection is also common.

(3) 5% incidence of true pancreatic abscess

(4) Pancreatitis occurs in 8% to 18% of these patients.

(5) Pancreatic pseudocysts can occur.

g. Organ injury scale (see Appendix A)

2. Duodenal injuries

a. Incidence. Most injuries are from penetrating trauma, predominantly GSW. Blunt mechanisms account for 20% to 25% of duodenal injuries; the duodenum can be compressed between the spine and steering wheel, lap belt, or handlebars. The second portion of the duodenum is most commonly injured. Delays in diagnosis are common and significantly increase morbidity and mortality. Duodenal injury rarely is an isolated abdominal injury; up to 98% have associated abdominal injuries. Commonly associated injuries include (in order of decreasing frequency): liver, pancreas, small bowel, colon, IVC, portal vein, and aorta.

b. Anatomy. The duodenum shares its blood supply with the pancreas. It extends from the pylorus to the ligament of Treitz (25 cm in length). There are four parts: the first portion (superior portion) of the duodenum is intraperitoneal; the second portion of the duodenum (descending portion) contains the orifices of the bile and pancreatic ducts; the third portion of the duodenum (transverse portion) extends from the ampulla of Vater to the mesenteric vessels, with the ureter, IVC, and aorta posteriorly and SMA anteriorly; the fourth portion of the duodenum (ascending portion) begins at the mesenteric vessels and ends at the jejunum, to the left of the lumbar column. Bile (1,000 mL/day), pancreatic juices (800–1,000 mL/day), and gastric juices (1,500–2,500 mL/day) mix in the duodenum.

c. Diagnosis

(1) Clinical suspicion is based on the mechanism of injury. With blunt injury, the patient usually has mid-epigastric or right upper quadrant pain or tenderness and can have peritoneal signs. The symptoms and findings can be subtle. Retroperitoneal air or obliteration of the right psoas margin may be seen on abdominal x-ray study. The diagnosis is generally made at laparotomy for associated injuries. With penetrating mechanisms, duodenal injury is found at laparotomy, usually for GSW.

(2) CT findings include paraduodenal hemorrhage and air or contrast leak; oral contrast and fastidious technique are important.

(3) With equivocal CT findings, an upper gastrointestinal (UGI) study may be essential. The contrast enhanced UGI study is first done with water-soluble contrast; if this is negative, barium is then used.

(4) DPL has a low sensitivity for duodenal injury but will often detect associated injuries.

(5) Adequate intraoperative exposure is vital; duodenal injuries are among the most commonly missed at laparotomy. They should be exposed in a manner similar to that used for the pancreas, including a wide Kocher maneuver. Bile staining, air in the retroperitoneum, or a central retroperitoneal hematoma mandates thorough exploration of the duodenum.

d. Treatment

(1) **Intramural duodenal hematoma** is more common in children than in adults; may be a result of child abuse. A "coiled spring" appearance is seen on UGI series. Follow-up UGI with Gastrografin should be obtained every 7 days, if the obstruction persists clinically.

(a) Treated nonoperatively with nasogastric suction and i.v. alimentation. Operation is necessary to evacuate the hematoma if it does not resolve after 2 to 3 weeks.

(b) Treatment of an intramural hematoma found at early laparotomy is controversial.

• One option is to open serosa, evacuate the hematoma without violation of the mucosa, and repair the wall of the bowel. The concern is that this may convert a partial tear to a full-thickness tear of the duodenal wall.

- Another option is to explore the duodenum to exclude a perforation, leaving the intramural hematoma intact and planning nasogastric decompression postoperatively.
- Consider placement of a jejunal feeding tube for postoperative enteral feeding.

(2) **Duodenal perforation** must be treated operatively. Many options are available, depending on injury severity.

(a) Transverse primary closure in one or two layers is applicable in 71% to 85% of duodenal injuries. This requires debridement of the edges of the duodenal wall and closure that avoids narrowing of the duodenal lumen. Longitudinal duodenotomies can usually be closed transversely if the length of the duodenal injury is <50% of the circumference of the duodenum. More severe injuries may require repairs using pyloric exclusion, duodenal decompression, or more complex operations. The risk factors with duodenal injury include:

- Associated vascular injury
- Associated pancreatic injury
- Blunt injury or missile injury
- >75% of the wall involved
- Injury in the first or second portion of the duodenum
- >24 hours since injury
- Associated common bile duct injury

(b) If the repair is considered to be tenuous, protect it by a retrograde jejunostomy drainage catheter or a lateral tube duodenostomy. If more protection is required, divert the stomach contents by pyloric exclusion with gastrojejunostomy. Oversew the pyloric outlet through a gastric incision (absorbable or non-absorbable suture) or staple, using the incision as the gastrojejunostomy site (Fig. 27.7). Vagotomy is usually not performed because the pyloric closure generally reopens in 2 to 3 weeks.

(c) If primary closure would compromise the lumen of the duodenum, use a jejunal mucosal patch duodenoplasty (rarely used) or a jejunal serosal patch.

(d) A three-tube technique may also be used. This consists of a gastrostomy tube to decompress the stomach, a retrograde jejunostomy to decompress the duodenum, and an antegrade jejunostomy to feed the patient.

(e) If complete duodenal transection or long lacerations of the duodenal wall are found, perform debridement and primary closure. If this cannot be accomplished without tension, a Roux-en-Y jejunostomy over the defect or closure of the distal duodenum and Roux-en-Y duodenojejunostomy proximally may be required.

(f) The uncommon circumstance of destructive combined injuries to the duodenum and the head of the pancreas may necessitate pancreaticoduodenectomy (Whipple procedure). In this rare circumstance, experienced help is essential.

e. Outcome

(1) The mortality rate reaches 40% if diagnosis is delayed >24 hours, but it is 2% to 11% if the patient has surgery within 24 hours of injury. Duodenal dehiscence with resultant sepsis accounts for nearly one half of the deaths. Complications occur in 64% of patients with duodenal injuries.

(2) Retrograde tube decompression of the duodenum can be associated with a decreased mortality rate (9% with tube decompression vs 19.4% without). The duodenal fistula rate was 2.3%

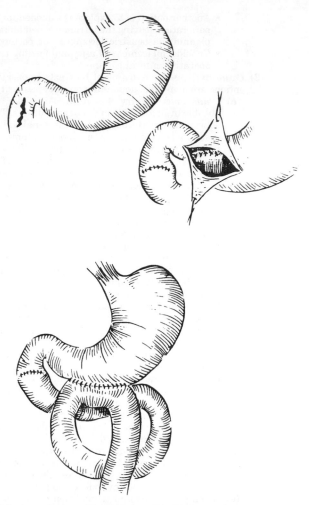

FIG. 27.7. Pyloric exclusion. (From Frame SB, McSwain NE. *Retroperitoneal trauma.* New York: Thieme, 1993:89, with permission.)

with decompression versus 11.8% without decompression in the same review. Pyloric exclusion can also provide adequate decompression of the duodenal closure if the repair is tenuous or a concomitant pancreatic injury is found.

     f. Organ injury scale (see Appendix A)

F. Liver

    1. Incidence. The liver is the most commonly injured intraabdominal organ; injury occurs more often in penetrating trauma than in blunt trauma. The mortality rate for liver injuries is 10%.

    2. Anatomy. An understanding of hepatic anatomy is essential to manage complex liver injuries. A saggital plane separates the right and left lobes of the liver from the IVC to the gallbladder fossa. The segmental anatomy of the liver is shown in Figure 27.8.

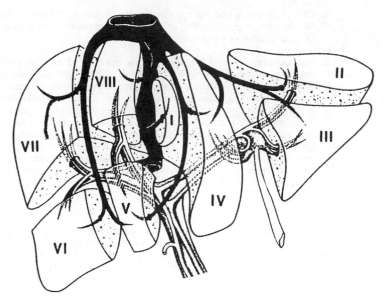

FIG. 27.8. Hepatic anatomy. (From Bismuth H. Surgical anatomy and anatomical surgery of the liver. *World J Surg* 1982;6(1):6, with permission.)

    a. The right and left hepatic veins have a short extrahepatic course before they empty directly in the IVC. The middle hepatic vein usually joins the left hepatic vein within the liver parenchyma. The retrohepatic IVC (8–10 cm in length) has multiple, small hepatic veins that enter the IVC directly; this area is exceedingly difficult to access and control.

    b. The portal vein delivers 75% of the hepatic blood flow and 50% of the oxygenated blood.

    c. The right and left hepatic arteries usually arise from the common hepatic artery. Anomalies are frequent and include the right hepatic artery originating from the SMA and the left hepatic artery originating from the left gastric artery.

    d. Adequate mobilization of the liver requires division of the ligamentous attachments.

        (1) The falciform ligament divides the left lateral segment of the liver from the medial segment of the left lobe.

        (2) The coronary ligaments are the diaphragmatic attachments to the liver (anterior and posterior leaflets); they do not meet on the posterior surface of the liver (the bare area). The triangular ligaments (left and right) are the more lateral extensions of the coronary ligaments. Injury to the diaphragm, phrenic veins, and hepatic veins must be avoided when mobilizing the liver.

3. Diagnosis

    a. Physical examination is often unreliable in the blunt trauma victim.

    b. The appropriate diagnostic modality depends on the hemodynamic status of the patient on arrival in the trauma resuscitation area. If the patient is hemodynamically stable with a blunt mechanism of injury, CT is preferred. CT is sensitive and specific in stable patients with a clinical suspicion of injury. Most hemodynamically stable patients with liver injuries can be treated nonoperatively.

    c. DPL is sensitive but not specific for liver injuries. Of liver injuries, 70% are no longer bleeding at the time of laparotomy for a positive DPL, depending on the patient population.

4. Treatment

    a. Management of blunt hepatic injuries has evolved substantially in the past several years. The hemodynamically stable patients with blunt injury of the liver, without other intraabdominal injury requiring laparotomy, can be treated nonoperatively, regardless of the grade of the liver injury. This may represent 50% to 80% of patients. The presence of hemoperitoneum on CT does not mandate laparotomy. **Arterial blush or pooling of contrast** on CT and high-grade (grade IV and V) hepatic injuries are most likely to fail nonoperative management. Nonetheless, embolization can circumvent the need for laparotomy; angioembolization has assumed an increasing role in the management of liver injury. The criteria for nonoperative management of blunt liver injuries include:

        (1) Hemodynamic stability

        (2) Absence of peritoneal signs

        (3) Lack of continued need for transfusion for the hepatic injury; bleeding can be addressed with angioembolization.

    b. Posterior right lobe injuries (even if extensive) and the split-liver type of injuries (extensive injury along the relatively avascular plane between the left and right lobes) can generally be managed successfully nonoperatively.

    c. The details of nonoperative management are institution- and provider-specific. No support is seen for frequent hemoglobin sampling, bedrest, and prolonged intensive care unit (ICU) monitoring. Similarly, the need to re-image asymptomatic hepatic injuries by CT scan is not documented. Practitioners should tailor monitoring practices to their institutional resources. Follow-up CT scanning can be deferred, except to document healing (at ~8 weeks) in physically active patients (e.g., athletes) before resumption of normal activities.

    d. Immediate laparotomy or angiographic intervention is required for those patients who fail nonoperative therapy by demonstrating enlarging lesions on CT scan, hemodynamic instability, or continual blood product requirement (<10%).

    e. If the patient is hemodynamically unstable or has indications for laparotomy, operative management is required. Management principles include the following:

        (1) **Adequate exposure of the injury is essential**. Exploration is through a long midline incision or bilateral subcostal incision. An extension to a median sternotomy or thoracotomy may be necessary for exposure of the injury. Use of a self-retaining retractor (Rochard, Thompson, or Upper Hand) to lift the upper edges of the wound cephalad and anteriorly facilitates exposure of the liver. Complete mobilization of the liver is performed, including division of the ligaments.

        (2) Most blunt and penetrating hepatic injuries are grade I and II (70% to 90%) and can be managed with simple techniques (e.g., electrocautery, simple suture, or hemostatic agents). Complex liver injuries can produce exsanguinating hemorrhage. Rapid, temporary tamponade of the bleeding by manual compression of the liver injury immediately after entering the abdomen allows the anesthesiologist to resuscitate the patient. After resuscitation, the liver injury can be repaired.

        (3) For complex hepatic injuries, occlude the portal triad with an atraumatic clamp (Pringle maneuver). This should reduce bleeding from the liver, except in retrohepatic venous injuries.

Studies suggest that up to 60 to 90 minutes of warm hepatic ischemia can be tolerated.

(4) Hepatorrhaphy with individual vessel ligation is recommended instead of large ischemia-producing mass parenchymal suturing.

(a) Glisson's capsule is incised with the electrocautery.

(b) The injury within the liver is approached by the finger fracture technique (Fig. 27.9) or by division of the liver tissue over a right-angled clamp with ligation of the hepatic tissue with 2-0 silk sutures.

(c) With gentle traction on the liver edges, expose the injury site. Blood vessels and bile ducts are directly visualized and ligated or repaired (Fig. 27.10).

(d) Debride nonviable liver tissue.

(e) Pack the defect in the liver with viable omentum.

(5) Perform closed-suction drainage of grade III to V injuries. Drains are probably not necessary for grade I and II injuries if bleeding and bile leakage are controlled.

(6) Perform resectional debridement of nonviable tissue rather than formal anatomic resections.

(7) Perform perihepatic packing in cases of hemorrhage, hypothermia, and coagulopathy. Approximately 5% of patients with hepatic injury require perihepatic packing (i.e., damage control laparotomy). Indications include coagulopathy, subcapsular hematomas, bilobar injuries, and hypothermia, or to allow transfer of the patient to a higher level of care. Pack the liver

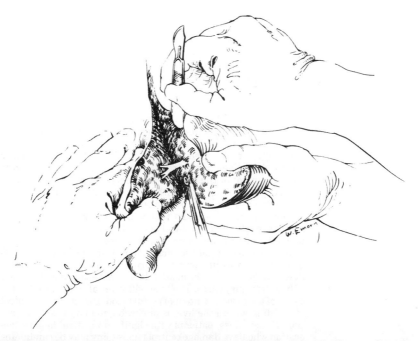

FIG. 27.9. Finger fracture technique. (From Lim RC. Injuries to the liver and extrahepatic ducts. In: Blaisdell FW, Trunkey DD, eds. *Trauma management, abdominal trauma.* New York: Thieme, 1982:141, with permission.)

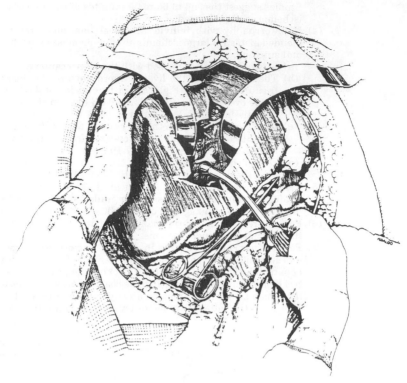

FIG. 27.10. Blood vessels and bile ducts are directly visualized and ligated or repaired. (From Feliciano DV, Moore EE, Mattox KL. *Trauma*, 3rd ed. Stamford, CT: Appleton & Lange, 1996:500, with permission.)

first by placing nonadhesive plastic on the liver, and placing laparotomy pads.

(8) Anatomic hepatic resection (segment or lobe) is not commonly required for liver injury; resectional debridement and direct suture control of the vessels and ducts can generally accomplish the same objectives, with lower mortality. Indications for formal hepatic resection include total destruction of a segment or lobe, an extensive injury that cannot be controlled with perihepatic packing, and control of bleeding that can be achieved only by anatomic resection. Planned, delayed anatomic resection is also an approach for major hepatic injury, if packing sufficiently controls hemorrhage during the initial laparotomy.

(9) Selective hepatic artery ligation has been reported in 1% to 2% of hepatic injury cases. The liver will generally tolerate this because of the oxygen content of portal blood. Direct suture control of bleeding within the liver is preferable to hepatic artery ligation. Nonetheless, patients with significant central hepatic laceration who have damage control laparotomy may be candidates for arteriography with possible embolization postoperatively.

f. Hepatic vascular isolation with occlusion of the suprahepatic and infrahepatic venae cavae, as well as application of the Pringle maneuver, may be required for major retrohepatic venous injury. If exposure is necessary, the midline incision can be extended to a median sternotomy, which will allow excellent exposure of the hepatic veins for retrohepatic venous injuries. Atrial-caval shunts have been recommended by some authors for retrohepatic caval injury. A 36F chest tube or 9-mm endotracheal tube, each with extra side holes, is inserted through the right atrial appendage. The side holes allow flow from the shunt into the right atrium. The distal end of the tube is at the level of the renal veins. Survival with this technique is dismal. Alternatively, complex retrohepatic vascular injury in which tamponade does not achieve hemostasis can be repaired in an avascular field on venovenous bypass with total hepatic vascular isolation. Survival depends on prompt recognition of this anatomic site of injury.

  g. Bleeding from penetrating wounds of the liver that are not easily accessed, at times, can be controlled with internal tamponade. This is accomplished by using Penrose drains tied at each end (as a balloon) over a red rubber catheter. The end of the Penrose drain is brought through the skin. Finally, in wounds where tamponade does not achieve hemostasis, consider repair under vascular isolation by experienced personnel.

5. Outcome. Mortality correlates with the degree of injury. Because most hepatic injuries are grade I or II, the overall mortality rate for liver injuries is 10%. However, the mortality rates for more severe liver injury are grade III, 25%; grade IV, 46%; grade V, 80%; and grade VI, fatal.

  a. Complications

  (1) With recurrent bleeding (occurs in 2% to 7% of patients) → return the patient to the OR or, in selected patients, obtain an angiogram and perform embolization. Recurrent bleeding is generally caused by inadequate initial hemostasis. Hypothermia and coagulopathy must be corrected. Preparations to control retrohepatic hemorrhage (i.e., vascular bypass) should be made.

  (2) Hemobilia is a rare complication of liver injury. The classic presentation is right upper quadrant pain, jaundice, and hemorrhage; one third of patients have all three components of the triad. The patient may present with hemobilia days or weeks after injury. Treatment is angiogram and embolization.

  (3) Intrahepatic or perihepatic abscess or biloma (occur in 7% to 40% of patients) can generally be drained percutaneously. Meticulous control of bleeding and repair of bile ducts, adequate debridement, and closed-suction drainage are essential to avoid abscess formation.

  (4) Biliary fistulas (>50 mL/day for >2 weeks) usually resolve nonoperatively if external drainage of the leak is adequate and distal obstruction is not present.

    (a) If >300 mL of bile drains each day, further evaluation with a radionucleotide scan, a fistulogram, ERCP, or a transhepatic cholangiogram may be necessary. Major ductal injury can be stented to facilitate healing of the injury, or as a guide if operative repair is required. Endoscopic sphincterotomy or transampullary stenting may facilitate resolution of the biliary leak.

  6. Organ injury scale (see Appendix A)

G. Extrahepatic biliary tract injury is uncommon. The gallbladder is the most common site; cholecystectomy is the usual treatment. Injury to the extrahepatic bile ducts can be missed at laparotomy unless careful operative inspection of the porta hepatis is performed. A cholangiogram through the gallbladder or cystic duct stump helps define the injury. The location and severity of the injury will dictate the appropriate treatment. Simple bile duct injury (<50% of the circumference) can be repaired with primary suture repair. Complex bile duct injury (>50% of the circumference) may require Roux-en-Y choledochojejunostomy or hepaticojejunostomy. Primary end-to-end anastomosis of the bile duct is not advised; the stricture rate approaches 50% (see Appendix A).

H. Spleen

1. **Incidence.** Blunt splenic injury is produced by compression or deceleration force (e.g., from motor vehicle crashes, falls, or direct blows to the abdomen). Penetrating injury to the spleen is less common.

2. **Anatomy and function.** The spleen is bounded by the stomach, left hemidiaphragm, left kidney and adrenal gland, colon, and chest wall. These relationships define the attachment of the spleen: gastrosplenic ligament, splenorenal ligament, splenophrenic ligament, splenocolic ligament, and pancreaticosplenic attachments. The spleen receives 5% of the cardiac output, primarily through the splenic artery. The splenic artery usually bifurcates into superior and inferior polar arteries. Further division of the blood supply is along transverse planes. The spleen has an open microcirculation without endothelium. It filters blood-borne bacteria, particulate matter, and aged cells. The spleen produces antibodies, properdin, and tuftsin.

3. **Diagnosis**

   a. The patient may have signs of hypovolemia with tachycardia or hypotension, and complain of left upper quadrant tenderness or referred pain to the left shoulder (Kehr's sign).

   b. Physical examination is insensitive and nonspecific in the diagnosis of splenic injury. The patient may have signs of generalized peritoneal irritation or left upper quadrant tenderness or fullness.

   c. Of patients with left lower rib fractures (ribs 9 through 12), 25% will have a splenic injury.

   d. In the unstable trauma patient, ultrasound or DPL will provide the most rapid diagnosis of hemoperitoneum, the source of which is commonly the spleen.

   e. In the stable patient suffering from blunt injury, CT imaging of the abdomen allows delineation and grading of the splenic injury (see Appendix A). The most common finding on CT in association with a splenic injury is hemoperitoneum.

   f. Angiography has been used as an adjunct in the management of splenic injury in highly selected patients, with therapeutic embolization of arterial bleeding.

4. **Treatment**

   a. The use of abdominal CT and an understanding of the importance of splenic function have resulted in the preservation of many injured spleens, by either nonoperative management or splenorrhaphy. Management of splenic injury depends primarily on the hemodynamic stability of the patient on presentation. Other factors include the age of the patient, associated injuries (which are the rule in adults), and the grade of the splenic injury.

      (1) Nonoperative management of splenic injury is successful in >90% of children, irrespective of the grade of splenic injury.

      (2) Nonoperative management of blunt splenic injury in adults is becoming more routine, with approximately 65% of adults ultimately managed nonoperatively for blunt injury to the spleen.

   b. If hemodynamically stable, adult patients with grade I or II injury can often be treated nonoperatively (Fig. 27.11). Patients with grade IV or V splenic injuries are often unstable. Grade III splenic injuries (certainly in children, and in selected adults) can be treated nonoperatively based on stability and reliable physical examination. The failure rate of nonoperative management of splenic injuries in adults increases with grade of splenic injury: grade I, 5%; grade 2, 10%; grade III, 20%; grade IV, 33%; and grade V, 75%. In adults (but

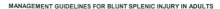

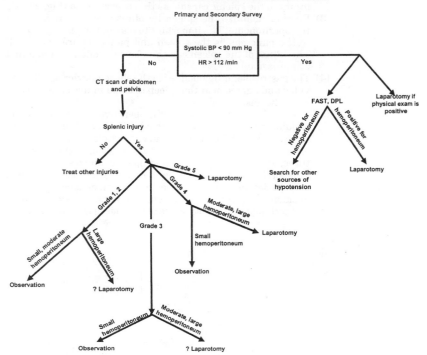

FIG. 27.11. Management guidelines for blunt splenic injury. (BP, blood pressure; HR, heart rate; CT, computed tomography; DPL, diagnostic peritoneal lavage; Hcts, hematocrits).

not children), risk of failure of nonoperative management of blunt splenic injury correlates with grade of splenic injury and quantity of hemoperitoneum. Most failures occur within 72 hours of injury.

c. Patients with significant splenic injuries treated nonoperatively should be observed in a monitored unit and have **immediate access** to a CT scanner, a surgeon, and an OR. Changes in physical examination, hemodynamic stability, ongoing blood, or fluid requirements indicate the need for laparotomy.

d. If the patient is not hemodynamically stable, operative treatment is required. The operative therapy of choice is splenic conservation where possible to avoid the risk of death from overwhelming postsplenectomy sepsis that can occur after splenectomy for trauma. However, in the presence of multiple injuries or critical instability, splenectomy is more rapid and judicious.

    (1) Exploration is through a long midline incision. The abdomen is packed and explored. Exsanguinating hemorrhage and gastrointestinal soilage are controlled first.

    (2) Mobilize the spleen to visualize the injury. The operator's nondominant hand will provide medial traction on the spleen to facilitate the operation. The splenocolic ligament can be vascular and require ligation. The splenorenal and splenophrenic

ligaments are avascular and should be divided sharply; avoid
injury to the splenic capsule as this is performed (Fig. 27.12).

(3) Further mobilize the spleen by bluntly freeing it from the
retroperitoneum. It is important to stay in the plane posterior
to the pancreas as the spleen and pancreas are mobilized.
The hilum of the spleen can then be controlled with manual
compression.

(4) The gastrosplenic ligament with the short gastric vessels is divided and ligated near the spleen to avoid injury or late necrosis of the gastric wall.

(5) Then mobilize the spleen into the operative field. Splenectomy
should be performed in unstable patients, and in those with
associated life-threatening injury, multiple sources for postoperative blood loss (pelvic fracture, multiple long-bone fractures, and so forth), and complex splenic injuries.

(6) Splenorrhaphy should be contemplated when circumstances
permit. Because of the increased reliance on nonoperative management of splenic injury, splenorrhaphy is rarely employed.
The technique is dictated by the magnitude of the splenic injury.

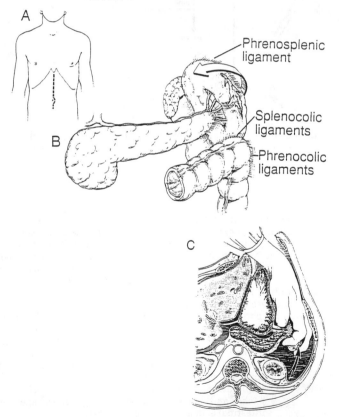

FIG. 27.12. A. Midline incision. **B.** Phrenosplenic, splenocolic, and phrenocolic ligaments. **C.** Mobilization of spleen. (From Beal SL, Trunkey DD. Splenic injury.
In: Blaisdell FW, Trunkey DD, eds. *Abdominal trauma*, 2nd ed. New York:
Thieme, 1993:239, with permission.)

(a) Nonbleeding grade I splenic injury may require no further treatment. Topical hemostatic agents, an argon beam coagulator, or electrocautery may suffice.

(b) Grade II to III splenic injury may require the aforementioned interventions, suture repair, or mesh wrap of capsular defects. Suture repair in adults often requires Teflon pledgets to avoid tearing of the splenic capsule (Fig. 27.13).

(c) Grade IV to V splenic injury may require anatomic resection, including ligation of the lobar artery. A small rim of capsule at the resection line may help reinforce the resection line. Pledgeted horizontal mattress sutures may also be necessary. Grade V splenic injury usually requires splenectomy.

(d) One third of the splenic mass must be functional to maintain immunocompetence. Thus, at least one half of the spleen must be preserved to justify splenorrhaphy.

(7) Drainage of the splenic fossa is associated with an increased incidence of subphrenic abscess and should be avoided. The exception is when concern exists about injury to the tail of the pancreas.

(8) Autotransplantation of the spleen has been reported and involves implanting multiple 1-mm slices of the spleen in the omentum after splenectomy. This technique remains experimental.

5. **Outcome**

a. The outcome is generally good; rebleeding rates as low as 1% have been reported with splenorrhaphy.

b. The failure rate of nonoperative therapy is 2% to 10% in children and as high as 18% in adults. It has been reported that adults >55 years of age are especially susceptible to failure of nonoperative therapy, although some question this.

c. Pulmonary complications, which are common in patients treated operatively and nonoperatively, include atelectasis, left pleural effusion, and pneumonia. Left subphrenic abscess occurs in 3% to 13% of postoperative patients and may be more common with the use of drains or with concomitant bowel injury.

d. Thrombocytosis occurs in as many as 50% of patients after splenectomy; the platelet count usually peaks 2 to 10 days postoperatively. The elevated platelet count generally abates in several weeks. Treatment is usually not required.

e. The risk of overwhelming postsplenectomy infection (OPSI) is greater in children than in adults. The mortality rate for OPSI approaches 50%. The common organism are encapsulated organisms: meningococcus, *Haemophilus influenzae*, and *Streptococcus pneumoniae*, as well as *Staphylococcus aureus* and *Escherichia coli*. After splenectomy, pneumococcal (Pneumovax), *H. influenzae*, and meningococcal vaccines should be administered. The timing of injection of the vaccine is controversial. Some authors recommend giving the vaccine 3 to 4 weeks postoperatively because the patient may be too immunosuppressed in the immediate postinjury period. Current recommendation is to repeat the pneumococcal vaccination at 5 years. The patient should be discharged from the hospital with a clear understanding of the concerns about OPSI, should wear a tag alerting healthcare providers of his or her asplenic state, and should begin penicillin therapy with the development of even mild infections.

6. **Organ injury scale (see Appendix A)**

VI. **Retroperitoneal hematomas**

A. **Management of retroperitoneal hematomas** depends largely on location and the mechanism of injury. Generally, all penetrating wounds of the

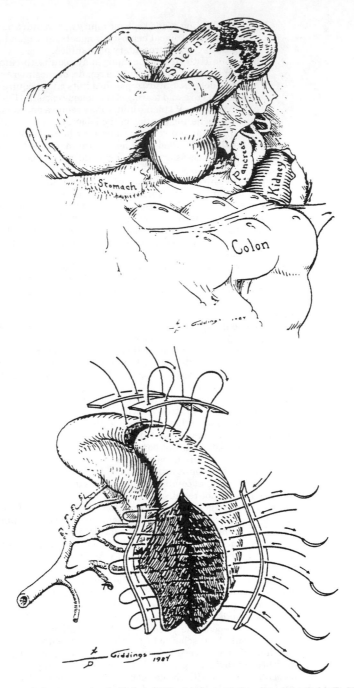

FIG. 27.13. Splenic repair. **A.** The mobilized spleen in the operative field. **B.** Horizontal mattress sutures with pledgets for splenic repair. (From Champion HR, Robbs JV, Trunkey DD. Trauma surgery, parts 1 and 2. In: *Rob and Smith's operative surgery*. London: Butterworth, 1989:370, with permission.)

retroperitoneum found at laparotomy require thorough exploration. Some simply observe nonexpanding perinephric hematomas. If the hematoma is large, expanding, or proximal to the retroperitoneal vessels (aorta, iliac artery, and so forth), first obtain proximal and distal control of the vessels.

B. Blunt trauma produces 70% to 80% of retroperitoneal hematomas; most are caused by pelvic fracture. In general, nonexpanding lateral (zone II) or pelvic (zone III) hematomas secondary to blunt trauma do not require exploration. Be certain that the overlying bowel (i.e., colon or duodenum) is intact (Fig. 27.14).

    1. Central hematomas (zone I) always require exploration to rule out a major vascular or visceral injury. In the case of ongoing hemorrhage, the aorta can be occluded at the diaphragmatic hiatus or above the diaphragm via a left thoracotomy, and the vascular structures approached by mobilizing the abdominal viscera from the retroperitoneum (right or left medial visceral rotation). Injury to the pancreas and duodenum must also be sought in exploration of a central hematoma.

C. Most retroperitoneal vascular injuries can be repaired with a lateral arteriorrhaphy or venorrhaphy. If a patch is required, prosthetic material can be used, except in the setting of gross contamination with colon contents, in which case an autologous patch should be used.

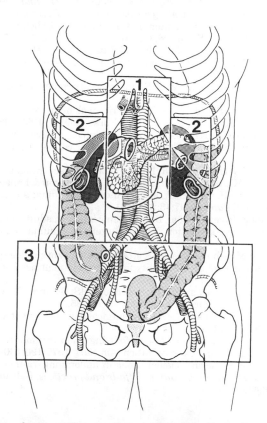

FIG. 27.14. Zones of retroperitoneum. 1: central-medial retroperitoneal zone; 2: lateral retroperitoneal zone; 3: pelvic retroperitoneal zone. (From Kudsk KA, Sheldon GF. Retroperitoneal hematoma. In: Blaisdell FW, Trunkey DD, eds. *Trauma management, abdominal trauma.* New York: Thieme, 1982:281, with permission.)

Bibliography

Asensio JA, Feliciano DV, Britt LD, et al. Management of duodenal injuries. *Curr Probl Surg* 1993;30:1021–1100.

Blaisdell FW, Trunkey DD, eds. *Abdominal trauma*. New York: Thieme, 1993.

Boone, DC, Federle M, Billiar TR, et al. Evolution of major hepatic trauma: Identification of patterns of injury. *J Trauma* 1995;39:344–350.

Buckman BF Jr, Miraliakbari, R, Badellino MM. Juxtahepatic venous injuries: a critical review of reported management strategies. *J Trauma* 2000;48:978–984.

Cogbill T, Moore EE, Feliciano DV, et al. Conservative management of duodenal trauma: a multicenter perspective. *J Trauma* 1990;30:1469–1475.

Cogbill TH, Moore EE, Jurkovich J, et al. Nonoperative management of blunt splenic trauma: a multicenter experience. *J Trauma* 1989;29:1312–1317.

Esposito TJ, Gamelli RL. Injury to the spleen. In: Feliciano DV, Moore EE, Mattox KL, eds. *Trauma*. Stamford, CT: Appleton & Lange, 1996:525–550.

Fabian TC, Croce MA. Abdominal trauma, including indications for celiotomy. In: Feliciano DV, Moore EE, Mattox KL, eds. *Trauma*. Stamford, CT: Appleton & Lange, 1996;441–459.

Feliciano DV, Jordan GL, Bitondo CG, et al. Management of 1000 cases of hepatic trauma. *Ann Surg* 1986;294:438–445.

Grossman, MD, Schwab CW, Reilly PR, et al. Determining anatomic injury with computed tomography in selected torso gunshot wounds. *J Trauma* 1998;45:446–456.

Hasson J, Stern D, Moss G. Penetrating duodenal trauma. *J Trauma* 1984;24:471–474.

Jurkovich GJ. Injury to the duodenum and pancreas. In: Feliciano, DV, Moore EE, Mattox KL, eds. *Trauma*. Stamford, CT: Appleton & Lange, 1996:573–594.

Mackersie RC, Tiwary AD, Shackford SR, et al. Intra-abdominal injury following blunt trauma—identifying the high-risk patient using objective risk factors. *Arch Surg* 1989;124:809–813.

McGrath V, Fabian TC, Croce MA, et al. Rectal trauma: management based on anatomic distinctions. *Am Surg* 1998;64:1136–1141.

Meyer AA, Kudsk KA, Sheldon GF. Retroperitoneal hematoma. In: Blaisdell FW, Trunkey DD, eds. *Abdominal trauma*. New York: Thieme, 1993:398–413.

Pachter HL, Knudson MM, Esrig B, et al. Status of nonoperative management of blunt hepatic injuries in 1995: a multicenter experience with 404 patients. *J Trauma* 1996;40:31–38.

Pachter HL, Liang HG, Hofstetter SR. Liver and biliary tract trauma. In: Feliciano DV, Moore EE, Mattox KL, eds. *Trauma*. Stamford, CT: Appleton & Lange, 1996:487–523.

Patton JH Jr, Lyden SP, Croce MA, et al. Pancreatic trauma: a simplified management guideline. *J Trauma* 1997;43:234–241.

Peitzman AB, Heil B, Rivera L, et al. Blunt splenic injury in adults: multi-institutional study of the Eastern Association for the Surgery of Trauma. *J Trauma* 2000;49: 177–189.

Rozycki G, Ochsner M, Schmidt J, et al. A prospective study of surgeon-performed ultrasound as the primary adjunct modality for injured patient assessment. *J Trauma* 1995;39(3):492–500.

Singer DB. Post-splenectomy sepsis. In: Rosenburg HS, Bolande RP, eds. *Perspectives in pediatric pathology*. Chicago: Year Book, 1973:285.

Snyder W, Weigelt J, Watkins WL, et al. The surgical management of duodenal trauma. *Arch Surg* 1980;115:422–429.

Stone HH, Fabian TC. Management of perforating colon trauma; randomization between primary closure and exteriorization. *Am Surg* 1979;190:430–438.

Wilson RF, Walt AJ. General considerations in abdominal trauma. In: Wilson RF, Walt AJ, eds. *Management of trauma. Pitfalls and practices*. Baltimore: Williams & Wilkins, 1996:411–431.

28. ABDOMINAL VASCULAR INJURY

Michael B. Shapiro

I. **Introduction.** More than 90% of abdominal vascular injuries are caused by penetrating wounds. These injuries are found at laparotomy in 25% of patients with gunshot wounds and in 10% of patients with stab wounds. They are rarely isolated, and multiple associated intraabdominal injuries, including multiple hollow viscus injuries, should be expected. Recent availability and popularity of semiautomatic weapons has led to a trend to multiple shot assaults, which has increased the incidence of these injuries.

II. **Mechanism of injury.** Abdominal vascular injury can result in a hematoma contained in the retroperitoneum or mesentery, or free intraperitoneal bleeding. This distinction is critical in defining a patient's status at initial presentation. Penetrating injuries cause through-and-through perforations or partial wall defects. Complete transection of abdominal vessels is likely to be immediately lethal and, therefore, is uncommonly seen. Blast effect injuries from tangential high-power gunshot wounds are uncommon in abdominal vessels, but they can present as an intimal flap. Blunt abdominal vascular injuries arise from a direct blow or rapid deceleration, often occurring in association with seatbelt injury, mesenteric avulsion, or pelvic fracture.

III. **Presentation and diagnosis.** Determination of trajectory is critical in establishing the diagnosis. A bullet that crosses the upper abdomen or violates the posterior abdomen or posterolateral pelvis frequently causes a vascular injury.

   A. **Normotensive patient.** With early presentation and a contained hematoma, a patient may have normal blood pressure and little pain. This usually occurs with wounds to the flank or back. Evaluation may include chest and supine abdominal radiographs, which should include metallic markers (e.g., paper clips, x-ray markers, metallic buttons) at wound sites to help determine trajectory. Local wound exploration can also help define trajectory, especially for tangential wounds. Triple-contrast (oral, rectal, and intravenous [i.v.]) computerized tomography (CT) may define the extent of a contained hematoma, assess trajectory, and establish the presence of retroperitoneal colon injury in a patient with flank or posterior wounds.

   B. **Hypotensive patient.** A patient with a penetrating abdominal injury and hypotension should be considered to have a vascular injury, which requires prompt laparotomy. Patients can also present with abdominal distention, gross hematuria, or loss of one or both lower extremity pulses. The patient with a contained hematoma can become normotensive with fluid resuscitation, whereas the patient with active hemorrhage will not. **The association of hypotension and a penetrating wound to the abdomen strongly suggests a major vascular injury in the abdomen or pelvis.**

   C. **Exsanguinated patient.** Some patients with abdominal injury present with profound hypotension, tachycardia or agonal rhythm, obtundation, and massive abdominal distention. These patients should be considered to have a major vascular injury with free intraperitoneal hemorrhage and >40% total blood volume loss. They require **immediate laparotomy** for control of hemorrhage, resuscitation, and definitive injury management.

IV. **Initial evaluation and resuscitation**

   A. **Normotensive and hypotensive patients**

      1. Establish airway control early and definitively; administer 100% oxygen by face-mask, bag-mask device, or endotracheal tube.

      2. Intravenous access should be promptly established with multiple large-bore lines in the upper extremities, subclavian or jugular veins. Avoid femoral lines if concern of abdominal vascular injury exists.

      3. Prewarmed fluids and fluid warmers should be used to avoid hypothermia. All fluids should be warmed to 38°C to 40°C.

4. Use blood transfusion for patients who do not rapidly respond to 2 to 3 L of crystalloid resuscitation or who are obviously actively bleeding. Blood is reconstituted with normal saline (250–500 mL) at 38°C to 40°C; this warms and dilutes the blood, decreasing viscosity and improving flow.
   a. Type O, universal donor blood, should be immediately available in the trauma room.
   b. Type specific blood (A, B, O, Rh) should be administered as soon as available.
   c. Crossmatched blood may require 40 to 60 minutes to be available. **Do not delay transfusion in the unstable patient**.
5. Blood components (fresh frozen plasma and platelets) should be transfused early in the patient with a major vascular injury; **avoid coagulopathy**. Immediately order blood components for those patients thought to have a major vascular injury (transfusion requirement is likely to exceed 4 to 6 units of packed red blood cells).
6. Blood bank notification is critical in the setting of abdominal vascular injury, as a massive transfusion requirement should be expected. Request immediate delivery of 10 units of type O, universal donor packed red blood cells, to the emergency department or operating room (OR). O-positive blood is given to male patients, O-negative to female patients. Also request immediate preparation of 10 units of fresh frozen plasma and 10 units of platelets for administration as soon as ready.
7. Use rapid infusion and cell-saver devices in the OR.
8. Administer tetanus prophylaxis and antibiotics preoperatively, with coverage of aerobic and anaerobic organisms.

B. **Exsanguinating patient**
1. Immediately perform endotracheal intubation; administer 100% oxygen.
2. Begin blood transfusion immediately with type O, universal donor blood, and notify the blood bank of massive requirements, as above.
3. **Immediate laparotomy; definitive control of injuries must be obtained promptly in the OR. Hemorrhage control and resuscitation occur simultaneously in the OR.**
4. Left anterolateral thoracotomy may be necessary to obtain aortic control. Consider this for the patient with agonal cardiac rhythm, systolic blood pressure <70 mmHg, and massive abdominal distension.
5. **Damage control** operative procedures are appropriate in this setting. The immediate goal with these patients is to prevent early death from exsanguination. This approach involves the following three phases.
   a. Rapid operative control of hemorrhage and contamination, followed by peritoneal packing and abdominal skin closure
   b. Ongoing resuscitation in the intensive care unit (ICU) until rewarming and reversal of coagulopathy and hypothermia are achieved. **If hemorrhage from solid visceral injury is controlled with packing, consider angiography evaluation after the patient is physiologically resuscitated, both for anatomic clarification and, if possible, therapeutic intervention, before returning to the OR.**
   c. Subsequent definitive reexploration

V. **Operation** (Table 28.1)
A. **Preparation**. To avoid hypothermia, place the patient on a warming blanket with head and extremities wrapped in a Baer hugger, and maintain room temperature at >27°C. Skin should be prepared and the patient draped from the chin to the knees and to the table laterally, to enable access to the chest or groin, or saphenous vein harvesting.
B. **Exploration**
1. Explore the abdomen through a midline incision, extending from the xiphoid process to the symphysis pubis. A large retroperitoneal hematoma can cause significant distortion of normal anatomy and tissue planes.
2. Compress visible active arterial hemorrhage with digital pressure or packs. Control active hemorrhage from within or beneath a hematoma in

Table 28.1. Conduct of the operation for major abdominal vascular injury

Preparation
–Identify trauma operating room in advance, with anesthesia and operating
  equipment in place
–Maintain operating room temperature >27°C
–Cell saver and rapid infusion devices in room
Position
–Patient supine, both arms out
–Multiple, large-bore intravenous lines above the diaphragm
–Urinary catheter with collection bag beneath head of bed
–Chest tubes, if present, to suction and in view of nurses and anesthesiologists
–Skin preparation from chin to knees, drape to expose torso and thighs,
  and laterally on the chest to allow thoracotomy
–Extra operating room help (i.e., scrub assistant or extra physician) to help
  operating surgeon
Incision
–Midline, xiphoid to symphysis pubis
–If patient is agonal and aortic control is needed, consider left thoracotomy
  with aortic occlusion first
First maneuvers: assessment
–Four-hand retraction, evacuate blood and clot, pack all four quadrants
–Look for bleeding; if easy, control large bleeding sites
–Note hematomas and sites of contamination
–Place large, self-retaining retractor (e.g., Bookwalter, Thompson)
Second maneuvers: exposure
–With retroperitoneal hematoma, perform right or left medial visceral rotation,
  or other necessary maneuvers to expose retroperitoneal vascular structures
Third maneuvers: control and repair
–Control hemorrhage: decide on the "best" approach for proximal and distal control,
  or for control of an active bleeding site directly or through a hematoma
–Control contamination: after arterial and venous control is obtained, control all
  hollow visceral injuries
–Vascular repair: reestablish vascular continuity with repair or graft. If patient is in
  extremis—cold, coagulopathic, acidotic—consider damage control (with intravascular
  shunt, if needed) or vessel ligation

the same fashion, after directly opening the hematoma. Proximal control
can be obtained with occlusive clamps or tourniquets, or if the injury is
visible, with side-biting vascular clamps that exclude the injury without
occluding the vessel. Select a Fogarty or Foley balloon catheter, which can
help control hemorrhage during local dissection, based on the size of
the injured vessel. **When the patient's condition warrants a "damage control" strategy, continuity of critical vessels (e.g., superior
mesenteric or common/external iliac arteries) can be maintained
with a temporary vascular shunt.** The decision to utilize a damage
control approach depends on the patient's complex of injuries and physiology (see Chapter 29).
   3. Venous hemorrhage may be controlled with finger or sponge stick com-
      pression while obtaining proximal and distal control. Allis or Babcock
      clamps can be used to coapt the edges of a venous injury to facilitate
      suture repair.
   4. Use cell-saving techniques from the outset to assure maximal blood
      salvage.
   C. **Midline injury (zone 1)** is associated with injuries to the aorta, vena cava,
      their bifurcations, central branches, and tributaries. Operative approach is

directed by findings of free hemorrhage versus hematoma, and its origin above or below the transverse mesocolon (Fig. 28.1).

1. **Exposure**

   a. If the hematoma is cephalad to the transverse mesocolon, obtain proximal control of the supraceliac aorta first. **Medial visceral rotation** of the left-sided viscera (spleen, tail of pancreas, colon, kidney) exposes the anterolateral aorta from the diaphragmatic hiatus to the bifurcation (Mattox maneuver) (Fig. 28.2). The distal descending thoracic aorta can be controlled in the posterior mediastinum by dividing the crural fibers of the diaphragm to the left of the aortic hiatus and the parasympathetic plexus surrounding it.

   b. Reflection of the right colon with extensive mobilization of the duodenum and head of the pancreas (**right-sided medial visceral rotation** or Cattell-Brasch maneuver) is commonly used to expose the infrahepatic vena cava, but it also effectively exposes the suprarenal aorta below the celiac axis and superior mesenteric artery, the distal aorta, and the right common iliac artery and vein (Fig. 28.3).

   c. In contrast to the stable hematoma, when active hemorrhage cephalad to the transverse mesocolon is encountered, control the bleeding immediately by manual compression. The aorta can be controlled at the hiatus after dividing the gastrohepatic omentum by retraction of the stomach and esophagus to the left, finger dissection to the aorta on the vertebral column, and applying an aortic clamp or man-

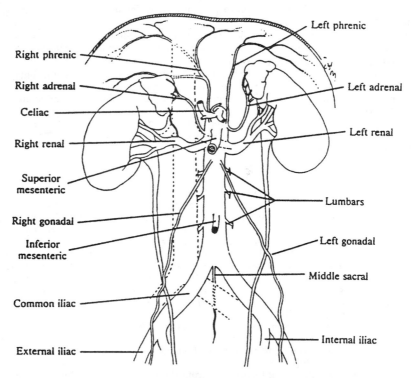

FIG. 28.1. Abdominal vascular anatomy. (From Frey W. Abdominal arterial trauma. In: Blaisdell FW, Trunkey DD, eds. *Abdominal trauma*, 2nd ed. New York: Thieme, 1993:345, with permission.)

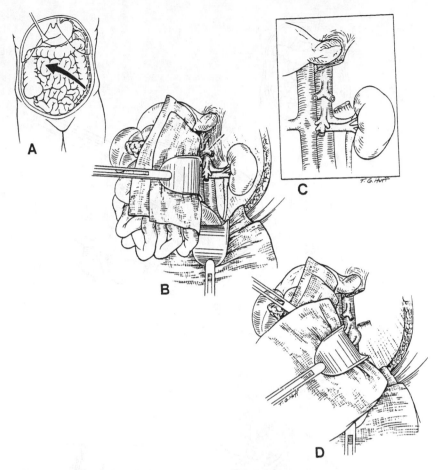

FIG. 28.2. Left-sided medial visceral rotation. (From Frey W: Abdominal arterial trauma. In: Blaisdell FW, Trunkey DD, eds. *Abdominal trauma*, 2nd ed. New York: Thieme, 1993:345, with permission.)

ual compression device. Exposure may require a thoracoabdominal incision into the left chest and takedown of the left hemidiaphragm.

   d. If a central hematoma extending laterally into the flanks or active arterial hemorrhage is present caudal to the transverse mesocolon, control of the infrarenal aorta is obtained. The transverse colon and small intestine are reflected superiorly and to the right, respectively, and the midline retroperitoneum is divided to expose the aorta and vena cava from the renal vessels distally.

   e. Hematoma or active venous bleeding from under the duodenum suggests a more proximal vena cava injury, which can be better visualized and controlled by the right-sided medial visceral rotation.

2. The aorta. Direct repair, in a transverse direction to limit narrowing, is performed with 4-0 polypropylene suture. In the event of a large lateral defect, narrowing may be avoided by a polytetrafluoroethylene (PTFE) patch. Extensive destruction may necessitate placement of a Dacron

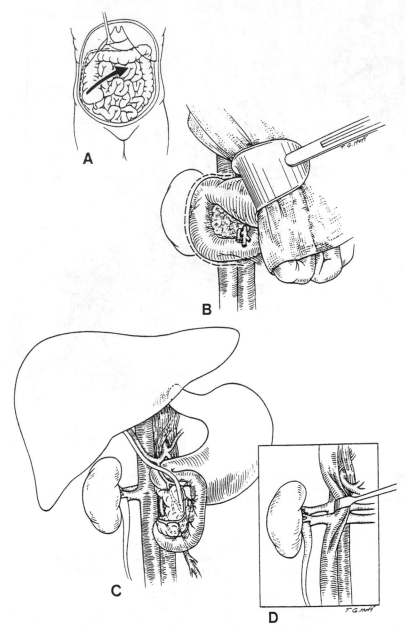

FIG. 28.3. Right-sided medial visceral rotation. (From Frey W: Abdominal arterial trauma. In: Blaisdell FW, Trunkey DD, eds. *Abdominal trauma*, 2nd ed. New York: Thieme, 1993:345, with permission.)

or PTFE graft. In desperate situations, the distal aorta, below the renal arteries, can be ligated, although lower extremity ischemia is likely and extraanatomic revascularization may be subsequently required (Table 28.2). Survival in this circumstance is unlikely.

3. **Celiac axis, superior mesenteric artery, and superior mesenteric vein.** The celiac axis is repaired with 5-0 or 6-0 polypropylene suture, but it can also be ligated without significant morbidity. Injury to the portal vein or proximal superior mesenteric artery or vein may require transection of the neck of the pancreas to visualize and control. Attempt primary repair with 5-0 or 6-0 polypropylene suture. Extensive injury to the superior mesenteric artery may require bypass with saphenous vein or PTFE graft to maintain midgut viability. Temporary shunting of the superior mesenteric artery with delayed reconstruction has been reported. In theory, this artery can be ligated, but collateral flow in the trauma patient in shock is usually inadequate. If ligation is performed, plan a second-look procedure within 24 hours. The superior mesenteric vein should be repaired, when possible; ligation is acceptable for the patient *in extremis*, but mesenteric viability will be jeopardized and a second-look operation is necessary within 24 hours.

4. **Mesentery** injuries are usually visible on direct inspection. These can be controlled directly with local dissection and ligation; avoid blind clamping into the hematoma. It is imperative to reassess bowel viability after ligation. Close the mesenteric defect to prevent internal hernia.

5. **Inferior vena cava** injuries can be repaired with 5-0 polypropylene suture. The infrarenal vena cava can be ligated, although measures must be taken to minimize lower extremity edema postoperatively, and

Table 28.2. Abdominal vessel ligation and expected complications

Vessel	Complication	Recommendations
Celiac axis	None	
Splenic artery	None if short gastric vessels intact	
Common hepatic artery	None if portal vein intact; possible gallbladder ischemia	Consider cholecystectomy
Superior mesenteric artery	Bowel ischemia	Second-look procedure
Superior mesenteric vein	Bowel ischemia	Second-look procedure
Portal vein	Bowel ischemia	Second-look procedure
Suprarenal inferior vena cava	Possible renal failure	
Infrarenal aorta	Lower extremity ischemia	Consider calf fasciotomies or extra-anatomic bypass
Infrarenal inferior vena cava	Lower extremity edema	Wrap and elevate legs
Left renal vein (proximal)	None	
Right renal vein	Renal ischemia	Nephrectomy
Common and external iliac artery	Lower extremity ischemia	Consider calf fasciotomies or extra-anatomic bypass
Common and external iliac vein	Lower extremity edema	Wrap and elevate legs
Internal iliac vein	None	

bilateral four-compartment calf fasciotomies are recommended. The suprarenal vena cava should be repaired or reconstructed to prevent possible renal failure, but it can be ligated in the patient *in extremis*.

D. Lateral injury (zone 2) is associated with injury to the renal artery and vein, and kidney. Penetrating injuries are always explored. With blunt injury, a stable hematoma should not be disturbed if a hollow viscus injury can be excluded, especially if a preoperative study shows intact blood flow and urine excretion. This is true even if the study shows urinary extravasation, provided this is contained within Gerota's fascia.

1. **Exposure**
   a. With penetrating injury and a perirenal hematoma, first obtain proximal control of the ipsilateral renal vessels through the midline retroperitoneum. Arterial control requires mobilization of the overlying left renal vein. Control of the right renal vein requires mobilization of right colon and duodenum. If hematoma extends from the lateral aspect to midline or beyond, then first obtain proximal and distal aortic control before disturbing the hematoma.
   b. Active bleeding from a renal injury precludes proximal vessel control. The kidney is manually compressed and elevated through Gerota's fascia laterally, and a vascular clamp placed across the renal hilum.
2. **Renal artery** injuries should be repaired directly or with end-to-end anastomosis with 5-0 polypropylene suture. Interposition grafting with autogenous vein is appropriate only when the patient is stable and the kidney is believed salvageable. If palpation determines that the contralateral kidney is present and of normal size, then nephrectomy is advisable if the patient is unstable and the renal artery cannot be easily repaired.
3. **Renal vein.** Perform lateral venorrhaphy in a transverse direction with 5-0 polypropylene suture. Right renal vein ligation necessitates nephrectomy. The left renal vein can be ligated in the midline, proximal to patent adrenal and gonadal veins.

E. Pelvic injury (zone 3)
1. **Exposure**. Full exposure of pelvic vascular injuries may require mobilization of the ipsilateral and contralateral colon from the pelvis.
   a. When a pelvic hematoma is identified over the iliac vessels, obtain proximal control of the common iliac artery and vein through the midline retroperitoneum at the aortic and inferior vena cava bifurcation or, preferentially, proximal to the area of injury on the iliac vessels themselves. Temporary transection of the right common iliac artery may be necessary to enable control of the proximal right common iliac vein. Obtain distal control of the external iliac artery and vein just proximal to the inguinal ligament on the up-slope of the pelvic floor. Injuries to the distal iliac vessels may necessitate control of the common femoral vessels through a groin incision. Expose the internal iliac artery after gaining control of the common and external iliac vessels and opening the hematoma.
   b. Deep pelvic arterial bleeding and venous bleeding from deep pelvic, presacral veins is best handled by tamponade and arteriography with embolization.
2. **The iliac artery**. Repair common and external iliac artery injuries with 5-0 polypropylene suture or an autogenous vein or PTFE graft when direct repair is not possible. Ligation of these vessels is associated with a 40% to 50% rate of subsequent amputation (ligation of the common iliac artery is better tolerated than the more distal external iliac artery). When ligation is necessary, consider a femoral-femoral, extra-anatomic bypass, or at minimum a four-compartment calf fasciotomy. Internal iliac artery repair can be done with 5-0 polypropylene suture, but ligation is well-tolerated.
3. **The iliac vein** injuries should be repaired with 5-0 polypropylene suture, when possible, but ligation is well-tolerated. Ligation of the exter-

nal or common iliac vein can lead to significant lower extremity edema in the early postoperative period. Anticoagulation after venous repair or ligation is controversial; the risk of iliofemoral thrombosis is nearly 30%.

F. Portal and retrohepatic injury

1. **Exposure**

   a. **Hematoma or hemorrhage** in the porta hepatis is controlled with a vascular clamp across the portal structures just above the duodenum (Pringle maneuver); a second clamp at the liver edge may also be helpful. The hepatic artery and portal vein are dissected and isolated, and the injury identified.

   b. Control of the retropancreatic portion of the portal vein can require transection of the neck of the pancreas.

   c. An expanding retrohepatic hematoma or active hemorrhage is initially controlled with manual compression of the overlying liver. Although direct repair may be feasible, control can also require vascular isolation of the liver with occlusion of the hepatoduodenal ligament, and suprahepatic and infrahepatic vena cava.

      (1) An atriocaval shunt, necessitating median sternotomy, can be used.

      (2) In some cases, when manual compression seems to control bleeding, firm packing may be appropriate (damage control) with subsequent angiographic embolization of bleeding arterial vessels or balloon control of the inferior vena cava.

2. **Hepatic artery.** Direct repair or end-to-end reanastomosis is performed with 5-0 polypropylene suture. Perform ligation in the presence of extensive injury or continued instability, which is well tolerated, but consider performing a cholecystectomy.

3. **Portal vein.** Perform direct transverse venorrhaphy with 5-0 polypropylene suture. The vein can be ligated in the presence of extensive injury, but hepatic and mesenteric viability can be compromised, and a second-look operation within 24 hours is necessary.

4. **Retrohepatic vena cava.** One attempt should be made to visualize the injury directly for control and repair. If this is impossible because of exsanguinating hemorrhage, resume compression of the overlying liver. Options for management include a direct transhepatic approach, vascular isolation of the liver, atriocaval shunt (usually performed with a 36F-chest tube or No. 8 or 9 endotracheal tube), or retrograde balloon catheter insertions through the femoral vein for occlusion above and below the injury. Repair the vena cava transversely with 4-0 polypropylene suture. Branches of the hepatic veins can be ligated.

Axioms

- The patient with abdominal vascular injury can present normotensive, hypotensive, or *in extremis* from exsanguination.
- Determination of trajectory is the key to anatomic diagnosis in penetrating injury.
- A patient in shock with a penetrating injury or distended abdomen has a major vascular injury until proved otherwise.
- In cases of suspected abdominal vascular injury, anticipate massive transfusion requirements. Begin blood transfusion early, including replacement of plasma and platelets.
- Expect major distortion of anatomy by hemorrhage and hematoma.
- Direct pressure with fingers or packs is the first maneuver to control bleeding. Hemorrhage control may require a direct approach through the hematoma, with finger dissection and sponge stick or clamp control. Proximal and distal control are preferred for controlled vascular repair, but may not always be possible initially.
- Patients who present *in extremis* with shock and exsanguinating injury benefit from a "damage control" approach, which emphasizes immediate control of hemorrhage and contamination, then resuscitation, with delayed, definitive reexploration.

Bibliography

Feliciano DV. Management of traumatic retroperitoneal hematoma. *Ann Surg* 1990; 211:109–123.

Feliciano DV. Abdominal vessels. In: Ivatury RR, Cayten CG, eds. *The textbook of penetrating trauma.* Baltimore: Williams & Wilkins, 1996:702–715.

Fry WR, Fry RE, Fry WJ. Operative exposure of the abdominal arteries for trauma. *Arch Surg* 1991;126:289–291.

Reilly PM, Rotondo MF, Carpenter JC, et al. Temporary vascular continuity during damage control: intraluminal shunting for proximal superior mesenteric artery injury. *J Trauma* 1995;39:757–760.

Rotondo MF, Schwab CW, McGonigal MD, et al. Damage control: an approach for improved survival in exsanguinating penetrating abdominal injury. *J Trauma* 1993; 35:375–383.

29. DAMAGE CONTROL

Michael F. Rotondo

I. **Introduction.** The damage control approach arose out of the necessity to rapidly stop cavitary bleeding, stage physiologic resuscitation, and reverse the death spiral. In select circumstances, the traditional approach to exsanguinating abdominal injury was often not appropriate or effective. This appeared particularly true in physiologically unstable patients with multiple penetrating wounds or blunt high-energy transfer with massive blood loss. During the struggle for surgical control of bleeding, repeated bouts of hypotension and physiologic instability frequently resulted in a lethal triad of metabolic acidosis, hypothermia, and coagulopathy. Historically, if the surgeon persisted with the traditional approach—completion of definitive laparotomy or thoracotomy—this vicious cycle of events killed the patient in many cases. In this situation, an alternative approach called "damage control" has been recommended as the procedure of choice.

For the trauma surgeon, damage control describes a technique of abbreviated laparotomy, with precise containment of bleeding and contamination, and temporary intraabdominal packing for initial injury control. Subsequently, the patient is moved to the intensive care unit (ICU) for physiologic restoration and later definitive repair of all injuries in the operating room (OR). For the practicing general surgeon caring for trauma patients, this approach can be useful to stabilize and transfer the trauma patient to a level I Trauma Center. For the general surgeon caring for the patient with an abdominal catastrophe, such as acute mesenteric ischemia or a ruptured abdominal aortic aneurysm, it may have important applicability in temporization and stabilization of the patient. In either case, damage control constitutes a premeditated, deliberate surgical exercise requiring careful judgment. Damage control is not surgical failure, but rather an aggressive move to break the pattern of physiologic failure.

A. **Definition.** Damage control is defined in three distinct phases.

1. **Phase I.** Immediate exploratory laparotomy to control hemorrhage and contamination using simple techniques. Definitive reconstruction is delayed. Intraabdominal packing is applied to all dissected surfaces and injured organs, followed by rapid closure of the skin or abdominal coverage. Damage control has been used in the chest and the extremities as a technique of abbreviated surgical control of hemorrhage.

2. **Phase II.** Secondary and continued resuscitation in the ICU characterized by maximization of hemodynamics aimed at optimization of oxygen delivery and consumption, lactate clearance, core rewarming, correction of coagulopathy, complete ventilatory support, monitoring for abdominal compartment syndrome, and continued injury identification.

3. **Phase III.** Reoperation for removal of intraabdominal packing, definitive repair of abdominal injury, and closure, if possible. Moreover, extraabdominal injury repair may ensue.

II. **Patient selection.** Success of damage control is dependent on judicious selection of patients based on the development of abnormal physiology from profound hypoperfusion. Although a number of studies have attempted to identify objective elements in the selection process in an effort to define strict criteria, none have successfully done so. However, a number of important factors have been identified. One simple method to remember these factors is to consider conditions, complexes, and critical factors.

A. **Conditions.** Pertinent mechanisms of injury and the presence of physiologic instability

1. High-energy blunt torso trauma
2. Multiple torso penetrations

3. Profound hemodynamic instability
4. Coagulopathy, hypothermia, or severe acidosis as a result of initial injury or comorbidity
- **B. Complexes**. Important injury patterns to consider:
  1. Major abdominal vascular injury with multiple visceral injuries
  2. Multiregional exsanguination with concomitant visceral injuries
  3. Multiregional injury in the presence of intraabdominal injury with competing priorities (e.g., severe closed head injury, widened mediastinum, pelvic fracture)
- **C. Critical factors**. Salient intraoperative considerations
  1. **Severe metabolic acidosis with pH < 7.30**
  2. **Hypothermia with temperature <35°C**
  3. **Coagulopathy**, as evidenced by the development of nonmechanical bleeding, elevation of both prothrombin time (PT) and partial thromboplastin time (PTT), thrombocytopenia, or massive transfusion (>10 units packed red blood cells) is a hallmark.
  4. **Resuscitation and operative time >90 minutes**
- **III. Technical considerations**. Elements of the damage control approach are contrary to traditional surgical teaching and, therefore, warrant special mention.
  - **A. Damage control, phase I**. Establishing control and knowing when to stop
    1. **Hemorrhage control**
       a. Establish initial control of vascular injuries using vascular clamps and suture ligatures. Simple lateral repairs may be possible; however, complex reconstruction is usually not achievable and should be avoided. Temporary vascular shunting can be another useful adjunct.
       b. Also avoid complex repairs of bleeding solid organ injury. Manage splenic and renal injuries by rapid resection. Hepatic injuries may require a variety of temporizing measures, including the Pringle maneuver, for arterial and portal venous exclusion; manual pressure, using the most experienced available surgical hands; packing, using laparotomy packs; and plugging, using Gelfoam and thrombin or balloon catheter tamponade. Avoid anatomic resection, complex debridement, lengthy finger fracture techniques, and mesh hepatorrhaphy. Interventional radiology for complex hepatic, renal, pelvic, and muscle bleeding is of paramount importance and should immediately follow the abbreviated surgical procedure, when necessary.
    2. **Contamination control**
       a. Control hollow viscus injuries with ligation (with umbilical tapes), simple repair (oversewing defects), rapid staple closure, or resection. Restoration of gastrointestinal continuity should be delayed as should stoma formation and placement of gastrostomy or jejunostomy tubes.
       b. Bile duct injuries are temporized by intraluminal tube drainage, ligation, end choledochostomy, or simple drainage; avoid complex reconstructions.
       c. Pancreatic injuries must be drained and, if necessary, simple resections performed to control pancreatic secretions. The unabated flow of pancreatic juice severely damages surrounding tissues and compromises later reconstructive efforts. **Critical is wide, laterally placed closed suction drainage of pancreatic injuries**.
    3. **Packing**. Apply laparotomy pads over all dissected surfaces and any solid organ injuries. It is possible to "overpack" the abdominal cavity. Packing should be tight enough to provide adequate tamponade without impeding venous return or arterial blood supply.
    4. **Abdominal closure**. Although some recommend towel clip closure of the skin for rapid abdominal wall closure, we recommend a running, continuous suture in the skin only. Closure of the fascia, at this juncture, takes time and leads to unnecessary fascial loss, which complicates definitive closure later. However, at times, even skin closure is not possible because

of massive bowel edema. In this setting, packing and closure with a layered nonadhesive and adhesive plastic membrane is recommended. With this technique, plastic (e.g., an x-ray cassette bag or intestinal bag) can be tailored and tucked under the fascial edges. Alternatively, a towel encased in plastic adhesive drape can be used. Place laparotomy pads over the plastic to maintain the intestines near the level of the fascia. Place closed suction drains in the lateral subcutaneous gutters and an adhesive plastic membrane over the skin with packs to seal and secure the dressing. Application of low continuous wall suction allows for a vac-pac seal and excellent wound management with minimal fistula formation.

   a. As an alternative approach, a nonadherent substance, such as a sterilized intravenous bags ("Bogota bag"), can be sewn to the skin or fascia.

5. Pitfalls. During the course of this technique, continually reassess the appropriateness of damage control. In this situation, it is important to remember that bleeding or contamination that is incompletely controlled will **not** respond to packing. Therefore, injury that is not adequately controlled or is missed will most certainly lead to the patient's death. As mentioned, in select circumstances, angiography is an important adjunct for injuries that are incompletely controlled in the OR. This may be particularly useful for hepatic, pelvic, or retroperitoneal bleeding.

On the other hand, if insufficient factors warrant damage control, the patient will be subjected to an unnecessary delay to definitive operation. Multiple factors influence the timing and application of damage control; experience and good judgment are essential in this decision.

B. Damage control, phase II. Secondary resuscitation: breaking the vicious cycle.

1. Maximization of hemodynamics. The key to resolution of metabolic acidosis and subsequent clearing of the accumulated lactic acid is restoration of adequate tissue perfusion, which can be directed by invasive monitors. Often these monitors are not placed during damage control phase I because of competing priorities during that phase of resuscitation. Placement of an arterial line and use of Swan Ganz catheter monitoring are essential in damage control phase II. Many institutions use oximetric Swan Ganz catheters to direct resuscitation on the basis of oxygen delivery and consumption curves. Moreover, clearance of lactic acid helps predict survival in these patients.

2. Core rewarming. Immediate and aggressive core rewarming not only improves perfusion, but it also helps reverse coagulopathy. A number of techniques have been suggested, including pleural and gastric lavage with warm fluids, increasing ambient room temperature, administration of warm fluids using rapid infusion devices, external warming devices, and extracorporeal circulation devices such as venovenous bypass and arterial-venous bypass (see Chapter 42). Inability to rewarm a patient correlates with increases in mortality; prolonged postoperative hypothermia correlates with increases in morbidity. The inability to warm a patient suggests that the patient may have ongoing bleeding. A combined approached of both active and passing warming measures is recommended.

3. Coagulopathy correction

   a. The factors causing coagulopathy in these patients include hypothermia, leading to both qualitative and quantitative alterations of the clotting cascade; platelet aggregation dysfunction; changes in fibrinolysis; persistent metabolic acidosis, leading to microvascular sludging and changes in red blood cell and platelet interaction; and dilution, caused by administration of large volumes of crystalloid and packed red blood cells, both devoid of clotting factors and platelets.

   b. Standard therapy to correct coagulopathy includes reversal of hypothermia and administration of fresh frozen plasma (FFP), which is rich in factors V and VIII. Repletion of clotting factors with FFP is directed by serial sampling for PTT and PT. Platelet levels can also be followed and platelets administered accordingly. Fibrinogen levels should also be measured and, if necessary, cryoprecipitate given. Most importantly, all repletion factors should be warmed before administration and, if necessary, **given as continuous infusions until the coagulopathy is reversed**.

4. **Complete ventilatory support**. During critical secondary resuscitation, patients should remain sedated and in synchrony with the ventilator. Often, chemical paralysis is necessary for maximal ventilatory support and control. Benefits of this approach outweigh the risks associated with the presumed delay in rewarming secondary to neuromuscular blockade. Maximization of perfusion cannot occur without excellent oxygen saturation.

5. **Continued injury identification**. Complete injury identification is essential during damage control phase II. Another complete physical examination, the tertiary survey, should include additional radiographic examinations of newly found fractures and completion of the spine survey. Additional computed tomography (CT) scanning should be obtained as needed.

6. **Monitoring for abdominal compartment syndrome**. Bladder pressures should be transduced every 4 to 6 hours to identify elevated intraabdominal pressures. Intraabdominal hypertension is classified and treated as follows: grade I (<15 mmHg)—normovolemic resuscitation; grade II (15–25 mm Hg)—hypervolemic resuscitation; grade III (25–35 mmHg)—hypervolemic resuscitation with opening of the abdominal closure or adjustment of the vac-pac dressing at bedside; and grade IV (>35 mmHg)—hypervolemic resuscitation with return to the OR for exploration.

7. **Pitfalls**
   a. **Abdominal compartment syndrome (ACS)** (see Chapter 30) is clinically characterized by increased ventilatory pressures (peak inspiratory pressure >60 cm H_2O), decreased PaO_2, increased $PaCO_2$, and decreased urine output (from decreased end-organ perfusion). Diagnosis can be made on these clinical grounds alone; however, many believe that these are the late signs of ACS. If acted on at this juncture, it is most likely that end-organ ischemia has been ongoing and considerable secondary insult has already occurred. It is clear that as intraabdominal pressure rises, venous return is impeded and end-organ perfusion is significantly diminished. Therefore, transduced bladder pressure monitoring is warranted. At higher grades of intraabdominal hypertension, open the abdomen to evacuate clot and to replace packs, as appropriate. This can be done in the ICU, but it is best accomplished in the OR, particularly if a persistent bleeding source or missed injury is suspected. Early descriptions of ACS included discussions of a lethal reperfusion syndrome that occurred at the time of abdominal release characterized by sudden death.
   b. **Abdominal compartment syndrome can be avoided by leaving the abdomen open at the initial damage control laparotomy and liberal application of the "vac-pac" technique**.
   c. **Reoperation for bleeding**. The need for immediate reoperation on the basis of ongoing, uncontrolled hemorrhage must continually be assessed. After hemodynamic maximization, core rewarming, and coagulopathy correction have been achieved, an ongoing blood requirement of more than 2 units of packed red blood cells (PRBCs) per hour may indicate the need for immediate reexploration. This decision is difficult and requires experienced judgment rather than absolute rules. If normal physiology cannot be achieved or if normal physiology has been restored and then deteriorates, reoperation is indicated.

Both ongoing bleeding and abdominal compartment syndrome can prevent physiologic restoration. Return to the OR is warranted for reinspection for missed or inadequately controlled injury and an additional attempt at definitive control of hemorrhage. If necessary, the abdomen can be repacked and left open using a vac-pac closure or other synthetic membrane to bridge the abdominal opening.

  d. Timing for return to the OR for definitive laparotomy is of utmost importance. It should be based on the reestablishment of normal physiology; average time for restoration of normal physiology is about 36 hours. At that time, little difficulty with recurrent coagulopathy or electrolyte imbalance will be encountered at the second operation. Furthermore, this allows ample time for a complete tertiary survey, additional radiographic examinations, and planning by consultants for definitive management of associated injuries. Although premature return to the OR can result in coagulopathy and repacking, prolonged, delayed return can lead to an increase in intraabdominal infection rate and missed opportunity for definitive repair of associated injuries.

C. **Damage control, phase III. Second operation**.
  1. **Reinspection and reconstruction**
     a. All areas previously packed must be carefully inspected and meticulous hemostasis obtained in areas that are still bleeding. Solid organs, which have been packed, require the most care and attention. Carefully remove the packs with copious amounts of irrigation and obtain hemostasis in a stepwise fashion. This can be done using electrocautery, argon beam coagulation, thrombin preparations, or other clot-promoting materials. Suture ligate other vascular injuries still oozing. If temporary shunting has been used, reconstruction can be done at this time using traditional vascular reconstructive techniques.
     b. Inspect all gastrointestinal repairs and resections. At this point, gastrointestinal continuity can be restored. If necessary, gastrostomy tubes, jejunostomy tubes, and end stomas can be created. If fascial closure has been unachievable, end stomas and enterostomy tubes should be avoided. In our experience with the open abdomen, these techniques are associated with an inordinately high complication rate as the relationship of the intraabdominal contents changes to the geometry of the anterior abdominal wall after damage control phase III. Instead, primary anastomoses should be created for gastrointestinal continuity and both nasogastric tubes and nasoduodenal tubes should be placed and directed intraoperatively for proximal decompression and feeding respectively. If at all possible, anastomosis should be tucked deep inside fascial edges or covered with omentum to afford a natural habitat and promote sealing.
  2. **Closure of the anterior abdominal wall and management of the open abdomen**. A number of choices exist for anterior abdominal wall closure. Primary fascial closure followed by skin closure is the best option, if possible. Separation of parts can mobilize the midline sufficiently to allow primary fascial closure. If fascial closure is not possible, skin closure only, with a planned ventral hernia repair is a viable choice. Some have advocated immediate placement of prosthetic material, followed by sequential closure of the fascia and skin, although we have not found this to be efficacious. Others have advocated application of vac-pac dressing for several days after damage control phase III in the patient who has persistent massive visceral edema and in whom abdominal closure is simply not possible. Meticulous reapplication of the vac-pac dressing is of utmost importance to minimize the risk of fistula formation. Fistula formation is extremely vexing and difficult to manage in this setting. Remember, these are not enterocutaneous fistulas, but rather

"enteroatmospheric" fistulas without a subcutaneous component and spontaneous closure without surgical intervention is impossible. Early reports on application of the vac-pac dressing indicate a fistula formation rate of <5%. When it is clear that both bowel and anterior abdominal wall edema will not resolve in a reasonable time frame (5–7 days), application of a tension free absorbable mesh fascial closure is indicated. After 7 to 14 days of local wound care over the absorbable mesh graft, a traditional split-thickness skin graft can be placed over an exuberant granulation bed. Interval repair of the subsequent abdominal wall hernia can be done at 6 to 9 months when the patient has sufficiently recovered. At this point, reconstruction can be accomplished through excision of the split-thickness skin graft, complete adhesiolysis between the small bowel mat and the parietal peritoneum, followed by anterior abdominal wall component separation technique.

3. **Pitfalls.** The second operation (damage control III) can be lengthy, on average 2 to 4 hours, but it is generally well tolerated. Some patients may redevelop metabolic acidosis and hypothermia and abrupt termination of operation and reapplication of packing may be necessary again. On average, blood product requirements can be as high as 6 to 8 units of PRBC, with a matching amount of FFP. If the second operation must be terminated, the same principles of judgment applied in damage control phase I should be used and the vac-pac applied to manage the open abdomen.

IV. **Morbidity and mortality. The damage control principle is founded on the fact that decrease in mortality is achieved at a cost of increased morbidity.**

   A. A careful review of the literature reveals that the overall survivorship of patients treated with the damage control approach is 50%; survival rates have been reported as low as 30% and as high as 77%. As the damage control technique is refined and applied more aggressively, survival rates continue to improve and may indeed be as high as 80% to 90%.

   B. The incidence of abdominal complications is approximately 35%. These complications include abscess, intraabdominal abscess, biliary and gastrointestinal fistula, hepatic necrosis, obstruction, anastomotic leak, pancreatic fistula, and abdominal wall failure. Precise rates for each of these complications are currently unknown. Furthermore, other complications (e.g., fever, pneumonia, renal failure, sepsis, systemic inflammatory response syndrome, adult respiratory distress syndrome, and multiple organ dysfunction syndrome) are common in these severely injured patients.

Axioms

- Damage control is a three-phase approach to the exsanguinating trauma patient. It includes:
  1. Abbreviated surgical control of hemorrhage and contamination
  2. Continued and complete resuscitation in the ICU
  3. Definitive repair and reconstruction
- Damage control requires exquisite surgical judgment.
- When attempting to resuscitate the patient in the ICU, recognition of failed surgical control of bleeding and the need for reexploration is essential.
- Abdominal compartment syndrome can be avoided by managing the abdomen open.
- Meticulous management of the open abdomen is warranted to avoid fistula formation.

Bibliography

Abou-Khalil B, Scalea T, Trooskin SZ, et al. Hemodynamic responses to shock in young trauma patients: need for invasive monitoring. *Crit Care Med* 1994;22(4):633–639.

Barker DE, Kaufman HJ, Smith LA, et al. Vacuum pack technique of temporary abdominal closure: a 7-year experience with 112 patients. *J Trauma* 2000;8:201–207.

Burch JM, Moore EE, Moore FA, et al. The abdominal compartment syndrome. *Surg Clin North Am* 1996;76:833–842.

Burch JM, Denton JR, Noble RD. Physiologic rationale for abbreviated laparotomy. *Surg Clin North Am* 1997;77:779–782.

Burch JM, Ortiz VB, Richardson RJ, et al. Abbreviated laparotomy and planned reoperation for critically injured patients. *Ann Surg* 1992;215:476.

Carrillo EH, Spain DA, Wilson MA, et al. Alternatives in the management of penetrating injuries to the iliac vessels. *J Trauma* 1998;44(6):1024–1030.

Cosgriff N, Moore EE, Sauaia A, et al. Predicting life-threatening coagulopathy in the massively transfused trauma patient: hypothermia and acidosis revisited. *J Trauma* 1997;42(5):857–862.

Cushman JG, Feliciano DV, Renz BM, et al. Iliac vessel injury: operative physiology related to outcome. *J Trauma* 1997;2(6):1033–1040.

Fabian TC, Croce MA, Pritchard FE, et al. Planned ventral hernia, staged management for acute abdominal wall defects. *Ann Surg* 1994;219(6):643–653.

Gubler KD, Gentilello LM, Hassantash SA, et al. The impact of hypothermia on dilutional coagulopathy. *J Trauma* 1994;36(6):847–851.

Hirshberg A, Mattox KL. Planned reoperation for severe trauma. *Ann Surg* 1995;222(1):3–8.

Ivatury RR, Diebel L, Porter JM, et al. Intra-abdominal hypertension and the abdominal compartment syndrome. *Surg Clin North Am* 1997;77:783–800.

Mayberry JC, Mullins RJ, Crass RA, et al. Prevention of abdominal compartment syndrome by absorbable mesh prosthesis closure. *Arch Surg* 1997;132:957–962.

Moore EE, Burch JM, Franciose RJ, et al. Staged physiologic restoration and damage control surgery. *World J Surg* 1998;22:1184–1191.

Morris JA, Eddy VA, Rutherford EJ. The staged celiotomy: damage control. *Trauma Quarterly* 1993;10(1):60–70.

Peitzman AB, Heil B, Rivera L, et al. Blunt splenic injury in adults: multi-institutional study of the Eastern Association for the Surgery of Trauma. *J Trauma* 2000;49(2):177–187.

Richardson JD, Polk HC. Reoperation for trauma. *Ann Surg* 1995;222(1):1–2.

Rotondo MF, Schwab CW, McGonigal MD, et al. Damage control: an approach for improved survival in exsanguinating penetrating abdominal injury. *J Trauma* 1993;35(3):375–383.

Rotondo MF, Zonies DH. The damage control sequence and underlying logic. *Surg Clin North Am* 1997;77:761–777.

Shapiro MB, Jenkins DH, Schwab CW, et al. Damage control: collective review. *J Trauma* 2000;49:969–978.

Sherck J, Seiver A, Shatney C, et al. Covering the "open abdomen": a better technique. *Am Surg* 1998;64:854–857.

Smith LA, Barker DE, Chase CW, et al. Vacuum pack technique of temporary abdominal closure: a four year experience. *Am Surg* 1997;63:1102–1107.

30. ABDOMINAL COMPARTMENT SYNDROME

Robert A. Maxwell and Marilyn J. Borst

I. **Introduction. Abdominal compartment syndrome (ACS)** is a clinical condition in which elevated intraabdominal pressure (intraabdominal hypertension) leads to impaired end-organ perfusion of the viscera. This results in respiratory, cardiac, and renal compromise, followed by multiple system organ dysfunction and death, if not appropriately diagnosed and treated. Onset can be insidious or fulminant and clinicians must be astute in making the diagnosis.

II. **Clinical scenarios.** ACS has been reported after ruptured abdominal aortic aneurysm repair, intraperitoneal hemorrhage, massive resuscitation for burns, pancreatitis, ileus, intestinal obstruction, postoperative bowel edema, pneumoperitoneum (e.g., secondary to barotrauma), septic shock, neoplasm, and liver transplantation; **the most common scenario is after major abdominal injury.** Two types of ACS have now been described, primary and secondary.

   A. **Primary ACS** occurs after laparotomy for major adominal trauma or other intraabdominal pathology. ACS can occur even when the abdomen has been left temporarily closed with prosthetics (e.g., "vac pacs," polyvinyl chloride bags, or mesh) and should be monitored in all patients requiring ongoing resuscitation after laparotomy. **In general, the most common cause of primary ACS is persistent hemorrhage**, ischemia or reperfusion injury, although visceral edema from third space losses is also an important factor. Hemorrhage can be either surgical (ongoing bleeding) or nonsurgical (coagulopathy or hypothermia). Hypothermia and coagulopathy need aggressive correction before returning for decompression, but this should not delay reexploration when bladder pressures exceed 30 mmHg.

   B. **Secondary ACS** develops in trauma or burn patients **without** intraabdominal injury who require aggressive resuscitation for massive extremity trauma, vascular injury, or severe burns (generally >50% total body surface area [TBSA]). The primary mechanism appears to be fluid sequestration within the viscera caused by reperfusion injury and increased capillary permeability.

III. **Clinical manifestations.** Diagnosis of ACS is clinical and should be considered in any trauma or intensive care unit (ICU) patient with oliguria and abdominal distention. Physical examination will generally reveal a **stone-hard** abdomen that is characteristic for ACS.

   A. **Pulmonary** effects occur via elevation of the diaphragm, which results in decreased thoracic compliance and elevated peak airway pressures (>40 cm H_2O). The end results are hypoxia, hypercapnia, and respiratory acidosis.

   B. **Cardiac** manifestations occur from elevated thoracic pressure, which causes **normal or falsely elevated filling pressures (central venous pressure and pulmonary capillary wedge pressure)**, decreased cardiac return, and decreased cardiac compliance. The end result is decreased cardiac output, particularly in the hypovolemic patient, and decreased end-organ perfusion.

   C. **Renal** effects occur from direct parenchymal and caval compression, and decreased cardiac output resulting in decreased perfusion and oliguria.

   D. **Gastrointestinal** effects occur from hypoperfusion of the splanchnic beds (direct compression and decreased cardiac output) leading to bacterial translocation and increased septic complications.

   E. **Neurologic** effects recently have been described as a consequence of ACS. The elevation in intrathoracic pressure presents a functional obstruction to jugular drainage and elevated intracranial pressure (ICP) results.

   F. **Ischemia to the abdominal wall**

IV. **Diagnosis** of ACS requires a high index of clinical suspicion. The clinical manifestations have been described above. Other supportive information may include measurement of bladder pressure. Any patient with ongoing fluid **resuscitation**

>10 L crystalloid or 10 U packed red blood cells (PRBCs) should have bladder pressure monitoring. In the early phases of ACS, when oliguria may be the only sign, measurement of intraabdominal pressure (IAP) may be useful.

A. **Bladder pressure,** the standard method for estimating intraabdominal pressure, can be measured at the bedside by an arterial line pressure transducer or water column manometer.

   1. **Clamp** the Foley catheter drainage tubing just distal to the aspiration port.
   2. **Inject** 50 to 100 mL of sterile saline into the bladder with a catheter-tipped syringe via the Foley catheter and reconnect to the drainage tubing.
   3. **Connect** a 16-gauge needle to the arterial line pressure tubing; flush and insert it into the aspiration port.
   4. **Zero** the system at the symphysis pubis while the patient is supine. Determine IAP with the transducer at the top of the symphysis pubis.

V. **Treatment** of ACS is based on the measured IAP and clinical suspicion. Intraabdominal pressure >30 mmHg is an indication for abdominal decompression, whereas management of pressures between 20 and 30 mmHg is controversial. Decompressive celiotomy should be considered with pressures between 20 and 30 mmHg with one or more of the following: (*a*) peak airway pressure >40 to 60 cm H_2O, (*b*) depressed cardiac output, or (*c*) oliguria.

A. **Decompressive celiotomy** for ACS is a surgical emergency.

   1. **Preoperative preparation.** Take the following actions during decompression of the abdomen to prevent hemodynamic decompensation: restore intravascular volume; maximize oxygen delivery; correct hypothermia; and correct coagulation defects.
   2. **Operative facilities.** Although a temptation exists to perform decompression at the bedside, generally avoid this in case ongoing bleeding or missed injury is discovered. Most ICUs are not the appropriate place to handle such problems.
   3. **Reperfusion syndrome.** Abdominal decompression results in the release of numerous toxic metabolites and acids into the systemic circulation that can lead to profound cardiac depression and hypotension. Some authors have recommended infusion of a 2-L solution consisting of 1 L of 0.45% normal saline with 50 g of mannitol and 50 mEq of sodium bicarbonate to avoid the decompensation, although the efficacy of this infusion is controversial.

B. **Abdominal closure.** A variety of techniques have been used for temporary abdominal closure and are usually institution specific.

   1. **Methods of temporary closure**
      a. Running continuous suture for closure of skin only. **Towel clip** closure is a universal technique for rapidly completing a damage control procedure, but is generally inadequate for decompressing ACS.
      b. **Prosthetic coverage.** No ideal way exists to deal with this issue; multiple options include "Bogota" (polyvinyl chloride) bags, "vac pacs," x-ray cassette covers, woven vicryl mesh, and fascial zippers, all **with the main risk being fistula formation.** Bogota bags and sterile x-ray cassette covers sewn to the skin are generally least expensive and usually adequate if early take-back is anticipated. Mesh sewn to the skin or fascia works well but can be a wound management problem in cases of large amounts of ascites. The vac pac works well under these circumstances.
      c. In all methods of temporary closure, an insert plastic material must be placed between bowel and sponges or towels.
      d. **Protect the fascia for definitive closure**
      e. Maintain abdominal domain as much as possible.
      f. Remove temporary closure as soon as possible and close fascia; diuresis can facilitate early closure. The patient is generally ready for attempted closure from postinjury day 3 to 7.
      g. Close skin, if the fascia cannot be closed.

      h. Do not use polypropylene mesh.
      i. Stomas and feeding tubes are created at the final abdominal exploration when the patient has stabilized.
    2. Methods of permanent closure
      a. Primary closure of the fascia. When visceral edema has sufficiently resolved, perform fascial closure. If primary closure cannot be performed by postoperative days 7 to 10, it will generally not occur because the abdomen becomes "socked-in" and staged reconstruction will be necessary.
      b. Split-thickness skin graft. If primary fascial closure cannot be performed and closure of skin only is not possible, the bowel will usually granulate through the absorbable mesh to accept a skin graft by 3 to 4 weeks postoperatively. This procedure generally permits the bowel edema to resolve and adhesions to subside.
      c. Delayed abdominal wall reconstruction. When the skin graft can easily be lifted off the underlying bowel, generally 6 to 9 months following grafting, abdominal wall reconstruction can be performed. Rectus sheath advancement (components technique) or permanent prosthetic placement is usually necessary because of loss of abdominal domain.
VI. Prevention of ACS
    A. Leave the abdomen open. It is now widely accepted to use temporary closure techniques after laparotomy in face of significant visceral edema, especially when further fluid sequestration can be expected.
    B. Correct coagulopathies and hypothermia. Coagulopathies and hypothermia lead to nonsurgical bleeding, which causes increased IAP and further resuscitation requirements.
VII. Morbidity and mortality
    A. Morbidity. Delayed diagnosis of ACS leads to bacterial translocation, increased rates of sepsis, and multiple organ dysfunction.
    B. Mortality of ACS ranges from 42% to 68% after detection and treatment and 100% in those **not** having decompression. Reduced rates of morbidity and mortality appear to hinge on early and aggressive detection and management.

Axioms
- Abdominal compartment syndrome should be suspected in any trauma or burn patient with abdominal distention and oliguria, despite normal or elevated filling pressures.
- As with any compartment syndrome, measurement of compartment (bladder) pressure is instrumental in establishing the diagnosis and should be routinely monitored in patients at risk.
- Patients with intraabdominal pressure >20 mmHg and signs of physiologic compromise should be decompressed.
- Forced fascial closure over swollen bowel or packs is generally contraindicated after trauma.

Bibliography
Bloomfield GL, Ridings PC, Blocher CK, et al. Effects of increasing intracranial pressure secondary to acute abdominal compartment syndrome upon intracranial and cerebral perfusion pressure before and after volume expansion. *J Trauma* 1996;40:936–943.
Eddy V, Nunn C, Morris JA Jr. Abdominal compartment syndrome: the Nashville experience. *Surg Clin North Am* 1997;77:801–812.
Fabian TC, Croce MA, Pritchard FE, et al. Planned ventral hernia: staged management for acute abdominal wall defects. *Ann Surg* 1994;219:643–650.
Ivatury RR, Diebel LN, Porter JM, et al. Intra-abdominal hypertension and the abdominal compartment syndrome. *Surg Clin North Am* 1997;77:783–800.
Meldrum DR, Moore FA, Moore EE, et al. Prospective characterization and selective management of the abdominal compartment syndrome. *Am J Surg* 1997;174:667–672.

31. GENITOURINARY INJURIES

Michael Rhodes and Fredrick Giberson

I. **Introduction**
   A. Most genitourinary (GU) injuries occur from blunt force. Improved imaging and subsequent staging of injury has resulted in a trend toward a more conservative approach to treatment. Hematuria is a key marker of urinary tract injury; extent of hematuria can guide the subsequent diagnostic evaluation. Once hematuria is identified, it is important to determine whether it is coming from the **upper** (kidney and ureter) or **lower** (bladder and urethra) **urinary tract**. History, physical findings, and trajectory (in penetrating injury) are important in guiding the priority of diagnostic evaluations.

II. **Hematuria** (Fig. 31.1)
   A. **Hematuria is either microscopic or macroscopic.**
      1. Although grossly bloody urine usually implies significant injury, **all macroscopic hematuria** (any blood, even light pink, seen with the naked eye) deserves further evaluation of the GU system.
      2. **Microscopic hematuria** (determined by urine dipstick or urinalysis) is nonspecific, but usually indicates the presence of injury or infection. Up to 15% of renal injuries will have **no** hematuria; however, most of these represent minor contusions. If possible, the first 5 mL of urine after catheter placement should be discarded to reduce catheter-related false-positive results.
      3. Although the urine dipstick and urinalysis quantification of red blood cells do not correlate well, their sensitivity and specificity as independent tests are equivalent. Absolute quantification of the numbers of red cells is not necessary.
   B. **Microscopic hematuria**
      1. Quantification of dipstick positivity (1+, 2+, 3+, 4+) has been used by some to determine the need for GU imaging. However, a **selective** approach has emerged recommending that **microscopic hematuria** of any amount should prompt further **imaging only** in patients with specific **physical findings** or **mechanism of injury** that suggests GU injury (i.e., blow to the flank, straddle injury). These include:
         a. Proximity penetrating injuries
         b. Children (<15 years of age)
         c. Adults with blunt injury and:
            • Flank pain or tenderness
            • Flank mass, fractured lower ribs, or spine fracture
            • History of hypotension (even if transient)
            • Multiple injuries
            • Straddle injury
            • History of high-energy impact (e.g., motor vehicle crash)

III. **Diagnostic tests**
   A. **Urethrogram**
      1. The urethrogram is indicated in any suspected urethral injury. The urethrogram is obtained by placing a small catheter approximately 2 cm into the distal urethra and instilling 10 mL of 30% contrast while occluding the urethral meatus. This can also be done through a partially advanced Foley catheter.
      2. The urethrogram should be performed at a 30° oblique angle.
   B. **Cystogram**
      1. After assuring no urethral injury is present, a Foley catheter is placed, through which a minimum of 300 to 400 mL of contrast (e.g., 30% Renografin) is infused by gravity. It is important to **fully distend the**

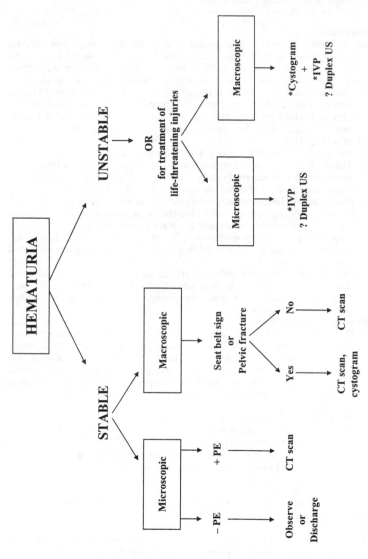

FIG. 31.1. Hematuria workup. PE, flank mass, flank pain, lower rib fractures, spine fracture, hypotension (even transient); *rapid portable study in trauma resuscitation area or operating room.

bladder to avoid missing small injuries. A radiograph of the full bladder is obtained, primarily looking for intraperitoneal tears and large extraperitoneal tears. A postvoid film is then obtained to detect small tears, especially with extraperitoneal or penetrating injury. Most cystograms are performed in the resuscitation area in patients with grossly bloody urine and obvious pelvic trauma. It may be efficient in these circumstances to obtain the cystogram as part of the original pelvic film. The concern of masking a pelvic fracture with the contrast is unrealized because the fractures are small, stable fractures that do not affect the immediate resuscitation and subsequently will be identified by pelvic computed tomography (CT).

  2. CT cystography, an alternative that can be used in stable patients, is usually accomplished by clamping the urethral catheter before performing an abdominal CT. However, if the bladder is not distended, contrast injection into the bladder may be necessary. CT cystography is most useful for identifying small tears, because large tears are usually present with grossly bloody urine and are identified on the pelvic or cystogram film in the resuscitation area.

C. CT scan

  1. The CT scan is the diagnostic test of choice for renal trauma. It is superior to the intravenous pyelogram (IVP) in that both vascular integrity of the kidney and any associated injury can be evaluated. CT is the gold standard for staging renal trauma. It is emerging as a useful test for ureteral and bladder injury in selected cases.

D. Arteriogram

  1. The arteriogram is used in renal trauma to delineate the vascular integrity of the kidney in clinical conditions in which the CT scan is indeterminate (e.g., nonfunctioning of the kidney on CT scan suggestive of traumatic renal artery thrombosis).

  2. Arteriogram followed by therapeutic stenting or embolization has been used in selected cases of renal trauma.

E. Intravenous pyelogram

  1. The CT scan for staging renal trauma has supplanted the IVP. The **one-shot IVP** (2 mg/kg of 50% intravenous [i.v.] contrast at wide-open drip, followed by a film in 10 minutes) has a **limited** role for the patient being transported to the operating room (OR) or in the OR for emergent laparotomy to delineate the presence of bilateral renal function.

  2. The IVP may be helpful in suspected/selected cases of ureteral trauma.

F. Ultrasound

  1. Ultrasound can rapidly outline the kidney parenchyma and surrounding tissues and provide evidence that an additional study (e.g., CT scan) may be necessary.

  2. It is an excellent technique to evaluate the injured transplanted kidney.

  3. Ultrasound is the test of choice to identify testicular injury.

  4. It can help identify renal blood flow intraoperatively when combined with Doppler (duplex).

IV. Renal injury (Fig. 31.2)

A. Mechanism

  1. Of renal injuries in the United States, 80% are from blunt trauma, resulting in a loss of the kidney in 5%. Penetrating injuries comprise 20%, resulting in a higher renal loss (40%).

B. Diagnosis

  1. The presence of hematuria, mechanism of injury, and physical findings (see section II. *Hematuria*)

  2. Staging of renal trauma is done by CT scan or at surgery (see Appendix A).

C. Treatment

  1. Nonoperative treatment of renal trauma (grades I to III) has become standard. If the injury is properly staged, nonoperative management is

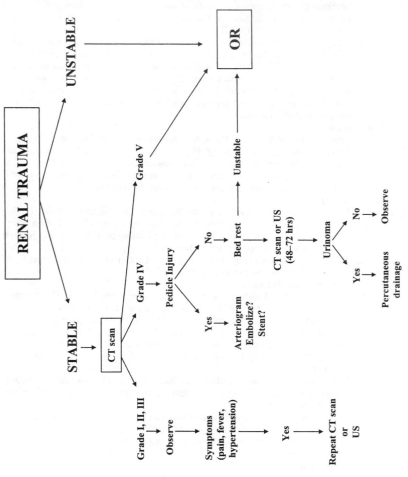

FIG. 31.2. Renal trauma workup.

successful for contusions, contained lacerations, most lesions with moderate extravasation of urine, or when blood is seen in **hemodynamically stable** patients.

2. Operative treatment is indicated for patients who are unstable, those who have suffered a hilar or pedicle injury, and patients with marked extravasation of urine or blood (grade IV). If the abdomen is explored for other reasons, a decision about renal exploration should be entertained for pulsatile or expanding retroperitoneal hematomas. An intraoperative IVP may be necessary to ascertain bilateral renal function. Palpation of the renal artery or intraoperative Doppler, ultrasound (Duplex), or both may be useful in determining renal blood flow.

3. In the stable patient, obtaining proximal vascular control before unroofing the perirenal hematoma may be helpful. Such control is best obtained by incising the mesentery just medial and inferior to the inferior mesenteric vein (Fig. 31.3). This allows access to both the left and right renal vessels.

4. In the **unstable** patient, it may be necessary to proceed with a **"scoop" nephrectomy**, wherein the hematoma is quickly mobilized followed by clamping of the renal hilum.

5. Proximal vascular control increases the rate of renal salvage. Repair of the renal parenchyma, with or without heminephrectomy, can have excellent results (Fig. 31.4). Reinforcement of the repair with omentum or mesh can be a useful alternative. Wide drainage is indicated.

6. Traumatic hilar vessel injury usually results in nephrectomy. However, the left renal vein can be ligated proximal to the gonadal vein without compromising renal salvage.

7. Traumatic **renal arterial thrombosis** usually results in renal loss. Although renal salvage has been obtained with arterial repair when the warm ischemia time was <4 hours, this is unusual without early operative intervention and repair. Nonoperative management is usually recommended for stable patients, except in the case of bilateral injury or absence of a contralateral kidney. Interventional radiographic thrombolysis and stenting has been reported. Spontaneous recanalization of part or the entire renal artery has been reported. Flank pain and hypertension are possible sequelae of renal arterial thrombosis, which can resolve spontaneously.

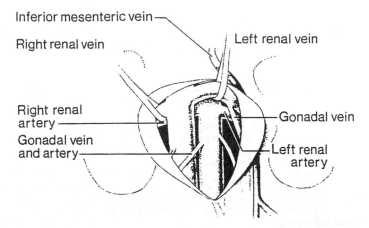

FIG. 31.3. Incision of the mesentery just medial and inferior to the inferior mesenteric vein. (From Carroll PR, Dixon CM, McAninch JW. The management of renal and ureteral trauma. In: Blaisdell FW, Trunkey DD, eds. *Trauma*, 2nd ed. New York: Thieme, 1993:260, with permission.)

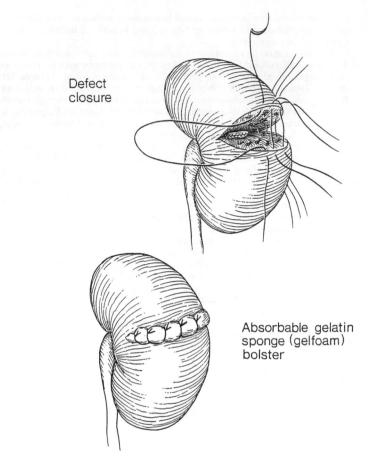

Defect
closure

Absorbable gelatin
sponge (gelfoam)
bolster

FIG. 31.4. Repair of the renal parenchyma. (From Carroll PR, Dixon CM, McAninch JW. The management of renal and ureteral trauma. In: Blaisdell FW, Trunkey DD, eds. *Trauma*, 2nd ed. New York: Thieme, 1993:260, with permission.)

8. A tiny intimal defect of the renal artery can be treated conservatively. Larger tears usually require repair or endovascular stenting.

D. Complications
1. The mortality of renal trauma is directly related to the associated injuries.
2. Postoperative urinoma or abscess can frequently be treated successfully with percutaneous drainage. Operation may be required for failure of percutaneous drainage.
3. Postinjury hypertension can occur in up to 5% of patients suffering renal trauma and may be delayed in onset up to 6 months after the injury. This is usually self-limited, but may require antihypertensive therapy. On rare occasion, late nephrectomy is required.

V. Ureteral injury
A. Mechanism
1. Most ureteral injuries are from penetrating trauma, mainly gunshot wounds. A high incidence is seen of associated injuries, and the treatment depends on the location, extent, and time from injury.

    a. Congenital abnormalities of the draining system are common (e.g., double collection system).

  2. Blunt injury of the ureter is rare and usually occurs at the renal pelvis as an avulsion injury. Rarely, ureteral compression can result from retroperitoneal hematoma or entrapment in a pelvic fracture.

B. Diagnosis

  1. IVP and CT scan can be complementary diagnostic tests for ureteral injury.

  2. In selected cases, a retrograde ureterogram is needed for diagnosis and treatment.

C. Treatment

  1. Most ureteral injuries are treated with primary repair and stenting. The ureter should be repaired with interrupted, absorbable sutures in a watertight fashion using spatulated ends. Diverting nephrostomies are sometimes necessary for large proximal ureteral injuries.

  2. A distal ureteral injury may require tunneling of the distal ureter into the bladder or mobilization of a small portion of the bladder to facilitate the anastomosis (psoas hitch, Boari flap).

  3. Transureteroureterostomy may be necessary in unusual circumstances in which a segment of ureter is lost or gross contamination is present.

  4. If a large segment of ureter is missing, autotransplantation of the kidney to the pelvis can be done.

  5. In patients who are profoundly unstable, particularly within the framework of damage control, the ureter can be exteriorized with a catheter as a ureterostomy or ligated with proximal diversion by nephrostomy (see Chapter 29).

D. Complications

  1. Complications of ureteral repair include leak, abscess, disruption, and stenosis.

VI. Bladder injury

A. Mechanism

  1. Most bladder ruptures are from blunt trauma; 80% are extraperitoneal and 20% are intraperitoneal. Extraperitoneal rupture is generally caused by pelvic fracture. Intraperitoneal rupture is associated with a full bladder at the time of impact, less often with pelvic fracture.

  2. Bladder injury from penetrating trauma may be occult and require more precise imaging. However, diagnosis is frequently made intraoperatively during exploration for other injuries.

B. Diagnosis

  1. Any patient with gross hematuria who has a seatbelt sign or pelvic fracture should have a cystogram. The cystogram should be done before a diagnostic peritoneal lavage (DPL) because identification of an intraperitoneal bladder rupture obviates the need for a DPL.

  2. In evaluating penetrating trauma, it is usually helpful to obtain an IVP or CT scan before a cystogram, so that the contrast does not obliterate a distal ureteral injury.

  3. A postvoiding cystogram is recommended for blunt injury to detect small lacerations. A properly performed cystogram (full bladder) will usually detect a clinically significant injury.

  4. It is important to differentiate between extraperitoneal and intraperitoneal injuries. An **extraperitoneal** bladder rupture is usually associated with fractures of the superior or inferior pubic rami. The cystogram has a characteristic **"sunburst"** appearance.

  5. Intraperitoneal ruptures are frequently associated with seatbelt injuries with rupture of the dome of the bladder. The cystogram has a characteristic appearance of **free dye outlining the loops of bowel**. Treatment of intraperitoneal bladder rupture requires a laparotomy, and further intraabdominal studies are usually not indicated.

C. Treatment
1. **Intraperitoneal bladder rupture** requires exploratory laparotomy and repair.
   a. Multiple layers, absorbable watertight sutures, bladder drainage
2. **Small extraperitoneal bladder ruptures** can be managed with bladder drainage alone, but tears with marked extravasation usually are repaired.
3. A suprapubic tube is placed if the patient is going to remain supine, whereas a urinary catheter may be all that is necessary for the mobile patient.

VII. Urethral injury
A. Mechanism
1. **The mechanism of urethral injury is usually blunt.** The posterior urethra is more commonly injured in males and is usually associated with pelvic fracture; the anterior urethra may be injured in penetrating trauma.
2. A straddle injury can cause urethral trauma in the absence of a pelvic fracture.
3. Injury to the female urethra is rare, except in open pelvic fractures.

B. Diagnosis
1. A high index of suspicion is necessary in males suffering blunt pelvic trauma with scrotal ecchymosis, swelling, or ecchymosis of the perineum; blood in the urethra; an indiscreet prostate on rectal examination; or inability to pass the urinary catheter.
2. The diagnosis is made by a urethrogram, which can be done through a partially advanced catheter (see III.A).

C. Treatment
1. Although immediate repair has been successfully performed in some centers, the traditional treatment is a suprapubic cystostomy and delayed repair of the urethral injury. On occasion and in experienced hands, a urinary catheter can be gently advanced to stent the urethral injury. This temporarily treats the injury and facilitates subsequent repair. Frequently, however, the urethral segments are distracted and cannot be reapproximated until swelling resolves.

VIII. Scrotal injury
A. Mechanism
1. The mechanism may be blunt or penetrating trauma.
B. A large scrotal hematoma is not uncommon from pelvic fracture and extravasation of blood. Although the scrotum may become large and tense, resolution is usual with conservative treatment of cleansing and elevation.
C. Testicular hematoma can be difficult to diagnose by physical examination.
1. Diagnosis is usually made with ultrasound. Early repair is indicated.
D. In wounds in which the scrotal sac is devitalized (e.g., blast injuries and avulsions), exposed testicles can be temporarily buried in the subcutaneous tissue of the thigh or abdomen until further wound repair is performed.

IX. Penile injury
A. Diagnosis
1. **Penile fracture** is usually diagnosed on history. It frequently occurs in the erect penis and is immediately followed by severe pain and deformity. Urgent urologic consultation is required.
B. Treatment
1. Lacerations or fractures of the penis require reconstruction by a urologist.

X. Vaginal injury
A. Mechanism
1. Usually occurs through blunt trauma and can be associated with pelvic fracture.
B. Diagnosis
1. **In females with pelvic fracture**, a pelvic examination with speculum inspection of the vaginal vault **is mandatory** to avoid missing occult injuries.

2. Examination is best obtained in the anesthetized patient in the lithotomy position.

C. Treatment

1. Treatment is simple closure and, occasionally, drainage.

Axioms

- All trauma patients with macroscopic hematuria require further evaluation.
- Evaluate microscopic hematuria by physical findings and mechanism of injury.
- In stable patients with renal injury, CT scan staging is essential for subsequent management strategies.
- Renal artery thrombosis is usually treated nonoperatively, unless bilateral or absence of a second kidney.
- Most ureteral injuries occur from penetrating trauma.
- Many extraperitoneal bladder injuries can be treated with bladder drainage alone.
- A urethrogram should be performed before placement of a urethral catheter in male patients with blood in the penile meatus, perineal ecchymosis, or an indistinct prostate on rectal examination.

Bibliography

Elliott DS, Barrett DM. Long-term follow-up and evaluation of primary realignment of posterior urethral disruptions. *J Urol* 1997;157(3):814–816.

Mee SI, McAninch JW. Indications for radiographic assessment in suspected renal trauma. *Urol Clin North Am* 1989;16:187–192.

Peterson NE. Genitourinary trauma. In: Mattox KL, Feliciano DV, Moore EE, eds. *Trauma*, 4th ed. New York: McGraw-Hill, 2000:839–878.

Santucci RA, McAninch JW. Diagnosis and management of renal trauma: past, present, and future. *J Am Coll Surg* 2000;191(4):443–451.

Villas PA, Cohen G, Putnam SG III, et al. Wallstent placement in a renal artery after blunt abdominal trauma. *J Trauma* 1999;46(6):1137–1139.

32. ORTHOPEDIC INJURIES

Bruce H. Ziran and Paul T. Freudigman

I. **General principles of dislocations and fractures**
  A. Fractures and dislocations occur in a significant number of trauma patients, resulting from indirect or direct force. Evaluation of a trauma patient with a fracture or dislocation always includes a complete musculoskeletal evaluation. Pay careful attention to the mechanism of injury, which aids in the treatment of the patient and provides prognostic information.
    1. **Dislocation** is defined as a complete loss of articular contact between two bones in a joint; this occurs with severe injury to ligamentous and capsular tissues. **Define the direction of the dislocation** with the distal piece described in relation to the proximal joint or bone. Most dislocations require urgent reduction to prevent complications. Dislocations should be identified during the secondary survey.
      a. Findings on examination with joint dislocation include pain, loss of motion, shortening of the extremity, and associated nerve or vascular injuries (Table 32.1).
      b. **Relocation of major joint dislocation must occur as soon as possible after completion of a secondary survey**. Relocation is performed generally with intravenous sedation and finesse rather than force. Occasionally, general anesthesia is necessary for relocation.
    2. **Subluxation** refers to the partial loss of articular congruity; sufficient capsular and ligamentous structures remain to prevent complete dislocation. On a continuum, subluxation represents less injury than dislocation, although a complete dislocation that has partially reduced from the elastic recoil of the soft tissue can deceptively appear to be a subluxation.
    3. **A fracture** is a structural break in bone continuity. Clinical signs include pain, displacement, shortening, swelling, and loss of function. Fractures are classified as either **open** (communicates with the external environment) or **closed**. Clinical deformity should be described as well as the status of soft tissues and neurovascular structures. **Fractures are described according to a universal scheme**.
      a. The distal piece is described in relation to the proximal piece.
      b. Fractures are classified with respect to the following:
        (1) **Pattern** (transverse, oblique, spiral, other)
        (2) **Morphology**: simple (two parts) or comminuted (three or more parts)
        (3) **Location** (proximal, middle, or distal; extraarticular or intraarticular)
        (4) Radiographic parameters (e.g., **displacement, angulation, rotation, shortening, apposition**)
      c. Degree of soft-tissue injury in closed or open fractures is important. Extensive soft-tissue injury increases the risk of the development of compartment syndrome.
    4. **Pediatric** fractures are further classified according to their **physeal (growth plate)** involvement (Salter-Harris classification).
      a. **Type I**: displaced or nondisplaced through growth plate
      b. **Type II**: small metaphyseal fragment
      c. **Type III**: intraarticular through epiphysis
      d. **Type IV**: through metaphysis and epiphysis
      e. **Type V**: severe crush to growth plate (cannot be determined acutely, only after growth arrest)

Table 32.1. Neurovascular injuries associated with fractures or dislocations

Orthopedic injury	Neurovascular injury
Anterior shoulder dislocation	Axillary nerve injury, axillary artery injury
Humeral shaft fracture	Radial nerve injury
Supracondylar humeral fracture	Brachial artery
Distal radius fracture	Median nerve injury
Perilunate dislocation	Median nerve injury
Posterior hip dislocation	Sciatic nerve injury
Supracondylar femoral fracture/ posterior knee dislocation/ tibial plateau fracture	Popliteal artery injury/thrombosis
Proximal fibular fracture	Peroneal nerve
Mangled extremity/tibial fracture	All neurovascular structures of the lower leg, compartment syndrome

B. The orthopedic **physical examination** focuses on the musculoskeletal system but assessment for concomitant injuries is also necessary. Be familiar with the events surrounding the injury and with the patient's underlying medical conditions and current complaints. After obtaining a history, proceed systematically with the examination. In the multiply injured patient, 15% to 20% of minor fractures (hand, foot, clavicle) are missed initially.
  1. Visually **inspect** for obvious soft-tissue abnormalities, including breaks in the skin, and deformities or asymmetry of the extremities.
  2. Palpate bone and soft tissues to evaluate tenderness, crepitus, and firmness of compartments.
  3. Test active and passive **range of motion** to detect bony injury, ligamentous injury, or weakness.
  4. A **neurovascular examination** records quality of peripheral pulses as well as sensory (pinprick, light touch), and motor function.
  5. We perform an additional **tertiary orthopedic survey** after the initial 24 to 48 hours or when the patient is more responsive.
C. Radiographic evaluation
  1. At least **two views at right angles** (generally anteroposterior and lateral views) are obtained of the extremity. Oblique views may be needed to adequately define fractures, particularly those involving joints. Joints above and below the fracture or dislocation must be visualized radiographically. Other views (e.g., stress views of the ankle or knee) may be necessary to assess joint stability.
D. Tests designed for specific conditions or anatomic injuries conclude the examination: tomography, arthrography, computed tomography (CT), or magnetic resonance imaging (MRI). These should be ordered by the orthopedist.
E. Initial treatment of fractures or dislocations
  1. Reduce the fracture or dislocation.
  2. Splint the extremity.
  3. Irrigate open fractures and cover with sterile saline-soaked gauze.
  4. Administer antibiotics for open fractures or perioperatively in patients who require open reduction and internal fixation (ORIF).
  5. Administer tetanus prophylaxis for open fractures or to patients who require ORIF.
F. Definitive treatment of fractures or dislocations. The goal in treatment of musculoskeletal injury is to restore normal anatomy and function and relieve pain as quickly as possible. The capability to perform early reduction and internal fixation in the multiply injured patient has significantly reduced morbidity and mortality. Stabilization of the spine, pelvis, and long bone fractures (femur, tibia) has allowed early mobilization of patients.

1. **Reduction** can be accomplished by either closed (external realignment) or open (direct operative approach).
2. **Immobilization of the extremity** by splint, cast, traction, orthosis, external fixation, or internal fixation.

G. **Open fractures** constitute a significant proportion of injuries to the musculoskeletal system. Open fractures communicate externally through a break in the skin, vaginal wall, or rectum; they pose a threat for infection and amputation. The tenets of care for open fractures include appropriate debridement along with skeletal stabilization. Prevention of infection is of paramount importance. Development of osteomyelitis because of inadequate debridement can be a devastating complication and will greatly increase the morbidity and potential for loss of function or limb. **Antibiotics cannot be a substitute for adequate debridement of necrotic and contaminated tissues.**
   1. **Classification of open fractures (Gustilo and Anderson)**
      a. **Grade I**: low energy, <1 cm wound caused by protrusion of the bone through the skin or a low-velocity bullet
      b. **Grade II**: moderate energy, >1 cm with flap or avulsion wound in the skin with minimal devitalized soft tissue and minimal contamination
      c. **Grade III**: high energy, extensive soft-tissue injury (usually >10 cm), barnyard
         (1) **IIIa**: adequate soft-tissue coverage
         (2) **IIIb**: significant soft-tissue loss with exposed bone that requires tissue transfer (muscle flap, rotation or free) for coverage
         (3) **IIIc**: vascular injury requiring repair for limb preservation; amputation rates reported from 25% to 50%. (Not all vascular injuries are limb threatening.)
   2. **Management**
      a. Early irrigation of gross contamination in the trauma resuscitation area. Wounds should be managed using sterile saline-soaked gauze and covered with dry, sterile rolled gauze.
      b. Splint the extremity as soon as the wound is covered to reduce hemorrhage, prevent further injury, and alleviate pain.
      c. Antibiotic prophylaxis includes tetanus toxoid, first-generation cephalosporin, and aminoglycoside for contaminated wound or grade III fracture. Penicillin should be added for barnyard injury. Organisms may be gram-negative or gram-positive bacteria.
      d. Orthopedic consultation should be obtained early.
      e. Wounds require urgent operative irrigation and debridement; the orthopedic standard is within 6 to 8 hours if the patient is physiologically stable.
      f. Wounds require repeated irrigation and debridement in the operating room (OR) every 2 to 4 days, until definitive soft-tissue coverage can be achieved (usually, 5–10 days), which can require pedicle-based or free tissue flaps. **Minimize multiple inspections of the wound outside the OR, except by the surgeon making critical management decisions.** Continue antibiotics until 48 hours after definitive coverage of soft tissue and wound.
      g. Antibiotic-impregnated bone cement "beads" have been shown to benefit delivery of antibiotics to dead spaces that do not receive the systemic antibiotics. This local delivery has few systemic effects and is efficacious. The general mix dose is three vials of tobramycin (1.2 g each, 3.6 g total), per bag of cement. The beads are strung on a stainless steel wire and, when hard, placed into the wound and covered with a liquid-sealed dressing (e.g., OpSite, Ioban). This "bead pouch" retains the fluid bathing the beads and is rich in antibiotic concentration. Tobramycin is used because in such high concentrations, it provides coverage of both gram-positive and gram-negative organisms.
      h. Internal fixation of grade I open fractures after adequate debridement and irrigation can be accomplished with infection rates of

<2%. If soft-tissue loss is minimal and coverage is adequate, selected grade II open fractures can be treated with intramedullary fixation. External fixation may be necessary to stabilize grade III open fractures (infection rates of 10% to 50%).

3. **Gunshot wounds**
   a. **Low-velocity gunshot wounds** cause less soft-tissue destruction than high-velocity gunshot wounds. Because of the splintering effect of gunshot injuries, bone is often unstable and requires operative fixation. Debride the skin wounds and treat the bone as in closed injury. Prolonged antibiotic use is controversial; our practice is to administer oral antibiotics for 5 to 7 days.
   b. **High-velocity gunshot wounds** and **close-range shotgun blasts** cause significant soft-tissue injury, and should be treated as severe grade III open fractures. These wounds often result in massive soft-tissue defects and require extensive reconstruction. Search for associated neural or vascular injuries.

II. **Specific injuries**
A. **Pelvis** (see Chapter 33)
B. **Acetabular (hip socket) fractures** are complex, and can be associated with a hip dislocation. Acetabular fractures represent significant injury to the hip that can be associated with lifelong disability. Acetabular fractures, which are often associated with injuries to the pelvic ring, are usually addressed before treatment of the acetabulum. Most acetabular fractures require temporary skeletal traction to maintain the reduction and prevent soft-tissue contracture. The acetabulum has anterior and posterior columns.
   1. **Types**
      a. **Central fracture** most often requires temporary skeletal traction.
      b. **Posterior fracture or dislocation** requires urgent reduction under anesthesia. Sciatic nerve injuries have been reported in 10% to 30% of patients. A careful neurologic examination must be performed before and following reduction of the dislocation. Superior gluteal artery injuries can occur, usually presenting when the fracture exits into the greater sciatic notch.
      c. **Anterior fracture or dislocation**, which is rare, is often associated with more severe acetabular fractures.
   2. **Radiographic evaluation** includes anteroposterior, lateral, and obturator oblique and iliac oblique views (collectively called Judet views) of the pelvis. After reduction of the dislocation, CT scan of the acetabulum is performed with 3-mm cuts.
   3. **Treatment**
      a. Temporary skeletal traction
      b. Delayed ORIF is the treatment of choice for displaced fractures. Definitive operative intervention is usually from 2 to 7 days postinjury, which reduces the chance for bleeding complications at the operative site.
      c. Posttraumatic arthritis, chondrolysis, and heterotopic ossification are the common complications. Postoperative radiation (single 700 Gy dose) or indomethacin (75 mg/day for 2 weeks) can be used to prevent heterotopic ossification.
C. **Hip dislocation**, with or without associated acetabular fracture, occurs through the capsular area containing the blood supply to the femoral head (Fig. 32.1).
   1. **Types** (based on orientation of the femoral head to the acetabulum)
      a. **Posterior dislocation** is most common. Sciatic nerve injuries occur (10% to 30%). The leg is usually flexed and adducted.
      b. **Anterior dislocation**. The femoral head sits on top of the pubis or in the obturator foramen. The leg is generally abducted and externally rotated.
   2. Radiographic evaluation in the trauma resuscitation area includes anteroposterior, lateral, and Judet views. CT scan is required postreduction.

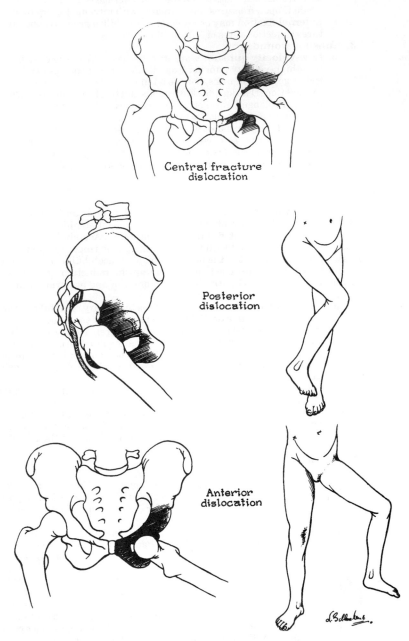

FIG. 32.1. Hip dislocation. (From Mick CA. Initial management of fractures and joint injuries. In: *Management of trauma.* Philadelphia: WB Saunders, 1985:673, with permission.)

3. **Treatment**. Dislocation of the hip requires urgent reduction because of the risk of avascular necrosis (AVN) of the femoral head. Delay in diagnosis and treatment increases the incidence of AVN, which can manifest years after injury. Reduction under intravenous sedation can be attempted (by an orthopedist) once the patient is in the trauma resuscitation area. If not achieved, perform urgent closed reduction under anesthesia. If closed reduction under anesthesia is unsuccessful after several attempts, open reduction is necessary.

   a. Postreduction CT scan (3-mm cuts) is obtained to exclude associated fracture or loose bodies.

   b. A careful neurologic examination testing femoral, posterior tibial, and peroneal nerve sensory and motor function is mandatory before and following reduction of the dislocation.

D. **Lower extremity fractures** play a significant role in the management of trauma patients. Early internal fixation has significantly reduced mortality and morbidity with these fractures. Stabilization of long bone fractures, including the femur and tibia, has allowed patients to mobilize early. Advances in orthopedic hardware, including the development of statically locked intramedullary nails, have significantly improved outcome. A variety of injuries or combination of injuries can be seen in the lower extremities. The most common injuries are discussed below.

1. **Femoral neck fractures** in young patients are the result of high-energy impact. They commonly occur in the elderly, often from low-energy injuries (falls from a standing position). Femoral neck fractures are generally displaced. Femoral neck fractures occur concurrently with 15% of femoral diaphyseal fractures. For this reason, radiographic evaluation of the hip is essential before femoral shaft fracture fixation.

   a. **Treatment**. Displaced femoral neck fractures require immediate orthopedic consultation and urgent ORIF to reduce the complication rates of AVN and nonunion. Elderly patients with significant medical problems may have hemiarthroplasty in a delayed fashion. Morbidity and mortality of hip fractures in the elderly are related to preinjury cognitive function and associated medical illnesses.

2. **Peritrochanteric femur fractures** are more common in elderly patients; in young patients, they result from high-energy trauma. Treatment is generally operative, but because the vascular supply is usually spared, ORIF is not as urgent as in femoral neck fractures; immediate or delayed ORIF is acceptable. Temporary skin traction is used for comfort before ORIF. Peritrochanteric femur fractures in the elderly have high morbidity and mortality because of comorbid diseases in this population.

   a. **Treatment** has traditionally been with plates and screws. However, we have used newer intramedullary implants that permit immediate weight bearing in most cases, which allows more independence and more efficient care postoperatively. Preoperative planning is essential for these fractures. If operative intervention is delayed, skeletal traction should be employed. A high rate of nonunion and hardware failure is found in these fractures.

3. **Femoral shaft fractures** are defined as 5 cm distal to the lesser trochanter and 8 cm proximal to the knee joint. They result from high-energy forces. Hip or pelvis radiographs should be taken to rule out an associated femoral neck fracture. Describe fractures based on location, soft-tissue injury, comminution, and angulation.

   a. **Treatment**. Early intramedullary nailing is the treatment of choice. This is generally performed without actual exposure of the fracture site. This operative approach reduces the incidence of malrotation, shortening, and pulmonary complications. Newer, minimally invasive techniques have been developed that allow rapid mobilization and earlier discharge. We supplement with intrafracture injection of local anesthesia, which allows mobilization and discharge as soon as 36 hours after surgery in certain isolated fractures.

4. **Supracondylar femur fractures** occur within 8 cm of the knee joint. They can be intraarticular or extraarticular, unicondylar or bicondylar. They can be associated with superficial femoral artery or popliteal artery injury.
   a. **Treatment.** Complex, intraarticular closed fracture requires careful preoperative planning and may be delayed. If delayed, use skeletal traction through the tibia or calcaneus.

5. **Knee dislocation** requires urgent reduction and immobilization. Injury to the popliteal artery is common (20%) because the artery can be tethered between the adductor hiatus proximally and the interosseous membrane distally. Arteriography or immediate operation is essential if asymmetry is found in the neurovascular examination. Even in the absence of clear signs of arterial injury, consider arteriography for documented knee dislocation because of the risk of undetected intimal injury with late occlusion. Tibial and peroneal nerve injuries occur frequently.
   a. **Types.** Anterior, posterior, medial, lateral, or rotatory
   b. **Treatment.** Early reconstruction is not necessary but can be performed. Acute treatment can be achieved with a splint or hinged brace. Prompt evaluation of the arterial system is mandatory.

6. **Patellar fractures**
   a. Usually result from direct blow to the flexed knee. Displacement results in loss of continuity of the quadriceps mechanism.
   b. Nonoperative treatment for nondisplaced fractures. Operation is necessary to restore quadriceps function and articular surface integrity. Repair requires ORIF or partial patellectomy. Patellar retinacula must be repaired.

7. **Tibial plateau fractures** involve the medial or lateral tibial plateau. They involve the presence or absence of articular surface depression and fracture location. They can be nondisplaced or displaced (4 mm). Associated knee ligament injury or vascular injury occurs. Compartment syndrome is seen in up to 25% of patients with high-energy tibial plateau fractures.
   a. **Treatment.** ORIF is preferred for displaced fractures. Treat nondisplaced fractures nonoperatively or with percutaneous screw fixation. In the elderly, tibial plateau fractures are usually minimally displaced and can often be treated nonoperatively. In young adults with high-energy injury, the fracture often extends to the tibial diaphysis.

8. **Tibial shaft fractures** occur as high-energy injuries (e.g., motorcycle crashes, pedestrian-automobile impact, crush injuries). Open tibial fractures occur commonly and are best treated by intramedullary nailing. Compartment syndrome occurs in 10% of tibia fractures, more commonly in proximal tibial fractures. Tibial fractures are described based on location (proximal one third, middle one third, distal one third), displacement, comminution degree, and open versus closed.
   a. **Treatment**
      (1) Closed fractures can often be treated with closed reduction and casting. Open reduction and internal fixation with intramedullary nailing may be required for unstable fracture patterns, segmental fractures, or tibial fractures associated with ipsilateral femur fractures unless severe soft-tissue injury is present.
      (2) Open tibial fractures are treated based on the grade of the open fracture and degree of soft-tissue injury. Consider external fixation in fractures with significant soft-tissue injury because it provides adequate stability, minimizes the foreign body burden

(metal implant), and allows access to the limb for soft-tissue reconstruction.

(a) Early soft-tissue coverage of open fractures has decreased the incidence of secondary infection. Flaps commonly used include (*a*) proximal one third fracture-gastrocnemius muscle, (*b*) middle one third fracture-soleus muscle, and (*c*) distal one third fracture-latissimus, gracilis, or rectus muscle.

(b) Early amputation may be indicated in severely crushed limbs or grade IIIc open fractures with anatomic disruption of the tibial nerve.

(c) **Mangled extremity** (Table 33.2). When the injured extremity has such severe injury that its salvageability is in question, decisions in management require input from the trauma surgeon and orthopedist; considerable judgment is necessary. Various scoring systems have been developed to help clinicians determine the benefit of early amputation versus attempts at limb salvage. The mangled extremity may be an open or closed fracture. Most scoring systems have been developed for the lower extremity; the most commonly used is the MESS system (mangled extremity severity scoring system). A limb with a MESS ≥7 is ultimately likely to undergo amputation of the extremity; whereas limbs with MESS <7 can generally be successfully salvaged. The scoring system should be used as a guide, not as a rule of clinical practice. The decision to perform a primary amputation as opposed to heroic attempts at limb salvage of the mangled extremity is difficult, because of the psychological, functional, and morbid effects of this decision. Ability to salvage an extremity depends on the status of the skin, bone, muscles, vessels, and nerves. If nerve injury is to the degree that ultimate function is unlikely, primary amputation should be considered. Prolonged attempts at limb salvage may

Table 32.2. Mangled extremity severity scoring system

Factor	Score
Skeletal/soft-tissue injury	
–Low energy (stab, fracture, civilian gunshot wound GSW)	1
–Medium energy (open or multiple fracture)	2
–High energy (shotgun or high velocity GSW, crush injury)	3
–Very high energy (above, combined with gross contamination)	4
Limb ischemia (double value if ischemia >6 hours)	
–Pulse reduced or absent, but normal capillary fill	1
–Pulseless, diminished capillary fill	2
–Limb is cool, paralyzed, insensate	3
Shock	
–Systolic blood pressure consistently > 90 mmHg	0
–Systolic blood pressure transiently < 90 mmHg	1
–Systolic blood pressure persistently < 90 mmHg	2
Age (years)	
<30	0
30–50	1
>50	2

also be inappropriate in the multiply injured patient with immediately life-threatening injuries of the chest, head, or abdomen.

   (d) **Damage control** principles have been applied to the unstable, multiply injured patient with orthopedic injury. This approach involves rapid external fixation of extremity fractures to temporarily stabilize them. Intramedullary nailing is done when the patient is stabilized.

9. **Tibial plafond (pilon) fractures** occur in the distal tibia, usually involving the articular surface from an axial load. CT scan or tomograms can be useful in defining the character of the fracture. The fibula may be involved. Pilon fractures generally involve significant concomitant soft-tissue injury with high risk of associated soft-tissue loss and infection.

   a. **Treatment** should be dictated by the status of the soft-tissue envelope as wound complication rates are high. Temporary skeletal stabilization with an external fixator may be necessary until the soft-tissue edema decreases at which time ORIF can be performed safely. Posttraumatic arthritis usually requires late ankle arthrodesis.

10. **Ankle fractures** are produced by external rotation with a fracture to the fibula or an injury to the interosseous membrane (Maseoneuve injury). Ankle fractures are classified based on fracture location of the lateral malleolus (fibula) and the presence (or absence) of a medial malleolus fracture.

   a. Radiographic evaluation includes anteroposterior, lateral, and mortise views, both initially and after reduction.

   b. **Treatment** requires ORIF if any subluxation (>1 mm) or incongruity of the ankle joint is found. Perform this immediately, before soft-tissue swelling is significant, or on a delayed basis (7–14 days).

11. **Calcaneus fractures** are usually the result of significant falls and are often bilateral. Associated spine injuries should be sought. Calcaneal fractures are very disabling injuries and patients are often unable to return to labor.

   a. **Radiographic evaluation** includes anteroposterior, lateral, and axial views. Obtain CT scan (3-mm cuts) in two planes (axial and coronal) for adequate delineation of the fracture and joint.

   b. **Treatment.** Displaced intraarticular fractures require ORIF, which should be done when the soft-tissue swelling subsides (7–14 days). Use elevation and a foot pump to reduce swelling. For fractures not reconstructible, use primary arthrodesis. If the soft-tissue injury is extensive, external fixation or simple percutaneous pinning can also be used. Late subtalar arthrodesis should be performed for posttraumatic arthritis. The complication rate with ORIF is 15% to 30% and often results in the need for muscle flaps and infection. This high risk of infection has prompted many to use only limited reductions and *in situ* pinning. This approach allows restoration of the hindfoot architecture and reconstructive procedures on a delayed basis, when less chance exists for soft-tissue complications.

12. **Talar neck fractures** are usually caused by forced hyperdorsiflexion of the foot on the ankle. Because of the precarious blood supply to the talar body, talar neck fractures require an anatomic reduction. Associated subtalar or talar dislocations **should be reduced immediately** to minimize risk of AVN, the incidence of which is related to fracture severity (as high as 85% to 100%). Displaced fractures require ORIF and nondisplaced fractures can be treated with percutaneous screw fixation.

13. **Tarsometatarsal (Lis Franc) fractures** are usually associated with significant midfoot swelling, and they are commonly missed at initial presentation. Foot compartment syndrome can occur and results in significant disability. ORIF is indicated for displaced fractures. These are devastating injuries and can be associated with significant injury to the

plantar ligamentous structures, which can result in late deformity (e.g., planovalgus). Post-traumatic degenerative joint disease (DJD) is common and requires delayed arthrodesis.

14. **Metatarsal fractures** can usually be treated in a short leg walking cast. Open reduction is indicated for intraarticular displacement. Closed reduction and pin fixation is indicated for significant plantar displacement.

E. **Upper extremity fractures** also have an impact on the outcome of trauma patients. Upper extremities are necessary for activities of daily living and as weight-bearing structures when the lower extremities are compromised.

1. **Sternoclavicular dislocation** can be anterior or posterior.

   a. Anterior dislocation is of minimal clinical significance. Perform a single attempt at closed reduction. However, reduction is usually unstable. Fixation and multiple attempts at relocation are contraindicated.

   b. Posterior dislocation of the clavicle can be associated with life-threatening mediastinal injuries. CT scan or arteriography may be necessary for evaluation. Closed reduction should be performed in the OR under general anesthesia. Open reduction is performed if closed reduction is unsuccessful. A general or thoracic surgeon should be on standby in the event complications arise.

2. **Clavicle shaft fractures** are generally of minimal clinical significance. They are classified according to location of the fracture: medial one third, middle one third (most common), and distal one third. Associated injuries include brachial plexus injury, pneumothorax, and sternoclavicular or acromioclavicular joint injury.

   a. **Treatment**. These fractures are generally treated symptomatically with a sling; expect healing in 6 to 8 weeks. Figure-of-eight straps tend not to be well tolerated. ORIF is indicated for open fractures, neurovascular compromise, and skin compromise. Also, selected fractures of the distal one third of the clavicle may require ORIF.

3. **Acromioclavicular joint sprains (separated shoulder)** are usually treated symptomatically with a sling. ORIF is indicated for severe displacement with trapezoid ligament entrapment. Late distal clavicle excision may be necessary for symptomatic arthritis.

4. **Scapula fractures**, which are produced by high-energy impact, are frequently associated with intrathoracic injuries. Symptomatic treatment in a sling is usually sufficient with early motion. ORIF is indicated for the following:

   a. Large, displaced coracoid or acromial fragments

   b. Ipsilateral, displaced glenoid neck and displaced clavicle fracture (floating shoulder)

   c. Intraarticular glenoid (subluxation of the glenoid >25% surface)

5. **Glenohumeral dislocation (shoulder)** is usually anterior. Posterior dislocations can occur with seizures, electrocution, and dashboard injuries. Careful neurovascular examination is needed to exclude axillary nerve or artery injury.

   a. **Radiographs** are obtained to assess concomitant fractures—anteroposterior and axillary lateral views.

   b. **Treatment**. Early closed reduction with adequate sedation followed by sling protection with supervised active range-of-motion when pain abates. Associated rotator cuff injuries are common in patients >40 years of age but do not change the initial management.

6. **Proximal humerus fractures** usually occur in elderly osteoporotic bone. When occurring in young patients, they are usually caused by high-energy trauma, and associated injuries are common.

   a. **Types**. Anatomic classification is based on four parts: head, greater tuberosity, lesser tuberosity, or metaphysis fractures. Displacement is defined as 1 cm of displacement or 45° angulation.

      (1) One-part fracture: all undisplaced fractures, regardless of the number of fracture lines

(2) Two-part fracture: fractures involving the anatomic neck, surgical neck, isolated lesser or greater tuberosity fractures
(3) Three-part fracture: fracture of the neck and a tuberosity fracture
(4) Four-part fracture: fracture of the neck, greater tuberosity fracture, and lesser tuberosity fracture

b. **Treatment**. In young patients, efforts are aimed at accurate reduction of the fracture, often surgically, to maximize function. In the elderly or less active individuals, nonoperative management or hemiarthroplasty allows adequate pain relief and function.
   (1) Stable, two-part impacted neck fractures → sling and swathe
   (2) Two-part neck or unstable → ORIF closed reduction, percutaneous pinning
   (3) Displaced greater tuberosity fracture → ORIF
   (4) Three-part in younger patients with good bone stock → ORIF
   (5) Hemiarthroplasty for the following:
      (a) Three-part in elderly patient
      (b) Three-part with poor bone stock
      (c) Four-part, except elderly debilitated patient or severe diabetic

7. **Humeral shaft fractures** have a high rate of union with nonoperative management using fracture braces. In the multiply injured patient, however, ORIF or intramedullary nailing may be indicated to facilitate nursing care or utilize the extremity for weight bearing and activities of daily living. Distal third fractures can be associated with a radial nerve palsy (usually a neuropraxia).

8. **Distal humerus fractures** are more common in children than in adults. The classification scheme is as complex as the fractures themselves, based on intraarticular versus extraarticular, degree of comminution, and displacement. Intraarticular fractures mandate an anatomic reduction.
   a. **Pediatric distal humerus fractures** are associated with neurovascular injury and compartment syndrome. Urgent (not emergent) closed reduction should be performed in the OR. Percutaneous pinning is necessary for unstable fractures or those with significant soft-tissue swelling. Open reduction is required if closed reduction is unsuccessful. Cubitus varus is a common complication.
   b. **Adult distal humerus fractures** require ORIF if displaced. Heterotopic ossification can occur, especially in head-injured patients. Stiffness and ulnar neuropathy can occur.
   c. **Capitellum and trochlea** fractures should be treated with ORIF for large, displaced fragments and excision for small, displaced fragments.

9. **Olecranon fractures** usually occur as traction injuries. ORIF with tension band techniques is indicated if displacement is >2 mm. For severely comminuted fractures, excise (≤50% of the olecranon). With associated dislocation, early excision is contraindicated.

10. **Coronoid fractures** are treated with early motion if <50% and ORIF if >50%. They are very common in elbow dislocations that remain unstable after closed reduction.

11. **Radial head fractures** occur from a fall on an outstretched hand.
   a. **Treatment**. Nondisplaced fractures should be treated with early motion. ORIF is performed if angulation is >30°, 3-mm displacement, or depression greater than one third of the articular surface. Early excision can be performed for severely comminuted fractures. Manage associated dislocations first; suspect distal radioulnar joint injury.

12. **Elbow dislocations** are common and most often posterior. Dislocations and fractures of the elbow usually result from a fall on an outstretched

arm or direct impact on the elbow. A careful neurovascular examination is performed to rule out injury to the ulnar, radial or median nerve, or the brachial artery; most nerve injuries are neuropraxia. Associated fractures of the coronoid, radial head, and medial epicondyle can occur; obtain radiographs to exclude an associated fracture. Treatment consists of immediate closed reduction and application of a posterior splint. Document median and ulnar nerve function before and after reduction; nerve entrapment can occur with reduction. The splint should be removed at 7 to 10 days and early active range of motion begun. In unstable cases, maintain suspicion of a coronoid or radial head fracture. A relocated elbow will demonstrate trochlear congruity on the anteroposterior radiograph, and congruence of the olecranon-humerus, and radius-capitellar articulations on the lateral radiograph.

13. **Combined radius and ulna fractures** in an adult should be treated with ORIF. Fractures of both bones in the forearm risk compartment syndrome. Posterior interosseous nerve injury is common with proximal third fractures. Severely contaminated open fractures may require external fixation.

14. **Ulnar shaft fractures** occur as a result of a direct blow. These fractures are generally treated with functional bracing, but delayed union is common. ORIF should be performed if angulation is >10° or displacement is >50%. Associated injuries to the wrist and elbow should be suspected. **Monteggia's fracture-dislocation** is a proximal ulnar fracture with an associated radial head dislocation; this mandates ORIF.

15. **Radius fractures** are treated in a long arm cast in supination if they are nondisplaced and in the proximal one fifth. Fractures distal to this in the radial shaft should be treated by ORIF. **Galeazzi fracture** is a radial shaft fracture, at the junction of the middle and distal third of the radius, associated with dislocation of the distal radioulnar joint. Treatment is forearm immobilization in supination for 6 weeks.

16. **Distal radius fractures** usually occur from a fall on an outstretched arm. Associated median or ulnar nerve injury, distal radioulnar joint disruption, and carpal instability can occur. Extensor pollicis longus rupture can also occur and is usually seen 5 to 8 weeks after injury. **Colles fracture** is a fracture of the distal radius with displacement of the carpus. **Smith's fracture** is a reversed Colles fracture—a fracture of the distal radius with the distal fragment and accompanying carpal row displaced volarly. **Barton's fracture** is a distal radius fracture with displacement of a palmar or dorsally based triangular segment from the radius.

    a. **Radiographic evaluation** includes anteroposterior, lateral, and oblique views. Also obtain radiographs of the hand and elbow.

    b. **Treatment** is initially with closed reduction and casting. Fracture involving an intraarticular step-off, shortening, or severe comminution requires accurate reduction and fixation with pins or plates, with or without external fixation. ORIF is required with large, displaced articular fragments.

17. **Scaphoid fractures** can be associated with other carpal injuries. For nondisplaced (<2 mm) fractures, treatment should consist of a long arm thumb spica. Treatment duration varies with fracture location, but ranges from 8 to 20 weeks. For displaced fractures, perform closed reduction and pinning or ORIF. An anatomic reduction is necessary to reduce the risk of nonunion and avascular necrosis. AVN and nonunion are more common with waist and proximal pole fractures.

18. **Perilunate dislocations** are commonly missed at initial presentation. Careful radiologic evaluation is mandatory. Associated scaphoid fractures are common. Reduction and pinning are necessary, and dorsal ligament repair may also be required. Associated median nerve injury is also common and early carpal tunnel decompression may be required.

19. **Hand** (see Chapter 34)

III. **Amputation injuries** can result in significant morbidity and potentially dysfunctional limbs. Therefore, amputation injuries should be handled only at institutions under the direction of a team whose care is directed by a microvascular surgeon. **Amputations are true limb- and life-threatening injuries and should be handled as such, with no delays in treatment.** Unsuccessful reimplantations can result in significant disability. Realistic expectations can only be provided to the patient after evaluation by the reimplantation surgeon.
   A. The physician responsible for replantation should be notified before acceptance. Acceptance is defined as evaluation for *possible* replantation.
   B. Necessary historical data on the patient includes the patient's name, age, occupation, handedness for upper extremity, **time of injury**, mechanism of injury, level of injury (bone, soft tissue), exact neurovascular status, concomitant injuries and associated medical conditions, and the location and telephone number of the nearest relative, especially if the patient is a minor.
   C. The OR should be prepared as soon as acceptance is made.
   D. Transport the patient expeditiously.
   E. Preserve amputated parts by wrapping in a sterile gauze moistened with sterile saline solution. Place in a watertight plastic container or resealable plastic bag, which should then be placed into an iced saline bath. **DO NOT use dry ice. DO NOT place the amputated part in direct contact with ice.** Clearly label the container with the patient's name and time placed.
      1. Administer tetanus and broad-spectrum antibiotics as for open fractures.
   F. The replantation team should be present at time of arrival to the emergency department; notify the OR. Perform primary and secondary surveys with resuscitation. Limbs and amputated parts should be evaluated and examined radiographically. Amputated parts are replaced in container (as above).
   G. Transfer the patient to the OR. A two-team approach is used if associated injuries require intervention.
   H. Factors associated with a poor outcome include crush injury, long ischemia time (>6 hours), proximal amputations, nerve injuries (axonotmesis), systemic hypotension, severe contamination, concomitant injuries or medical conditions, and whether the patient is elderly, has poor nutrition, or psychological compromise or decompensation.
IV. **Basic splinting.** Splinting of extremity injuries is a practice about which all physicians should have some knowledge. Creativity is useful in constructing splints for various body parts and conditions. Splinting should never be harmful, and adequate knowledge of relevant anatomy and potential complications is necessary. Follow the principles of splinting described below.
   A. The **purpose for splinting is immobilization**. This provides temporary stabilization of bone and soft tissue, aids in control of hemorrhage, and helps reduce pain and prevent further injury.
   B. **Principles** of splinting include splinting open fractures as they lie. Gross angulation in closed fractures should be reduced by longitudinal traction. When commercial splints are unavailable, use your ingenuity. Neurovascular status must **always** be reassessed after the splint is applied. If neurovascular compromise is present, remove or loosen the splint. When splinting, include the joint above and joint below, and make sure the splint is rigid enough to provide immobilization. It should not be circumferentially compressive unless excessive hemorrhage is present.
   C. **Types of commercial splints**
      1. Military antishock trousers (MAST) can be used for pelvic fractures and lower extremity fractures. Be aware they can induce compartment syndrome. Rigid cervical orthosis should be used for cervical spine (C-spine), and backboard should be used for the spine.
         a. Air splints for extremity fractures can induce compartment syndrome.
         b. Structural aluminum malleable (SAM) splints consist of semirigid cardboard; they are useful for upper extremity, ankle, and foot fractures.

    c. Silicone splints function similar to air splints, but with less chance for compartment syndrome. They are useful for distal extremities.

    d. Hare and Thomas traction splints are useful for femur fractures, and they provide longitudinal traction from foot to ischial tuberosity. Other commercial splints include knee immobilizers, sling, or sling and swathe for shoulder and proximal humerus, and aluminum splints for fingers.

D. Other types of splints include plaster of paris, which is the gold standard for the orthopedist. It is readily available, relatively inexpensive, and easy to use. Newer premade fiberglass splints may be more rigid than the plaster counterpart and provide no added advantage. Pillow splints are easy to use, and they can be secured with ace wrap or roll gauze. They are effective, comfortable, and an excellent choice for distal extremities. Splints can also be fashioned with cardboard, blankets or towels, and aluminum.

E. Specific areas

  1. C-spine may require a cervical collar and sandbags.

  2. The spine may require a backboard and logroll.

  3. The shoulder may require a sling, sling and swathe, and ace wrap arm to chest.

  4. Splints for the humerus are the same as for the shoulder and also may include a SAM splint or plaster U-splint.

  5. Elbows should be splinted at a 90° angle with a posterior plaster splint.

  6. Splinting of the forearm, wrist, and hand should include the elbow at a 90° angle. Plaster U-splint or pillow splint can also be used.

  7. MAST may be used initially to splint pelvic fractures.

  8. Splinting of the proximal femur and femoral shaft should include Hare traction, posterior plaster splint, pillow splints, and MAST.

  9. Splinting of the distal femur, knee, and proximal tibia may require a knee immobilizer, posterior plaster splint, pillow splints, and MAST.

  10. Splinting of the tibial shaft should include posterior plaster or U-splint, pillow splints, silicone splints, and MAST.

  11. Ankle and foot splinting can be performed with posterior plaster or U-splint, pillow splints, and silicone splints.

Bibliography

Browner B. *Skeletal trauma*. Philadelphia: WB Saunders, 1992.

Crenshaw A. *Campbell's operative orthopaedics*. St. Louis: Mosby, 1992.

Feliciano DV. Patterns of injury. In: Feliciano DV, Moore EE, Mattox KL, eds. *Trauma*. Stamford, CT: Appleton & Lange, 1996:85–103.

Frymoyer J. *Orthopaedic knowledge update 4*. Rosemont: American Academy of Orthopaedic Surgeons, 1990.

Gustilo RB, Anderson JT. Prevention of infection in the treatment of 1025 open fractures of long bones. *J Bone Joint Surg* 1976;58A:453–459.

Johansen K, Daines M, Howey T, et al. Objective criteria accurately predict amputation following lower extremity trauma. *J Trauma* 1990;30:568–573.

Jones AL. Principles of fractures and dislocations. In: Lopez-Viego MA, ed. *The Parkland trauma handbook*. St. Louis: Mosby, 1994:415–418.

Poss R. *Orthopaedic knowledge update 3*. Rosemont: American Academy of Orthopaedic Surgeons, 1990.

Rockwood C. *Rockwood and Green's fractures in adults*. Philadelphia: JB Lippincott, 1991.

Rockwood C. *Rockwood and Green's fractures in children*. Philadelphia: JB Lippincott, 1991.

Scalea TM, Boswell SA, Scott JD, et al. External fixation as a bridge to intramedullary nailing for patients with multiple injuries and with femur fractures: damage control orthopedics. *J Trauma* 2000;48:613–621.

33. PELVIC FRACTURES

Michael J. Prayson and Gary S. Gruen

I. **Incidence and mechanism of injury.** Fractures of the pelvic ring account for approximately 3% of all fractures. Many pelvic fractures result from low-energy trauma, and can be managed through conservative methods. Unstable pelvic ring disruptions are generally caused by high-energy events such as motor vehicle and motorcycle crashes, pedestrians struck by motor vehicles, and falls from heights. Such injuries can present with life-threatening hemorrhage or result in long-term pain and disability. The fractured pelvis is the primary cause of death in 10% to 15% of patients with pelvic fractures. Pelvic fractures have a high incidence of associated injuries (43% to 74%) to the abdomen, thorax, and head, which contribute significantly to the overall morbidity and mortality of multiply injured patients. Aggressive volume resuscitation and expedient treatment of associated injuries are imperative.

II. **Examination.** History and clinical examination of the pelvis, which are important for diagnosis of suspected injury, should be done concurrently with resuscitation, especially in the hypotensive patient. Early orthopedic consultation is important.

    A. The awake and communicative patient with a pelvic fracture may complain of pelvic pain, which guides further examination. Patients with urethral disruption may complain of an inability to void (urethral tears are uncommon in females).

    B. Inspection of the soft tissue around the pelvis is essential to identify a laceration or skin degloving. **Open fractures**, which occur in approximately 5% of pelvic fractures, contribute to 50% of the mortality. Patients with open pelvic fractures often require urgent exploratory laparotomy and a diverting colostomy. Temporarily cover open wounds with sterile compressive dressings. The posterior pelvis can be evaluated by logrolling the patient to inspect for lacerations or hematoma.

        1. In males, examine the scrotal contents for testicular displacement and inspect the urethral meatus for blood. The absence of blood does not exclude a urethral injury. Palpate the anterior pubic symphysis and rami for diastasis or crepitus, respectively.

        2. In females, appropriate evaluation of the external genitalia should include a visual and bimanual pelvic examination for lacerations that may involve the urethra, vagina, or rectum. If an adequate examination is not possible in the emergency department, thorough examination under anesthesia should be done as soon as possible. Vaginal lacerations should be irrigated and closed, if the tissues appear healthy. Perineal lacerations are generally managed open with serial debridement and delayed closure.

        3. Perform rectal examination before inserting the Foley catheter (check for a displaced prostate in males, which is indicative of urethral disruption). Urethral tears are more frequent in males and commonly occur below the urogenital diaphragm. Blood on the examining finger with rectal examination requires direct visualization of the anus and rectum; anoscopy and proctoscopy are indicated. A rectal tear in the setting of a pelvic fracture is a contaminated open fracture. Diverting colostomy and irrigation of the wound are indicated. Maintain a high suspicion of rectal injury in all cases of displaced pelvic fractures. Rectal tears can result from perforation by bony fragments, crush injury to the rectum, or ischemic injury to the rectum from mesenteric vessel injury. **Consider proctoscopy for all patients with significantly displaced pelvic fractures.**

4. An open pelvic fracture with active bleeding through a soft-tissue defect represents a difficult management problem. The fracture is no longer contained and the patient can rapidly exsanguinate (Fig. 33.1). Major vascular disruption occurs in only 1% of pelvic fractures, but has a 75% mortality rate. Management includes:

    a. Airway control and multiple-site, large bore, intravenous (i.v.) access; early blood transfusion

    b. Pressure tamponade of soft-tissue bleeding in the trauma room

    c. Transfer to the operating room (OR) for laparotomy, control of bleeding from extrapelvic sources, and simultaneous control and packing of pelvic bleeding. Control of pelvic bleeding may require suture ligation of obvious bleeding sites through both the abdomen and perineal wound.

    d. External fixation with diverting colostomy if the perineal wound involves the anus or rectum

    e. Arteriogram with embolization if possible

    f. Serial operative debridement with delayed definitive fracture management and wound closure

  C. The mechanical stability is often difficult to assess manually. Repetitive stressing of the pelvis is not advisable as this can exacerbate bleeding and increase patient discomfort. Direct manipulation of the pelvis in compression is a test of rotational stability, whereas the push-pull maneuver of the lower leg is a clinical sign of vertical displacement.

  D. Perform a detailed motor and sensory examination of the lower extremities to evaluate for associated neurologic injury, particularly of the lumbosacral plexus. The examination should include sphincter tone, perineal sensation, as well as lower extremity function and sensation. The nerve roots may be injured through stretch or laceration. Perform and document the examination both before and after fracture reduction.

III. Radiographic analysis. All patients involved in high-energy trauma, and those complaining of pelvic pain after low-energy trauma require an anteroposterior (AP) radiograph of the pelvis. It is important to note that displacement occurring at the time of injury can be greater than that visualized on the radiograph because of the elastic recoil of the pelvis.

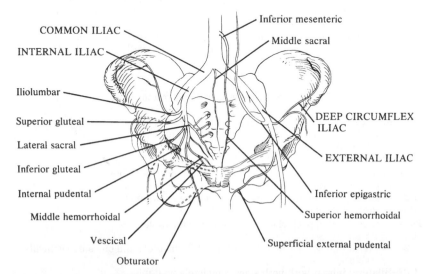

COMMON ILIAC

INTERNAL ILIAC

Iliolumbar

Superior gluteal

Lateral sacral

Inferior gluteal

Internal pudental

Middle hemorrhoidal

Vescical

Obturator

Inferior mesenteric

Middle sacral

DEEP CIRCUMFLEX ILIAC

EXTERNAL ILIAC

Inferior epigastric

Superior hemorrhoidal

Superficial external pudental

FIG. 33.1. Arterial supply to the pelvis. (From Kudsk KA, Sheldon GF. Retroperitoneal hematoma. In: Blaisdell FW, Trunkey DD. *Trauma management, abdominal trauma.* New York: Thieme 1982:284, with permission.)

    A. If pelvis asymmetry or fracture is identified, obtain pelvic inlet and outlet views to determine AP and vertical displacement of the hemipelvis, respectively.

    B. Obtain a **Judet** oblique radiographs in patients with suspicion of acetabular fractures.

    C. Evidence of significant posterior or vertical instability includes displacement of the posterior pelvic complex by >5 mm.

        1. Obtain a **computed tomography (CT)** scan of the pelvis, with 3-mm contiguous cuts, in patients with evidence of a pelvic fracture (when the patient is hemodynamically **stable**). The CT scan provides information on the extent of injury, magnitude of fracture or joint displacement, and foraminal compression of the sacrum. The CT scan is especially helpful in evaluating the posterior pelvic ring in comparison with plain radiographs. Information obtained from the CT defines the anatomic pattern in greater detail and may change what the orthopedic surgeons do operatively.

    D. Evaluate the genitourinary tract in patients with hematuria, blood at the urethral meatus, or inability or urinate.

        1. A retrograde urethrogram or cystogram is required to evaluate for potential urethral injury or bladder injury. Genitourinary injuries associated with pelvic fractures are missed in 23% on initial evaluation.

IV. Types of pelvic fractures. Mechanisms of injury and force vectors involved determine the pelvic fracture pattern, as well as associated injuries. Numerous classification systems exist to describe the injured pelvis and deformity patterns. However, the most commonly used classification system is that of Tile, stratified on the instability of the bony injury (Table 33.1).

    A. Stable, minimally displaced pelvic ring fractures are usually associated with low-energy trauma. These injuries are characterized by pubic rami fractures, avulsion fractures or simple, transverse sacral or coccygeal fractures (Fig. 33.2A).

    B. Rotationally unstable fractures consist of anterior and posterior pelvic ring injuries resulting in rotational laxity (through AP compression or lateral compression mechanisms) but vertical stability (Fig. 33.2B). The symphysis, rami, or both are involved anteriorly, whereas the sacrum, sacroiliac joint, or both are involved posteriorly. Both ipsilateral and contralateral injuries are represented (Fig. 33.2C).

    C. Vertically and rotationally unstable fractures are characterized by disruptions in the anterior and posterior elements, with vertical displacement of

Table 33.1. Types of pelvic fractures

Type A: Stable
-**A1**—Fractures not involving the ring; avulsion injuries
-**A2**—Stable, minimal displacement
-**A3**—Transverse fractures of the sacrum or coccyx

Type B: Rotationally unstable; vertically and posteriorly stable
-**B1**—External rotation instability; open book injury
-**B2**—Internal rotation instability; lateral compression injury
-**B3**—Bilateral rotationally unstable injury

Type C: Rotationally, posteriorly and vertically unstable
-**C1**—Unilateral injury
-**C2**—Bilateral injury, with one side rotationally unstable and one side vertically unstable
-**C3**—Bilateral injury, with both sides completely unstable

(From Tile M. Pelvic ring fractures: should they be fixed? *J Bone Joint Surg* 1988; 70:1, with permission.)

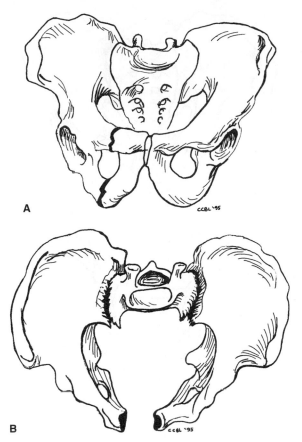

FIG. 33.2. A. Stable, minimally displaced pelvic ring fracture. **B.** Rotationally unstable pubic symphysis diastasis.

either one or both hemipelves, either with or without associated acetabular fractures (Fig. 33.2D).

   D. The mechanism of injury determines associated injuries:

      1. Lateral compression fractures: closed head injury, lung, spleen, liver

      2. Anteroposterior compression (open book fractures): bladder, urethra, rectum, lower extremities, chest injuries

      3. Vertical shear fractures: neurovascular injury, calcaneal fractures, thoracolumbar spine fractures

V. Resuscitative treatment. A team approach, including simultaneous evaluation by multiple trauma specialists, is essential (Fig. 33.3).

   A. Hypotension (systolic blood pressure <90 mmHg) in the patient with pelvic fracture requires prompt, aggressive treatment. **The source of bleeding in such a patient is more commonly from the chest or abdomen than from the pelvic fracture**. Major blood loss in the multiply injured patient with a displaced pelvic ring fracture can occur from the following five major areas:

      1. Intrathoracic bleeding may be detected on the screening chest radiograph obtained immediately on arrival to the emergency department (e.g., massive hemothorax).

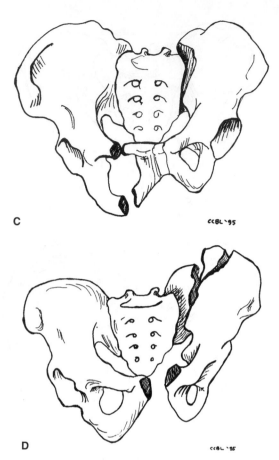

C

CCBL '95

D

CCBL '95

FIG. 33.2. *Continued.* **C.** Rotationally unstable pubic ramus fracture and concomitant sacral injury. **D.** Vertically and rotationally unstable fracture with disruption of anterior and posterior elements and vertical displacement of the hemipelvis.

2. Intraperitoneal bleeding can be evaluated by **diagnostic peritoneal lavage (DPL) or ultrasound**, especially in the hemodynamically unstable patient. Assume hypotension is from an intraperitoneal injury rather than the pelvic fracture. Common abdominal injuries causing major bleeding include the spleen, liver, mesenteric tears, and lacerations to the iliac vessels. A **supraumbilical incision for DPL** decreases the rate of false-positive findings. If the patient requires laparotomy, or suprapubic tube, place the **incision as cephalad and central as possible** to avoid compromise of the surgical incisions required for open reduction and internal fixation (ORIF) of the pelvis. Assess peripheral pulses from the femoral artery to the dorsalis pedis.

a. On rare occasion, the patient with a pelvic fracture presents with exsanguinating hemorrhage. The patient must be transferred immediately to the OR. The bleeding can be caused by major vascular injury (iliac or femoral arteries), intraperitoneal bleeding, or from the pelvis. Once in the abdomen, if the bleeding is from the pelvis and can

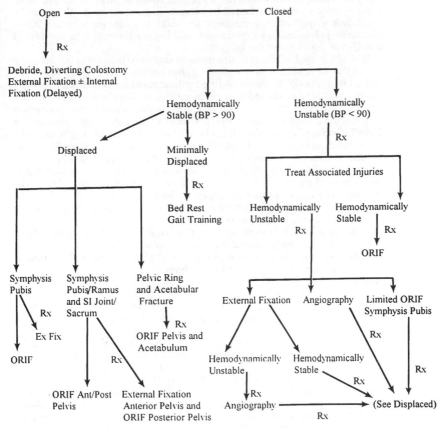

FIG. 33.3. Algorithm for the treatment of the multiply injured patient with a pelvic ring fracture.

be controlled with pressure, pack the pelvis and **transfer the patient promptly for pelvic angiography and embolization.** Initial stabilization with external fixation is also considered.

   3. Retroperitoneal bleeding, generally caused by the pelvic fracture
   4. External wounds are usually obvious and controlled with direct pressure.
   5. Extremity fractures: multiple, open, or closed
B. Pelvic hemorrhage occurs from exposed bone fracture surfaces, venous plexus disruption, and arterial tears, particularly the superior gluteal artery. The retroperitoneal space can accommodate many liters of blood before tamponade occurs.
C. Some pelvic fractures need immediate pelvic ring stabilization. This can be accomplished rapidly with readily available hospital equipment and supplies. Consider these temporary, noninvasive, pelvic immobilization maneuvers in **hemodynamically unstable** patients who meet clinical or radiographic criteria of pelvic instability: 1) clinical: the bony pelvis is mobile on physical examination or 2) radiographic: significant widening of the anterior or posterior pelvic ring on AP radiograph of the pelvis. Under these conditions,

temporary noninvasive pelvic immobilization can be achieved with the military antishock trousers (MAST), a vacuum splint or large "bean bag" mattress or even a standard folded bed sheet. Regardless of the device to be used, before application, complete a thorough physical examination of the abdomen, pelvis, buttocks, perineum, and lower extremities to identify all significant injuries or wounds.

If MAST is used, all three compartments should be inflated to low pressure levels (30–40 mmHg; firm to squeezing, but not hard). If a "bean bag" is acquired from the OR, it should be lined with a standard bed sheet, manually shaped about the pelvis and lower extremities, held in place, and suction applied until rigid. This serves as a shell for the pelvis and lower extremities and has the advantage of splinting fractures in the legs as well (as does the MAST). The application of the folded bed sheet is universally applicable. The sheet is folded length-wise in widths of approximately 18 inches. The sheet is placed about the patient's pelvis and crossed anteriorly at the level of the symphysis pubis. As the sheet is crossed and tension created, a second person "closes" the pelvis by pressing inward and firmly on the lateral buttocks just posterior to the anterior iliac spines. The sheet is then secured by knotting or with large clamps. Regardless of the device selected, the application of these temporary immobilizers:

    a. Must be done with the spine in the neutral position; logrolling, lifting the entire body without axial flexion or extension

    b. Used for a short period of time as a bridge to external fixation or angiographic control of hemorrhage

D. Angiographic evaluation and embolization is indicated in patients with persistent hemodynamic instability who have had adequate volume resuscitation, correction of coagulopathy, treatment of extrapelvic sources of bleeding, and persistent bleeding, despite external or limited internal fixation. Hemodynamic instability from the pelvis is defined as ongoing resuscitation of >6 units of packed red blood cells (PRBC) in a 4-hour time span. Broader indications for angiography include >6 units PRBC in 48 hours because of pelvic bleeding; hemodynamic instability in a patient with a negative focused abdominal sonography for trauma (FAST) or DPL; large pelvic hematoma seen on CT or at laparotomy; and active extravasation noted on pelvic CT. Displaced pelvic fractures through the sciatic notch have a high incidence of associated vascular injury (superior gluteal artery). **Prompt recognition of patients who require angiography and embolization to control bleeding associated with pelvic fractures is essential**; minimizing time to definitive control of bleeding is as critical in this setting as with cavitary hemorrhage requiring operative control.

    1. Obvious bleeding is seen in<40% of pelvic angiograms (3% of all pelvic fractures).

VI. Hemodynamically unstable patients. Acute stabilization of pelvic fractures in hemodynamically unstable trauma patients with associated extrapelvic injuries is controversial.

    A. Pneumatic antishock garment (PASG) or MAST is useful in the prehospital setting.

    B. External fixation has certain advantages and disadvantages in the treatment of the patient with an unstable pelvic ring fracture.

        1. Advantages. Simple, uniplanar frames are advocated, with the bars positioned to allow 90° of hip flexion to allow sitting and not obstruct genitourinary or abdominal access. In addition, resuscitative C-shaped clamps have been utilized in the emergency department for pelvic stabilization.

        a. Restoration of the spherical bony anatomy of the disrupted pelvic ring is believed to tamponade and decrease hemorrhage, as well as stabilize the blood clot formed around the bleeding vessel or fractured bone.

        b. Transfusion requirements may be reduced as well as the duration of shock.

   c. The pelvic stability provided allows for easier intrahospital transport.

   d. Mobilization of the patient is facilitated, along with improved nursing care and diminished narcotic requirements.

   e. External fixation remains as the initial treatment of choice for open pelvic fractures (through skin, vagina, or rectum).

  2. Disadvantages

   a. Certain fracture patterns (e.g., fractures of the iliac wing) are not amenable to external fixation.

   b. Lateral compression fractures with disruption of the sacrum or sacroiliac joints are not adequately stabilized by standard anterior external fixation alone.

   c. Use of the C-clamp in osteopenic patients has been associated with additional comminution of the fracture.

   d. External fixation for definitive care can be associated with loss of fracture reduction.

   e. The incisions used for pin placement, as well as pin tract infections, can preclude a surgical approach to the pelvis at the time of ORIF.

C. Limited ORIF of the anterior pelvis (e.g., pubic symphysis disruption) can be performed acutely as part of the resuscitation effort, especially with laparotomy. Either extend the laparotomy incision or use a preferred Pfannenstiel incision. This same incision can be used to repair bladder and other genitourinary injuries.

VII. Definitive ORIF of the displaced pelvic ring fracture with posterior disruption is often necessary. Recent biomechanical studies indicate that internal fixation improves overall stability, particularly when all disrupted elements are stabilized.

A. ORIF of the anterior pelvis, including pubic symphysis or rami, with a plate can be done acutely, as noted above, or on a delayed basis in the hemodynamically stable patient.

B. Posterior pelvic ring fractures of either the sacrum or sacroiliac joint are definitively treated with ORIF. Anterior and posterior approaches have been described. Iliosacral lag screws placed under fluoroscopic or CT guidance stabilize the posterior pelvis with minimal dissection. Displaced sacral fractures with nerve root impingement may require a posterior approach with foraminal decompression.

C. Acetabular fractures can be associated with pelvic ring fractures. Stabilization of the pelvic ring is the first priority, especially if the patient is in shock. If the iliac wing is fractured in association with the acetabular fracture, internal fixation is required. In stable patients, acetabular and pelvic ring fractures are often addressed simultaneously.

D. Internal stabilization of open fractures can be undertaken after serial irrigation and debridement produce a clean wound.

Axioms

- Pelvic fractures have a high incidence of associated injuries that contribute significantly to morbidity and mortality.
- The hypotensive patient with a pelvic fracture frequently has active bleeding from the abdomen or chest as the primary cause for hypotension.
- The mechanism and vector of injury determine the pelvic fracture pattern, as well as associated injuries.
- Carefully inspect the perineum, rectum, and vagina to detect open pelvic fractures.
- Active bleeding in association with pelvic fracture requiring angiography and embolization must be recognized and controlled expeditiously.

Bibliography

Burgess AR, Eastridges BJ, Youung JWR, et al. Pelvic ring disruptions: effective classification system and treatment protocols. *J Trauma* 1990;30:858.

Flint L, Babikian G, Anders M, et al. Definitive control of mortality from severe pelvic fractures. *Ann Surg* 1990;211:703.

Goldstein A, Phillips F, Scalfani SJA, et al. Early open reduction and internal fixation of the disrupted pelvic ring. *J Trauma* 1986;26:325.

Gruen GS, Leit ME, Gruen RJ, et al. The acute management of hemodynamically unstable multiple trauma patients with pelvic ring fractures. *J Trauma* 1994;36:706.

Panetta T, Scalfani SJ, Goldstein AS, et al. Percutaneous embolization for massive bleeding from pelvic fractures. *J Trauma* 1985;25:1021.

Poole GV, Ward EF, Muakassa FF, et al. Pelvic fractures from major blunt trauma: outcome is determined by associated injuries. *Ann Surg* 1991;213:532.

Riemer BL, Butterfield SL, Diamond DL, et al. Acute mortality associated with injuries to the pelvis: the role of early patient mobilization and external fixation. *J Trauma* 1993;35:671.

Shuler T, Boone DC, Gruen G, et al. Percutaneous iliosacral screw fixation: optimal treatment for unstable posterior pelvic ring disruption. *J Trauma* 1995;38:453–458.

Tile M. Pelvic ring fractures: should they be fixed? *J Bone Joint Surg* 1988;70:1.

34. HAND TRAUMA

Steven L. Bernard, Ramon Llull, and N. Ake Nyström

I. **Introduction**. The hand is injured more often than any other part of the body. The open position and constant use of our hands puts them in jeopardy whenever we work or play. Fortunately, most of the injuries are minor and few require emergency department treatment. Fewer still require the expertise of a hand specialist. This chapter provides information to help confidently diagnose injuries of the hand, and to recognize which injuries require the care of a specialist.

Once a trauma patient is stabilized, the evaluation of the hand can begin. An initial examination of both upper extremities should take <10 minutes to determine whether the patient requires operative intervention, the problem requires immediate attention, or it can be treated in a more elective manner. The assessment in the emergency department is important because delay in treatment can result in greater permanent disability.

Hand injury can be the cause of significant morbidity from blood loss. Peripheral bleeding should be controlled with direct pressure, and tourniquet use is discouraged, other than the controlled environment of an operating room (OR).

II. **Evaluation**
  A. **History**
    1. Patient's name, age, sex, occupation
    2. Handedness (which hand is dominant)
    3. When the injury occurred
    4. Where the injury occurred (e.g., a farm)
    5. Mechanism of injury (e.g., fall on dorsiflexed hand)
    6. Referring physician's diagnosis
    7. Treatment initiated by referring physician
       a. Dressing
       b. Drugs (antibiotics, analgesics, tetanus toxoid)
       c. Nerve blocks
    8. Estimated time of arrival; estimate cold and warm ischemia times
    9. Medical history
       a. Previous hand injuries
       b. Current medication
       c. Smoking history
       d. Allergies
       e. Diabetes mellitus, cardiac or peripheral vascular diseases, and so forth
  B. **Physical examination**
    1. **General considerations**. Examine the patient while sitting, and explain each step of the examination. It is often helpful to demonstrate (on the patient's uninjured hand) the various diagnostic maneuvers. Assume injury to deep structures (nerve, vessel, tendon, muscle, bone) in the presence of a laceration, swelling, or ecchymosis. The assumption is particularly important if the patient is unconscious. Encourage the patient to look at the injured hand, to better participate in planning treatment.
    2. **Skin**
       a. Note **location**, and estimate **area** and **depth** of lacerations or burns.
       b. Note **color** and **temperature** of the injured extremity.
    3. **Circulation**
       a. Palpate **pulses** in the radial, ulnar, and digital arteries.
       b. Perform a **Doppler** examination, if pulses are not palpable.

    c. Allen's test: with the patient making a tight fist, occlude both the radial and ulnar arteries with digital pressure. When the patient opens the fist, release pressure over one of the arteries. The entire hand should quickly become an even pink. The test is repeated with the opposite artery. Brisk refill indicates patency of the respective artery and the palmar arch. Slow, absent or partial refill can indicate an arterial injury.

4. Nerve

    a. Two-point discrimination (**2PD**): normal is <5 mm (Fig. 34.1). Pinprick testing has little or no value in the emergency room.

    b. Sudomotor function (sweat): dry finger pulp can indicate nerve injury: compare injured to the uninjured side, particularly in pediatric patients.

    c. Motor function: test muscle function distal to the laceration; compare injured to the uninjured side.

5. Tendon (see details under *Nerve Injuries* and *Tendon Injuries*)

    a. Finger cascade (Fig. 34.2A). At rest with the wrist in a neutral position, the fingers normally assume a slightly flexed position: the "cascade" of the hand. A flexor tendon laceration can disrupt the cascade (Fig. 34.2B).

    b. Tenodesis (Fig. 34.3). On dorsiflexion of the wrist, the fingers flex, unless a tendon is injured. Likewise, on palmar flexion, the fingers extend in the uninjured hand.

    c. Squeeze the flexor or extensor compartments of the forearm to cause the fingers to flex or extend.

    d. Active motion. Inability to actively move a supple joint can indicate injury to tendon, muscle, or nerve. A partial tendon laceration

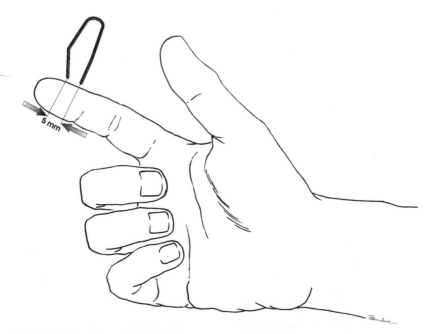

FIG. 34.1. Two point discrimination.

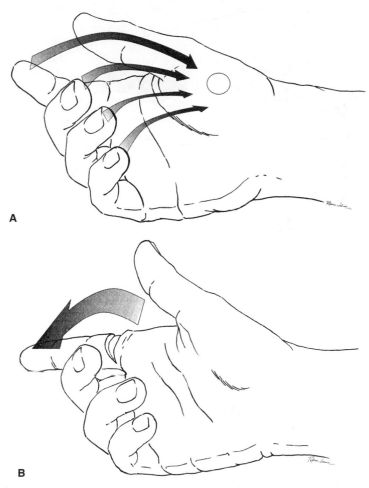

FIG. 34.2. A. Cascade. **B.** Loss of cascade.

does not result in loss of active motion, but can cause pain on attempted movement.

   6. **Bone and joints**
      a. Palpate and look for deformities
      b. Passive and active **range of motion**
      c. Stability
      d. **Open vs closed** dislocations or fractures
C. **Diagnostic tests**
   1. **Plain radiographs** for fractures, dislocations, foreign bodies, or gas
      a. **Standard views**: posteroanterior, lateral, and oblique
      b. **Bilateral views in children** to avoid confounding epiphyseal plates
         with fractures
      c. Stress views (clenched fist, radial or ulnar deviation), especially for
         the wrist

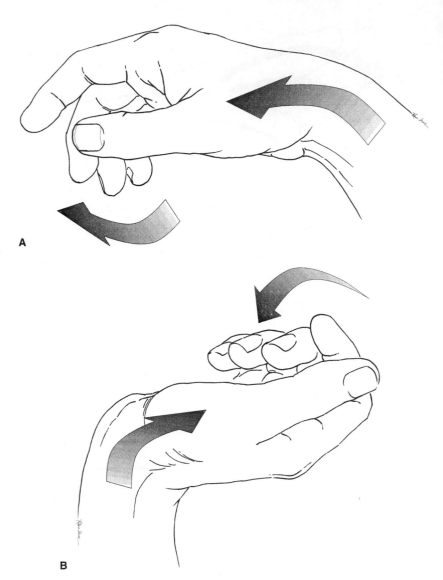

FIG. 34.3. A. Tenodesis (volar flexion). **B.** Tenodesis (dorsal flexion).

2. **Angiography** or **Doppler examination** to assess arterial integrity
3. **Sonogram** to identify non-radiopaque foreign body (wood, glass)
4. **Compartment pressure measurements** can be performed with a sphygmomanometer, intravenous (i.v.) tubing, three-way stopcock, and an inline bubble. A pressure >40 mmHg is an indication for fasciotomy, whereas a normal reading (i.e., pressure <25 mmHg) does not exclude a compartment syndrome or the need for surgery.
5. **Wound cultures** should be obtained before treatment with antibiotics.

D. Analgesia and anesthesia
  1. **General considerations**
     a. Only a pain-free patient can make rational decisions about care. Pain relief is most effectively achieved with local anesthetic. Therefore, consider a regional block once the neurologic examination is complete.
     b. Use 25- to 27-gauge needle on a 10-mL syringe. The smaller needle causes less pain.
     c. Use **lidocaine** (0.5%) or **bupivacaine** (0.25%, for a longer lasting block). **Do not use epinephrine in the hand.**
  2. **Wrist block**
     a. **Technique.** For a complete block of the hand, inject 5 to 7 mL of the local anesthetic to each of the four injection sites illustrated in Fig. 34.4. Aspirate to confirm that the tip of the needle is not intravascular. Little resistance should be encountered with the injection of local anesthetic. If the patient complains of sharp, shooting pain—**STOP**; you may be injecting into the nerve rather than around it. Injecting into a nerve can cause permanent loss of function, and chronic disabling pain. **Wait** for 10 minutes or until the block is complete. **Do not** inject a second time around a partially anesthetized nerve. Instead, use longer acting local anesthetic.
  3. **Digital block**
     a. Injection of local anesthesia inside the **tendon sheath** is a simple and effective method that provides circumferential anesthesia with one needle-stick; particularly valuable in children. In the midline of the proximal phalanx, push the needle through the flexor tendon, and back off just slightly from the bone. Slowly inject 3 to 5 mL of local anesthetic.
     b. **Finger base.** Inject 3 mL of local anesthetic into the web space on each side of the digit. A third injection to the dorsal aspect of the finger completes the block.

III. Specific injuries
  A. **Vascular compromise** can represent a true emergency and must be dealt with promptly, whether requiring fasciotomy, vascular repair, replantation, reduction of fracture or dislocation, or bypass surgery.
  1. **Arterial insufficiency**
     a. **Signs.** Pale, cold extremity with slow or absent capillary refill, decreased skin turgor; slow, often dark bleeding from pin prick
     b. **Diagnosis** is based on clinical findings, supported by laboratory studies (x-ray, Doppler) as needed.
     c. **Treatment** is surgical (vascular reconstruction, thrombectomy), conservative (reduce fracture), or pharmacologic (thrombolysis), depending on cause.
  2. **Venous insufficiency**
     a. **Signs.** Bluish-purple, cold extremity with quick capillary refill (<2 seconds), increased skin turgor; brisk, dark-colored bleeding from pinprick
     b. In the severely ill or injured patient with evidence of venous insufficiency, always suspect venous gangrene and consult with a hematologist. **Consider HITT-syndrome** (heparin induced thrombocytopenia and thombosis syndrome).
  3. **Compartment syndrome**
     a. **Signs.** The diagnosis is almost always clinical. Suspect when passive stretching (most commonly the flexors in the forearm) is restricted and painful in a patient with a history of trauma. Surgical fasciotomy is diagnostic as well as therapeutic. Arterial pulses, paresthesias, and so on **do not** confirm or rule out compartment syndrome.
     b. Causes are legion and include any acute disturbance of muscle circulation: crush or extended pressure (e.g., unconscious person laying on the arm), arterial thrombosis, embolization, dislocation, fracture

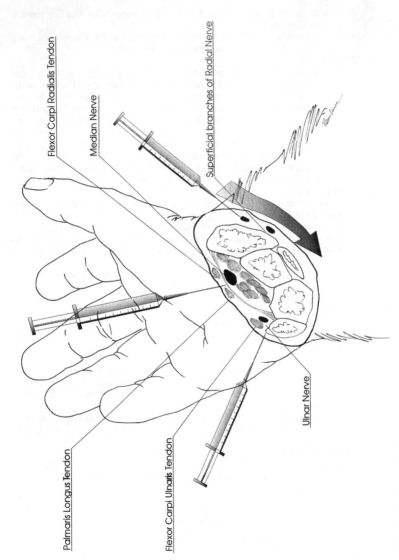

Flexor Carpi Radialis Tendon

Median Nerve

Superficial branches of Radial Nerve

Palmaris Longus Tendon

Flexor Carpi Ulnaris Tendon

Ulnar Nerve

FIG. 34.4. Nerve block.

(supracondylar humerus fractures), intramuscular bleeding (stab wound), pressure injection, snake bite, and burn (does not have to be circumferential).

    c. Treatment is surgical and consists of urgent decompression through fasciotomy. The flexor compartment of the forearm is most commonly affected. The operation, in selected cases, may include the carpal tunnel, Guyon's canal, the extensor compartment in the forearm, and the intrinsic muscles in the hand (Fig. 34.5).

B. Nerve injury (Fig. 34.6)

    1. Classification of nerve injuries to guide treatment and prognosis.

        a. Neurapraxia is usually caused by blunt trauma or pressure (e.g., "Saturday night palsy"). Axons are intact and full recovery is the rule, usually within days to months. Support with splint as indicated.

        b. Axonotmesis is usually caused by crush or stretch injury. Epineurium is intact, but the axons are disrupted. Prognosis is relatively good, and recovery can be complete. Support with splint as indicated.

        c. Neurotmesis involves a severed nerve. Requires surgical repair for optimal recovery, which rarely is complete.

    2. Signs. Assess level of injury by examining sensory and motor function (see above). The clinical examination can confirm loss of nerve function, but not necessarily the potential for recovery (usually better in children). Always consider surgery in cases of possible nerve laceration (neurotmesis).

        a. Median nerve. Motor function: flexor carpi radialis (FCR), flexor digitorum superficialis (FDS), flexor digitorum profundus (FDP) to index, flexor pollicis longus (FPL), abductor pollicis brevis (APB). **Sensory** function (2PD): palmar aspect of the thumb, index, middle, and radial half of the ring finger. A crossover of fibers between the median and ulnar nerves in the forearm ("Martin-Gruber") or the

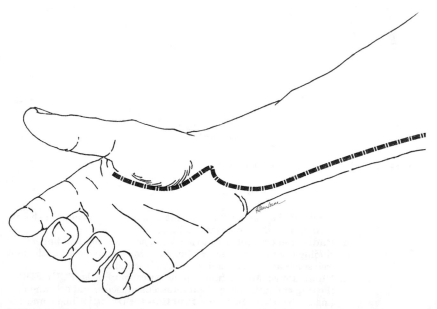

FIG. 34.5. Fasciotomy.

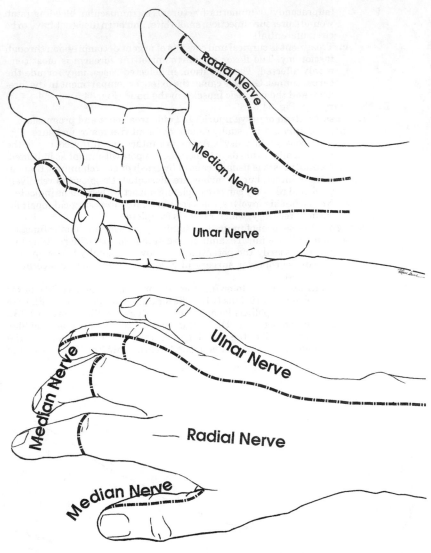

FIG. 34.6. A. Sensory fields (volar). **B.** Sensory fields (dorsal).

hand ("Riche-Canneu") can result in subtle differences in the examination from that described here.

b. Radial nerve. **Motor** function: extensors of wrist and fingers, including the thumb. **Sensory** function: the dorsal aspect of the first web space and dorsal radial aspect of the hand.

c. Ulnar nerve. **Motor** function: flexor carpi ulnaris (FCU), FDP to the ring and fifth finger, the interosseus muscles, and first and fifth finger abduction. **Sensory function** (2PD): little finger and the ulnar half of the ring finger.

3. **Treatment**. If possible, treat a lacerated nerve in the OR, with direct repair or nerve graft within 10 days of the injury. Optimal conditions require the use of an operating microscope. If a nerve injury is recognized in the emergency department, the skin can be sutured and the patient safely referred to a hand surgeon.

C. **Flexor tendon injury**
   1. **Anatomy**
      a. **The tendon sheath** is a fiber-osseous tunnel that contains the flexor tendons along the ventral aspect of the fingers. An isolated injury to the tendon sheath rarely requires surgical repair.
      b. **Tendons**. Two long flexors (FDS and FDP) run in the tendon sheath of each finger, in the thumb only one (FPL) (Figs. 34.7 and 34.8).
      c. **Zones** (Fig. 34.9). The choice of surgical technique and the prognosis depend on several factors, including the anatomic level of the tendon injury. Zone II (distal palmar crease to the mid-middle phalanx) injuries tend to have the poorest functional prognosis, and require specialist repair and rehabilitation.
      d. A "jersey" injury is an avulsion of the FDP (ring finger in 75%) from the distal phalanx (e.g., from grasping a football jersey during a tackle). A sliver of bone, corresponding to the avulsed bony insertion of the tendon, may be seen on x-ray.
   2. **Signs**. Assume tendon injury when the patient is unable to move a joint through a full active range of motion, and the attempted movement is painful. The integrity of the tendons must be tested individually (Figs. 34.7 and Fig. 34.8).
   3. **Treatment**. Surgical repair should be performed under optimal conditions in the OR.

D. **Extensor tendon injury**
   1. **Anatomy**
      a. The long extensor tendons act primarily on the metacarpophalangeal (MP) joints, whereas the intrinsic muscles are primary extensors to the interphalangeal joints. In addition to the common

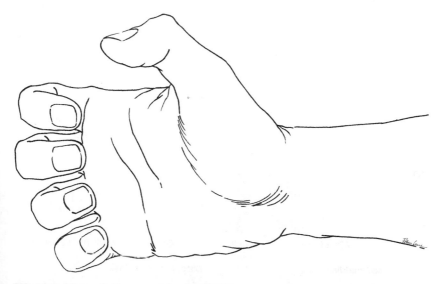

FIG. 34.7. Flexor digitorum profundus (FDP).

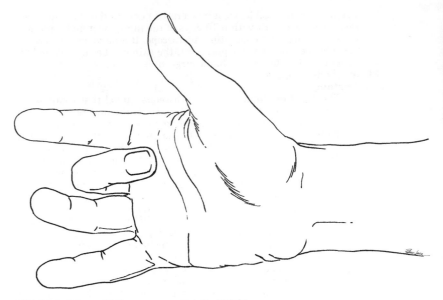

FIG. 34.8. Flexor digitorum superficialis (FDS).

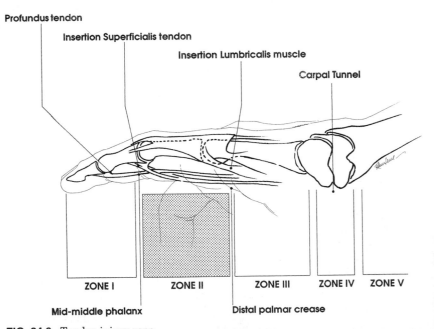

FIG. 34.9. Tendon injury zone.

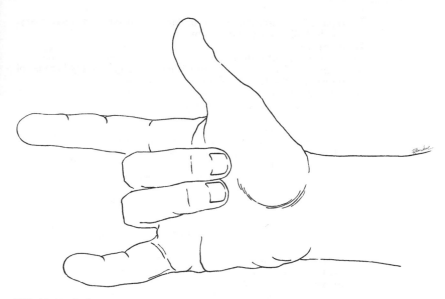

FIG. 34.10. Independent extrinsic extensors.

digital extensor, extensor digitorum communis, and the index and little fingers each have an independent extrinsic extensor: extensor indicus proprius and extensor digiti minimi (Fig. 34.10).
  b. *Juncturae tendineae* are connections between the extensor tendons proximal to the MP joint.
  c. A lacerated long extensor of the thumb can retract into the forearm, whereas this rarely is the case for extensors to the four fingers.
2. **Signs**
  a. Loss of active range of motion can indicate a tendon injury. Through function of the intrinsics, the interphalangeal joints still extend after an injury to the long extensor tendon proximal to the MP joint. Note, that juncturae tendineae initially can mask an extensor tendon laceration proximal to the MP joints.
  b. **Drop finger (Mallet finger)** is caused by an avulsion of the extensor tendon from the distal phalanx, and results in an inability to actively extend the distal interphalangeal (DIP) joint.
  c. **Boutonnière deformity** (proximal interphalangeal (PIP) flexed and DIP extended) is the late result of an isolated laceration of the extensor tendon insertion to the middle phalanx. Treatment is conservative (splinting) or surgical, depending on the nature of the injury.
3. **Treatment**. Surgical repair, with the exception of most mallet fingers (and sometimes boutonnière) deformities. Most surgeons prefer to keep the hand or finger immobilized for a period of 4 to 6 weeks after the repair, depending on the level, or zone of injury. Mallet finger (in the absence of a fracture with a large displaced fragment) is treated conservatively: splint the distal interphalangeal joint in full extension for 6 weeks.
E. **Joints**
  1. **Ligament injury**
    a. **Fingers**. Splint for comfort, or "buddy tape" to an adjacent finger. Surgical repair is rarely indicated.
    b. **Thumb**. A rupture of the thumb's ulnar collateral ligament at the MP (Stener lesion, Gamekeeper's thumb) usually requires surgical

repair. Test lateral stability, under local anesthesia if necessary, and look for an avulsion fracture on x-ray.
2. **Dislocation**
   a. **Simple**. Anesthetize and reduce
   b. **Complex**. Cannot be reduced without surgery, usually because of interposed soft tissue (volar plate or tendon).
   c. X-ray study both before and after reducing a dislocated joint, to assess the presence of a fracture.
   d. DIP joint
      (1) Usually dorsal
      (2) Dorsal block splint with immediate movement if stable
   e. PIP joint
      (1) Usually dorsal. In palmar dislocation, the head of the proximal phalanx may be caught between the lateral bands and require surgery.
      (2) Splint with dorsal block and move immediately if stable.
   f. MP joint
      (1) Usually dorsal
      (2) Dorsal block splint in 20° to 30° of flexion, mobilize if stable.
   g. CMC (carpometacarpal) joint
      (1) Usually dorsal, usually associated with fracture
      (2) Usually requires surgical reduction and K-wire fixation
   h. Scapholunate dissociation
      (1) A ligament rupture between the scaphoid and lunate should be suspected if the distance between the two bones is >4 mm on posteroanterior radiograph. Requires treatment in the OR, with (early) ligament reconstruction.
F. **Fractures**
   1. **Classification** of fractures to define treatment and prognosis
      a. Open or closed
      b. Simple or comminuted
      c. Transverse, oblique, or spiral
      d. Intraarticular or extraarticular
      e. **Translation** (off axis), **angulation** (palmar, dorsal radial, or ulnar apex)
      f. **Rotation** can usually not be assessed from radiographs.
      g. **Epiphyseal**: Salter-Harris classification (Fig. 34.11)
      h. **Stable** fractures hold reduction, whereas **unstable** fractures do not, and therefore often require surgery.
   2. Phalanges (see also fingertip injuries)
      a. **Nondisplaced, stable** fractures are buddy taped or splinted for 3 weeks.
      b. **Unstable fractures** are treated with closed reduction and K-wire fixation, if possible, or with open reduction and internal fixation through plate or K-wires.
      c. **Intraarticular** fractures must be reduced to minimize the risk for posttraumatic arthritis. Surgery or treatment with dynamic traction may be indicated.
   3. Metacarpals
      a. **Neck** fracture (Boxer's fracture) can be treated with 2 weeks of splinting for comfort, or be mobilized immediately.
      b. **Shaft** fractures can be splinted, if stable, or K-wired or plated open if grossly unstable.
   4. Thumb
      a. **Bennett's fracture** is an intraarticular fracture of the first CMC joint. By definition, it is unstable and often requires surgical fixation after reduction.
      b. **Rolando's fracture** involves both the palmar (as in a Bennett's fracture) and the dorsal aspect of the first metacarpal. The fracture may be unstable and require surgical treatment.

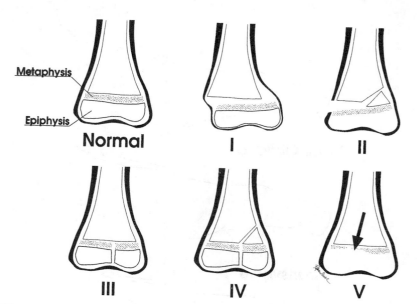

FIG. 34.11. Salter-Harris fracture classification.

5. Scaphoid; >50% of all carpal fractures
    a. **Signs**. Tenderness in the "anatomic snuff box" between the abductor pollicis longus (APL) and extensor pollicis longus (EPL) tendons distal to the radial styloid at the wrist. If initial x-ray films do not confirm a clinical suspicion of scaphoid fracture, immobilize and repeat radiographs after 3 weeks or consider an early bone scan. Delay in treatment of a scaphoid fracture significantly increases the rate of nonunion.
    b. **Treatment**. Immobilize in short arm cast or thumb spica splint until radiologically healed, usually 6 to 12 weeks. Displaced or unstable fractures may require primary surgery.
6. Hook of hamate
    a. Unusual
    b. Diagnosis by clinical examination (tender) and x-ray study: hamate view or computed tomography (CT)
    c. Refer for elective surgical treatment
G. Fingertip
    1. Nailbed injury
        a. **Signs**. Suspect nailbed injury if fracture of distal phalanx is seen on x-ray film.
        b. **Treatment**. Drain subungual hematoma to reduce pain (use heated paper clip). Repair nailbed lacerations with 6-0 chromic. Reposition the nail under the nailfold to function as a splint. Fractures of the distal phalanx are usually stable and rarely require immobilization other than for comfort.
    2. **Amputation**
        a. **Signs**. The key element is the nail, in particular the germinal matrix.
        b. **Treatment**. If the germinal nail matrix is intact, avoid surgery for the best functional and cosmetic result. Instead, allow the fingertip to heal by **secondary intention**. Treatment does not represent a risk for acute or chronic infection, even if bone initially is left exposed. **Do not shorten the distal phalanx** unless it protrudes several mil-

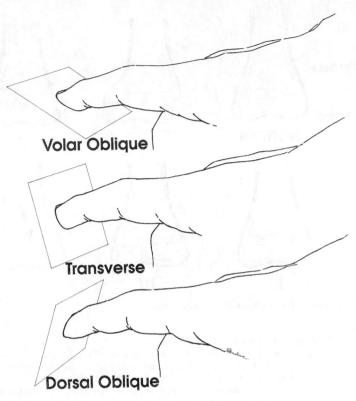

FIG. 34.12. Fingertip injuries.

limeters beyond the level of soft-tissue amputation. Skin **flaps** can occasionally be used to cover oblique amputations (Fig. 34.12). Avoid direct suture or skin grafts.

H. **Proximal amputations**
1. **General considerations**. Any amputation to the upper extremity should be considered a potential indication for replantation. For transport, store the part on saline-moistened gauze in a plastic bag and place in a container with ice and water. Avoid direct contact between the part and the ice. Provide pain relief (regional block, whenever possible).
2. **Inform** the replantation surgeon of the type and level of trauma, time and place of the incident, patient's age, gender, profession, and medical history.
3. If properly **cooled**, a part without muscle can still be replanted >24 hours after injury.
4. In the absence of specific contraindications, the decision to attempt a replantation should be made jointly by the patient and the replantation surgeon. Replantation adds little if any demonstrable function to the hand. However, the level of patient satisfaction after replantation surgery tends to be extremely high.
5. Relative contraindications
   a. Multiple levels of injury, crush, burn, and so on
   b. Unstable patient
   c. Psychological problems
   d. Proximal forearm and above after 6 hours of ischemia

6. Sequence of surgery
   a. **Two or more team approach**. One team prepares the stump, second team prepares the part (tags vessels and nerves), third team harvests graft tissues.
   b. **Throw nothing away**; all tissues may be used as grafts.
   c. **Fix bone**, repair tendons, vessels, and finally nerves.
   d. Provide soft-tissue coverage or skin graft.

I. **Burn** (see Chapter 46)
   1. **Immerse** the hand in cool water; provide pain relief.
   2. Assess depth, area, and need for surgery.
      a. **Debride** broken blisters and apply 1% silver sulfadiazine cream twice daily.
   3. **Debride** deeper burns in OR, using tourniquet to control blood loss.
   4. **Skin grafting** may be indicated to avoid secondary complications.
   5. **Splint** in position of safety if risk for contractures.
   6. **Chemical burns** are treated as in other parts of the body.

J. Infection
   1. The most important treatment to prevent infection is adequate **debridement**.
   2. **Farm injuries** are notorious for infection and should receive prophylactic antibiotics.
   3. **Human bite wounds**, such as those sustained during a fist fight in which an MP joint is opened by a tooth (Fig. 34.13), can cause multiple organism infections. Treat aggressively with a combination of surgery, cephalosporin, and penicillin.
   4. Operations on the hand generally do not require antibiotic coverage; however, consider prophylactic treatment in patients with open fractures or extensive soft-tissue damage, severely contaminated wounds, and so forth.

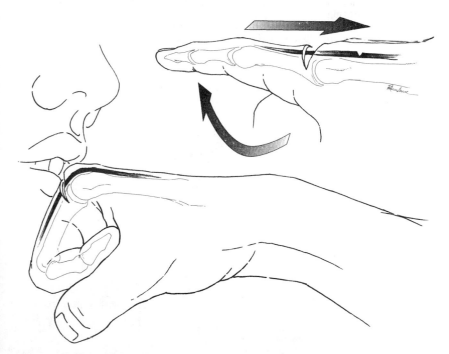

FIG. 34.13. Human bite wounds.

DIP and PIP extension

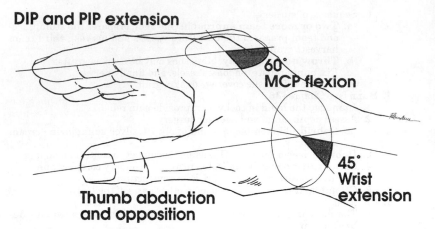

FIG. 34.14. Position of safety.

K. Dressings. Use splints in order to:
1. Protect wound
2. Promote healing and decrease pain
3. Prevent stiffness
4. Position of safety: wrist extended (30°–40°), MP joints flexed (>70°), interphalangeal joints straight (flexion <15°), and thumb radially and palmarly abducted (>45°) (Fig. 34.14).
5. Place fluffed gauze between fingers for comfort, and to avoid skin maceration.
6. Postoperative pain, until proved otherwise, is always caused by a tight dressing; split or change the dressing.

35. COMPARTMENT SYNDROME AND RHABDOMYOLYSIS

Preston R. Miller, III and John M. Kane, III

I. **Compartment syndrome** occurs when increased tissue pressure within a limited anatomic space compromises perfusion. Compartment syndrome of the arm, leg, or thigh is frequently encountered in trauma patients, most commonly following vascular or orthopedic injury. Left untreated, this syndrome leads to myoneural necrosis and permanent loss of function or amputation. The degree of damage depends on the degree of compartmental pressure elevation as well as the length of time that pressure is elevated. Concomitant shock increases the degree of damage for any given pressure and time.

A. **Etiology.** Any injury that leads to severe tissue edema within the fascial compartments can cause compartment syndrome.

1. **Vascular injury with limb ischemia** leads to tissue edema. Reperfusion produces toxic oxygen metabolites and increased capillary permeability, which worsens this swelling. Bleeding within a closed space from disrupted vessels can also lead to the syndrome.

2. **Crush injury.** Direct injury of tissues by crushing leads to edema with subsequent compartment syndrome.

3. **Fractures** account for approximately 50% of compartment syndromes. Tibial fractures are the most common fracture causing the syndrome, but any extremity fracture can lead to increased compartment pressure. Compartment syndrome can occur in the absence of fracture with soft-tissue injury, ischemia with reperfusion, prolonged compression, burns, and operative osteotomies.

4. **Trauma situations with high risk for the development of compartment syndrome** include reperfusion after >4 to 6 hours of ischemia, significant crush injury, and combined venous and arterial injury in a limb.

B. **Pathophysiology.** Local tissue injury, whether secondary to direct injury or as a result of ischemia or reperfusion, is the initiating factor in the development of compartment syndrome. With distensible vessels (e.g., veins), increased intracompartmental pressure translates directly into increased local venous pressure. Subsequent decrease in arteriovenous pressure gradient leads to local tissue hypoperfusion and anoxia. Anoxia produces more edema, which further increases intracompartmental pressure. This cycle continues until tissue necrosis occurs.

C. **Diagnosis.** As the signs and symptoms of compartment syndrome develop, ischemia can rapidly lead to irreversible damage. Diagnosis of compartment syndrome can be difficult.

1. **Symptoms.** Pain out of proportion to physical findings is usually seen in patients with compartment syndrome who are awake and alert. Paraesthesias followed late in the progression of the syndrome by paralysis may also be present.

2. **Signs** of compartment syndrome include a tensely swollen compartment and pain on passive stretch of the muscles in the affected compartment. Other important signs include sensory deficit in the nerve traversing the affected compartment, which can be followed by progressive motor weakness. **Loss of function may be the earliest sign.** Loss of peripheral pulse may be seen, but this is a late finding usually accompanied by irreversible damage.

   a. Compartment syndrome occurs most frequently in the lower leg, but can occur in the forearm, thigh, foot, or hand. **The lower leg** is composed of four compartments and their respective components.

      (1) **Anterior compartment**: tibialis anterior and great toe extensor muscles and the deep peroneal nerve.

336 The Trauma Manual

(2) **Lateral (peroneal) compartment**: peroneus longus and brevis muscles and the superficial peroneal nerve.

(3) **Superficial posterior compartment**: gastrocnemius and soleus muscles and the sural nerve.

(4) **Deep posterior compartment**: tibialis posterior and great toe flexor muscles and the tibial nerve.

b. The **forearm** is composed of three compartments with their respective components:

(1) **Volar compartment**: wrist and finger flexor muscles and the ulnar and median nerves.

(2) **Dorsal compartment**: wrist and finger extensor muscles and the posterior interosseous nerve.

(3) **Mobile wad**: extensor carpi radialis longus, extensor carpi radialis brevis, and brachioradialis muscles.

3. **Compartment pressures**. Elevated compartment pressure, by definition, will precede symptoms of compartment syndrome. For this reason, pressure measurement is an important adjunct to diagnosis. This is especially true in the patient with decreased mental status in whom physical examination is less reliable. Although disagreement exists to the cutoff between normal and abnormal compartment pressure, most consider compartment pressures >30 mmHg an indication for fasciotomy. Pressures between 20 and 30 mmHg in the symptomatic patient or in the face of prolonged hypotension also warrant fasciotomy. If question exists to the diagnosis, err on the side of fasciotomy rather than observation.

a. **Measurement devices** commonly available include the needle catheter and the Stryker handheld monitor. Needle catheters can produce inaccurately high pressures if not used correctly, but are universally available. A measurement system of this type can be made by attaching an 18-g needle to a length of pressure tubing. This tubing is connected to a pressure transducer as used for arterial line pressure measurement. The Stryker monitor is easily portable and accurate.

b. **Technique**: the skin overlying the compartment to be measured is prepared in a sterile fashion and infiltrated with local anesthetic, if necessary. The needle for the system to be used is then advanced into the muscle compartment. A small amount of saline is flushed through the catheter to ensure that plugging of the catheter does not interfere. The pressure is recorded. Correct needle position can be confirmed by noting a brief increase in pressure with compression of the compartment being measured. Measurements should be repeated to confirm elevated pressures.

D. **Treatment** of compartment syndrome is based on returning compartmental pressures to normal to restore adequate tissue perfusion—surgical fasciotomy of the affected limb. At the time of fasciotomy, debridement should be reserved for only frankly necrotic tissue. If tissue viability is questionable, the compartment should be reassessed to determine viability. **Whenever doubt exists whether compartment syndrome is present, fasciotomy should be performed**.

1. **Lower leg fasciotomy** (Fig. 35.1). Fasciotomy of the leg should release all four compartments (anterior, lateral, superficial, and deep posterior). This is easily accomplished with a double incision technique. Make an incision on the lateral leg from just below the head of the fibula to just above the ankle, approximately 1 cm anterior to the fibula. Identify the septum dividing the anterior and lateral compartments and open the fascia on either side of this septum to release these compartments, taking care to avoid the superficial peroneal nerve located along the intercompartmental septum in the lateral compartment. Make a second incision of similar length on the medial side of the leg, 2 cm posterior to the tibia. Open the fascia here to release the superficial posterior compartment. Here, partially detach the proximal soleus from the back of the tibia and incise the fascia, which releases the deep posterior compartment.

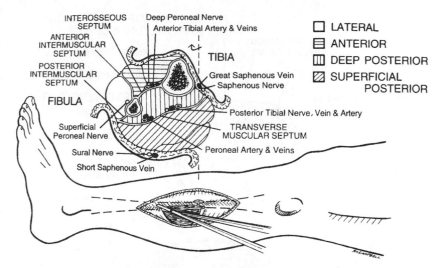

FIG. 35.1. Technique for calf fasciotomy. (From Ombrellaro MP, Steven SI. Compartment syndrome: a collective review. In: Maull KI, Cleveland HC, Feliciano DV, et al. (eds). *Advances in trauma and critical care*. St. Louis: Mosby-Yearbook, 1995;10:100, with permission.)

    2. **Thigh fasciotomy** involves the release of three compartments. Access the quadriceps compartment through an anterolateral incision on the thigh. Then, decompress the hamstring compartment by dividing the intermuscular septum posteriorly. Release the adductor compartment through a separate incision medially along the length of the compartment.

    3. **Forearm fasciotomy** (Fig. 35.2). Release the volar compartment through an incision along the volar aspect of the forearm, curving across joint spaces to avoid contracture with healing. Most authors suggest carpal tunnel release with this procedure. At this point, measure the dorsal compartment pressures and, if they remain elevated, perform dorsal fasciotomy. Release the dorsal compartment through a single straight incision on the back of the forearm from the lateral epicondyle to the wrist.

    4. **Closure.** These wounds can be closed 5 to 10 days later with primary closure or skin grafting, if needed, to avoid closing the wound under undue tension.

  E. **Complications.** The major complications of compartment syndrome include infection and rhabdomyolysis.

    1. Infection occurs secondary to the presence of necrotic muscle. Control of the process requires aggressive debridement of all nonviable tissue, which can lead to significant limitation of function of the affected limb.

    2. **Rhabdomyolysis** may be seen as a sequela of compartment syndrome and is discussed in detail below.

II. **Rhabdomyolysis** occurs when muscle damage from traumatic or nontraumatic causes releases toxins into the systemic circulation, which can lead to renal failure and even death. Early recognition and treatment of this disease reduces the incidence of renal dysfunction and other complications.

  A. **Etiology.** The causes of rhabdomyolysis are broadly divided into two categories, traumatic and nontraumatic.

    1. **Traumatic.** Crush injuries, ischemia or reperfusion, and compartment syndrome with muscle death all lead to release of myoglobin and other toxins into the circulation. Electrical injury, extreme exertion, and prolonged compression from surgical positioning can also create muscle injury. In addition, epidemic forms of rhabdomyolysis are seen in some

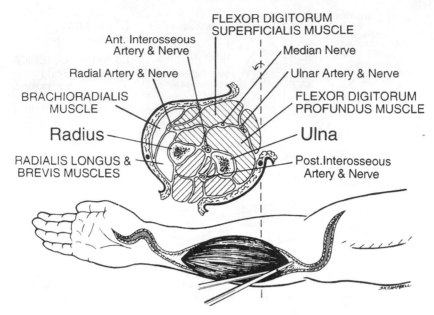

Ant. Interosseous
Artery & Nerve

FLEXOR DIGITORUM
SUPERFICIALIS MUSCLE

Median Nerve

Radial Artery & Nerve

Ulnar Artery & Nerve

BRACHIORADIALIS
MUSCLE

FLEXOR DIGITORUM
PROFUNDUS MUSCLE

Radius

Ulna

RADIALIS LONGUS &
BREVIS MUSCLES

Post.Interosseous
Artery & Nerve

FIG. 35.2. Technique for forearm fasciotomy. (From Ombrellaro MP, Steven SL. Compartment syndrome: a collective review. In: *Advances in trauma and critical care*. St. Louis: Mosby-Yearbook, 1995;10:100, with permission.)

mass casualty settings (e.g., the devastating earthquakes in Armenia in 1988). Over half of all patients admitted to hospitals during this disaster suffered from rhabdomyolysis.

2. **Nontraumatic**. Rhabdomyolysis is seen in conjunction with alcohol intoxication as well as with use of drugs such as cocaine, heroin, or others. Muscle damage is also well described in the setting of viral or bacterial infections as can be seen in the surgical patient. Hereditary causes of rhabdomyolysis include several of the glycogen storage diseases and the neuroleptic malignant syndrome. **Neuroleptic malignant syndrome (NMS)** occurs in patients receiving any neuroleptic drug, especially phenothiazine, haloperidol, dibenzoxepine, or dopamine-depleting drugs. NMS presents as fever, muscular rigidity, tachypnea, tachycardia, dystonia, or diaphoresis. **Malignant hyperthermia** is another cause that is pertinent to the surgical patient. Malignant hyperthermia is a hereditary hypermetabolic state of skeletal muscle resulting in high fever, rigidity, tachyarrhythmias, and rhabdomyolysis. It is generally associated with inhalation anesthetics.

B. **Pathophysiology**. Damaged muscle releases myoglobin, which normally assists in oxygen storage. This protein is filtered in the glomerulus and rapidly reabsorbed in the proximal tubules. As myoglobin is degraded here, iron is released which acts as an electron donor or acceptor, leading to the production of toxic oxygen metabolites and subsequent renal injury. This injury is compounded by the formation of myoglobin-protein casts that can clog the tubules. Cast formation is accelerated in an acid environment. The damaged muscle becomes edematous, leading to reduced extracellular or intravascular volume and, thus, reduced glomerular filtration rate. In addition, large amounts of potassium and other ions are released with further detrimental effects.

C. **Diagnosis**. A combination of clinical and laboratory findings in the appropriate clinical setting is the key to the diagnosis of rhabdomyolysis.

1. **Signs and symptoms**. Patients can have severe muscle pain and weakness. In addition, the urine can become dark and appear to contain blood. Physical examination can be normal in up to 50% of patients with rhabdomyolysis.
2. **Laboratory findings**. Urinalysis shows large blood on dipstick with few or no red blood cells on microscopic examination. Urine myoglobin is usually positive and pigmented casts can also be seen. On serum analysis, **elevated creatine phosphokinase** is the most sensitive marker of muscle damage in rhabdomyolysis. Muscle cell death leads to hyperkalemia, hyperuricemia, and hyperphosphatemia. Hypocalcemia secondary to production of calcium phosphate salts commonly follows hyperphosphatemia.

D. **Treatment** of rhabdomyolysis centers on prevention of renal dysfunction and correction of electrolyte abnormalities. It is also imperative to attempt to find and correct the underlying cause of rhabdomyolysis (e.g., compartment syndrome, dead tissue, infection).
   1. **Prevention of renal dysfunction**
      a. **Volume expansion**. The cornerstone of the treatment of rhabdomyolysis is expansion of intravascular volume, which ensures adequate renal perfusion. This has been experimentally shown in both animals and human subjects to prevent renal failure in rhabdomyolysis. The optimal level of intravascular volume expansion to prevent renal failure is not known, but preload should be adequate to maintain urine flow at least 1 to 2 mL/kg/h.
      b. **Sodium bicarbonate**. Some nonrandomized data suggest that alkalinization of the urine using sodium bicarbonate prevents the formation of pigmented casts and, thus, decreases the incidence of renal failure. Sodium bicarbonate can be given as a bolus or as continuous infusion with the goal of maintaining urine pH of 6 to 7.
      c. **Diuretics**. Although forced diuresis can be useful in maintaining urine flow, no prospective evidence proves that diuretics (e.g., mannitol or furosemide) are helpful in preventing renal failure in rhabdomyolysis. If diuretics are used, extreme care must be taken to avoid intravascular volume depletion, which has been shown conclusively to increase the incidence of renal failure in this syndrome.
      d. **Prognosis in renal failure**. If patients go on to develop renal failure and dialysis dependence, the prognosis is generally good, with most patients regaining baseline renal function in 3 to 4 weeks.
   2. **Correction of electrolyte abnormalities**
      a. **Hyperkalemia** is the most dangerous electrolyte abnormality seen with this disease and must be treated aggressively. Sodium bicarbonate and insulin administered with dextrose help drive potassium into the intracellular compartment. Calcium stabilizes the myocardium, making the heart more resistant to arrhythmia; use potassium binders following these therapies. Emergency dialysis may be necessary for refractory hyperkalemia.
      b. **Hypocalcemia**. Although commonly seen in rhabdomyolysis, hypocalcemia is rarely associated with adverse clinical events and generally requires no specific therapy.
      c. **Hyperphosphatemia** can become a problem in acute renal failure associated with rhabdomyolysis. Hyperphosphatemia responds to phosphate binding antacid administration.

Axioms
- Loss of function can be the earliest sign in the development of compartment syndrome.
- Loss of pulse is a late finding in the time course of compartment syndrome.
- Whenever doubt exists whether compartment syndrome is present, perform fasciotomy.
- Serum creatine phosphokinase is the most sensitive marker for muscle injury.
- Prevention of renal failure in association with rhabdomyolysis is critical.

36. PERIPHERAL VASCULAR INJURIES

Louis H. Alarcon and Ricard N. Townsend

I. **Introduction**. Prompt diagnosis of peripheral vascular injury requiring operation is crucial to optimal outcome. Delay in recognition and treatment are the leading causes of preventable limb loss. Vascular injuries result primarily from penetrating trauma, with injuries to the brachial vessels of the upper extremity and superficial femoral vessels of the lower extremity being the most common requiring surgical repair in civilian trauma practice. Mandatory operative exploration is no longer the routine for all potential vascular injuries. Selective evaluation using noninvasive vascular testing and angiography has become well established. To prevent limb loss, early diagnosis and treatment is mandatory (Table 36.1). Unnecessary arteriography is a leading cause of treatment delay.

II. **Etiology**

    A. Penetrating vascular trauma can be caused by stab wounds, low-velocity gunshots (including long-range shotgun wounds), or high-velocity gunshots by hunting weapons or close-range shotgun wounds (destructive wounds). The mechanism is critical to determine the risk of vascular injury from the knife, projectile, or blast effect.

    B. Blunt trauma is a less common cause of vascular injury but results in a higher amputation rate because of delay in diagnosis and therapy. Blunt vascular trauma is commonly associated with orthopedic injures (Table 36.2).

III. **Arterial injuries**

    A. Diagnosis. All injured extremities must be carefully evaluated. Delays in diagnosis or therapy can be prevented through careful history and physical examination and appropriate use of noninvasive vascular testing and angiography. A diagnostic algorithm for vascular trauma should be used (Fig. 36.1).

        1. History. Details of the event, mechanism of injury, type of projectile, prehospital estimation of blood loss, and the vital signs during prehospital care are important clues to identify major vascular injury. A history of pulsatile blood loss before treatment is important diagnostic information. As always, stabilization of the patient with a primary survey takes priority.

        2. Physical examination. Three important elements of the physical assessment are detailed vascular, neurologic, and soft-tissue or skeletal examinations. These elements will determine the potential for vascular injury and the risk for limb loss.

        a. Vascular examination

            (1) Palpate all pulses proximal and distal to the potential area of injury; record them in detail. Compare injured with uninjured extremity. Note any differences in pulses.

            (2) Record the color, capillary refill, skin temperature, and the neurologic examination (motor and sensory) of the affected extremity.

            (3) Hard or soft signs of arterial injury. The relative possibility of a vascular injury based on history and physical examination are summarized in these according to hard or soft signs (Table 36.3). Most patients with "hard" signs require vascular repairs.

                (a) Hard signs of arterial injury. Any hard sign findings mandate immediate surgical exploration, as virtually all will have injuries requiring operative repair. In general,

Table 36.1. Factors associated with higher rates of limb loss in vascular trauma

Treatment delay >6 hours
Blunt mechanism of injury
Lower extremity injuries, especially of the popliteal artery
Associated injuries: nerve, vein, bone, soft tissue loss
High velocity gunshot wounds and close range shotgun wounds
Preexisting atherosclerotic disease
Failure or delay in performing fasciotomy

sending these patients to the radiology department for formal arteriography should be avoided.

(b) **Soft signs of arterial injury.** These patients can be evaluated with serial physical examination, noninvasive vascular studies, or angiography; management of this group of patients is controversial.

b. Perform and carefully record the details of the motor and sensory examination of the affected extremity and compare it with the uninjured extremity.

c. Describe the associated soft-tissue injury and skeletal injury. Complete exposure of the patient and meticulous search for all bullet holes is critical. The presence of an odd number of sites of penetration implies that at least one projectile remains in the patient.

3. **Noninvasive tests.** These adjuncts can be useful in the patient with soft signs of arterial injury, but are inappropriate in the evaluation of patients with hard signs of arterial injury.

a. Systolic blood pressure using Doppler (ankle-brachial index). Use a portable, handheld Doppler probe to identify the arterial signal proximal and distal to injury.

(1) Record the phase and, if appropriate, systolic pressure (use appropriate size cuff).

(2) Compare ABI (ankle brachial index) of injured versus uninjured extremity (injured or uninjured) or with another uninjured extremity.

(3) If ABI is <0.90, a vascular injury that requires surgical repair is likely.

b. Duplex imaging

(1) With skilled technical hands, duplex imaging is a useful tool.

c. Transcutaneous oxygen measurement can be a useful adjunct to the physical examination and also to monitor the vascular supply to the injured extremity.

d. Plain radiography is useful in detecting fractures and location of retained projectiles.

Table 36.2. Vascular injuries associated with specific orthopedic injuries

Orthopedic injury	Associated vascular injury
Knee dislocation	Popliteal artery
Femur fracture	Superficial femoral artery
Supracondylar humerus fracture	Brachial artery
Clavicular fracture	Subclavian artery
Shoulder dislocation	Axillary artery

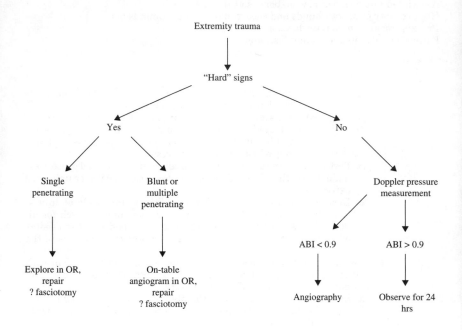

ABI = ankle/brachial index

FIG. 36.1. Algorithm for peripheral vascular trauma.

Table 36.3. Signs of arterial injury

Hard signs	Soft signs
Absent or diminished distal pulses	Proximity of wound or blunt injury to artery
Pulsatile bleeding	Small, nonpulsatile hematoma
Expanding or pulsatile hematoma	Extremity neurologic deficit
Palpable thrill or bruit	Prehospital history of arterial bleeding
Signs of distal ischemia: pain, pallor, paresthesias, paralysis, coolness.	

Peripheral Vascular Injuries 343

4. **Arteriography** is the most accurate test in establishing the presence of vascular injury. Suspicion of an arterial injury based on proximity of a wound is not an indication for angiography unless a shotgun has caused the wound. Angiography can exclude vascular trauma and help plan operation if vascular injury exists. Angiogram in the presence of hard signs of vascular injury is unnecessary unless the site of injury cannot be determined on physical examination (more likely in blunt arterial injury). Unstable patients should not be sent to the radiology department. An alternative to the formal angiogram is the on-table or emergency center angiogram. The technique for this procedure is as follows:

   a. Use a short 16- to 20-g catheter in the proximal vessel.

   b. Just before and during hand injection of full-strength contrast, manually compress inflow.

   c. Image during injection.

   d. Inject 20 to 30 mL of full-strength contrast.

B. **Blunt vascular injury**

1. History. Examine the extremity, documenting change in examination over time. Obtain a full history from the prehospital providers (e.g., Did they reduce a joint dislocation in the field?).

2. Delay in the diagnosis and treatment of blunt vascular injury can result in ischemia, compartment syndrome, and limb loss.

3. Angulated fractures and joint dislocations can cause temporary vascular compromise. Perform careful vascular examination before and after manipulation, splinting, or relocation of joints.

4. Persistent pulse deficit mandates immediate vascular evaluation, either noninvasively or angiographically.

5. Dressings, wraps, or splints can restrict venous or arterial flow. Swelling and edema can increase over time, leading to constriction by dressings.

C. **Operative management**. Arterial injuries should be repaired immediately, unless more life-threatening injuries have priority. Restore flow to an extremity within 6 hours to maximize limb salvage.

1. No attempts should be made to blindly clamp bleeding vessels before obtaining adequate surgical exposure in the operating room (OR). Use direct pressure to arrest hemorrhage en route to surgery. In general, tourniquets should be avoided. However, a blood pressure cuff placed proximal to the injury may control hemorrhage during stabilization and transport to the OR. Inflate the blood pressure cuff just above systolic blood pressure.

2. Give perioperative antibiotics to cover gram-positive organisms.

3. Prepare and drape the uninjured extremity to harvest a vein conduit.

4. In general, fix vascular injuries before associated injuries in the extremity. Restoration of blood flow takes priority. In combined orthopedic and vascular injury, the use of temporary shunts allows skeletal stabilization before definitive arterial repair.

5. Gain proximal and distal vascular control before entering hematoma or removing foreign bodies (e.g., knife) that may be tamponading the injured vessel.

6. Systemic heparin can be given, especially in case of isolated injury. This may not be appropriate with massive blood loss, extensive soft-tissue injury, or multiple injuries. Local heparin can be flushed proximally and distally in the injured vessel in these settings.

7. Debride injured vessel to remove areas of contused arterial wall or intimal flap.

8. Perform proximal and distal balloon catheter thrombectomy before completing repair.

9. Primary repair is the preferred method for arterial repair. However, because of loss of the injured arterial segment from injury or appropriate debridement, primary repair without undue tension is infrequently

possible. Therefore, a reversed interposition saphenous vein graft harvested from the **opposite** extremity is generally necessary. Other conduit options include basilic or cephalic vein and polytetrafluoroethylene (PTFE) (avoid in heavily contaminated areas). Repair arterial injuries distal to the knee or elbow with interrupted sutures, at least on the anterior wall of the vessel.

10. Perform completion arteriography via cannulation with a small catheter proximal to the repair, proximal occlusion during the injection of full strength contrast, and obtain the film during active injection. Image intensification provides superior images.

11. Consider fasciotomy if ischemic time approximates 4 to 6 hours or a simultaneous venous injury in the extremity. **Prophylactic rather than therapeutic fasciotomy offers the best opportunity for limb salvage and preservation of limb function.**

12. Close postoperative monitoring for the development of thrombosis or compartment syndrome.

D. **Outcomes and complications**

1. Long-term outcome for successful arterial repair is good (>95% salvage rates). Limb loss increases with delay in diagnosis and in restoration of flow (>6 hours), high-velocity or destructive gunshot wounds, preexisting peripheral vascular disease, injury to smaller (more distal) vessels, and in patients who suffer multiple injuries or are hemodynamically unstable.

2. Orthopedic injuries with vascular injuries have higher rates of infection, and amputation (70%) in some series (e.g., open tibia or fibula fractures with trifurcation injury are associated with high incidence of limb loss).

3. **Management of arteriographically "minimal" injury.** Selected injuries to arteries in the extremities without hard signs of vessel injury have been increasingly managed nonoperatively. These minimal injuries include minimal vessel irregularities, small intimal flaps, small pseudoaneurysms, and small, arteriovenous fistulae.

4. Most **preventable** complications relate to prolonged ischemic times or failure to perform fasciotomy. Complications include:

   a. **Early**: thrombosis, most often related to technical problems; bleeding; compartment syndrome; infection; limb loss; rhabdomyolysis, associated with renal failure, disseminated intravascular coagulation (DIC), myocardiopathy; death; venous thromboembolism, related to immobility or venous injury.

   b. **Late**: pseudoaneurysm, arteriovenous fistula, infection, and occlusion.

IV. **Venous injuries**. In general, venous injuries are recognized at the time of exploration for arterial injury. Management of venous injury is controversial: repair or ligate. Some benefit is found in repair of venous injury, especially if the popliteal vein is injured. Consider repair rather than ligation of the venous injury if evidence of venous hypertension is seen on completion of the arterial repair.

A. **Diagnosis**

1. Clinical signs of venous injury include hemorrhage, venous engorgement, and swelling of the extremity.

B. **Treatment**

1. Venous injury without active bleeding or hematoma does not require operation. Venous injury found at the time exploration can be repaired by lateral venorrhaphy if no pressing associated injuries exist; on occasion, interposition graft is necessary for venous injury. Lateral venorrhaphy is preferred, if possible, although long-term patency results are lower than arterial repair. Nonetheless, short-term patency reduces the postoperative complications of swelling and edema. In the extremities, ligation remains acceptable treatment of venous injury. If

ligation is needed, fasciotomy or leg elevation and compression stockings should be used.

V. Controversial areas

A. Immediate amputation—the mangled extremity (see Chapter 32). Indications for immediate amputation without attempting arterial repair include the following:

1. Nerve destruction, resulting in an insensate and paralyzed extremity, confirmed by direct examination at exploration to exclude simple nerve contusion.
2. Extensive bone and soft tissue loss
3. Arterial injury in a patient with more immediately life-threatening injury

B. Use of temporary conduits as a "damage control" bridge (i.e., shunts) and external fixation of skeletal injuries may allow rapid restoration of distal blood flow and provide the option to take the multiply injured patient to the intensive care unit (ICU) for further hemodynamic stabilization.

C. Whereas the conduit of choice for vascular repair is the autogenous saphenous vein, associated injuries can preclude its use. Vein grafts have the highest long-term patency rates and lowest infection risk. PTFE may be necessary in contaminated fields; consider extraanatomic bypass in this situation.

D. Damage control for vascular injury should be considered in all patients with multisystem trauma. The use of temporary shunts and synthetic materials for grafting has become accepted in patients with complex injuries. Although the risks of infection are significant, the long-term results are better in all patients who have rapid restoration of arterial blood supply.

E. Optimal sequence of repair: artery → vein → bone. Reestablishment of distal perfusion takes precedence in most cases. In the patient with combined bony and vascular injuries, good judgment is essential. At times, an arterial shunt is needed to temporarily restore flow, while the fracture is realigned. The trauma or vascular surgeon should be present during the orthopedic procedure to assist in the manipulation of the repaired vessels.

VI. Management of specific arterial injuries

A. Axillary artery

1. A continuation of the subclavian artery starts at the lateral border of the first rib and ends at the inferior border of the teres major muscle. The axillary artery has three parts from which six branches originate (Fig. 36.2). Axillary vein and brachial plexus run with the axillary artery.
2. Of arterial trauma, 3% to 9% are usually penetrating trauma; 50% are with associated nerve injury and 40% with venous injury.
3. Entire arm, neck, and chest should be included in the operative field. Expose the axillary artery via an S-shaped incision, starting at the middle of the clavicle, following the deltopectoral groove and continuing to the groove between biceps and triceps muscles. Perform primary repair or resection with primary anastomosis, if possible. Do not sacrifice collaterals to complete primary repair; place an interposition graft in this setting.

B. Brachial artery

1. Begins at the border of the teres major muscle and ends 1 cm below the antecubital fossa. Major branches are the profunda brachii, ulnar, and radial arteries (Fig. 36.3). Degree of ischemia depends on whether injury is proximal or distal to the profundus brachii; ischemia and ultimate amputation rate is higher for proximal injury. Median nerve courses with the brachial artery; radial and ulnar nerves are also in proximity.
2. Injuries are caused by penetrating trauma, including iatrogenic; comprises 20% of civilian vascular injury. Supracondylar humerus fracture can result in Volkmann's ischemic contracture.
3. Operative approach is along the groove between the triceps and biceps muscles, via an S-shaped extension, if the incision crosses the antecubital fossa. End-to-end repair is generally possible; may require a saphenous vein interposition graft.

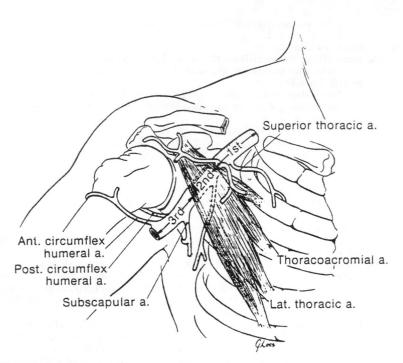

Superior thoracic a.

Ant. circumflex
humeral a.
Post. circumflex
humeral a.

Thoracoacromial a.

Subscapular a.

Lat. thoracic a.

FIG. 36.2. Anatomy of axillary artery. (From Rich NM, Spencer FC. *Vascular trauma.* Philadelphia: WB Saunders, 1978:331, with permission.)

C. Forearm vascular injury
   1. One inch below the antecubital fossa, the brachial artery divides into radial and ulnar arteries (85% of hands have a dominant ulnar artery); 10% of patients have incomplete palmar arch; 60% have concomitant nerve injury.
   2. Operative repair is through a longitudinal incision overlying the artery. If only the radial or ulnar artery is injured and distal neurologic function is intact, perform ligation. Even with early successful repair, long-term patency of a repaired single vessel is only 50%.
D. Common, profunda, and superficial femoral arteries (Fig. 36.4)
   1. Commonly injured in civilians, comprise 20% of vascular injuries. Mechanism is usually penetrating, can be iatrogenic.
   2. Operative approach involves preparing the abdomen, entire injured leg, and proximal contralateral leg in case saphenous vein is needed. Proximal control may require splitting the inguinal ligament or retroperitoneal control of the external iliac artery. Make a longitudinal incision over the course of the femoral vessels. Approach to the superficial femoral artery involves a longitudinal incision along the anterior border of the sartorius muscle. Repair all arterial injuries except for distal injuries to the profunda femoral artery.
E. Popliteal artery
   1. Begins at the hiatus of the adductor magnus muscle, as a continuation of the superficial femoral artery. Proximally, the popliteal artery runs behind the femur and distally behind the capsule of the knee joint (Fig. 36.5). The popliteal vein courses from lateral to medial side

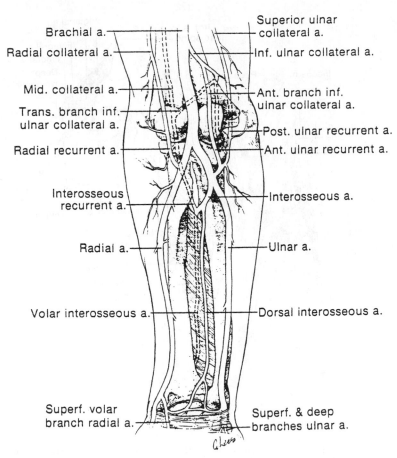

FIG. 36.3. Anatomy of brachial artery. (From Rich NM, Spencer FC. *Vascular trauma.* Philadelphia: WB Saunders, 1978:331, with permission.)

of the artery in its midportion. Both artery and vein are commonly injured.

2. Comprises 5% to 10% of civilian vascular trauma 25% to 50% caused by blunt mechanism of injury. Amputation rates up to 25% for blunt injury, 4% of gunshot wounds result in amputation. With blunt injury, the magnitude of the bony and soft tissue injuries often dictates ultimate amputation.

3. Operative approach is generally via medial exposure (Fig. 36.6). The contralateral leg must be prepared so that saphenous vein can be harvested. Preserve the ipsilateral saphenous vein during the operation; this may be the only venous drainage from the injured extremity. The medial head of gastrocnemius muscle can be detached to provide adequate distal exposure. Fix venous injuries if at all possible. Plan to perform fasciotomies; more than 60% of patients will require fasciotomy. Perform completion arteriography.

F. Anterior tibial, posterior tibial, and peroneal arteries

1. Anterior tibial artery is generally the first branch; tibioperoneal trunk bifurcates into the peroneal artery and posterior tibial artery.

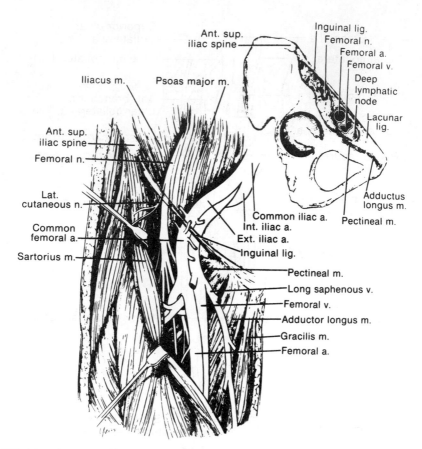

FIG. 36.4. Anatomy of femoral artery. (From Rich NM, Spencer FC. *Vascular trauma.* Philadelphia: WB Saunders, 1978:331, with permission.)

2. Mechanism of injury is two-thirds penetrating, one-third blunt. Amputation rate >50% with injury to the tibioperoneal trunk or all three vessels. A single vessel injury does not require repair. An ischemic limb, injury to the tibioperoneal trunk, or injury to multiple vessels requires restoration of flow through at least one trifurcation vessel.

Axioms
- Physical examination is the cornerstone for the diagnosis of vascular injury.
- Hard signs of arterial injury mandate immediate operation; formal arteriography in the radiology department is dangerous and unnecessary in this setting.
- "Proximity" alone is not an indication for arteriography.
- Harvest saphenous vein from the contralateral uninjured extremity.
- Most preventable amputations are associated with delayed or inadequate fasciotomy.
- Optimal sequence of repair with combined bony and vascular injury is artery, vein, bone. In most cases, reestablishment of flow takes precedence.

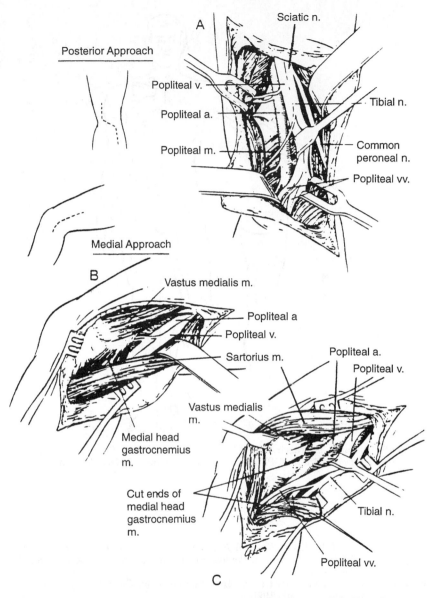

FIG. 36.5. Anatomy of popliteal artery. (From Rich NM, Spencer FC. *Vascular trauma*. Philadelphia: WB Saunders, 1978:331, with permission.)

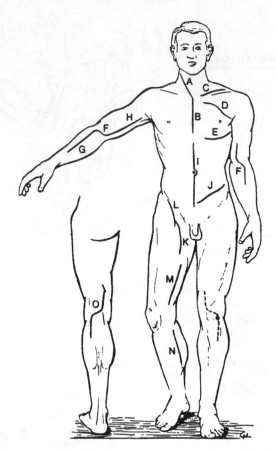

FIG. 36.6. Operative approach to peripheral vascular trauma. (From Rich NM, Spencer FC. *Vascular trauma*. Philadelphia: WB Saunders, 1978:331, with permission.)

Bibliography

Arrillaga A, Nagy K, Frykberg ER, et al. *Practice management guidelines for the management of penetrating trauma to the lower extremity*. Eastern Association for the Surgery of Trauma, 1999.

Aucar JA, Mattox KL. Vascular trauma. In: Cameron JL, ed. *Current surgical therapy*. St. Louis: Mosby-Year Book, 1998.

Frykberg ER. Advances in the diagnosis and treatment of extremity vascular trauma. *Surg Clin North Am* 1995;75(2):207–224.

Frykberg ER, Dennis JW, Bishop K, et al. The reliability of physical examination in the evaluation of penetrating extremity trauma for vascular injury: results at one year. *J Trauma* 1991;31(4):502–511.

Gillespie DL, Woodson J, Kaufman J, et al. Role of arteriography for blunt or penetrating injuries in proximity to major vascular structures: an evolution in management. *Ann Vasc Surg* 1993;7(2):145–149.

McCready RA. Upper-extremity vascular injuries. *Surg Clin North Am* 1988;68(4): 725–740.

Perry MO. Vascular trauma. *Adv Surg* 1995;28:59–70.

Rich NM. Management of venous trauma. *Surg Clin North Am* 1988;58(4):809–821.

Rutherford RB. Diagnostic evaluation of extremity vascular injuries. *Surg Clin North Am* 1988;68(4):683–691.

Schilling J. Extremity vascular trauma. In: Lopez-Viego MA, ed. *The Parkland trauma handbook*. St. Louis: Mosby-Yearbook, 1994.

Thal ER, Snyder WH, Perry MO. Vascular injuries of the extremities. In: Rutherford RB, ed. *Vascular surgery*. Philadelphia: WB Saunders, 1995.

37. SOFT-TISSUE TRAUMA

Kimberly A. Davis

I. **Mechanism of injury**
  A. **Blunt**
    1. **Shear**. This is the most common mechanism of injury, resulting in laceration of tissues.
    2. **Crush**. An injury as a result of compressive forces, creates wounds that are often stellate. Because of their devitalized nature, crush wounds are at high risk for complications and should be **debrided**.
  B. **Penetrating**
    1. Knife stab wounds: low velocity, minimal tissue damage.
    2. Gunshot wounds
      a. **Low** velocity: induced by all handguns (except .44 magnum). Damage to surrounding tissues ("cavitation") causes wound morbidity.
      b. **High** velocity: caused by velocities >2,500 feet/second, associated with military weapons and some hunting rifles. Large amount of associated soft tissue injury often requires massive debridement in the operating room (OR). These are rarely closed primarily.
    3. Shotgun wounds
      a. **Close** range: considered a high-velocity wound, with associated devitalization of tissue. These are contaminated wounds because of retained wadding and clothing, and must be debrided aggressively.
      b. **Far** range: multiple, small low-velocity wounds that often do not require intervention.
II. **Initial management**
  A. **Assessment of tissue viability**
    1. **General**. Assessment of wound viability is difficult early after trauma and requires repeated examination.
    2. **Skin**. Assess by color, capillary refill, presence of dermal bleeding, and sensory examination.
    3. **Subcutaneous tissues**. Fat is difficult to assess, but can readily be debrided, as long as care is taken not to devascularize the overlying skin.
    4. **Muscle**. The most difficult tissue to assess; examine muscle for color, bleeding, and contractile response.
    5. **Nerve**. Visual inspection and electrical stimulation are the best methods to assess nerve viability. If primary repair is not indicated (e.g., contaminated wound or other more important issues), tag nerves for later identification.
  B. **Threats to wound healing**
    1. **Ischemia and necrosis**. Wound hypoxia results in decreased collagen deposition and impairs the functioning of immunocompetent cells.
    2. **Hemorrhage**. Inadequate hemostasis can create a wound hematoma; this reduces the quantity of bacterial contamination necessary to produce infection. If adequate hemostasis is not possible because of coagulopathy, delay the wound closure.
    3. **Bacterial contamination**. Sources of contamination include both the patient's normal bacterial flora and external contamination at the time of the trauma.
    4. **Foreign material contamination**. A foreign body in the wound impairs phagocytosis and reduces the inoculum necessary to cause infection. In addition to "hand debridement" of materials, it is important to irrigate wounds with large-volume, pressurized (5–8 lb/in^2, produced by using ≤19-g needle tip) and pulsatile lavage for heavily contaminated wounds to prevent wound infection.

    5. Systemic factors. Shock, malnutrition, and preexisting immuno-compromise can impair wound healing and foster infection.

  C. Tetanus prophylaxis. Assess the need for and type (active and passive versus active alone) of tetanus prophylaxis for all wounds (see Appendix B).

  D. Decision-making. Factors influencing the decision regarding management of a wound in the emergency department or the OR include the size of the wound, the degree of contamination, the presence of devitalized tissue, the anatomic location of the wound, and the presence of associated injuries.

III. Treatment

  A. Anesthesia

    1. Local. Lidocaine with epinephrine (0.5% to 1.0%) can be administered to a maximal dose of 7 mg/kg of body weight. Avoid epinephrine in wounds of the nose and digits, tissues with poor perfusion or recently grafted, and in extremity wounds of those patients with peripheral vascular disease. The maximal dose of lidocaine without epinephrine is 4 mg/kg body weight. The addition of bicarbonate (1 mL from standard resuscitation ampule added to 10 mL anesthetic), warming to body temperature, and slow proximal to distal injections can minimize the pain of injection. Bupivacaine (0.25%, with or without epinephrine) is an alternative to lidocaine; it lasts longer, has a similar onset of action for infiltration or small nerve block, and causes less irritation.

    2. Regional. This is an extremely useful and underutilized technique for wounds of the distal extremities and the face.

    3. Systemic analgesics. These (especially opioids) can be powerful adjuncts or alternatives in complex cases (see Chapter 41).

  B. Antibiotic prophylaxis. Prophylactic antibiotics are not indicated in simple wounds (uncontaminated, noncrush, minimally devitalized, and of low depth) in a healthy patient because the underlying risk of infection is small. Additionally, antibiotics are not a substitute for adequate debridement and local wound care. However, most surgeons recommend the use of preventive antibiotics in the following situations:

    1. Open fractures and joint spaces

    2. Wounds with heavy contamination or requiring extensive debridement

    3. Patients with immunocompromise, peripheral vascular disease, or cardiac valvular disease.

  C. Debridement

    1. Sharp debridement remains the *sine qua non*, allowing the removal of dead skin, muscle, and fat.

    2. Mechanical (pulsatile lavage). High-pressure irrigation (minimum 5–8 lb/in^2—using a ≤19-g needle or irrigation exit port) is the best method of clearing debris and bacteria, especially in wounds containing specialized tissues (nerves, tendons and vessels) not amenable to sharp debridement.

  D. Closure

    1. Primary closure is appropriate for class I (simple, no contamination or devitalized tissue) and class II (minimal contamination or devitalized tissue) wounds, as long as the wound is closed within the first 8 hours of injury.

    2. Secondary closure (also known as secondary intention) allows the wound to heal by granulation and subsequent contraction.

    3. Delayed primary closure (also known as tertiary closure) is used for class III (contaminated) and class IV (infected) wounds. Wound edges are left open for up to 5 days, and packed with damp to dry sterile saline dressings. Thereafter, the wound is reapproximated with suture, staples, or sterile tapes.

    4. Skin grafting, either split thickness or full thickness, can be used for the closure of traumatic wounds with tissue defects. In general, full-thickness grafts are used for the face and hands, with split-thickness grafts used elsewhere.

      5. Tissue transfer involves the use of either myocutaneous rotational flaps (for truncal wounds) or free flaps, used predominantly in the reconstruction of lower extremity defects.

E. Suture removal
1. Face: 3 to 5 days
2. Abdominal wall: 7 to 10 days
3. Scalp: 10 days
4. Wounds crossing joints: 2 weeks
5. Vertical torso wounds: 2 weeks

F. Difficult wounds
1. **Scalp**. The scalp can bleed extensively, and require urgent hemostasis, using either Raney clips or temporary closure with heavy nylon sutures, incorporating the galea aponeurotica. Formal closure depends on the extent of the injury, but should always involve a layered closure, with careful approximation of the galea aponeurotica. For large lacerations, it is occasionally beneficial to place a closed suction drain for 24 hours. Shaving or clipping hair around the wound edges is helpful to avoid entangling hair and suture lines.
2. **Face**. Repair can be delayed for up to 24 hours while the patient is stabilized. A good examination is necessary to identify facial fractures and intraoral lacerations. It is important to carefully reapproximate the vermillion border of the lip. Plastic surgical consultation for extensive lacerations may be warranted. Finally, treat exposed cartilage with prophylactic antibiotics.
3. **Perineal degloving injuries** are complex injuries associated with mortality rates approaching 30%, usually caused either by hemorrhage or pelvic sepsis. Early sigmoidoscopy, complete fecal diversion with distal rectal washout, early aggressive debridement, and subsequent daily debridement with pulsatile lavage for at least 5 days postinjury has markedly reduced the incidence of late pelvic sepsis. Allow the wounds to heal by secondary intention, with delayed split-thickness skin grafting or closure with myocutaneous flaps.
4. **Closed internal degloving injuries** are most commonly associated with pelvic and acetabular fractures (Morel-Lavallee lesions) in which the subcutaneous tissues tear away from the underlying fascia, resulting in a cavity filled with hematoma and liquefied fat. It occurs most commonly over the greater trochanter, but can also occur in the flank and lumbodorsal regions. These wounds require aggressive debridement either before or at the time of fracture fixation. Leave these wounds open, followed by repeated debridement, as needed, with delayed closure (using either split-thickness skin grafts or myocutaneous flaps) ultimately.

IV. Bites and stings
A. **Human bite** wounds are considered contaminated and devitalized, and at high risk for subsequent soft-tissue infection. Common infecting organisms include *Streptococcus viridans, Staphylococcus* spp., *Eikenella corrodens, Bacteroides* spp., and microaerophilic *Streptococcus* spp. Treat these by using aggressive irrigation, systemic antibiotics (recommended is ampicillin combined with a β-lactamase inhibitor) and elevation. Aside from face or other cosmetically sensitive wounds, leave all others open.
B. **Cat bite and scratch** wounds also tend to be heavily contaminated, with scratches that penetrate the skin assuming the same high risk as a bite. Common infecting organisms include *Pasteurella multocida* and *Staphylococcus* spp. Again, principles are the same as those noted for humans—use of empiric ampicillin plus a β-lactamase inhibitor antibiotic. Assess the need for rabies and tetanus immunization in all of these wounds.
C. **Dog bites**. Because of the enormous force generated by the muscles of mastication, these wounds are often associated with massive soft-tissue injury. Infection is not as common as in human and cat bites but still seen more often than in simple nonmammalian-associated wounds. Again, the princi-

ples of wound care are the same as noted for humans and cats—copious, high-pressure irrigation, and debridement, leaving open, if possible. Antibiotic choices are same as with cats, although *Pasteurella* is less commonly cultured from infected wounds. Also, assess rabies and tetanus prophylaxis needs for all these wounds.

D. Snake bites. Initial field therapy should involve immobilization, neutral positioning, and a lightly compressive dressing. The use of local suctioning and tourniquets are controversial and not currently recommended. Severe envenomations (severe or progressive extremity involvement, coagulopathy, or systemic signs) can be treated with antivenin. Supportive treatment with intensive care unit (ICU) monitoring and replacement of blood factors are the mainstays of therapy in extreme cases.

E. Spider bites. Two common species of spiders are dangerous to humans in the continental United States, the brown recluse and the black widow. The brown recluse (*Loxosceles reclusa*) is most common, and has a violin-shaped carapace on its body. Bites are painless initially, and then can result in a hemorrhagic blister with progression to a necrotic area. Treatment is supportive—early debridement of clearly dead tissue is helpful. Other therapies, including early aggressive debridement, and dapsone or hyperbaric oxygen use are all of unproved value and some risk. The black widow (*Lactrodectus macrotans*) has a red hourglass on the ventral surface of the abdomen. Bites are characterized by a toxic systemic reaction, including pain, muscle rigidity, altered mental status, and seizures. Treatment is supportive, although an equine antivenin is available for severe cases.

Bibliography

Hak DJ, Olson SA, Matta JM. Diagnosis and management of closed internal degloving injuries associated with pelvic and acetabular fractures: the Morel-Lavallee lesion. *J Trauma* 1997;42(6):1046–1051.

Hobbs GD, Anderson AR, Greene TJ, et al. Comparison of hyperbaric oxygen and dapsone therapy for Loxosceles envenomation. *Acad Emerg Med* 1996;3:758–761.

Kudsk KA, McQueen MA, Voeller GR, et al. Management of complex perineal soft-tissue injuries. *J Trauma* 1990;30(9):1155–1160.

Stewart RM, Page CP. Wounds, bites and stings. In: Feliciano DV, Moore EE, Mattox KL, eds. *Trauma*, 3rd ed. Stamford: Appleton & Lange, 1996:917–936.

Sullivan JB. The past, present and future of immunotherapy of snake venoms. *Ann Emerg Med* 1987;16(9):938–944.

38. PRIORITIES IN THE ICU CARE OF THE ADULT TRAUMA PATIENT

Keith D. Clancy and Joseph M. Darby

I. **Introduction**. Early in the care of the trauma patient in the intensive care unit (ICU) shock, respiratory failure, and intracranial hypertension are the main concerns, whereas infectious complications and multiple organ dysfunction syndrome (MODS) develop later.

A. **Trauma mortality in the ICU**. Most in-hospital trauma mortality occurs in the ICU during the first few days of admission because of closed head injury, respiratory failure, or refractory hemorrhagic shock; these deaths are largely not preventable. The remainder, many of which may be preventable, occur late, usually because of MODS. Technical, monitoring, and critical care management errors have been reported in up to half of preventable trauma deaths.

B. **Role and goals of trauma ICU care**. Trauma care in the ICU is best provided by a multidisciplinary team focused on resuscitation, monitoring, and life support. For patients admitted with lethal brain injury, the trauma ICU also plays a vital role in the support and maintenance of potential organ donors. **Fundamental goals of ICU management of the seriously injured trauma patient include early restoration and maintenance of tissue oxygenation, diagnosis and treatment of occult injuries, and prevention and treatment of infection and MODS**.

C. **ICU admissions**. The decision to admit the trauma patient to an ICU depends on the patient's age, injury severity, comorbid conditions, and availability of both ICU beds and intermediate level care beds (Table 38.1).

D. **Phases of ICU care**. Management of critically injured patients in the ICU can be divided into the following four phases:

1. **Resuscitative phase (the first 24 hours postinjury)**. Management focuses on fluid resuscitation; the goal is to maintain adequate tissue oxygenation. Concomitantly, seek occult life-threatening injuries.

2. **Early life support phase (24 to 72 hours postinjury)**. Treatment focuses principally on the management of posttraumatic respiratory failure and progressive intracranial hypertension in those patients with severe head injury. Diagnostic evaluation for occult injuries should be completed. Evidence of early MODS may become apparent during this phase.

3. **Prolonged life support (>72 hours postinjury)**. The duration of this phase depends on injury severity and associated complications. During this phase, many critically injured patients can be successfully weaned from life support. The more seriously injured patient enters a phase in which ongoing life support for organ system failure is needed. Infectious complications become predominant clinical concerns that can lead to the development of late MODS or death.

4. **Recovery phase (deintensification, separation from the ICU)**. During this phase of care, patients are transitioned from full ventilatory support to spontaneous breathing and invasive monitoring devices are removed. Patient and family are prepared for the transition to the general patient unit or intermediate care unit; plans for further convalescence and rehabilitation are developed.

II. **Multisystem organ dysfunction syndrome**. A clinical syndrome characterized by progressive dysfunction of multiple and interdependent organs, MODS is a continuum of progressive organ dysfunction rather than one of absolute failure; lungs, liver, and kidneys are the principal target organs. Failure of the cardiovascular and central nervous systems may also be prominent. In trauma patients, the principal inciting factors are hemorrhagic shock and infection. As

Table 38.1. Posttraumatic injuries or problems requiring initial ICU admission

Injuries
–Multisystem trauma
–Severe head injury (GCS ≤8)
–Cervical spinal cord injury
–Severe pulmonary contusion or flail chest
–Facial or neck trauma with threatened airway
–Postoperative, repair major vascular injuries
–Severe pelvic fracture with retroperitoneal hemorrhage
–Blunt cardiac trauma with ongoing dysrhythmia or hypotension
–Crush injuries
–Severe burns or smoke inhalation

Problems
–Respiratory failure requiring mechanical ventilation
–Ongoing shock or hemodynamic instability
–Massive blood or fluid resuscitation
–High base deficit
–Hypothermia
–Seizures
–Pregnancy

Posttraumatic injuries or problems suitable for intermediate care*
–Isolated liver or splenic injuries
–Uncomplicated blunt anterior chest trauma
–Isolated multiple rib fractures or pulmonary contusion with adequate oxygenation
–Isolated thoracic spinal cord injury
–Head injury (GCS 9–14)
–Minor injuries with high risk of alcohol withdrawal syndrome
–Isolated vascular injuries to the extremities

* Patients aged > 65 years, those with comorbidity or any hemodynamic instability should be considered for ICU admission.
ICU, intensive care unit; GCS, Glasgow Coma Scale score.

techniques for life support and resuscitation have improved, the incidence of MODS has increased (frequency of 8% to 25% of critically injured patients with overall mortality as high as 50% to 60%). MODS developing early (<3 days postinjury) is usually a consequence of shock or inadequate resuscitation, whereas late onset MODS is usually a result of severe infection.

A. Pathophysiology. MODS develops as a consequence of an uncontrolled systemic inflammatory response to inciting factors (e.g., severe injury, shock, or infection). Two basic models of MODS have emerged. In the "one-hit" model, a single insult (e.g., sepsis, shock) initiates a systemic inflammatory response syndrome (SIRS) that results in progressive MODS (see Chapter 4). In the "two-hit" model, sequential insults (e.g., a period of shock followed by a subsequent infection) can lead to MODS. In this model, the initial insult may prime the inflammatory response such that a second, even modest insult (e.g., infection) results in an exaggerated inflammatory response and subsequent organ dysfunction. Several hypotheses have been advanced to explain the development of organ dysfunction.

   1. **Macrophage or mediator hypothesis.** Activated macrophages release proinflammatory cytokines, resulting in the release of secondary mediators, which then activate neutrophils and vascular endothelial cells, promoting disturbances in the microcirculation leading to ischemia and tissue injury.

   2. **Microcirculatory hypothesis.** Organ damage occurs consequent to inadequate tissue oxygen delivery or ischemia-reperfusion with the

generation of oxygen-free radicals, or as a result of microcirculatory disturbances brought about by endothelial cell and leukocyte interactions.

3. **Gut hypothesis.** Increased intestinal permeability, impaired mucosal integrity, and reduced intestinal IgA production may promote systemic translocation of bacteria or endotoxin, resulting in SIRS or MODS.

B. **Identification of patients at risk for MODS.** Factors increasing the risk for MODS include persistent and refractory shock with lactic acidemia and elevated base deficit, high injury Severity Score (ISS), and the need for multiple blood transfusions. Advanced age can increase the risk of developing MODS because of comorbid disease.

C. **Clinical diagnostic criteria** for MODS are not yet standardized. A Multiple Organ Dysfunction score has recently been developed that uses the following variables to derive a composite score: PaO_2/FIO_2, platelet count, serum creatinine ($\mu mol/L$), serum bilirubin ($\mu mol/L$), Glasgow Coma Scale (GCS) score, and the pressure-adjusted heart rate (HR × [central venous pressure (CVP)/mean arterial pressure (MAP)]) (Table 38.2). In this model, the number of significant organ failure score, >3, is correlated with ICU mortality (Table 38.3). Before this model is widely applied, prospective validation is necessary.

D. **Prevention of MODS.** Other than treatment of infection and general ICU supportive care, specific therapy for established MODS is currently limited. Therefore, strategies to prevent MODS are paramount; they include appropriate fluid resuscitation that is effective in establishing and maintaining tissue oxygenation, debridement of devitalized tissue, early fracture fixation and stabilization, early enteral nutritional support, when possible, and prevention and treatment of nosocomial infections.

III. **Priorities in the resuscitation phase (first 24 hours postinjury)**

A. **Recognition and treatment of inadequate tissue oxygenation.** Deficient tissue oxygen delivery in the acutely traumatized patient is usually caused by impaired perfusion (hypovolemia, shock) or severe hypoxemia (respiratory failure).

Table 38.2. The multiple organ dysfunction score

Organ/System	Score				
	0	1	2	3	4
Respiratory* (PaO_2/FIO_2 ratio)	>300	226–300	151–225	76–150	≤75
Renal[†] (serum creatinine)	≤100	101–200	201–350	351–500	>500
Hepatic[‡] (serum bilirubin)	≤20	21–60	61–120	121–240	>240
Cardiovascular[§] (PAR)	≤10.0	10.1–15.0	15.1–20.0	20.1–30.0	>30.0
Hematologic[‖] (platelet count)	>230	81–120	51–80	21–50	≤20
Neurologic[¶] (Glasgow Coma Scale score)	15	13–14	10–12	7–9	≤6

* The PaO_2/FIO_2 ratio is calculated without reference to the use or mode of mechanical ventilation, and without reference to the use of positive end-expiratory pressure.
[†] Creatinine in $\mu mol/L$.
[‡] Bilirubin in $\mu mol/L$.
[§] Pressure-adjusted heart rate (PAR) is calculated as the product of the heart rate minute/(HR) multiplied by the ratio of right atrial pressure (RAP) to the mean arterial pressure (MAP):PAR = HR × RAP/MAP.
[‖] Platelet count in platelets/mL10^{-3}.
[¶] Glasgow Coma Scale (GCS) score as scored conservatively (for the patient receiving sedation or muscle relaxants, normal function is assumed, unless evidence if found of intrinsically altered mentation).
(Reprinted from Marshall JC, Cook DJ, Christou NV, et al. Multiple organ dysfunction score: a reliable descriptor of a complex clinical outcome. *Crit Care Med* 1995;23:1638–1652, with permission.)

Table 38.3. ICU mortality as a function of the number of failing organ systems as defined by an organ dysfunction score of ≥ 3

Number of failing systems	Number of patients	Deaths	Mortality (%)	Multiple organ dysfunction score (mean ± SD)
0	396	3	0.8	2.8 ± 1.8
1	177	12	6.8	6.4 ± 2.2
2	61	16	26.2	10.1 ± 2.2
3	33	16	48.5	13.4 ± 1.5
4	16	11	58.8	16.6 ± 2.1
5	6	5	83.3	19.2 ± 1.3
6	3	2	66.7	22.3 ± 1.7

ICU; intensive care unit; SD, standard deviation.
(Reprinted from Marshall JC, Cook DJ, Christou NV, et al. Mutliple organ dysfunction score: a reliable descriptor of a complex clinical outcome. *Crit Care Med* 1995;23:1638–1652, with permission.)

1. **Posttraumatic shock**. The following causes of shock are germane in the acute postinjury phase (see Chapter 5). **Hypovolemic shock** caused by incomplete resuscitation, ongoing third-space fluid losses, or active hemorrhage is the usual cause of hypotension or occult hypoperfusion in the trauma patient early after ICU admission. Volume replacement is the principal therapy, titrated to restore normal perfusion, with restoration of urine output and correction of base deficit and lactic acidosis as endpoints. When patients fail to respond to volume replacement, consider ongoing hemorrhage or other causes of shock.

   a. In the patient who is unresponsive to volume resuscitation, consider **ongoing blood loss** as the most likely cause or obstructive shock (cardiac tamponade, tension pneumothorax, or tension pneumopericardium) as a possible cause.

   b. Posttraumatic **cardiogenic shock** is usually caused by blunt myocardial injury or underlying cardiac disease. Right ventricular function can be impaired with blunt myocardial injury. Treatment is initiated with volume expansion, followed by inotropic support, if cardiac output is still inadequate. Valvular injury is uncommon in patients surviving severe chest trauma, but it may require immediate surgical repair. Myocardial ischemia and underlying valvular heart disease should be suspected in older trauma patients who appear to be in cardiogenic shock. Management may require inotropic support, ventricular unloading, or intraaortic balloon counterpulsation.

   c. **Neurogenic shock** can occur with high spinal cord injury or brain death.

   d. **Vasogenic shock** (distributive shock). Although septic shock is the prototypic form of vasogenic shock, it does not occur immediately after injury. Although not well described in the literature, severely injured trauma patients can demonstrate a hyperdynamic state early after injury, similar to SIRS, presumably caused by trauma-induced release of vasoactive mediators. These patients are characterized by a hyperdynamic circulation (high cardiac index), low blood pressure and, therefore, low calculated systemic vascular resistance. Hypotension may not completely respond to fluid resuscitation, and it may require vasopressor use for up to 24 hours before blood pressure stabilizes. Preliminary studies using vasopressin drip to decrease the amount of vasopressors have demonstrated some efficacy in the trauma population.

   e. **Clinical assessment**. Unless the patient is hypotensive, it is often difficult to recognize occult impairment in tissue perfusion. Lactic acidemia or persistent base deficit indicates ongoing tissue hypoperfusion. Additional monitoring is necessary to optimize oxygen delivery to the tissues when clinical uncertainty exists, or when refractory hemodynamic instability or other factors confound the clinical evaluation and response to therapy.

f. **Pulmonary artery catheterization.** Pulmonary artery (PA) catheterization allows determination of oxygen delivery and consumption (utilization). These data are used as diagnostic and therapeutic adjuncts in the critically injured patient with refractory shock, persistent lactic acidosis, suspected cardiac tamponade, complicated myocardial contusion, preexisting cardiopulmonary disease, high spinal cord injury, adult respiratory distress syndrome (ARDS), massive hemorrhage, or old age.

(1) Modified PA catheters are available to monitor mixed venous oxygen saturation continuously and measure right ventricular end-diastolic volume (RVEDV). These catheters can be useful in trauma patients with ARDS or high intraabdominal pressure. RVEDV can be a better reflection of preload than the wedge pressure under these circumstances.

(2) Hemodynamic endpoints associated with improved survival in trauma patients have been suggested: cardiac index >4.5 L/min/m^2, systemic oxygen delivery index (DO$_2$I) >600 mL/min/m^2, and oxygen consumption index (VO$_2$I) >160 to 170 mL/min/m^2. These hemodynamic parameters can be reasonable endpoints, with other evidence of hypoperfusion (e.g., persistent lactic acidosis). However, such goal-directed therapy is controversial.

(3) **The key principle is that blood pressure alone as an endpoint in fluid resuscitation is inadequate. Other indices of tissue perfusion must be monitored. Correction of base deficit or lactic acidosis and maintenance of adequate urine output can be monitored easily.**

g. **Gastric tonometry.** One of the pitfalls of using systemic oxygen delivery and consumption indices is that they are global measures and may not reflect the adequacy of tissue oxygenation in vital organ beds. Gastric tonometry, an estimate of gastric mucosal pH (pHi), is reflective of tissue oxygen delivery to the gastrointestinal tract. Preliminary data suggest that resuscitation guided to achieve and maintain pHi >7.3 within the first 24 hours is associated with reduced incidence of MODS. Further prospective studies using pHi as a resuscitative endpoint are necessary before normalization of pHi becomes a standard resuscitative endpoint.

2. **Posttraumatic respiratory failure.** The lung is the most common organ to fail in patients with severe injuries. Thus, respiratory failure or insufficiency is the most common indication for admission of the trauma patient to the ICU.

a. **Etiology.** The principal causes of acute respiratory failure in the early postinjury phase are detailed below.

(1) **Chest trauma.** Direct chest trauma, including multiple rib fractures, pulmonary contusion or laceration, and flail chest, frequently causes respiratory failure requiring ventilatory support. Multiple rib fractures alone identifies a population of trauma patients who frequently require ICU admission. Less commonly, injury to the tracheobronchial tree poses major difficulties in providing adequate gas exchange because of massive air leak. Signs suggesting a major tracheobronchial injury include subcutaneous emphysema, massive bronchial pleural fistula, pneumomediastinum, or hemoptysis. If tracheobronchial disruption is suspected, use bronchoscopy. Most tracheal ruptures occur at

or above the fourth tracheal ring. Most blunt major airway injuries occur within 2.5 cm of the carina. Chest tube drainage, ventilation with minimal airway pressures, and operative repair are needed for major tracheobronchial disruption. Independent lung ventilation using a double lumen tube may be necessary until the injury is repaired.

(2) **Fluid overload.** Massive fluid resuscitation often is accompanied by acute pulmonary edema. A positive fluid balance of >3 L during the first 24 hours may predict patients developing respiratory failure. In some patients, a positive fluid balance can be an unavoidable consequence of extensive resuscitation.

(3) **Shock.** Any form of shock can indirectly cause respiratory failure, as the work of breathing becomes excessive because of severe metabolic acidosis or inadequate oxygen delivery to the respiratory muscles.

(4) **Aspiration.** Maxillofacial injury, impaired consciousness, and endotracheal intubation are factors predisposing the patient to aspiration. Hypoxemia results both from airway obstruction or collapse with food or particulate aspiration and from diffuse lung injury with acid aspiration. Pulmonary infection is a late consequence of gastric aspiration. Antibiotics are best reserved for patients with clinical evidence of pneumonia.

(5) **Posttraumatic ARDS.** Extreme impairment in gas exchange is seen in ARDS.

   (a) **ARDS is characterized by:**
   - Severe hypoxemia ($PaO_2/FIO_2 \leq 150-200$)
   - Diffuse bilateral pulmonary infiltrates
   - Low or normal wedge pressure (or absence of heart failure)
   - Low lung compliance

   (b) **Risk factors for posttraumatic ARDS** include female sex, ISS >20, multiple transfusions, pulmonary contusion, and multiple fractures (multiple long bones or long bone and major pelvic fractures). Of those trauma patients with risk factors, approximately 25% will develop ARDS.

(6) **Spinal cord injury.** Isolated high thoracic or cervical spinal cord injury can lead to respiratory failure, as mechanical lung function is impaired consequent to the functional loss of innervation to respiratory muscles. Although overt respiratory failure may not be evident within the first 24 hours, these patients are at high risk for decompensation as a result of progression of the spinal injury (ascension) or the development of retained secretions and atelectasis.

(7) **Fat embolism syndrome.** Multiple long bone fractures or their stabilization and repair (using rod or nail) are associated with fat embolism. However, the clinical fat embolism syndrome (altered sensorium, petechiae, thrombocytopenia, pulmonary infiltrates) is uncommon. In the multiply injured patient, diagnosis is usually one of exclusion, with treatment being supportive. The clinical scenario is often suggestive of pulmonary embolism, which must be investigated. In fat embolism syndrome, fat generates an inflammatory response with end-organ responses seen remote from the initial injury: confusion (central nervous system), hypoxemia (pulmonary), and hematologic (thrombocytopenia).

(8) **Miscellaneous.** Intubation and mechanical ventilation are often necessary for patient recovery following long operative procedures or for the control of ventilation and oxygenation in the head-injured patient.

b. **Assessment and monitoring**. Respiratory failure is a clinical diagnosis based on the physical examination and arterial blood gases. Although arterial blood gases are helpful in establishing the diagnosis, clinical signs of respiratory failure (e.g., diaphoresis, tachypnea, use of accessory muscles of respiration, or paradoxic breathing) are more useful in deciding need for mechanical ventilatory support.

(1) **Respiratory monitoring**. All patients require continuous pulse oximetry, supplemented with arterial blood gases, in those circumstances where acid-base disorders are suspected or are being actively treated.

(a) **Capnography should be considered in those patients with severe head injury or intracranial hypertension to detect inadvertent hypoventilation**.

(b) Lung mechanics (negative inspiratory force [NIF], vital capacity [VC]) should be measured for the first few days after admission in patients with spinal cord injury to assess baseline respiratory muscle strength to determine if progressive weakness present might warrant continued ICU observation or institution of mechanical ventilatory support.

(c) In those patients with ARDS, PA catheterization with continuous mixed venous oximetry is useful as resuscitation and ventilatory support are being titrated.

(2) **Bronchoscopy**. Fiberoptic bronchoscopy is indicated in patients with massive air leaks, hemoptysis, refractory lobar atelectasis, or when foreign body aspiration is suspected.

(3) **Ventilatory support modes**. Ventilatory support is provided to patients with respiratory failure to reduce the mechanical work of breathing and to facilitate oxygenation and ventilation.

(a) **Volume-cycled ventilation**. Most trauma patients with respiratory failure can be managed by conventional volume-cycled ventilation using either **intermittent mandatory ventilation (IMV)** or **assist control (AC)** modes. IMV is a volume-controlled mode that allows for spontaneous breathing between ventilator cycled breaths. The AC mode is similar to IMV in providing volume-cycled breaths at the set rate, but it also delivers volume-cycled breaths for each additional breath above the set rate that is initiated by the patient. Although the IMV mode can be used for most patients requiring routine ventilatory support, the AC mode is an alternative for spontaneously breathing patients with high minute ventilation demands to minimize the work of breathing.

Initial ventilator settings should provide a tidal volume of 7 to 10 mL/kg at a base range of 10 to 12 breaths/minute. Recent literature suggests that lower tidal volumes (4–6 mL/kg) for patients with ARDS reduces barotrauma and volutrauma to the lung. FIO_2 should initially be set at 90% to 100% and titrated down to "nontoxic" oxygen concentrations (40% to 60%) using pulse oximetry. Positive end-expiratory pressure (PEEP) is usually applied starting at 5 cm H_2O and subsequently increased, if necessary, to reduce FIO_2 to "nontoxic" levels within the first 24 hours if hemodynamic stability permits. If increases in PEEP are associated with impairment in hemodynamic status, consider insertion of a pulmonary artery catheter to monitor cardiac function and titrate fluid therapy.

(b) **Inverse ratio ventilation (IRV)**. Barotrauma and inflammation consequent to high airway pressures or high tidal volumes can exacerbate acute lung injury and complicate therapy. For patients with severe impairment in oxygenation on conventional volume cycled ventilation, use a strategy that employs low tidal volumes (4–7 mL/kg) with a prolonged inspiratory phase (IRV). Use either conventional volume-cycled ventilation with low inspiratory gas flow rates (40–50 L/min) or pressure-controlled ventilation to minimize peak pressures (<40 cm H_2O) while increasing mean intrathoracic pressure to facilitate oxygenation.

If severe head injury is not present, minute ventilation can be adjusted to allow hypercapnia (**permissive hypercapnia**) when necessary to minimize the untoward hemodynamic effects of high mean intrathoracic pressures that result from this ventilator strategy. This also reduces need for high ventilatory frequencies, which can also cause hemodynamic instability and mechanical lung injury. Sodium bicarbonate may be necessary initially to control acidemia, if severe.

(c) **Pressure support ventilation (PSV)** is a mode of positive-pressure ventilation frequently used in combination with IMV to reduce the work of breathing associated with the endotracheal tube and ventilator circuit or as a method of weaning from mechanical ventilation. The ventilator is triggered by the patient's spontaneous breathing efforts, is limited by the set pressure above PEEP, and is cycled off when the inspiratory gas flow reaches a predetermined flow rate. Ordinarily, pressure support levels of 5 to 10 cm H_2O are satisfactory to eliminate the work of breathing associated with the ventilator circuit. PSV may also be advantageous in providing full ventilatory support to patients who have difficulty synchronizing with the ventilator or to those with bronchopleural fistulas to minimize airway pressures.

(d) **Noninvasive ventilatory support.** Selected patients (i.e., isolated pulmonary contusion or flail chest) with mild or moderate respiratory failure can occasionally be successfully managed without endotracheal intubation and standard mechanical ventilation. In such cases, **face mask continuous positive airway pressure (CPAP), nasal bilevel positive airway pressure (BiPaP), or pressure support ventilation** with a full face mask can be used to reduce the work of breathing and provide satisfactory oxygenation provided that aggressive pain control is used as an adjunct.

B. **Recognition and treatment of hypothermia.** Hypothermia should be anticipated in injured patients who have suffered exposure or shock or had massive fluid and blood resuscitation or prolonged operative courses (see Chapter 42). Patients having damage control operations, by definition, have problems with hypothermia and coagulopathy. These patients are admitted to the ICU from a truncated operative resuscitation for secondary resuscitation, normalization of body temperature, and correction of coagulopathy. Return to the OR for definitive repair of major intraabdominal injuries usually occurs at 24 to 48 hours. The critical temperature in injured trauma patients that profoundly influences mortality appears to be approximately 32°C.
  1. **Classification.** Hypothermia is classified as mild (32°C to 35°C), moderate (28°C to 32°C), or severe (<28°C).
  2. **Complications of hypothermia.** Major complications are coagulopathy, platelet dysfunction, impaired cardiac function, and dysrhythmias. Clotting factor function, which is temperature dependent, is reduced

under hypothermic conditions. Platelet function, which is also impaired under hypothermic conditions, prevents platelet plugging.

3. **Management** (see Chapter 42). Methods used for rewarming depend on severity of hypothermia, ongoing hemorrhage and coagulopathy, hemodynamic stability, and availability of equipment and technical support.
   a. **Warmed resuscitation fluids and blood products**
   b. **Passive rewarming**
   c. **Active external rewarming**
   d. **Active core rewarming**
      (1) **Airway warming**
      (2) **Peritoneal and pleural lavage**
      (3) **Continuous arteriovenous rewarming (CAVR)**
      (4) **Partial cardiopulmonary bypass**

C. **Correction of coagulopathy and thrombocytopenia.** Clotting factor deficiency and thrombocytopenia are commonly seen in trauma patients with hemorrhagic shock requiring massive transfusion. Contributing factors include ongoing hemorrhage, shock, acidosis, hypothermia, and intraoperative blood salvage techniques.
   1. **Microvascular bleeding** refers to bleeding in the setting of massive transfusion and shock (once surgical bleeding is controlled). Microvascular bleeding is nonsurgical bleeding that appears as petechia, enlarging ecchymoses or hematomas, and oozing from mucous membranes, puncture sites, and raw surfaces. It is not usually observed until the patient has received at least one to two blood volume transfusions.
   2. **Management. Normalize body temperature.** Normalization of body temperature in hypothermic patients is essential to ensure functional clotting factors and platelets.
      a. **Evaluate for macrovascular bleeding (bleeding from a source that requires operative control). Search for ongoing occult bleeding that requires operative intervention (surgical bleeding) if the patient remains in refractory shock.**
      b. **Blood component therapy** (see Chapter 43). In the setting of microvascular bleeding with evidence of thrombocytopenia, prolongation of the prothrombin time (PT) and partial thromboplastin time (PTT), and low fibrinogen levels, give appropriate component therapy.

D. **Recognition and treatment of increased intracranial pressure** (ICP). Head injury is the major cause of early mortality in blunt trauma patients admitted to the ICU. The fundamental goal in ICU management of the severely head injured patient is to prevent secondary neuronal injury. Increased ICP is an important factor that can contribute to secondary brain injury. Therefore, monitoring and control of ICP and cerebral perfusion pressure (**CPP** = MAP – ICP) in severely head injured patients (GCS ≤8) is a high priority in the early phase after resuscitative ICU care. Other insults that are known to worsen neurologic injury include hypotension, hypoxia, hypercarbia, and elevated body temperature (see Chapter 19).
   1. **Control of elevated ICP.** The threshold for treatment of raised ICP is 20 to 25 mmHg. ICP is controlled by the sequential use of sedation, pharmacologic paralysis, cerebrospinal fluid (CSF) drainage, mannitol, hyperventilation, and, finally, barbiturates for refractory intracranial hypertension.
      a. Empiric use of hyperventilation and mannitol are avoided unless evidence is seen of impending herniation or routine measures have failed to control ICP.
      b. Extreme degrees of hypocapnia ($PaCO_2$ <25 mmHg) should be avoided unless therapy is guided by cerebral blood flow measurements or other indices of brain oxygenation (e.g., jugular venous oximetry).
      c. High doses of barbiturates are reserved for those patients who are refractory to conventional management.
   2. Prevention of other secondary insults. Mean arterial blood pressure, arterial oxygen saturation, $PaCO_2$ (end-tidal CO_2), and body temperature

are closely monitored to avoid secondary insults to the injured brain. MAP is supported to between 90 and 100 mmHg to provide a cerebral perfusion pressure of at least 70 to 80 mmHg. When volume expansion is unsuccessful in achieving these endpoints, vasopressors can be employed. Antipyretics and other cooling techniques can be applied in those patients with fever to minimize further neuronal loss.

E. **Recognition and prevention of acute renal failure**. Injured patients are at high risk for the development of acute renal failure (ARF) because of hypotension, rhabdomyolysis, use of iodinated contrast for diagnostic tests, and preexisting conditions such as diabetes. However, the frequency of ARF is relatively low. Approximately one third of cases of acute posttraumatic renal failure are caused by inadequate resuscitation. The remainder appear to develop as a component of MODS. Development of ARF complicates the overall ICU management of the patient, increases length of stay, and is associated with a mortality of approximately 60%. Oliguria in the early ICU phase of care should prompt a search for reversible causes of ARF.

1. **Hypovolemia**. Oliguria in the early ICU phase of care is most commonly caused by hypovolemia or inadequate fluid resuscitation. Use fluid boluses guided by measurements of central pressure to augment urine output. If urine output fails to respond to fluid boluses, consider PA catheterization to fully evaluate hemodynamics and filling pressures while other causes of oliguria are evaluated.

2. **Rhabdomyolysis** (see Chapter 35). Patients sustaining crush injuries, severe extremity injuries, compartment syndromes, or vascular injuries to the extremity with ischemia or reperfusion are at high risk for myoglobinuric ARF. Total creatine phosphokinase (CPK) >15,000 IU increases the risk for development of myoglobinuric ARF. Laboratory data that suggest severe rhabdomyolysis include a low blood urea nitrogen (BUN):creatinine ratio, myoglobinuria, hypocalcemia, or hyperphosphatemia. Cloudy urine that is dipstick positive for protein or blood, but without red blood cells on microscopic examination, suggests rhabdomyolysis. When CPK is high or brown tea-colored urine is noted, start vigorous fluid resuscitation with the goal of maintaining a high urinary flow (100–300 mL/hour). For patients who are oliguric, mannitol or loop diuretics can be used to establish urine flow. Early alkalinization of urine (pH >6) has proved successful in some studies but it is unclear whether this effect is additive to the benefit of maintaining high urinary flow.

3. **Abdominal compartment syndrome** (see Chapter 30). Severely traumatized patients having laparotomy, especially when associated with shock and massive volume resuscitation, can develop increased intraabdominal pressure (IAP). When IAP reaches 20 to 25 mmHg, oliguric acute renal failure can result. Other consequences of increased IAP include decreased mesenteric blood flow, decreased cardiac output, increased airway pressures, and increased ICP. Measurements of IAP can be obtained by measuring bladder pressure.

4. **Obstruction**. Although uncommon, patients with severe pelvic fractures can develop retroperitoneal hematomas that obstruct the ureter or bladder outlet. Sonography or computed tomography (CT) scan should be considered to evaluate the possibility of obstruction causing acute oliguria. Irrigate or change the catheter to exclude obstruction of the urinary drainage catheter by blood clot.

F. **Evaluation and correction of acid-base and electrolyte disturbances**. During the first 24 hours of ICU admission, disturbances in acid-base and electrolyte balance can be anticipated in patients in shock or in those who have received massive transfusions.

1. **Acid-base disorders**. Lactic acidemia, which is common and often multifactorial, is caused by shock, hypothermia, limb ischemia, and metabolic response to trauma.

    a. Persistent lactic acidosis requires determination of cause and consideration of invasive hemodynamic monitoring if impaired tissue oxygen delivery is suspected. Lactic acidosis that fails to clear within the first 24 hours of ICU admission identifies a group of patients at high risk of mortality.

    b. Direct treatment of persistent metabolic acidosis at the underlying cause. Reserve administration of sodium bicarbonate or other buffers for those patients with severe metabolic acidosis or evidence of cardiovascular instability.

    c. Other metabolic acid-base disorders may be seen in the acute phase of management, including hyperchloremic metabolic acidosis caused by large volume saline resuscitation. In recipients of massive transfusion, metabolic alkalosis can be consequent to the metabolism of the large citrate load from transfused blood products. Specific therapy is usually unnecessary.

2. Electrolyte disorders

    a. Hypokalemia. The most common electrolyte disturbance in the injured patient is hypokalemia. Excessive renal losses of potassium occur as a result of diagnostic and therapeutic use of osmotic diuretics, high doses of glucocorticoids (e.g., methylprednisolone in spinal cord injury), and high aldosterone levels in patients who are hypovolemic. Alkalosis, high catecholamine levels, and hypothermia can also cause intracellular K+ shift. Hypokalemia can be especially prominent in patients who have had massive transfusions, particularly when alkalosis is present. Because of transcellular shifts in potassium that cause hypokalemia, potassium salt administration should be judicious and closely monitored to avoid inadvertent hyperkalemia.

    b. Hyperkalemia. Hyperkalemia is uncommon except in those patients with severe metabolic acidosis or concomitant rapid blood transfusion of red blood cells (RBC) >100 to 150 mL/minute. Treat severe hyperkalemia that persists after correction of acidosis aggressively to prevent cardiac arrest.

    c. Hypocalcemia. Hypocalcemia occurs frequently in the severely injured patient, and it is usually caused by a reduction in total calcium from dilutional hypoalbuminemia (~50% of total calcium is bound to albumin). Hypocalcemia can occur in patients with severe rhabdomyolysis.

        (1) Ionized hypocalcemia. Despite the common occurrence of hypocalcemia, it is only clinically important with the physiologically active, ionized fraction (40%) is reduced. Clinical manifestations of ionized hypocalcemia are generally not evident until ionized calcium concentration is <0.7 mmol/L (normal = 1.0–1.25 mmol/L) and include hypotension, impaired ventricular function, bradycardia, bronchospasm, laryngospasm, and impaired response to catecholamines. Ionized hypocalcemia is seen in trauma patients with respiratory alkalosis or as a result of massive transfusion or with a concomitant impairment in hepatic citrate metabolism. Measure ionized calcium in patients at risk for severe hypocalcemia or those who remain hemodynamically unstable.

        (2) Treatment. Hypocalcemia should be empirically treated with intravenous (i.v.) calcium salts if the ionized calcium is low (<0.7 mmol/L) or when hemodynamic instability or other complications of hypocalcemia are recognized.

    d. Hypomagnesemia. Hypomagnesemia is also a common electrolyte disorder in critically ill surgical patients. Excessive renal or gastrointestinal losses and transcellular shifts (e.g., alkalosis) are general causes of hypomagnesemia. Complications of hypomagnesemia include hypocalcemia, refractory hypokalemia, peripheral and diaphragmatic muscle weakness, tetany, cardiac dysrhythmias, tremor, hyperreflexia, agitation, confusion, and seizures. Plasma magnesium measurement does not accurately reflect the ionized fraction (55% of total), which is the physiologically active form. Total plasma magnesium levels <1 mEq/L are associated with hypokalemia and increased mortality and, thus, serve as a practical threshold for initiating aggressive therapy.

  (1) **Treatment**. Severe hypomagnesemia is treated with magnesium salts i.v. Symptomatic hypomagnesemia (e.g., refractory cardiac dysrhythmias or seizures) can by treated with magnesium sulfate (2–5 g) (1 g = 8 mEq Mg^{+2}) administered slowly over 2 to 3 minutes while arterial blood pressure and heart rhythm are monitored. Following the initial bolus, a continuous infusion (2 g/hour for 5 hours followed by 1 g/hour for 10 hours) has been successfully used. For patients with asymptomatic but severe hypomagnesemia, $MgSO_4$ (6 g) is administered over 3 hours followed by 10 g administered continuously over the remainder of the day. Additional doses of 6 g/day for the next 2 to 5 days can be given as necessary to correct residual deficits. Less severe degrees of hypomagnesemia can be treated as indicated by supplements added to total parenteral nutrition (TPN) or by enteric administration of magnesium oxide.

G. **ICU tertiary survey**. Concomitant with measures that maintain adequate tissue oxygenation, reexamine the patient for occult injuries and obtain a medical history to determine comorbid disease.

  1. **Initial ICU evaluation**
     a. **Airway**. For patients with an artificial airway, evaluate the airway to confirm that it is properly positioned and secured with tape or a tube fixation device. Trauma patients are at high risk for self-extubation, especially if agitated. Ongoing direct observation of the patient, especially as emerging from anesthesia, sedation, or recovery from alcohol intoxication, is an important preventive strategy. Patients with a native airway should also be reevaluated to determine if the airway is still patent or is threatened.
     b. **Breathing**. Evaluate lungs, ventilator settings, oxygen saturation, and blood gases to determine that air entry is symmetric and that oxygenation, ventilation, and acid-base balance are satisfactory. Evaluate chest tubes to confirm that they are functional and whether ongoing air leak or bleeding is present.
     c. **Circulation**. Measure blood pressure, CVP and other available hemodynamic parameters to determine the need for additional resuscitative intervention or invasive hemodynamic monitoring. Also determine adequacy and patency of existing vascular access.

  2. **Evaluation for occult injuries**. In the early postinjury phase, the search for occult injuries is a high priority. The incidence of injuries missed during the initial trauma room evaluation has been reported as high as 20%, depending on the mechanism of injury. Missed injuries in blunt trauma victims are generally orthopedic in nature, whereas vascular and visceral injuries are most frequently missed in patients with penetrating trauma.
     a. **Factors predisposing to missed injuries**. Hemodynamic instability, spinal cord injury, closed head injury, intoxication, shock, abbreviated surgical exploration, and inability to communicate with the patient predispose the patient to undetected injuries. Miscommunication, technical problems, and a low index of suspicion are also factors that predispose to undetected injuries.
     b. **High priority occult injuries**. The search for occult injuries is prioritized to detect injuries that threaten life, limb, or organ system

function. Evaluation is continued with a complete head to toe physical reexamination, supplemented by a repeat chest x-ray on admission and diagnostic tests as indicated by clinical conditions. These high priority occult injuries may be previously undetected injuries or new neurologic deficits, systemic hypoperfusion, or limb ischemia caused by injury progression.

(1) **Brain and spinal cord injury.** Unrecognized neurologic injuries are most common when patients are admitted to the emergency department in hemorrhagic shock requiring operative intervention. Once in the ICU, a neurologic examination should be performed. Neuromuscular blockers should be held to permit examination. CT scan of the brain should be performed in those patients with newly recognized neurologic abnormalities or increasing ICP to establish the diagnosis of traumatic brain injury, or to determine if delayed hematoma formation is present in those patients with an identified brain injury. Evaluate neurologic abnormalities suggesting spinal cord injury with x-ray study directed at the level of the clinically suspected injury.

(2) **Vascular injuries**
  (a) **Thoracic aortic injury** (see Chapter 26a)
  (b) **Intraabdominal or pelvic vascular injury.** Vascular injury should be suspected in patients with penetrating wounds to the abdomen or those with pelvic fractures who demonstrate signs of ongoing hemorrhage.
  (c) **Vascular injuries to the extremities.** Examine all extremities, especially those that are injured or casted, to determine the state of perfusion. Numbness in an injured extremity suggests a compartment syndrome.
  (d) **Cerebrovascular injuries.** Injuries to the extracranial or intracranial circulation should be suspected in patients with penetrating injuries to the neck or brain, severe direct neck trauma, cervical spine (C-spine) fractures, fractures through the carotid or vertebral canal, and in those patients with delayed (>12 hours after injury) focal neurologic deficits.

(3) **Cardiac injuries.** Persistent hypotension or cardiac dysrhythmias suggest the possibility of blunt myocardial injury or cardiac tamponade in patients with chest trauma.

(4) **Aerodigestive tract injuries.** Injuries to the aerodigestive tract are likely in patients with penetrating injuries in proximity to the neck or mediastinum. Subcutaneous, mediastinal, or cervical air suggests injury.

(5) **Occult pneumothorax.** Plain supine x-rays of the chest can miss up to 50% of pneumothoraces in trauma patients. Review chest x-ray and CT scan of the abdomen for evidence of new or occult pneumothorax. Patients on mechanical ventilation with occult pneumothorax should have chest tubes placed to reduce the risk of progression.

(6) **Compartment syndrome** (see Chapter 35). Direct trauma, ischemia, and venous injury are common causes of compartment syndrome in the trauma patient. In addition, compartment syndrome can occur in uninjured extremities after massive fluid and blood resuscitation.

(7) **Eye injuries.** Approximately 13% of patients admitted with major trauma manifest some form of ocular trauma. Contact lenses should be removed, eyes and adnexa examined, and visual acuity tested when possible.

    c. Other occult injuries. Other injuries that may be evident in the early ICU phase of care include basilar skull fractures with cerebrospinal fluid (CSF) leak, scalp lacerations, facial and mandibular fractures, dental injuries, extremity fractures, and diaphragmatic tears.

3. **Assess comorbid conditions.** Obtain a thorough history from the patient or family to document prior medical conditions, medications, and allergies. Comorbid conditions increase mortality and morbidity following trauma. The most important conditions affecting trauma mortality include cirrhosis, congenital coagulopathies, ischemic heart disease, malignancy, pulmonary disease, renal disease, diabetes, and severe obesity. Also evaluate the patient for conditions that may have predisposed to injury, such as sleep apnea, acute myocardial infarction, cardiac arrhythmia, stroke, seizures, ruptured intracranial or abdominal aneurysm, hypoglycemia, and alcohol or drug intoxication.

H. Pain control (see Chapter 41). Inadequately treated pain has a number of adverse consequences including increased O_2 consumption, increased minute volume demands, psychic stress, sleep deprivation, and perhaps most importantly, impaired lung mechanics with associated pulmonary complications. Subjective pain assessment is documented and subsequently reevaluated after initiation of treatment. Inadequate pain relief can be determined objectively by the failure of the patient to achieve adequate volumes on incentive spirometry, persistently small radiographic lung volumes, or reluctance to cough and cooperate with chest physiotherapy. The mainstay of pain control in the ICU is i.v. opioids. Complications of opioid administration include oversedation, ileus, urinary retention, nausea, and pruritus.

1. **Bolus opioids.** Bolus doses of opioids (e.g., morphine, fentanyl) are useful in those patients with mild, intermittent pain, especially when the chest is uninjured.

2. **Patient-controlled analgesia (PCA).** In patients with multisystem trauma, chest wall injuries, or those after laparotomy, PCA frequently provides satisfactory pain relief. Typically, a morphine PCA is initiated with a loading dose of 0.5 to 3 mg followed by bolus doses of 1 mg with a lockout interval of between 5 and 20 minutes. If pain is not adequately controlled with this regimen, the bolus dose can to titrated up to 2 mg/dose or a continuous low dose infusion of morphine (1 mg/hour) can be added.

3. **Epidural analgesia** is considered for patients with severe chest trauma, especially when respiratory status is marginal, excessive sedation occurs with i.v. narcotics, or the patient has failed a trial at PCA. Bolus or continuous epidural infusion of opioids is usually used. Epidural morphine is commonly used in bolus doses of 1 to 6 mg, depending on patient age and catheter location (lower doses for elderly patients, higher doses for lumbar placement). Usual dosing interval is every 12 hours, but dosing may be required as often as every 6 to 8 hours. Continuous infusion of epidural morphine at 0.1 to 1.0 mg/hour can also be used. Local anesthetics (e.g., bupivacaine) can also be used alone or in combination with opioids.

4. **Interpleural anesthesia.** Another technique that can be useful in controlling pain in patients with severe chest trauma is the instillation of local anesthetics directly into the pleural space, either via existing chest tubes or following placement of a standard epidural catheter in the pleural space. A 20-mL dose of 0.5% bupivacaine (100 mg) with 1:200,000 epinephrine is injected and allowed to dwell at least 30 minutes (with chest tube clamped). Dosage can be repeated every 6 hours with the maximal dose not to exceed 400 mg/day of bupivacaine.

5. **Extrapleural analgesia.** A technique similar to interpleural analgesia uses a standard epidural catheter placed in the extrapleural space at the site of the most superior rib fracture. Injections of 20 mL of 0.25%

bupivacaine with epinephrine (1:200,000) are administered every 6 hours, as needed, for pain control.

6. **Intercostal nerve blocks.** Local anesthetic administration for rib fractures can provide adequate pain relief. However, they are somewhat impractical in patients with multiple fractures because of the need for repeated injections.

I. **Preventive measures in the ICU**

1. **Stress ulceration**

   a. **Risk factors.** Trauma patients at increased risk for stress ulceration include those with multisystem trauma (ISS >16), shock, respiratory failure, coagulopathy, preexisting ulcer disease, closed head and spinal cord injuries, severe burns, and patients who develop sepsis or MODS.

   b. **Preventive therapy.** Prophylactic agents are initiated on admission to the ICU and continued until the risk has abated (i.e., resolution of respiratory failure, normalization of ICP) or until the patient is receiving intragastric feedings. Small bowel feedings do not appear to have the same protective effect as intragastric feedings. H_2 blockers should be used in those patients at highest risk for stress bleeding. Sucralfate is a reasonable alternative prophylactic agent in patients with intermediate risk for stress bleeding (ISS ≥10 ≤16). Patients at low risk (ISS <10) probably do not require routine prophylaxis. Routine neutralization of gastric pH can result in an increased incidence of nosocomial pneumonia.

2. **Deep venous thrombosis (DVT)** (see Chapter 51). All patients with major injury are at risk for DVT and pulmonary embolism. Overall incidence of proximal DVT in trauma patients is approximately 18% without prophylaxis.

   a. **Risk factors.** Independent predictors for the development of DVT include need for blood transfusion or surgery, lower extremity and pelvic fractures, closed head injury, and spinal cord injury (SCI). Other high-risk conditions include age >60 years, prolonged immobility, injury severity score (ISS) >30, injuries to the vena cava or iliofemoral venous system, and prolonged retention (>24 hours) of large bore resuscitation catheters in the femoral veins.

   b. **Prophylaxis.** Some form of DVT prophylaxis should be implemented on admission to the ICU. Even with prophylaxis, DVT still occurs in high-risk trauma patients with a frequency of approximately 7% to 10% (see Chapter 51).

3. **Early infectious concerns.** Infectious morbidity increases ICU length of stay and late mortality.

   a. **Vaccinations.** Review the vaccination status of the patient to ensure that tetanus vaccination is up to date. Vaccinations to be given following splenectomy include *Streptococcus pneumoniae, H. influenzae,* and *Neisseria meningitidis* vaccines.

   b. **Wound debridement and closure.** Debride, irrigate, and close superficial lacerations. Ideally, wounds should be closed within 6 hours. Clean and dress abrasions. Treat large abrasions similar to a burn wound and use antibiotic ointment.

   c. **Removal and replacement of field i.v. catheters.** Intravenous catheters and central venous lines that were placed in the field or under suboptimal conditions during resuscitation should be removed as soon as possible.

   d. **Respiratory care.** Pulmonary infections are frequent in the later phases of ICU care. Interventions should be initiated within the first 24 hours to help minimize the risk of their development. These include rapid extubation in those patients not requiring mechanical ventilation or airway protection, pain control, upright posturing when possible, handwashing, incentive spirometry with encouragement of cough, active treatment to expand atelectatic lung segments (bronchoscopy, chest percussion, intermittent positive pressure breathing [IPPB]), and bronchodilators to facilitate mucociliary clearance. Lung volumes and chest physiotherapy regimens are optimized in the 35° head-up position in quadriplegic patients.

   e. Antibiotics. Options for antibiotic use in patients with contaminated wounds are shown in Table 38.4. Controlled data on the optimal antibiotic strategies for contaminated wounds in trauma patients are generally unavailable except for penetrating abdominal wounds.

 J. Family contact and support. Establish early contact with family members, explain the injuries, current clinical condition, and prognosis to provide essential information to the family under stress and to establish a therapeutic relationship between the ICU care team and family. Explain unit operations, ICU procedures, visiting hours, and available services.

IV. Priorities in the early life support phase (24 to 72 hours). Problems developing during this phase include intracranial hypertension, systemic inflammatory response syndrome, early multiple organ dysfunction syndrome, and continued respiratory insufficiency. **Maintenance of tissue oxygenation, control of ICP, ongoing search for occult injuries, and the institution of nutritional support are the main priorities.**

 A. Hemodynamics. Reevaluate the physical examination, hemodynamic parameters, vital signs, urine output, cardiac output, oxygen delivery and consumption, blood gases, and tonometrically measured gastric mucosal pH, when available, to assess the state of perfusion. In patients with normal blood pressure, indicators suggesting incomplete resuscitation include persistent lactic acidemia or uncorrected base deficit, oliguria, flow-dependent oxygen consumption, high oxygen extraction ratio, and gastric mucosal pH <7.3. Additional volume resuscitation or inotropic support guided by invasive hemodynamic monitoring is used to establish and maintain adequate systemic and organ perfusion. Occult injuries or ongoing blood loss should be suspected in patients who do not stabilize.

 B. Gas exchange and ventilatory support. Gas exchange frequently worsens the second day after trauma, especially in those patients who have been aggressively fluid resuscitated and those with severe chest injuries. Reevaluate clinical assessment, chest x-ray study, blood gases, chest tubes, and ventilatory support. Clinical signs of fatigue, deteriorating oxygenation or ventilation, high minute volume demands, worsening lung compliance, or pulmonary infiltrates all indicate need for institution or continuation of mechanical ventilation.

   1. A patient with a GCS ≤9 or a patient with an alveolar-arterial oxygen difference of >175 mmHg on the second day of ventilatory support helps to identify those patients likely to require prolonged ventilatory support (>14 days). For patients with persistent and severe respiratory failure, ventilator support is adjusted as possible to reduce the F_{IO_2} to "nontoxic" levels (40% to 60%) while maintaining low airway pressures as discussed above. Patients likely to be easily extubated during this phase of care are shown in Table 38.5.

 C. Intracranial pressure. Increasing ICP is usually most problematic during this phase of ICU care. Delayed hematoma formation or hemorrhagic expansion of contusions should be excluded with repeat CT scanning. Most commonly, however, increasing blood volume is causing intracranial hypertension. Thus, interventions that reduce cerebral blood volume (e.g., therapeutic hyperventilation) may have their greatest utility during this phase of care. Treatment is best guided by measurements of cerebral perfusion pressure, cerebral blood flow, or cerebral oxygen metabolism.

 D. Fluid and electrolyte balance. Fluid balance is usually positive in multiply injured patients. Total fluid administration is reduced to maintenance requirements. If pulmonary edema is present or lung water is increased in areas of contusion, maintenance fluids can be temporarily withheld and

Table 38.4. Options for preventive antibiotic strategies in injured patients

Site	Antibiotic	Duration	Comments
Abdomen			
Penetrating injury	ES Pen or 2nd generation Ceph or Flagyl + AG	24 hours, if bowel injured	Single preoperative dose adequate if no bowel injury
Thorax			
Penetrating esophageal	1st generation Ceph	24 hours, if minimal contamination	
	ES Pen	10–14 days	Mediastinal soiling
Penetrating lung	1st generation Ceph	24 hours	
Chest tube	1st generation Ceph	Until tube removed	Controversial
Orthopedic			
Closed fractures	1st generation Ceph	24 hours	Preoperative and after open reduction
Open fractures Grade I and II	1st generation Ceph	24–48 hours	Continue for 48–72 hours following soft tissue coverage
Open fractures Grade III	1st generation Ceph + AG or ES Pen		
Vascular			
	1st generation Ceph	24 hours	Extend treatment for extensive contamination or soft-tissue injury
Facial fractures			
Communication with skin	1st generation Ceph	Continue until fracture repaired	
Communication with oral cavity	Penicillin or clindamycin	Continue until fracture repaired	
Neck			
Larynx/Trachea/ Esophagus	ES Pen or 1st generation Ceph	Continue for 24 hours following repair	
Head			
Penetrating injury	Antistaphylococcal penicillin or vancomycin	5–7 days	Optimal antibiotics and duration uncertain
Open depressed skull fracture	Antistaphylococcal penicillin or vancomycin	24–48 hours following debridement and wound closure	
Basilar skull fracture	None		
Urologic Injury			
Extraperitoneal bladder rupture	ES Pen	3–5 days	Optimum duration uncertain
Upper tract injuries	1st generation Ceph	24 hours after repair	

Ceph, cephalosporin; ES Pen, extended spectrum penicillin; AG, aminoglycoside.

Table 38.5. Trauma patients typically requiring only
short-term mechanical ventilation

Alcohol intoxication with minor injuries
Postoperatively following repair of multiple orthopedic injuries
Postoperatively following isolated abdominal or thoracic trauma
Head injury: Glasgow Coma Scale score >9
Isolated chest trauma

diuretics administered to facilitate oxygenation and reduce ventilatory support needs. Common electrolyte abnormalities include hypokalemia, hypomagnesemia, hypocalcemia, and hypophosphatemia. Hypernatremia is common in patients requiring osmotic diuretics for the control of ICP or in those patients who develop diabetes insipidus.

E. **Hematologic parameters.** Patients with severe head injury, pelvic fracture with retroperitoneal hematoma, and those who have had massive resuscitation should have coagulation parameters (PT/PTT) and platelet counts remeasured. Ongoing coagulopathy suggests ongoing hemorrhage, preexisting liver disease, or severe ischemic liver injury. Administer blood component therapy, as indicated, for patients with ongoing bleeding. Thrombocytopenia (platelet count 50,000–100,000/mm³) is frequently seen during this phase of care, and it suggests either ongoing hemorrhage or is an expected finding in patients who have received massive transfusions. Thrombocytopenia following massive transfusion usually persists for 3 to 4 days before returning toward counts of 100,000 mm³. Withhold platelet transfusion therapy unless clinical evidence is found of ongoing bleeding. A platelet count <100,000 mm³ in patients with severe head injury should prompt early platelet transfusion therapy.

F. **Occult injuries.** Detection of missed injuries continues to be a high priority in the early life support phase of ICU care.

1. **Delayed intracranial hematoma formation.** Most patients with head injury who manifest delayed hematoma formation or an expansion of previously diagnosed contusions do so within 3 days after injury. Repeat CT scan of the brain is indicated in patients who continue to demonstrate severe neurologic dysfunction, deterioration in neurologic examination, or an increase in ICP.

2. **Intraabdominal injuries.** Frequency of missed intraabdominal injuries depends on the mechanism of injury and diagnostic modalities used initially to evaluate the abdomen. Patients developing early signs of infection or peritoneal signs should be rapidly evaluated for occult bowel perforation, pancreatic injury, or injury to the genitourinary (GU) tract.

3. **Cervical spine injury.** Radiologic survey of the C-spine may need to be completed in the ICU.

4. **Thoracic and lumbar spine injury.** For patients who are at risk for thoracic and lumbosacral spine injury, complete the radiologic survey.

5. **Extremity injury.** Reexamine the upper and lower extremities, especially the hands and feet. Radiographs are obtained based on physical findings including swelling, ecchymosis, and tenderness not appreciated during the initial resuscitation.

6. **Nerve injuries.** Repeat the neurologic examination with attention to injured extremities to determine if any missed cranial or peripheral nerve injuries are present.

G. **Initiation of nutritional support** (see Chapter 44). Nutritional support is usually initiated during the early life support phase once it is determined that the patient is fully resuscitated and is unlikely to resume normal dietary intake in 5 to 7 days. In general, initiate nutritional support as soon as possible after injury.

1. **Identify patients at risk**. Patients at risk for the development of malnutrition as a result of injury include those with multisystem trauma, severe respiratory failure, burns, severe head or spinal cord injuries, or those with injuries that restrict the patient's ability to consume a normal oral diet.
2. **Determine energy and protein requirements**. Calories are administered to meet resting energy expenditure (REE) demands. In most critically ill trauma patients, REE is in the range of 25% to 30% above energy expenditure as predicted by the Harris-Benedict equation (see Chapter 44).
3. **Determine route of administration**. The preferred route of nutritional support is enteral. Although transpyloric feedings are favored because of concern for aspiration with gastric feedings, this is still controversial. Use TPN in cases of contraindications to enteral feedings or intolerance (abdominal distension, vomiting).
4. **Monitoring nutritional support** (see Chapter 44)

H. **Prevention of complications**
   1. **Infections**
      a. **General measures**. General interventions directed at preventing nosocomial infection include good handwashing practice, removal of all unnecessary invasive monitoring tubes and lines, and avoiding unnecessary antibiotic therapy. Intermittent bladder catheterization is preferred in patients with spinal cord injury who no longer require continuous monitoring of urinary output.
      b. **Pulmonary infections**. In addition to general measures, early stabilization of long bone and pelvic fractures is thought to reduce pulmonary infectious morbidity by allowing earlier mobilization and upright positioning. Enteral feedings should be administered through small-bore feeding tubes to minimize the risk of aspiration. Removal of nasogastric (NG) tubes also helps minimize the risk of otitis and sinusitis.
      c. **Fungal infections**. Risk factors for yeast colonization include use of three or more antibiotics, Acute Physiology and Chronic Health Evaluation (APACHE) score >10, TPN, operations on the gastrointestinal tract, malignancy, and mechanical ventilation >48 hours. Prophylactic regimens directed against yeast have not been shown conclusively to be effective in reducing colonization or infection.
   2. **Agitation**. Agitated patients should first be evaluated for immediately life-threatening causes (hypoxemia, hypercarbia, hypoperfusion, expanding intracranial mass lesion). Then, treat the patients to relieve stress, prevent unplanned extubation, and limit unnecessary energy expenditure. Short-term sedation can be accomplished with midazolam or propofol, whereas lorazepam can be used in patients requiring more prolonged sedation. Haloperidol is also useful in controlling agitation, especially when accompanied by delirium. These drugs can be administered as intermittent i.v. boluses or as a continuous infusion. Treat agitated patients at risk for **alcohol withdrawal** with benzodiazepines if no contraindications exist. Clonidine and β-blockers can be used adjunctively to treat the hyperadrenergic state associated with alcohol withdrawal.
   3. **Neuromuscular blockade**. Prolonged neuromuscular blockade predisposes the patient to the development of pulmonary infections and muscle weakness. Neuromuscular blockers should be discontinued when not absolutely necessary for management of intracranial hypertension or ventilatory support. When neuromuscular blockers are necessary, titrate therapy using a nerve stimulator.

I. **Identification of potential organ donors**. Most potential organ donors are victims of head injuries. Most patients destined to die as a result of head injury (blunt or penetrating) will do so within the first 24 to 72 hours

after admission to the ICU. The main goals of management are to maintain organ perfusion and prevent complications to optimize the potential for the recovery of viable organs (see Chapter 45).
V. **Priorities in the prolonged life support phase (>72 hours postinjury).** The duration of this phase depends on injury severity and the development of complications. Prolonged respiratory failure and infectious complications are the most important concerns during this phase. For patients developing MODS, the main objective of management is to provide support for failing organ systems while attempting to isolate and eliminate inflammatory foci that may be perpetuating organ system failure.
   A. **Respiratory failure** that persists into the prolonged life support phase is usually caused by development of pneumonia, other systemic infections, impaired lung mechanics (flail chest, spinal cord injury) with attendant complications (atelectasis, retained secretions), muscle weakness consequent to prolonged neuromuscular blockade, or persistent ARDS. At this stage, treatment of respiratory failure is largely supportive (mechanical ventilation) while therapy is directed at resolving infections, atelectasis, and excess lung water.
      1. **Unexplained respiratory failure** should be evaluated to exclude occult heart failure, hypothyroidism, adrenal insufficiency, electrolyte imbalance, infection, diaphragmatic paralysis, and polyneuropathy.
      2. **Tracheostomy.** After 3 to 4 days of intubation, the following patients should be considered for early tracheostomy: head-injured patients who remain comatose, high spinal cord injuries, elderly patients with severe chest trauma, and patients anticipated to require >14 days of ventilatory support.
   B. **Infectious complications.** Trauma patients requiring prolonged ICU support invariably develop fever during the course of their stay. Infections are major complications of trauma that prolong ICU length of stay, cause and perpetuate MODS, and are associated with increased mortality. Differentiating noninfectious causes of fever (e.g., SIRS, pancreatitis, drugs) can be difficult.
      1. **Infectious causes of fever.** Common nosocomial infections in the ICU include pulmonary, urinary tract, and indwelling vascular catheters.
         a. **Nosocomial pneumonia.** Hospital-acquired pneumonia is the most common infectious complication diagnosed in trauma patients admitted to the ICU; the incidence of nosocomial pneumonia in trauma patients ranges from 20% to 40%. Risk factors include emergency intubation, hypotension on admission, blunt mechanism, severe head injury, high ISS, age >55 years, surgery of the head or chest, and combined abdominal and thoracic injury.
            (1) **Diagnosis.** Traditional diagnostic criteria (fever, leukocytosis, new radiographic infiltrate, purulent sputum) are nonspecific and lead to an incorrect diagnosis of nosocomial pneumonia approximately 40% of the time. Diagnosis may require quantitative cultures using the protected specimen brush (PSB) or bronchoalveolar lavage (BAL). Diagnostic cutoff for the PSB technique is 10^3 colony-forming units (CFU)/mL; whereas for bronchoalveolar lavage, it is in the range of 10^4 to 10^5 CFU/mL.
            (2) **Microbiology.** Organisms commonly isolated from trauma patients with pneumonia include *H. influenzae* and *Staphylococcus aureus*. Pneumonia with these isolates is commonly considered to be early onset pneumonia (occurring within 4 days after injury) as these organisms are aspirated into the tracheobronchial tree at the time of injury. Gram-negative isolates, typical of **ventilator-associated pneumonias** (late onset), are also common pathogens in trauma patients developing pneumonia.
            (3) **Antibiotic therapy.** Empiric antibiotic therapy with a single antibiotic that covers the isolates of concern can be initiated and later modified as indicated by culture results. Antibiotic therapy

using a combination of a β-lactam and aminoglycoside should be considered in patients with severe pneumonias caused by *Pseudomonas, Acinetobacter, Serratia,* and *Enterobacter* species. Volume of distribution of aminoglycoside is increased in trauma patients; thus, higher doses are necessary to achieve therapeutic levels.

b. Lung abscess and empyema. Patients sustaining chest trauma are at risk for empyema and occasionally lung abscess in the form of infected traumatic pneumatoceles. Risk factors for development of empyema are retained hemothorax, improper chest tube placement, pneumonia, and chest injury. CT scan and thoracentesis are useful in establishing these diagnoses.

c. Urinary tract infection (UTI). UTI is one of the most common causes of nosocomial infection and, thus, should be suspected in all patients who have had or have indwelling urinary drainage catheters. Risk factors for UTI include instrumentation of the genitourinary system, GU injury, age, duration of catheterization, and a break in the sterile system.

d. Wound infection. Inspect all surgical wounds for evidence of local infection. Surgical wound infection requires incision and drainage.

e. Catheter sepsis. Invasive monitoring device or catheter use for TPN administration is a major risk factor for nosocomial bacteremia. Catheter colonization is defined using semiquantitative catheter tip cultures growing >15 CFU of bacteria or fungi. Recent studies demonstrate an increased incidence of catheter-related bloodstream infection with standard catheters left in >7 days. The use of antibiotic-coated catheters reduces the rate of both catheter colonization and catheter-related bloodstream infection, and this reduction seems to continue after 7 days. If the catheter is changed in a fever workup, a single guidewire exchange of central lines is acceptable (with culture of the catheter tip). If the culture is positive, the catheter must then be removed.

f. Intraabdominal abscess abscess is a major diagnostic consideration in patients who have had exploratory laparotomy. Physical examination occasionally reveals peritoneal signs. Other signs of intraabdominal infection include fever, intolerance of tube feedings, ileus, or glucose intolerance; generally, a failure to thrive. CT scan is the diagnostic test of choice in patients who have had laparotomy. CT scan allows accurate diagnosis of the intraabdominal abscess and directed therapy—either percutaneous or operative drainage.

g. Acalculous cholecystitis. Risk factors associated with developing acute acalculous cholecystitis in trauma patients include fasting, TPN, transfusions, narcotic administration, sepsis, shock, and age. Signs and symptoms include fever, right upper quadrant pain, nausea, and vomiting. Initial diagnostic tests are liver function tests and a right upper quadrant ultrasound. Ultrasound may identify inflammatory changes, a thickened gallbladder wall, or pericholecystic fluid. Radionuclide imaging is nonspecific when abnormal and is helpful in excluding acalculous cholecystitis when normal gallbladder function is seen. Percutaneous drainage or cholecystectomy is the principal treatment.

h. Antibiotic-associated colitis. Widespread antibiotic use in trauma patients increases the risk of colitis with approximately 20% of antibiotic-associated diarrhea caused by *Clostridium difficile.* Stool should be assayed for *C. difficile* toxin in patients with fever and diarrhea. The patient may complain of abdominal pain. Currently, oral metronidazole for 10 days is the preferred therapy. Oral vancomycin is also effective.

i. Sinusitis and otitis media. Head injury, air-fluid levels in the maxillary sinuses on the admission CT scan, and use of various tubes in the nasal passages predispose patients to the development of purulent sinusitis and otitis media. When the cause of fever or infection is not apparent, examine the ears and sinuses for evidence of infection. Presence of otitis media helps select patients for further diagnostic study. The best diagnostic test for sinusitis is the CT scan. Although radiographic evidence of sinusitis may be present, other intercurrent infections are usually present, with sinusitis rarely the sole cause of fever. Tap and drain maxillary sinuses that are packed with fluid if the tap is purulent. Treatment includes removal of all large tubes from the nasopharynx, drainage, decongestants, and antibiotics.

j. Ventriculitis and meningitis. Ventriculitis and meningitis should be considered in patients with indwelling ventriculostomy catheters used for ICP monitoring or in patients who have basilar skull fractures. Gram stain and culture of the CSF establish the diagnosis. Empiric therapy should include vancomycin and a third generation cephalosporin until organisms have been identified and sensitivities reported.

k. Endovascular infection. Although relatively uncommon, septic thrombophlebitis or endocarditis should be considered in patients with persistent bacteremias.

2. Noninfectious causes of fever. Consider drug fever (β-lactam antibiotics, anticonvulsants), superficial and DVT and pancreatitis in the differential diagnosis of fever. Posttraumatic pancreatitis is increasingly recognized as a cause of fever. Noninfectious fevers can also be observed in hyperadrenergic states associated with head injury or alcohol withdrawal syndrome.

C. Multisystem organ dysfunction. Early shock and late sepsis can result in MODS, the major cause of late trauma deaths in the ICU. Identification and treatment of inflammatory foci, especially intraabdominal infection, is a high priority that is essential to survival. Adjust pharmacologic therapy for renal and hepatic failure.

D. Immobility (see Chapter 50). Cardiovascular deconditioning, muscle weakness, contractures, and skin breakdown can develop, especially in those patients with multiple orthopedic injuries, pelvic fractures, or central nervous system injuries. Passive and active range of motion should be initiated early in the patient's ICU course, when possible. Use wrist and ankle splints to prevent contractures, as necessary. Frequent turning and low air-loss beds are helpful in preventing decubitus ulcers.

VI. Priorities in the recovery phase of ICU care. Recovery from critical illness in the trauma patient requiring prolonged ICU care is imminent when signs of infection, respiratory failure, or multisystem failure abate.

A. Withdrawal of ventilatory support. The most important transition made during this phase of care is the transition from mechanical ventilation to unassisted breathing (weaning or liberation from the ventilator). Weaning begins when the causes of the respiratory failure have resolved. The process of weaning can be broken down by individually considering oxygenation, ventilation, mental status, and airway status and ability to clear secretions.

1. Oxygenation. FIO_2 and PEEP are first decreased to minimal settings that achieve acceptable arterial oxygenation. In general, if the PaO_2/FIO_2 ratio is ≥ 200 on minimal PEEP (≤ 5 cm H_2O), oxygenation should be adequate when the patient is spontaneously breathing on supplemental oxygen.

2. Ventilation. The essential determination to be made is whether the patient can meet the imposed ventilatory demands without developing ventilatory fatigue. Fatigue develops with excessive workload, respiratory muscle pump (diaphragm) weakness, lack of endurance, or, most commonly, a combination of these factors.

a. Fatigue. Ventilatory fatigue is clinically manifest initially as tachypnea at low tidal volumes. Other signs of excess ventilatory demand include use of accessory muscles of respiration, paradoxic breathing,

respiratory alternans (alternating diaphragmatic and chest wall breathing), hypertension, tachycardia, diaphoresis, and hypercapnia.
   b. **Limiting factors.** Other factors that can hamper the weaning process include pain, fever, metabolic acidosis, bronchospasm, pulmonary edema, lobar atelectasis, severe anemia, electrolyte abnormalities (hypokalemia, hypomagnesemia, and hypophosphatemia), malnutrition, and sleep deprivation.
3. **Weaning criteria.** No single parameter or combination of parameters is sufficiently accurate to predict successful weaning. Clinical assessment of the factors that might impede weaning is essential. Criteria helpful in predicting difficulty in the transition to spontaneous breathing include tachypnea (respiratory rate [RR] >30 breaths/minute), weakness (NIF <~20 cm H_2O), high minute ventilation demands (Ve >10–15 L/minute), high dead space (Vd/Vt >0.6), low static lung compliance (<35 mL/cm H_2O), low spontaneous tidal volume (Vt <4 mL/kg), and a high spontaneous frequency:tidal volume (L) ratio (>100)(referred to as the Rapid Shallow Breathing Index).
   a. **Weaning methods.** Many methods have been advocated for making the transition to spontaneous breathing (e.g., IMV, T-piece, pressure support ventilation).
      (1) **Short-term ventilation.** For patients requiring only short-term mechanical ventilation, the weaning method is probably inconsequential to success or failure. In such circumstances, positive pressure ventilation can be withdrawn relatively rapidly to either T-piece or minimal support settings (e.g., pressure support of 5–8 cm H_2O) and the patient assessed for signs of fatigue. These minimal settings will compensate for the imposed work of breathing caused by the endotracheal tube and ventilator circuit. If no signs are seen of fatigue and blood gases demonstrate adequate oxygenation and ventilation, extubation can proceed, provided no contraindications are found to extubation. In some cases, pulse oximetry can be used to guide weaning *in lieu* of arterial blood gases.
      (2) **Long-term ventilation.** Patients who have required prolonged mechanical ventilation are likely to demonstrate signs of ventilatory fatigue when initiating the withdrawal of positive pressure. The traditional method (T-piece or tracheal mask) of gradually increasing periods of spontaneous breathing interposed with gradually diminishing periods of complete or near complete ventilatory support is relatively simple and efficacious. Pressure support weaning may provide better chest wall stability in patients with flail chest, whereas the gradual reduction in ventilatory support via the IMV method may be preferred in those patients with left ventricular dysfunction. For any weaning method that is used in patients with chronic respiratory failure, adequate sleep and ventilatory rest must be assured.
4. **Airway assessment.** Once ventilatory support is no longer required, extubation should proceed unless contraindicated (i.e., coma, inability to clear secretions, or anatomic or injury-related considerations that threaten airway patency). In such patients tracheostomy is performed.
B. **Deintensification.** Goals of deintensification are to prepare the patient and family for the transition to a non-ICU environment. All nonessential invasive monitoring devices are removed, sedatives are titrated, and efforts are made to reestablish normal sleep-waking cycles. The patient and family who have developed a sense of security in the highly monitored environment of the ICU may find it difficult to adjust to the non-ICU environment. Informed preparation and support facilitates the transition for all involved.

Bibliography

Abou-khalil B, Scalea TM, Trooskin SZ, et al. Hemodynamic responses to shock in young trauma patients: need for invasive monitoring. *Crit Care Med* 1994;22(4):633–639.

Abramson D, Scalea TM, Hitchcock, et al. Lactate clearance and survival following injury. *J Trauma* 1993;35(4):584–589.

Bishop MH, Shoemaker WC, Appel PL, et al. Prospective, randomized trial of survivor values of cardiac index, oxygen delivery, and oxygen consumption as resuscitation endpoints in severe trauma. *J Trauma* 1995;38(5):780–787.

Caplan ES, Hoyt NJ. Identification and treatment of infections in multiply traumatized patients. *Am J Med* 1995;79(Suppl 1A):68–76.

Darouiche RO, Raad II, Heard SO, et al. A comparison of two antimicrobial-impregnated central venous catheters. *N Engl J Med* 1999;340(1):1–8.

Davis JW, Hoyt DB, McArdle MS, et al. An analysis of errors causing morbidity and mortality in a trauma system: a guide for quality improvement. *J Trauma* 1992; 32(5):660–666.

Davis JW, Hoyt DB, McArdle MS, et al. The significance of critical care errors in causing preventable death in trauma patients in a trauma system. *J Trauma* 1991; 31(6):813–819.

Eddy AC, Rice CL. The right ventricle: an emerging concern in the multiply injured patient. *J Crit Care* 1989;4(1):58–66.

Gattinoni L, Brazzi L, Pelosi P, et al. A trial of goal-oriented hemodynamic therapy in critically ill patients. *N Engl J Med* 1995;333(16):1025–1032.

Geerts WH, Code KI, Jay RM, et al. A prospective study of venous thromboembolism after major trauma. *N Engl J Med* 1994;331(24):160–166.

Gentilello LM, Moujaes S. Treatment of hypothermia in trauma victims: thermodynamic considerations. *Journal of Intensive Care Medicine* 1995;10:5–14.

Hirshberg A, Wall MJ, Allen MK, et al. Causes and patterns of missed injuries in trauma. *Am J Surg* 1994;168:299–303.

Hoyt DB, Simons RK, Winchell RJ. A risk analysis of pulmonary complication following major trauma. *J Trauma* 1993;35(4):524–531.

Ivatury RR, Simon RJ, Havriliak D, et al. Gastric mucosal pH and oxygen delivery and oxygen consumption indices in the assessment of adequacy of resuscitation after trauma: a prospective, randomized study. *J Trauma* 1995;39(1):128–136.

Livingston DH, Mosenthal AC, Deitch EA. Sepsis and multiple organ dysfunction syndrome: a clinical-mechanistic overview. *New Horizons* 1995;3(2):257–266.

Maki DG, Stolz SM, Wheeler S, et al. Prevention of central venous catheter-related bloodstream infection by use of an antiseptic-impregnated catheter. *Ann Intern Med* 1997;127(4):257–266.

Malangoni MA, Jacobs DG. Antibiotics prophylaxis for injured patients. *Surgical Infections* 1992;6(3):627–642.

Malay MB, Ashton RC, Landry DW, et al. Low-dose vasopressin in the treatment of vasodilatory septic shock. *J Trauma* 1999;47(4):690–705.

Marshall JC, Cook DJ, Christou NV, et al. Multiple organ dysfunction score: a reliable descriptor of a complex clinical outcome. *Crit Care Med* 1995;23(10):1638–1652.

Morris JA, MacKenzie EJ, Edelstein SL. The effect of preexisting conditions on mortality in trauma patients. *JAMA* 1994;263(14):1942–1946.

Richardson JD, Adams L, Flint LM. Selective management of flail chest and pulmonary contusion. *Ann Surg* 1992;196(4):481–487.

Rutherford EJ, Morris JA, Reed GW, et al. Base deficit stratifies mortality and determines therapy. *J Trauma* 1992;33(3):417–422.

Sauaia A, Moore FA, Moore EE, et al. Epidemiology of trauma deaths: a reassessment. *J Trauma* 1995;38(2):185–193.

Shackford SR. Blunt chest trauma: the intensivists perspective. *Journal of Intensive Care Medicine* 1986;1:125–136.

Simons RK, Hoyt DB, Winchell, et al. A risk analysis of stress ulceration after trauma. *J Trauma* 1995;39(2):289–292.

39. COMMONLY MISSED INJURIES AND PITFALLS

Gerard J. Fulda

I. **Introduction**
   A. The **incidence** of missed injuries varies from 2% to 50%, depending on the definition of a missed injury. Most authors define a missed injury as one that is discovered either after the initial resuscitation or >24 hours after admission
   B. Missed injuries, which can lead to increased morbidity, are the major causes of preventable trauma deaths and litigation.
   C. After completion of the primary and secondary surveys advocated by the Advanced Trauma Life Support course sponsored by the American College of Surgeons (see Chapter 13), a **tertiary survey** involves a head-to-toe examination of the stable patient before ambulation, after clearing the sensorium. Using this approach, which can be a delayed process in a patient who is initially unstable, an injury will be detected in 10% to 50% of patients on tertiary survey.
   D. Inform patients and their families on admission of the potential for missed injuries. For example, **"Our initial goal is to deal with the most obvious immediate threats to life and limb. It is not unusual to find additional injuries as time goes on."**
II. **Factors that contribute to missed injuries**
   A. Several **patient factors** can lead to missed injuries. When a patient presents with one of these factors, it is necessary to repeat evaluations following the resolution of the conflicting factor to avoid missing injuries.
      1. **Altered mental status** (from head injury, alcohol, or medications) is the most common reason for missed injuries.
      2. Pain or distress from **multiple injuries** can distract the physician from detecting additional injuries.
      3. **Nonavailability for frequent evaluation**. Patients who have prolonged operative procedures or lengthy diagnostic studies may be unavailable for frequent examination.
         a. When an **unstable patient** presents with an obvious life-threatening injury requiring operative intervention, complete a tertiary survey after stabilization to detect additional injuries.
      4. **Elderly patients** have little physiologic reserve and can deteriorate rapidly. Conversely, children, athletes, and pregnant patients have well-developed compensatory mechanisms and initially may not appear to be severely injured.
   B. **Physician factors**
      1. **Experience**. Trauma care is provided by physicians with varied training and experience. The inexperienced physician may obtain information correctly but misinterpret the significance of the finding. Subspecialty consultation can increase the injury detection rate, especially for injuries to the neurologic, musculoskeletal, and maxillofacial systems.
      2. **Fatigue**. Despite adequate training and experience, a fatigued physician is more likely to miss injuries. Members of the trauma team need to be physically and mentally prepared for each shift and to plan for adequate rest.
      3. **Information transfer**. Information is often lost when the care of a patient is transferred from one physician to another. Because the new physician is dependent on the medical record to guide the current evaluation and therapy, documentation must be accurate and complete. When documentation is inadequate, the new physician must approach the patient as if the patient is being evaluated for the first time.

4. **Clinical examination errors**
   a. **Incomplete history**. The initial history should include information on **A**llergies, **M**edications, **P**ast illness and **P**regnancy, **L**ast meal, and **E**vents of the injury (AMPLE). A more complete history should be part of the tertiary examination.
   b. **Unfamiliarity with injury patterns**. Be aware of several injury patterns that can increase the chances of detecting additional injuries. These include infrequent injuries with (a) high morbidity, (b) a high frequency, and (c) those associated with other injuries (some of which are listed below).
   c. **Failure to perform a tertiary survey**. Failure to expose, inspect, auscultate, palpate, and percuss every major body region can result in missed injuries. Smell can be important in uncovering wounds, injuries, and preexisting medical conditions. In some cases, it is not physically possible to examine the patient completely (e.g., facial swelling can prevent adequate examination of the eye), and a complete examination is delayed.
5. **Failure to understand the limitations and sensitivity of diagnostic studies** can result in injuries being overlooked.
   a. **Injuries missed with computed tomography (CT)**. Despite use of high-resolution CT scanners and an experienced radiologist, small bowel and some pancreatic injuries may not be detected.
   b. **Injuries missed with focused abdominal sonography for trauma (FAST)**. FAST is operator-dependent and is intended only to detect fluid in one of four spaces. Diagnostic limitations include the inability to diagnose bowel, mesenteric, pancreatic, diaphragmatic, and some solid organ injuries. Hemoperitoneum may not be present in 29% of patients with proven abdominal injuries. Bowel gas can obstruct critical portions of the image, thus obscuring an injury.
   c. **Injuries missed with diagnostic peritoneal lavage (DPL)**. DPL is extremely sensitive but not specific for the detection of intraperitoneal hemorrhage requiring operative control. DPL does not allow evaluation of retroperitoneal structures and can be difficult to interpret in the presence of a major pelvic injury because of contamination of the peritoneal space. Diaphragmatic injuries are also difficult to detect with DPL.
C. **Miscellaneous factors**
   1. **Nonoperative management** relies on diagnostic studies and physical examination to exclude significant injuries. Hollow organ injuries can be undetected by this approach until a perforation changes the findings on physical examination.
   2. During laparotomy, **failure to adequately examine** the bowel, explore the pancreas, or feel and visualize the diaphragm can lead to missed injuries. **Central retroperitoneal hematomas** can conceal major injuries and need to be completely evaluated during laparotomy.
   3. Half of all missed fractures are not imaged at the time of admission because of attention to primary injuries; another 23% of missed fractures are visible on radiograph, but not appreciated.
      a. **Image quality**. Radiographs taken in the trauma room may be suboptimal, accounting for 10% of missed fractures. Although such films can exclude immediately life-threatening conditions, it may be necessary to obtain additional radiographs in the radiology department after the patient has been stabilized.
      b. **Inadequate or incomplete** views can obscure significant findings. In imaging extremities, injuries can be missed without the inclusion of at least two views and visualization of the joint above and below the suspected injury.
      c. **Findings missed on review**. Many radiographic findings are subtle and may not be recognized on initial review. Obtain follow-up films for persistent complaints of pain.

III. **Commonly missed injuries by region**
   A. **Head and neck**
      1. **Occipital condyle and odontoid fractures** are usually associated with high-energy collisions. Their diagnosis can be enhanced with thin-slice CT images from C2 to the foramen magnum with three-dimensional reconstruction.
      2. **Orbital floor fractures** are difficult to assess in the presence of significant soft-tissue swelling. Sagittal and coronal CT views are often necessary to detect these injuries.
      3. **Carotid injury in blunt neck trauma** classically presents with a focal neurologic deficit with a normal initial CT scan of the head. Bruising (e.g., a seatbelt injury to the neck) should prompt either duplex ultrasonography or arteriography, even without a neurologic deficit.
      4. **Cavernous sinus fistulas** may be occult until symptoms appear. Proptosis and an orbital bruit may be present. Although a CT scan may suggest a lesion, definitive diagnosis is made with angiography or magnetic resonance angiography (MRA).
      5. Suspect **hyoid or laryngeal injury** when a patient with blunt trauma to the neck presents with hoarseness and subcutaneous emphysema.
      6. **Cervical spine fracture-dislocations**. A cervical spine injury should be assumed in any patient with maxillofacial trauma. The lateral cervical spine radiograph may detect only 74% of fractures. Of patients with false-negative radiographs, 30% may be treated subsequently for unstable fractures. The three-view cervical spine series, combined with flexion-extension plain films, CT, or magnetic resonance imaging (MRI), has an accuracy approaching 100%. Carefully review initial radiographs because C1-C2, C7-T1, and unilateral facet fracture-dislocations are cervical injuries that can be easily missed.
      7. **Cord syndromes**. Central or posterior cord syndromes can occur without a spinal fracture. The neurologic symptoms are often attributed to hysteria, intoxication, head injury, or associated injuries.
   B. **Thorax**
      1. **Traumatic rupture of the diaphragm** is unrecognized on presentation in 50% to 69% of patients. This injury can be missed on chest radiograph, CT, ultrasonography, and DPL. Diagnosis can be improved by placing a nasogastric tube, using gastrointestinal contrast, and repeat imaging, thoracoscopy, or laparoscopy.
      2. **Esophageal injury** can be easily missed following a transmediastinal gunshot wound, because early symptoms may not be present. Contrast study with dilute barium, when combined with esophagoscopy, has a 97% diagnostic accuracy.
      3. **Thoracic aortic disruption** can be missed on plain chest radiograph because the mediastinum may be normal in 15% of patients. Rapid, high-resolution spiral CT of the chest in blunt chest injury will identify either an aortic injury or a mediastinal hematoma, which requires arteriography. Transesophageal echocardiography (TEE) can also be useful, especially for the patient in the operating room for other injuries.
      4. **Pneumothorax on supine films** is difficult to appreciate and requires careful review of the radiograph for air density over the diaphragm or an erect image as a follow-up radiograph. These injuries are easily identified on CT of the abdomen or chest.
      5. **Cardiac wounds**. One third of patients with penetrating cardiac wounds present without overt signs and symptoms of cardiac injury. Pericardial ultrasonography or a pericardial window may be required for diagnosis.
      6. **Rib fractures** are frequently missed on conventional radiographs and are often clinically insignificant. However, undiagnosed rib fractures are associated with persistent thoracic wall pain.
      7. **Scapular fractures and acromioclavicular separations** can be detected with careful attention to the physical examination and bony struc-

ture on the chest radiograph. Although early therapy may not be mandatory, early recognition is important as a determinant of high-energy trauma.

C. **Abdomen and pelvis**
  1. **Traumatic abdominal wall hernias** are usually detected by CT; however, they can be missed during urgent laparotomy for other injuries.
  2. **Hollow viscus injuries** to the duodenum, small bowel, and colon can be missed or delayed because abdominal CT is not 100% accurate and physical findings can be delayed or masked. Unexplained fever, tachycardia, leukocytosis, abdominal distention, and abdominal tenderness, when assessable, require repeat or additional studies, including laparoscopy or laparotomy.
  3. **Pancreatic ductal injuries** can be missed on CT, DPL, FAST, and laparotomy. The mortality rate associated with missed pancreatic ductal injuries is ~50%. Completely inspect the pancreas during laparotomy in the presence of a peripancreatic hematoma or suspected injury.
  4. **Biliary duct disruption** can be missed in both blunt and penetrating trauma. When these injuries are missed, patients usually present with either biliary ascites or peritonitis. Diagnosis can be suggested by CT or ultrasonography and confirmed with a hepatic imidoacetic acid (HIDA) scan, percutaneous transhepatic cholangiography (PTC), or endoscopic retrograde cholangiopancreatography (ERCP).
  5. Suspect **rectal injuries** following proximity wounds to the buttocks. Proctoscopy or sigmoidoscopy is necessary to evaluate the rectum, even after a negative exploratory laparotomy.
  6. **Traumatic renal artery occlusion** can be occult because 10% to 15% of cases occur without hematuria. High-resolution CT or angiography is required to diagnose before a laparotomy. At laparotomy, duplex ultrasonography or Doppler ultrasonography may be helpful. Repair is indicated only if the injury is bilateral or in a patient without two kidneys, unless the lesion is detected intraoperatively with a warm ischemia time of <4 hours.
  7. **Ureteral injuries** can be missed in penetrating trauma without complete visualization during exploratory laparotomy.
  8. **Abdominal compartment syndrome (ACS)** requires a high index of suspicion for detection. The patient with multiple injuries who has had massive resuscitation should be assessed for ACS (Chapter 30).
  9. **Adrenal insufficiency** can occur in the intensive care unit following resuscitation in elderly patients, steroid-dependent patients, and those unresponsive to pressor therapy. Hyponatremia, hyperkalemia, and unexplained eosinophilia are diagnostic clues. Diagnosis is made with a cosyntropin stimulation test.

D. **Extremities and spine**
  1. **Fractures and dislocations**. The most commonly missed fractures in the emergency department include those of the wrist, elbow, calcaneus, ribs, and phalanges.
     a. **Radioulnar dislocation**. Up to 50% of these injuries are missed initially because of inadequate radiographic views.
     b. **Posterior dislocations of the shoulder** are uncommon, but frequently missed injuries associated with posterior glenoid rim fractures and anterior compression fractures of the humeral head.
     c. **Carpal bone fractures or dislocations** are frequently missed on radiographs because of soft-tissue swelling, their irregular contour, bony overlap, and the presence of distracting fractures of the metacarpals and distal arm bones. Multiple specialized views and knowledge of fracture patterns increase the detection rate.
     d. **Lisfranc joint injuries**, which are complex fracture-dislocations of the tarsometatarsal apparatus that are frequently overlooked, can lead to chronic disability.

   e. **Multilevel spinal fractures**. During evaluation of a patient with a spinal fracture, a second fracture will be discovered at another level in 15% to 25% of cases.

   f. **Knee fractures**. Most fractures involving the knee are seen on anteroposterior and lateral films. Some types of knee fractures are more difficult to detect by standard views.

    (1) **Tibial plateau fractures** can be seen on tangential or tunnel views.

    (2) Fibular head dislocations can be seen on the lateral view.

  2. **Ligamentous injuries** surrounding the large joints will not be detected on radiographs. A complete examination and selected use of CT or MRI can detect these missed injuries. Small chip fractures can be a clue to a significant ligamentous or tendon injury.

  3. **Arterial injuries**. Color-flow duplex ultrasonography is highly specific (99%) but less sensitive (50% to 95%) compared with angiography for detecting arterial injuries. However, its sensitivity for detecting arterial injuries that require surgical intervention is between 90% and 100%. False aneurysms and arteriovenous fistulas are the most commonly missed injuries. Interpret negative studies with caution, particularly in carotid, axillary, and brachial arteries.

  4. **Lumbosacral root avulsions** are usually missed on initial examination. Patients often have a neurologic deficit that involves varying degrees of lower-extremity motor and sensory loss. MRI may assist in the diagnosis.

  5. **Pelvic fractures**. Sacral, pubic rami, and nondisplaced acetabular fractures frequently are not appreciated on plain films. Thin-slice pelvic CT scans can detect these injuries. A patient with pelvic pain with movement on ambulation has a fracture until proved otherwise by CT.

  6. **Vaginal laceration** can be associated with pelvic fractures and may require speculum examination under anesthesia for diagnosis.

 E. **Pediatrics**

  1. **Child abuse** patterns of injury may not be appreciated by the casual observer (Chapter 47).

  2. **Spinal cord injury without radiologic abnormality (SCIWORA)** is more common in children. Often attributed to head injury or masked by multiple injuries, delay in initiating steroid therapy and stabilizing the spine can increase morbidity.

  3. **Hollow viscus injuries**. A delay in the diagnosis of small bowel injuries occurs in >50% of children with blunt abdominal trauma. Early DPL and CT are not sensitive. On CT scan, pneumoperitoneum, bowel thickening, and unexplained free fluid may be indications of bowel injury. Delayed DPL may help diagnose bowel injury following a nondiagnostic CT scan.

  4. **Monteggia fractures** of the elbow are missed by trauma physicians and attending radiologists 25% to 50% of the time.

  5. **Nondisplaced lateral condyle** elbow fractures are frequently missed.

IV. **Commonly associated injuries**

 A. **Significant brain injury in patients with a Glasgow Coma Scale (GCS) score of 13 to 15**. Although most patients with minor head injury will not develop significant problems, a small percentage (2% to 9%) will have an intracranial lesion that may require neurosurgical intervention, and about 10% to 35% will have posttraumatic findings on CT scan (Chapter 19). Soft-tissue injury, focal defects, basilar skull fracture, and advanced age all increase the likelihood of significant pathology.

 B. **Ocular injuries and orbital fractures**. Patients presenting with facial fractures, especially those involving the orbital bones, have an increased incidence of associated ocular injury and should have an ophthalmologic evaluation. When an orbital injury is associated with impaired visual acuity, an 80% chance exists of ocular injury.

 C. **Nerve root avulsions in traction injuries**. Motorcycle crashes often involve traction injuries to the upper extremities. When associated with head

injury, the underlying traction injury to the cervical nerve roots or brachial plexus may go undetected. MRI or CT myelography assists in this diagnosis.
D. **Seatbelts.** A patient wearing a seatbelt has an increased incidence of sternal fractures, hollow viscus injury, and hyperflexion fracture of the lumbar spine (Chance fracture).
E. **Calcaneal and spinal column fractures** are common in patients who fall from heights. Presence of either fracture should prompt an investigation for the other.
F. **Dislocation of the knee with popliteal artery injury** can occur in the presence of normal pulses. Failure to recognize this injury is a major cause of amputation. Because of the associated high morbidity, evaluate the popliteal artery following knee dislocation.
G. **Elbow dislocation** is an orthopedic emergency because it can compromise the **brachial artery**.

Axioms
- Musculoskeletal injuries are the most commonly missed injuries in trauma patients.
- A tertiary survey, including a careful review of all admitting imaging studies, is the best method of detecting missed injuries.
- Central retroperitoneal hematomas require exploration.
- Tell patients and families on admission that other injuries may be discovered during the patient's hospital course.
- Clear documentation and communication among members of the trauma team are essential to avoid missed injuries.
- Correct life-threatening problems as they are discovered.
- Neck veins may not be distended in the hypovolemic patient with tamponade.
- Presence of Doppler signals and palpable pulses does not exclude vascular injury.
- Before discharge, personally observe the patient standing and ambulating.
- Do not rely on "wet readings" of radiologic studies without personal review.

Bibliography
Enderson BL, Reath DB, Meadors J, et al. The tertiary trauma survey: a prospective study of missed injury. *J Trauma* 1990;30:666–669.

Enderson BL, Maull, KI. Missed injuries. *Surg Clin North Am* 1991;71:399–418.

Hirshberg A, Wall MJ Jr, Allen MK, et al. Causes and patterns of missed injuries in trauma. *Am J Surg* 1994;168:299–303.

Janjua KJ, Sugrue M, Deane SA. Prospective evaluation of early missed injuries and the role of tertiary trauma survey. *J Trauma* 1998;44:1000–1006.

Robertson R, Mattox R, Collins T, et al. Missed injuries in a rural area trauma center. *Am J Surg* 1996;172:564–567.

Scalea TM, Phillips TF, Goldstein AD, et al. Injuries missed at operation: nemesis of the trauma surgeon. *J Trauma* 1988;28:962–967.

Sung CK, Kim KH. Missed injuries in abdominal trauma. *J Trauma* 1996;41:276–282.

40. ANESTHESIA FOR THE TRAUMA PATIENT

Michael Rodrick, James W. Krugh, and C. William Hanson, III

I. **Introduction.** Anesthetic management of the trauma patient begins in the trauma resuscitation area and continues into the Operating Room (OR) and the Intensive Care Unit (ICU). The specific role for the anesthesiologist varies according to local practice, but it may include initial airway evaluation and management, assistance in the primary survey, intraoperative management and postoperative intensive care management.

II. **Evaluation**

A. **Airway.** All patients arriving in the trauma resuscitation area are treated with supplemental oxygen by facemask. The patient's response to simple questions provides meaningful information about mentation and airway competence. The airway should be examined immediately for foreign bodies, vomitus or blood, and suctioned as needed. Continuous reassessment of the airway is mandatory.

B. **Breathing.** Inspection and auscultation of the chest is an integral part of the primary assessment. Tracheal deviation, paradoxical chest wall motion or chest wall injuries may be visualized. Immediately life-threatening injuries include tension pneumothorax, open pneumothorax, massive hemothorax, flail chest, pulmonary contusion and cardiac tamponade; these injuries require immediate intervention.

C. **All victims of blunt trauma** must be presumed to have a cervical spine injury. Cervical spine immobilization should be maintained with a cervical collar until the cervical spine is cleared.

D. **If the airway** is patent and breathing is adequate, continue with the primary survey. If gas exchange is inadequate, support the patient with mask ventilation and prepare for endotracheal intubation.

E. **Endotracheal intubation** (see Chapter 14).

1. If time permits, a quick evaluation of the patient's airway may alert the clinician to the possibility of a difficult airway.

a. **Gross evaluation.** Evaluate dentition, jaw opening, micrognathia or macrognathia. Temporomandibular joint disruption may make an otherwise routine airway very difficult because of limited jaw opening.

b. **Thyromental distance.** A length of less than 6 cm. (three finger breadths) from the lower edge of the mandible to the thyroid notch is predictive of difficult intubation.

c. **Mallampati test.** Inability to visualize the uvula when a patient protrudes their tongue (Mallampati Class III or IV) is a sensitive but nonspecific indicator of a difficult airway.

d. **Atlantoaxial joint.** Movement of this joint is important in aligning the pharyngeal and laryngeal axes. However, cervical spine immobility must be maintained in the trauma patient; this makes intubation more difficult.

2. **All necessary equipment** should be ready prior to induction. A back up laryngoscope handle, several blades of varying size, endotracheal tube with stylet, and a functioning suction device with a Yankauer tip must be available.

3. **As discussed** in Chapter 14, as many as three people are required for intubation: the individual intubating the patient, a person to hold cricoid pressure and a third person to provide cervical spine immobilization. Cricoid pressure (Sellick maneuver) is a necessity, because all trauma patients are assumed to have a full stomach. Cricoid pressure must be maintained until the endotracheal tube is placed, the cuff is inflated and

correct position is confirmed by auscultation of breath sounds and detection of carbon dioxide in the exhaled gas.

4. **A blind nasotracheal intubation** may be used in awake, spontaneously breathing patients only if performed by someone with skill with the technique. Due to its higher failure rate, more frequent complications (epistaxis), and longer average time to intubation, the nasotracheal route is not the preferred method to achieve a secure airway when alternative approaches are feasible. However, in certain situations, such as the entrapped patient, nasotracheal intubation may be the only possible approach and therefore lifesaving.

5. **Fiberoptic intubation** is a useful alternative approach to the difficult airway. In an emergency setting, however, this technique of airway management is not encouraged. Drawbacks include the time required to perform fiberoptic intubation, difficulty visualizing anatomy in the presence of blood and secretions, possible precipitation of vomiting in the patient with a full stomach and a high failure rate in uncooperative patients.

6. **Excessively** combative patients are best handled with orotracheal intubation after induction and paralysis. Ketamine and succinylcholine are readily absorbed after intramuscular administration and are quite useful in controlling patients in whom intravenous access cannot be obtained. After a definitive airway is established the patient may be more effectively evaluated.

7. **Laryngeal mask airways** (LMA) may prove lifesaving in an emergency situation. An LMA is very quickly and easily placed in most patients, requires minimal training for use, and may be used as a bridge to a definitive airway. Its major drawback in the trauma patient is that it does not protect against aspiration; thus, the LMA represents a temporary airway.

F. **Intubated patients**. Endotracheal tubes placed prior to arrival in the trauma receiving area must be carefully checked for proper position. Determination of the presence of end-tidal carbon dioxide is essential. The most commonly malpositioned tubes are in the right mainstem bronchus, although esophageal intubations are not uncommon. Esophageal obturator airways (EOA) are not in common use, and should be converted promptly to an endotracheal tube.

G. **Surgical airway**. The inability to obtain a definitive airway using conventional techniques is a clear indication for a surgical airway. Severe maxillofacial injury may warrant a surgical airway as the initial means of airway control. In addition, multiple failed attempts at laryngoscopy may convert a patient who can be ventilated into a patient who cannot, creating the need for immediate surgical airway. The preferred method to obtain a surgical airway is a cricothyroidotomy. As access for an urgent airway, cricothyroidotomy is faster and easier to perform than tracheostomy.

III. **Circulation**

A. **The unstable** trauma patient should have two large bore intravenous (IV) lines (at least 16 gauge) secured in the trauma resuscitation area. If antecubital veins are not available, femoral, subclavian or internal jugular veins may be used. Meticulous attention to aseptic technique is often not possible in the trauma resuscitation area; therefore, these lines should be changed within 24 hours.

B. **Intraosseous puncture** may be used for administration of volume and medications in children under six years of age in whom IV access cannot be obtained (see Chapter 47).

C. **In the patient** with profound or persistent hypovolemia from bleeding, early blood transfusion is essential. Crossmatched blood is optimal; however type specific blood may be used if crossmatched blood is delayed. In the case of exsanguination, type O blood (Rh negative for females of childbearing age) may be used.

D. **Hypothermia** (see Chapter 42). Many patients are hypothermic on arrival in the trauma resuscitation area. All IV fluids should be warmed to prevent further loss of body temperature. Techniques to warm fluids include the following.

　　1. **A supply** of prewarmed crystalloid should be kept on hand in the trauma resuscitation area.

　　2. **Standard blood** and fluid warmers. In the event of hypovolemic shock these are of limited utility because of low flow rates.

　　3. **Level I warmer**. (Level I Technologies, Rockland, MA.) This device incorporates large-bore tubing to allow high flow rates. A wide bore stopcock is positioned near the patient to allow for quick changes in the OR.

　　4. Active infusion units that provide rapid delivery of warmed fluids are commercially available. The Rapid Infusion System (RIS) (Haemonetics Corporation, Braintree, MA) combines a 3L reservoir, heater, pumps, and alarms. The reservoir allows mixing of nonsanguinous fluids, blood components, and drugs. The **RIS** allows up to 1.5 to 2.0L/min transfusion through two 8.5 F introducers with pressures <250 mmHg.

IV. History

A. **Attempt** to obtain a past medical history. This may be obtained from the patient or from accompanying family members. A medic alert bracelet may also be invaluable in identifying premorbid disease processes. Past medical problems, drug allergies, medications and time of last meal are all-important pieces of data. Beta-adrenergic blocker or calcium channel blocker agents may blunt the normal tachycardic response to hypovolemia.

B. **Mechanism of injury**. Paramedics can often provide a concise description of the mechanism of injury.

C. **Street drugs**. The trauma patient is frequently under the influence of intoxicants prior to the accident.

　　1. **Alcohol**. Acute intoxication reduces anesthetic drug requirements. Chronic alcohol use leads to a cross-tolerance among anesthetic agents and therefore a higher requirement. The cirrhotic patient may have decreased drug metabolism, an altered volume of distribution and a pre-existing coagulopathy.

　　2. **Cocaine**. Acute intoxication can induce volume contraction, metabolic acidosis, hypertension, myocardial ischemia or infarction, dysrhythmias, seizures or stroke. Volume expansion will correct the metabolic acidosis. Chronic abuse has been associated with delusions and hypotension from depletion of catecholamines.

　　3. **Marijuana**. Acute intoxication can produce hypertension and tachycardia. Chronic use depletes catecholamines and leads to cardiovascular instability.

　　4. **Opioids**. Acute intoxication can produce hypertension and tachycardia. Chronic use will necessitate increased dosages of anesthetic agents. With chronic IV drug abuse, vascular access is a problem, in addition to risk of blood borne infections such as human immunodeficiency virus (HIV) and viral hepatitis. Opioid antagonists (i.e. naloxone) can cause acute withdrawal. Be prepared to treat withdrawal postoperatively.

　　5. **Ketamine**. Ketamine is a phencyclidine derivative which has recently gained popularity as a street drug. Acute intoxication is associated with graphic dreams and behavioral disturbances. Physiologic effects include hypertension, tachycardia, and an increase in cerebral blood flow.

V. Laboratory

A. **Trauma blood work**. Laboratory work should be sent from the trauma resuscitation area. A complete blood count (CBC), chemistry panel, type and screen or type and cross, beta human chorionic gonadotropin (in all females of childbearing age), drug screen and arterial blood gas may be useful.

B. **Electrocardiogram** (ECG) may be useful in evaluating blunt cardiac injuries as well as dysrhythmias and ischemia.

C. **Radiographs** (see Chapter 16.)

VI. Operating room management

A. Intraoperative monitoring is determined by the patient's condition. Insertion of invasive monitors should not delay definitive surgery.

1. **Standard monitors.** ECG, noninvasive blood pressure monitor, pulse oximetry, capnograph or multigas analyzer, oxygen analyzer and temperature should be monitored in the operating room.

2. **Arterial line.** An arterial line is useful in the hemodynamically unstable patient. It allows continuous monitoring of blood pressure as well as reliable access for serial blood gases and laboratories. The radial artery is the preferred site for placement of an arterial line.

3. **Central venous pressure** (CVP). Central veins provides reliable venous access and may be all that is available in a hemodynamically compromised, vasoconstricted patient. CVP may be helpful in assessing volume status in an ongoing resuscitation.

4. **Pulmonary artery catheter** (PAC). May prove useful in the patient with depressed ventricular function, valvular disease, persistent acidosis or unclear volume status.

5. **Transesophageal echocardiography** (TEE). Can be used to evaluate the heart for tamponade, effusion, wall motion abnormalities, ejection fraction, intracardiac air, valve function and volume status. The descending thoracic aorta may be visualized to diagnose aortic rupture or dissection.

6. **Temperature.** Trauma patients are often hypothermic because of exposure at the scene, open injuries, and ongoing resuscitation. Hypothermia causes decreased drug metabolism, impaired coagulation, increased incidence of wound infections and dehiscence as well as increased oxygen consumption from postoperative shivering. Core temperature may be measured via the esophagus, bladder or rectum. Measures to correct or minimize heat loss are as follows:

   a. **Warm OR.** Raising the operating room temperature to 30°C minimizes convective heat losses and is essential to prevent hypothermia. After the patient is normothermic and the patient is systemically well resuscitated, the room temperature may be lowered for OR personnel comfort.

   b. **Warm preparation** and irrigation solutions.

   c. **Warm** all IV fluids.

   d. **Use** a forced air warmer such as the Bair Hugger (Augustine Medical, Eden Prarie, MN) on any part of the patient that is not draped.

   e. **Wrap the head** or exposed limbs with blankets or plastic.

   f. **Heated** humidifier in the anesthetic circuit

7. **Neurological monitoring**

   a. **Intracranial pressure** (ICP) monitoring. An epidural or subarachnoid bolt or equivalent can be used to monitor ICP.

   b. **A ventriculostomy** can be used to monitor ICP as well as to drain cerebrospinal fluid (CSF) for ICP control.

   c. **Patients** with head injuries may be monitored with an electroencephalogram (EEG), brainstem auditory evoked responses or somatosensory evoked potentials.

   d. **Bispectral analysis** (BIS) of the electroencephalogram (EEG) may be used to judge depth of anesthesia and to avoid intraoperative recall.

8. **Coagulation** can be monitored by prothrombin time (PT), partial thromboplastin time (PTT), activated coagulation time (ACT), platelet count and thromboelastogram (TEG). Coagulation should be carefully monitored in patients with severe closed head injury, massive resuscitation, hypothermia or liver dysfunction.

B. Anesthetic induction agents. Thiopental, etomidate, or ketamine are the drugs most commonly used for anesthesia induction. Tables 40.1 through 40.3

Table 40.1 Induction doses and characteristics

Drug	Dose (mg/kg)	Onset (sec)	Duration (min)	Excitation	Pain
Thiopental	3–5*	30	5–8+	+	+
Etomidate	0.2–0.4	15–45	3–12	+++	+++
Propofol	1.5–3.0	15–45	5–10	+	++
Midazolam	0.2–0.4	30–60	15–30	0	0
Ketamine	1–3	45	10–20	+	0

0, None; + minimal; ++, moderate; +++, marked.
* Decrease for suspected hypovolemia.

list induction doses, durations and respiratory as well as cardiovascular side effects of these agents.

If the patient is brought to the OR still hypovolemic or in shock, small doses of an amnestic agent (scopolamine 0.2–0.4 mg, midazolam 1–2 mg or a small dose of ketamine) are used to prevent recall until bleeding is controlled and the blood volume returns toward normal.

1. **Thiopental**
   a. **Dose**: 3–5 mg/kg IV (decrease for hypovolemic patients).
   b. **Respiratory**: moderate depression.
   c. **Cardiovascular**: decreases contractility, cardiac output, and mean arterial pressure (MAP); causes venous dilation.
   d. **Central nervous system** (CNS): cerebral protective by decreasing cerebral metabolic rate (CMR) O2 and ICP.
   e. **Elimination** action ends by redistribution in the body. It is then metabolized by the liver.
   f. **Duration of action**: 5–10 minutes.
   g. **Side effects**: hypotension in the hypovolemic patient. May precipitate acute intermittent porphyria.
2. **Etomidate**
   a. **Dose**: 0.2–0.4 mg/kg IV.
   b. **Respiratory**: mild depression.
   c. **Cardiovascular**: no significant change in any cardiovascular parameter in a normovolemic patient.
   d. **CNS**: cerebral protective by decreasing cerebral metabolic rate (CMR) O2 and ICP; probably not as protective as thiopental.
   e. **Elimination**: action ends by redistribution in the body, then metabolism by the liver.
   f. **Duration of action**: 5–10 minutes.

Table 40.2 Cardiovascular and respiratory effects of induction drugs

Drug	Respiratory depression	MAP	HR	CO	Contractility	SVR	Venous dilatation
Thiopental	++	—	+	—	—	–	++
Etomidate	+	0	0	0	0	0	0
Propofol	++	—	–	–	–	—	++
Midazolam	+	0/–	–/+	0/–	0	–/0	+
Ketamine	0/+	++	++	+	+/–	+/–	0

—, Marked decrease; –, mild decrease; 0, no change, +, mild increase; ++, marked increase.
MAP, mean arterial pressure; HR, heart rate; CO, cardiac output; SVR, systemic vascular resistance.

Table 40.3 Central nervous system effects of common induction drugs

Drug	CMR O$_2$	CBF	CPP	ICP
Thiopental	—	—	–/0	—
Etomidate	—	—	0/+	—
Propofol	—	—	–/–	—
Midazolam	–	–/0	0	–
Ketamine	+	++	–/0/+	+

—, Marked decrease –, mild decrease; 0, no change; +, mild increase; ++ marked increase.
CMR, cerebral metabolic rate; CBF, cerebral blood flow; CPP, cerebral perfusion pressure; ICP, intracranial pressure.

      g. Side effects: causes excitement on induction. Pain on injection may be decreased by IV lidocaine prior to injection. Inhibits adrenocortical functions.

  3. Propofol

      a. Dose: 1.5–3.0 mg/kg.

      b. Respiratory: moderate depression.

      c. Cardiovascular: large decrease in systemic vascular resistance and increased venous dilatation; may have marked decrease in blood pressure with induction dose.

      d. CNS: Mild decrease in ICP.

      e. Elimination: action ends by redistribution in the body, then metabolism by the liver.

      f. Duration of action: 5–10 minutes.

      g. Side effects: causes mild excitement on induction. Pain on injection may be decreased by IV lidocaine prior to injection. Cardiovascular depression with resultant hypotension is common with propofol administration.

  4. Midazolam

      a. Dose: 0.2–0.4 mg/kg.

      b. Respiratory: mild depression.

      c. Cardiovascular: little or no change in the cardiovascular system with normovolemic patient.

      d. CNS: mild decrease in ICP.

      e. Elimination: action ends by redistribution in the body, then metabolism by the liver.

      f. Duration of action: 15–30 minutes. Major problem in the head injured patient because a neurological examination may not be repeated quickly.

      g. Side effects: minimal.

  5. Ketamine

      a. Dose: 1–3 mg/kg IV, 5 mg/kg intramuscularly (IM).

      b. Respiratory: minimal depression, is a bronchodilator (useful in asthmatic patients).

      c. Cardiovascular: increased heart rate, contractility, cardiac output and MAP.

      d. CNS: increases CMR O2, cerebral blood flow (CBF), and ICP. Should not be used in head injured patients or in patients with coronary artery disease.

      e. Elimination: action ends by redistribution in the body, then metabolism by the liver.

      f. Duration of action: 10–20 minutes.

      g. Side effects: good analgesic; excitement postoperatively, possible hallucinations (structurally related to phencyclidine).

Table 40.4 Doses and durations of neuromuscular drugs

Drug	Relaxant dose (mg/kg)	Intubation dose (mg/kg)	Duration in minutes (after intubating dose)
Succinylcholine		1.0–2.0	5–10
Rocuronium	0.3–0.4	0.6–1.0	45–75
Rapacuronium	0.5	1.5–2.0	10–20
Cisatracurium	0.1	0.15–0.2	45–90
Vecuronium	0.05	0.1–0.2	45–90
Pancuronium	0.05	0.08–0.12	60–120

   h. May be given IM in the combative patient to provide safe contact with the patient.
  C. Neuromuscular blocking agents. See Table 40.4 for doses and Table 40.5 for a summary of cardiovascular effects.
   1. Succinylcholine. The only clinically used depolarizing agent.
     a. Dose: 1.0–2.0 mg/kg. If pretreated with a nondepolarizer, dose is increased to 1.5–2.0 mg/kg. Double the dose if given intramuscularly.
     b. Duration: excellent intubating conditions in 45 seconds, duration 5–10 minutes.
     c. Elimination: metabolized by plasma cholinesterase (pseudocholinesterase). Pseudocholinesterase levels may be abnormally low because of a genetic defect or liver dysfunction, either of which will prolong duration of action of succinylcholine.
     d. Cardiovascular effects: stimulates nicotinic receptors in sympathetic and parasympathetic ganglia, and muscarinic receptors in the sinoatrial node of the heart. Dysrhythmias such as bradycardia, sinus arrest and junctional arrhythmias may follow succinylcholine administration, particularly after repeated doses.
     e. Complications
       (1) Hyperkalemia: serum potassium rises 0.5 mEq/L in normal patients. A marked rise in serum potassium, sufficient to cause cardiac arrest may be seen in burn patients (after 24 hours), massive crush injury (usually after several days), patients with neuromuscular diseases or upper motor neuron lesions and in renal failure patients.
       (2) Increased intraocular, intragastric and intracranial pressures: may be due to fasiculations and may be partially attenuated by pretreatment with a nondepolarizer. Use carefully with open globe injury.
       (3) Postoperative myalgias: associated with fasciculations.

Table 40.5 Autonomic effects of neuromuscular agents

Drug	Autonomic ganglia	Cardiac muscarinic receptors	Histamine release
Succinylcholine	Stimulates	Stimulates	Slight
Rocuronium	None	None	None
Rapacuronium	None	None	Slight
Cisatracurium	None	None	None
Vecuronium	None	None	None
Pancuronium	None	Blocks moderately	None

(4) **Malignant hyperthermia**: succinylcholine is a known trigger of malignant hyperthermia.
  f. **Recommendations:** 1.0–2.0 mg/kg intubating dose is the gold standard for a rapid sequence induction (if not contraindicated).
2. **Rocuronium**
  a. **Dose:** intubation dose 0.6–1.0 mg/kg.
  b. **Onset:** excellent intubating conditions in 60 seconds with a dose of 1.0 mg/kg.
  c. **Duration:** 30–45 minute duration of action.
  d. **Elimination:** eliminated in bile or stored in the liver.
  e. **Cardiovascular effects:** none.
  f. **Complications:** none.
  g. **Recommendations:** 1 mg/kg of rocuronium has been used with good results for a rapid sequence induction.
3. **Rapacuronium**
  a. **Dose:** intubation dose 1.5–2.0 mg/kg.
  b. **Onset:** excellent intubating conditions in 60–90 seconds.
  c. **Duration:** less than 20 minute duration with a dose of up to 2.0 mg/kg.
  d. **Elimination:** metabolized by liver and excreted by the kidney.
  e. **Cardiovascular effects:** causes histamine release which may result in hypotension and tachycardia.
  f. **Complications:** bronchospasm from histamine release, prolonged duration of action in renal failure from build up of a pharmacologically active metabolite.
4. **Cisatracurium**
  a. **Dose:** 0.15–0.20 mg/kg intubation dose.
  b. **Onset:** excellent intubating conditions in 2–3 minutes.
  c. **Duration:** 60 minute duration of action.
  d. **Elimination:** degraded by Hoffman elimination in the plasma. Elimination is independent of hepatic and renal function.
  e. **Cardiovascular effects:** none.
  f. **Complications:** none.
5. **Vecuronium**
  a. **Dose:** intubation dose of 0.1–0.2 mg/kg.
  b. **Onset:** excellent intubating conditions 2–3 minutes.
  c. **Duration:** 45–60 minute duration of action.
  d. **Elimination:** metabolized in the liver and excreted unchanged in the kidney.
  e. **Complications:** none.
  f. **Recommendations:** may be used for rapid sequence induction. To speed onset of adequate intubating conditions, 0.01 mg/kg followed after 3 minutes by 0.15 mg/kg will provide sufficient relaxation within 60–90 seconds.
6. **Pancuronium**
  a. **Dose:** intubation dose of 0.08–0.12 mg/kg.
  b. **Onset:** excellent intubating conditions in 3 minutes.
  c. **Duration:** 60 + minute duration of action.
  d. **Elimination:** eliminated by the kidneys with slight hepatic metabolism.
  e. **Cardiovascular effects:** mildly vagolytic.
  f. **Complications:** tachycardia.
D. **Maintenance of anesthesia**
  1. **Standard inhalation** agents can be used after restoration of intravascular volume and correction of acidosis. Judicious doses of agents with minimal hemodynamic effects (scopolamine, benzodiazepines, ketamine) can be used in the unstable patient to prevent intraoperative awareness. Drugs are chosen based on the postoperative plan for the patient. Short acting agents may be preferred if the patient is to be awakened rapidly

postoperatively. If continued ventilator support is necessary because of associated injuries, then a larger dose or longer acting opioids and neuromuscular agents should be used.

E. Common intraoperative problems. Continuous communication with the surgeon is essential in caring for the multiply injured patient. Sudden changes in vital signs must be communicated so that potentially occult injuries can be diagnosed. Similarly, the surgeon should be expected to give some notice when major bleeding can be expected to occur (i.e. before unclamping a vessel). In the event of persistent hypotension due to hypovolemia, the surgeon may pack off an area of uncontrolled bleeding or clamp a vessel until volume may be restored.

   1. Hypothermia. See discussion above on temperature monitoring and treatment. Mild hypothermia (34°C) has a cerebral protective effect in the event of cerebral ischemia. A damage control closure of the abdomen may be appropriate in the event of uncontrolled bleeding in a hypothermic patient.

   2. Massive transfusion (see Chapter 43).

      a. Type O and type specific blood must be available for immediate use in any trauma center. Crossmatched blood should be available within an hour of the patient's arrival at the trauma center. Rapid acquisition of fresh frozen plasma and platelets must be assured. Close communication with the blood bank is essential.

      b. Use of intraoperative blood salvage techniques can markedly reduce the amount of banked blood required. Contamination with intestinal contents is a contraindication to blood salvage procedures.

      c. Coagulation parameters such as PT, PTT and platelet count must be monitored. TEG and ACT may also be utilized.

   3. Hypoxemia may develop because of pulmonary contusion, pulmonary edema, pneumothorax (simple or tension), or misplaced endotracheal tube. This may occur at any time during an operative procedure. Patients with displaced rib fractures, subcutaneous emphysema or pneumothorax should have a chest tube inserted prior to receiving positive pressure ventilation.

   4. Hypotension: even transient drops in blood pressure have been shown to have adverse effects on survival in patients with head injury.

   5. Abdominal hypertension. Massive transfusion or significant abdominal injuries can result in intra-abdominal hypertension and abdominal compartment syndrome. This may manifest as elevated peak inspiratory pressures, decreased urine output, hypotension and decreased cardiac output. The condition is often observed on closure of the abdominal fascia. If abdominal compartment syndrome is suspected, a damage control closure should be employed.

F. Extubation. Timing of extubation should be discussed with the surgeon.

   1. It may be appropriate to extubate the stable trauma patient in the OR at the end of the operation. All trauma patients are considered to have a full stomach, so extubation should not occur until the stomach is emptied and the patient is able to protect his airway.

   2. In the multiply injured patient, extubation may be delayed until the patient has been stabilized and ongoing issues have been resolved. With a history of substance abuse, comorbid conditions, or in the elderly, delayed extubation may be more appropriate. In the severely head injured patient or in the event of significant maxillofacial trauma, an early tracheostomy should be considered.

G. Transfer to postoperative care. At the completion of operative procedures the patient is taken to either the postanesthesia care unit (PACU) or an ICU. A complete report and plan should be communicated to the receiving caregiver. This report should include the following:

   1. History: A brief description of the mechanism of injury, allergies, medical problems and pre-operative medications should be given.

2. **Procedure.** Describe the operative procedure and significant findings. Were there any surgical or anesthetic complications?
3. **Airway.** If the patient is still intubated, discuss the plan for ventilation and extubation. A difficult intubation must be communicated to avoid a problem after extubation. Any difficulty with ventilation in the OR must be described.
4. **Fluids.** Describe blood and fluid losses in the OR as well as all replacement fluids. Fresh frozen plasma, platelets and any other coagulation products administered must be mentioned. Report how much blood is still available in the blood bank.
5. **Medications.** Muscle relaxants, sedatives and amnestic agents used as well as time of administration are important. Postoperative neurologic checks may be important and administration of certain medications may delay these examinations. Communicate when the next dose of antibiotics or steroids is due.
6. **Laboratory data.** Communicate the most recent hemoglobin, blood gas and any other pertinent laboratory data.
7. **Lines.** Describe chest tubes, central lines, volume lines, etc. Were the lines placed in the OR or trauma resuscitation area? Were radiographs obtained after line placement?

Bibliography

Advanced trauma life support for doctors, 6th ed. Chicago: American College of Surgeons, 1998.

Barash, PG, Cullen, BF, et al. *Clinical anesthesia*, 2nd ed. Philadelphia: JB Lippincott, 1996.

Miller RD, ed. *Anesthesia*, 5th ed. Philadelphia: Churchill Livingstone, 2000.

Rodricks MB, Deutschman CS. Emergent airway management. *Crit Care Clin* July 2000.

41. TRAUMA PAIN MANAGEMENT

Kimberly K. Cantees and Donald M. Yealy

I. **Basic principles of analgesia**. Six basic principles of analgesia apply in all types of pain management.
   A. **Individualize the route and dose of analgesic.**
      1. Patients respond differently to painful stimuli based on the type and severity of injury, psychological make-up, and ethnic bias. In addition, individual analgesic requirements vary based on the time of day and previous use of analgesics or recreational substances. Although starting doses are offered (Table 41.1), the amount and timing should be altered based on the response.
      2. Patients may have expectations of being completely pain-free, or insensate; these expectations are often unrealistic. Provide adequate analgesia, defined as enhancing comfort to a tolerable level without side effect. The expected level of relief should be discussed with each patient to ensure understanding by both the provider and receiver.
      3. Intramuscular injection offers little analgesic advantage over oral or intravenous administration due to erratic absorption and pain on injection. The variable absorption with IM injection (due to hydration, sympathetic tone, muscle site and time of day factors) limits the ability to titrate analgesia to need in a timely fashion, forcing the physician to estimate the correct dose (which is inaccurate in up to two-thirds of cases). This route should rarely be used and can be replaced with subcutaneous injections (which are less painful) in those who cannot tolerate oral medicines or without intravenous access.
   B. **Offer analgesics on a time-contingent basis**.
      1. Time-contingent dosing affords steady blood levels of analgesia, avoiding the wide fluctuations with prn dosing. It also avoids making the patient request medication, still allowing for refusal if not needed; this increases the sense of empowerment and satisfaction, augmenting the perceived analgesia.
      2. Time-contingent dosing is suggested for all analgesic preparations, including NSAIDs, acetaminophen and opioid analgesics. When providing oral analgesics, offer the medication based on the pharmacologic profile (e.g., hydrocodone or oxycodone every 4–6 hours around the clock instead of prn), particularly in the acute phase of injury. Parenteral opioids should be administered on a time-contingent basis as well, by hourly infusion (e.g., morphine, 1–2 mg/hr in opioid naive patients) or via patient-controlled analgesia (PCA) device.
   C. **Opioids are the cornerstone of acute severe pain management**.
      1. Intravenous opioids offer the best opportunity to deliver rapid, titrated, adequate analgesia. Opioids, given in small increments every 5–10 minutes (e.g. morphine 2–5 mg or fentanyl 50–100 mcg for most adults), based on the pain and physiologic responses, remain the best agents for severe injury or initial postoperative pain. Oral opioids are inexpensive, effective, and tolerated well by patients with ongoing moderate to severe pain after the initial injury or postoperative period.
   D. **Combination therapy affords the best analgesia, especially in mild to moderate pain syndromes and after acute severe pain is initially controlled**.
      1. Include a NSAID preparation with an opioid whenever possible to provide analgesia by two different and synergistic methods. All NSAID have similar effects when given in equipotent doses, and the least expensive drug and route should be used for most patients (Table 41.2).

Table 41.1 Opioid analgesics

Name	Equianalgesic dose (mg) Oral (mg and hour interval in adults)	IV* (mg and hour interval in adults)	Starting oral dose Adults (mg and hour interval)	Children (mg/kg)
Pure agonists				
–Morphine	30 q 3–4	5 q 1–2	15–30 q 3–4	0.3
–Meperidine (Demerol)	300 q 2–3	75 q 2–3	Not recommended	
–Hydromorphone (Dilaudid)	4–6 q 3–4	1 q 3–4	2–4 q 4–6	0.06
–Codeine†	120–130 q 3–4	—	30–60 q 3–4	0.5–1
–Oxycodone (Roxicodone, Percocet, others)	30 q 3–4	—	10–20 q 3–4	0.3
–Hydrocodone (Lortab, Lorcet, Vicodin, others)	30 q 3–4	—	10–20 q 3–4	—
–Methadone	20 q 6–8	5 q 6–8	5–10 q 6–8	0.2
–Levorphanol (Levo-Dromoran)	4 q 6–8	1 q 6–8	2–4 q 6–8	0.04
–Fentanyl	—	0.05 q 0.5–1 (50 µg)	—	—
Mixed agonist-antagonists				
–Nalbuphine (Nubain)	—	5 q 3–4	—	—
–Butorphanol (Stadol)	—	1 q 2–4	—	—

* After initial titration, which is done using this dose at 10-minute intervals based on response; these are not recommended final doses but equipotent intial doses.
† Sedating and constipating in doses > 60–90 mg; oxycodone and hydrocodone preferred.
q, every.

    a. Ketorolac (30–60 mg i.m. or 15–30 mg i.v.) is the only NSAID available for parenteral use. It is no more potent than oral ibuprofen (800 mg) or indomethacin (50 mg), although much more expensive than these NSAID and generic morphine or meperidine. Ketorolac should be reserved for short-term use (<3 days) in those patients who are unable to take an inexpensive NSAID orally.

    b. Newer selective oral NSAID (termed **COX-2 inhibitors**) offer analgesic and antiinflammatory effects similar to traditional NSAID with a lower frequency of GI side effects and less anti-platelet effects. Celecoxib (100 mg BID initially) and **rofecoxib** (12.5–25 mg once daily to start, maximum 50 mg/daily) are available currently although with limited FDA sanctioned use (primarily arthritis treatment). Aside from dosing differences and the known cross-allergic potential shared with sulfonamides and celecoxib, both COX-2 inhibitors are effective in inflammatory based pain syndromes. However, they are more expensive that traditional NSAID, and do not avoid GI or renal side effects; they should be reserved for those patients intolerant of traditional NSAID or at high risk for complications.

2. Similarly, **acetaminophen** may augment opioid and NSAID analgesia, allowing greater pain relief with less toxicity. When using acetaminophen/

Table 41.2 Non-opioid analgesics/NSAID

Drug	Usual adult dose	Usual pediatric dose	Comments
Oral			
-Acetaminophen	650–1000 mg q 4 h	10–15 mg/kg q 4 hr	Acetaminophen lacks anti-inflammatory activity
-Aspirin	650–1,000 mg q 4 h	10–15 mg/kg q 4 h*	The standard against which other NSAIDs are compared. Inhibits platelet aggregation irreversibly (lasts 2 weeks); may cause postoperative bleeding
-Ibuprofen (Motrin, others)	400–600 mg q 4–6 h	10 mg/kg q 6–8 h	Available as several brand names and as generic
-Naproxen (Anaprox, Naprosyn others)	500–550 mg initial dose followed by 250–275 mg q 6–8 h	NA	Available as several brand names and as generic
Parenteral			
-Ketorolac tromethamine (Toradol)	30–60 mg i.m. or 15 mg i.v. initial dose followed by 15 or 30 mg q 6 hr		Parenteral use should not exceed 5 days

* Contraindicated in presence of fever or other evidence of viral illness.
† With the possible exception of trisalicylate and salsalate, all NSAID exhibit reversible antiplatelet effects. Also, these doses are associated with peak analgesic effects, although increased doses cause increased anti-inflammatory affects along with more side effects.
NSAID, nonsteroidal anti-inflammatory drug.

opioid combination preparations, attention to the daily acetaminophen dose is required to avoid toxicity, especially in patients with liver disease.

3. Antiemetics and phenothiazine/butyrophenone[s1] **do not** augment analgesia and may increase side effects (especially sedation and hypotension). These agents should be used to treat specific conditions but not routinely added to analgesic regimens.

4. **Benzodiazepines** (midazolam, diazepam, lorazepam) are pure sedatives. These drugs lessen anxiety, produce amnesia and cause skeletal muscular relaxation, augmenting the perceived analgesia. However, pure sedatives should not be used alone to treat pain because of their lack of analgesia; if used in combination with an opioid (e.g., during orthopedic manipulation), the dose of each should be lowered to avoid clinical respiratory depression or hypotension.

E. **Recognize and treat side effects of analgesic therapy.**

1. NSAID drugs are associated with platelet aggregation inhibition, gastrointestinal dysfunction ranging from dyspepsia to gastrointestinal bleeding, renal insufficiency, and (rarely) mental status changes ranging from somnolence to confusion. These complications occur irrespective of the route (i.e., parenteral ketorolac causes similar side effects to any equipotent dose of an oral NSAID); and are treated by discontinuation of the drug.

2. Opioid analgesia is associated with nausea (up to 40% of patients), sedation, itching, constipation, urinary retention and hypotension. Treatment of opioid induced side effects includes decreasing the dose or changing the route of administration of the drug, as well as treating the side effect.

   a. Opioid induced hypotension is the result of diminished peripheral sympathetic tone, histamine release and vasodilation. This usually is mild and transient, but can be dramatic in the sympathetically depleted or hypovolemic patient. Hypotension is best avoided by optimizing volume status and delivering the drug in titrated, small doses. If hypotension occurs, further doses should be withheld and crystalloid bolus infusions given. Opioid antagonists do not reverse opioid induced hypotension.

   b. Itching after an opioid is poorly understood but may be the result of histamine release or opioid receptor activity. Itching occurs with all agents to varying degrees, especially when given intravenously or in the epidural space. Antihistamines may be effective in relieving itching, with opioid antagonists (naloxone 0.1–0.2 mg) used for refractory or severe cases.

   c. Respiratory depression and sedation occur together, with sedation usually preceding clinical respiratory depression. Both can be reversed with incremental doses of an opioid antagonist. We recommend naloxone 0.04 mg every minute if lowered respiratory rate—prepared with 0.4 mg ampule diluted up to 10 cc with saline and given 1 cc at a time—to reverse the excessive effect but maintain analgesia. **For patients with profound coma or apnea, a full dose of naloxone 0.4 mg IV should be given immediately.**

F. **Pain is better treated early rather than later.**

1. There is evidence that "pain begets pain", probably secondary to peripheral and central neuromodulation that occurs after a prolonged painful stimulus such as injury.

2. Early treatment of pain can decrease the overall need for analgesics and improve patient satisfaction. Similarly, avoiding periods of inadequate analgesia will also help avert up-regulation of pain receptors and thus, improve pain relief.

3. Early *titrated* pain therapy can alter the sympathetic responses to injury and improve regional blood flow, further aiding resuscitation. Overzealous analgesic administration can produce the opposite response.

II. Overview: trauma pain management

A. The principles of pain management in the trauma patient include the basic analgesic principles outlined and principles of acute postoperative pain management.

B. Certain trauma patients present with special needs: patients with severe pain during resuscitation, those with substance abuse issues, and those with psychological issues either at the time of the injury or during the rehabilitation phase.

C. A small number of trauma patients will require analgesia for a prolonged period of time, or may develop a chronic pain syndrome as a result of injury. These patients are best managed with a multidisciplinary approach that includes the trauma and primary care physicians, a physician pain specialist, physical therapists and psychosocial clinicians.

III. Analgesia during resuscitation

A. Analgesia should not be withheld during the resuscitation unless one of three conditions exist:

- Hemodynamic instability
- Respiratory depression
- Profound sedation or coma

   In patients without these contraindications, titrated intravenous opioids should be given to attenuate pain with close attention to the physiologic response (especially blood pressure and level of consciousness.) **Any opioid or systemic sedative/induction agent can cause hypotension**, with the frequency and degree being the important difference between regimens.

B. **Fentanyl** causes the least hemodynamic effects and is the agent of choice for pain relief during resuscitation. In doses of 0.25 to 0.50 mcg/kg (50–100 mcg for average adults) every 5 to 10 minutes, it produces safe clinical analgesia up to 60 minutes in most patients. Side effects are treated as noted above. Chest wall rigidity is a rare occurrence, seen mostly with larger doses (>6 mcg/kg boluses). This can compromise ventilation, but is extremely rare in the doses recommended here. It is treated with positive pressure ventilation, opioid reversal agents and (in severe cases) neuromuscular blockade with endotracheal intubation.

C. Other inexpensive opioids (**morphine** 2–5 mg, **meperidine** 50–100 mg, **hydromorphone** 1–2 mg i.v. increments) produce longer analgesia but are associated with more hemodynamic effects. These drugs are best used in well-resuscitated patients. Other synthetic opioids (alfentanil, sufentanil, remifentanil) offer little advantage at a higher cost.

IV. Procedural sedation and analgesia

A. Patients usually require pharmacologic assistance when painful or anxiety-provoking procedures are planned. A continuum exists between mild sedation and systemic analgesia to general anesthesia. **In general, the deeper the intended or potential reflex and responsiveness change, the more closely the patient must be monitored by trained experts**.

B. Environmental and other adjuncts will ease the painful perceptions and anxiety. These include:

1. Comfortable surroundings (dimmed lights, quiet area, music if possible)
2. A calm, clear manner of communication, educating the patient of expected responses and asking for feedback to help improve care (e.g. "If you feel more pain, let me know and I will give more medicine").
3. Splinting and minimal or gentle handling of injured parts.
4. Family or friend presence (if possible, safe and desired).
5. Attempts to distract patient or help him/her think of other soothing or pleasing settings.
6. Local or topical anesthetics to ease nociceptive stimuli.

C. Most procedures can be safely and comfortably performed with mild sedation (no pain involved but anxiety provoking, e.g., radiologic studies) or conscious sedation/systemic analgesia (pain and anxiety anticipated, e.g., wound debridement, joint or fracture care). Monitoring of responses, vital signs, pulse oximetry can be performed by either a physician or a nurse with physician supervision.

1. Opioids are the cornerstone of pain relief during procedures. Titrated fentanyl (0.25–0.5 mcg/kg—often 50–100 mcg in adults) every 2 to 3 minutes based on the response is a common method. Other opioids—morphine or meperidine—are alternates, though the duration and hemodynamic effects differ from the limited amount seen with fentanyl.

2. Benzodiazepines, especially midazolam (1–2 mg increments in adults) or diazepam (2.5- to 5-mg increments), are best for procedures requiring sedation or muscular relaxation. These drugs do not relieve pain, though patients may lack recall of the pain.

3. Combination of opioids and benzodiazepines are often used for procedures that require pain and anxiety relief or pain relief and muscular relaxation. It is best to deliver the benzodiazepine first, and then add titrated doses of the opioid. Care to the effect is critical, since an additive or synergistic effect can occur, risking airway or hemodynamic complications.

4. Other agents can be used, including ketamine (0.25 mg/kg i.v. increments, creating a 'dissociative state' with rare emergence reactions or laryngospasm) and etomidate (0.05–0.1 mg/kg increments, creating good sedation but a small risk of deep sedation).

D. **General anesthesia is not sought in the trauma bay, emergency department or floor outside of rapid intubation**. Procedures requiring this are best performed in the operating room.

E. In the rare instance **when deep sedation is planned** (e.g., for hip relocation or cardioversion), **it should be done where continuous monitoring equipment** (ECG, automated blood pressure and pulse oximeter mandatory, capnography helpful) **are available, with a physician and nurse dedicated solely to delivering drugs and monitoring the patient**. Those two individuals must be expert in recognizing complications and treating them, from knowledge of reversal agents and cardiac drugs through airway support and endotracheal intubation. **The physician performing the procedure cannot safely be responsible for this monitoring.**

1. Because of the needs for close monitoring, deep sedation is often carried out in the operating room, though the emergency department and ICU are acceptable if the proper personnel (skilled in recognizing and treating complications, especially airway related) resources are available.

F. During procedural sedation/systemic analgesia of any level, create a record to document:

1. Immediate preprocedural exam (including noting review of previous exam, allergies, medications and last meal if after initial evaluation).

2. Serial measurement of vital signs, responses to stimuli, oximetry reading and any interventions. This is best done every 5 minutes.

3. Complications, including (but not limited to) vomiting, loss of consciousness or respirations, rhythm changes, rashes, dyspnea, agitation or any involuntary activity.

4. Clear timing of drugs and doses, including route.

5. Recovery period, including return to pre-procedural state or age appropriate functioning and ability to sit up, walk (if permitted) and take oral liquids.

V. **Special analgesic needs**

A. **Rib fractures/chest wall pain**

1. Rib fractures are in the category of severe pain syndromes; inadequate analgesia may lead to pulmonary compromise and pneumonia. Systemic opioids, especially via scheduled parenteral administration or PCA/continuous drip, are effective in most patients.

2. These patients may benefit from **continuous epidural analgesia.**

a. Indications: moderate to severe pain uncontrolled by systemic opioids, in those with preexisting or impending pulmonary compromise.

   b. Contraindications: Coagulopathy, hypovolemia, spinal fracture or
      skin infection at site of intended placement, and dural tear. Low
      molecular weight heparin should not be used in patients with an
      epidural catheter because of increased risk of epidural hematoma.
   c. Methods: Injection followed by continuous infusion of opioids (preser-
      vative free, usually morphine or fentanyl) and local anesthetics
      (lidocaine or bupivacaine), alone or together. These allow good
      pain relief at lower doses due to placement of the drug near the
      active site.
   d. Success is measured by adequate pain relief and improved pul-
      monary mechanics (or preservation of near normal in those without
      impairment). When a local anesthetic is infused, the dermatomal
      level of block can be estimated from a light tough/pin prick exam.
   e. Duration of therapy depends on the clinical response; generally,
      catheters are removed after 3 to 5 days (although longer intervals
      are acceptable in the absence of complications or infection). Most pa-
      tients can be converted to other systemic regimens within 48 hours.
   f. Epidural catheters should be removed immediately if signs of in-
      fection develop (erythema, drainage) or if they no longer function
      properly.
   g. Respiratory depression is rare compared to equipotent systemic
      doses but can occur early (minutes from injection due to systemic
      absorption) or late (hours after injection from rostral spread).
   h. Itching is common with epidural opioids. Antihistamines or opioid
      antagonists (at low doses) can be used to reverse pruritus from
      epidural opioid administration, with the latter often added in low
      doses to the infusion.
3. Individual intercostal nerve blocks (using 0.25% to 0.5% bupivacaine
   with epinephrine) can also be effective in patients with three or fewer
   rib fractures.
4. Pleural administration of a local anesthetic (e.g., bupivacaine 10–15 mL
   of a 0.25% to 0.5% solution) can afford good pain relief for 6 to 12 hours.
   Although it can be instilled through a thoracostomy tube, this is not recommended in the initial phases of management since the tube must be
   clamped for 20 to 30 minutes to allow contact with the pleura. More
   commonly, a small bore catheter can be placed in the extrapleural space
   during an open chest procedure and used postoperatively as a route for
   pleural anesthesia.
B. Nerve injury
   1. Any trauma may result in direct injury to nerves.
   2. Those patients complaining of pain described as burning, electrical in
      nature, or those patients with pain complaints that seem out of propor-
      tion to the magnitude of traumatic injury, may have neuropathic injury
      (pain from nerve injury).
   3. Opioid analgesia alone is often not beneficial for long term treatment.
      The use of adjuvants are common, including antidepressants and mem-
      brane stabilizers (anti-seizure medications).
      a. Cyclic antidepressants are best for those with this pain and sleep
         disturbance, taking advantage of their sedative effects. Amitripty-
         line (10–25 mg), nortriptyline (25–50 mg) and trazodone (25–50 mg)
         are the commonly used agents. These are usually started at bedtime
         and increased in dose and frequency based on the responses, with
         the lower doses used in the elderly.
      b. Selective serotonin reuptake inhibitor antidepressants can be used
         for others without sleep disturbance (e.g., fluoxetine 20 mg or ser-
         traline 50 mg once daily initially).
      c. Carbamazepine (100–200 mg three times daily) and dilantin (1 g
         initially followed by 100–200 mg twice daily) are also useful, with
         doses adjusted upward as needed.

4. Often, the advice of physicians that deal with advanced pain management is necessary to help with the analgesic plan and titration. Blood levels of these various agents generally do not predict success. Monitoring for side effects is necessary (e.g., serial blood counts and liver function studies in those on carbamazepine and ECG for elderly patients or those with conduction abnormalities in those on a cyclic antidepressant).

C. **Long-term opioid therapy**
1. Those patients requiring multiple surgical procedures, or those with extensive orthopedic injuries (external fixators, pelvic fractures) may require opioid therapy for extended intervals, with the development of opioid tolerance.
2. Patients receiving opioid therapy on a regular basis for more than two weeks are at risk for withdrawal if the opioid is abruptly discontinued. Mixed or partial opioid agonists/antagonists (e.g., butorphanol, pentacozine, nalbuphine) may produce withdrawal and should be avoided.
3. Signs of opioid withdrawal include hypertension, tachycardia, tearing, salivation, piloerection and anxiety.
4. Opioid withdrawal may be avoided by ensuring that opioid therapy is discontinued according to a taper schedule that decreases the amount of opioid by 20% each 24 to 48 hours.

Axioms
- Pain is best treated early and continuously; do not require awake patients to ask for relief.
- Intravenous opioids are the cornerstone of acute severe pain management. NSAIDs and acetaminophen are useful adjuncts in moderate to severe pain, and often adequate in mild to moderate pain syndromes. Morphine is inexpensive and predictable, while fentanyl offers limited hemodynamic effects at a higher (albeit still relatively low) cost and shorter duration of action.
- Intramuscular analgesics should be avoided.
- Analgesic regimens must be tailored to each individual, with variation of 5–10 fold seen in opioid naive patients and even higher in those using these drugs or other sedatives chronically.
- The ideal dose of opioid is the one that creates analgesia without excessive sedation or hemodynamic effect, with ceiling doses based on side effects rather than absolute amounts. Switching between opioids before adequate titration offers little benefit.
- When providing procedural sedation and systemic analgesia, watch for excessive effects (especially respiratory drive and protective reflexes); mishaps are usually related to failure to seek, recognize, or quickly treat excessive sedation.

Bibliography
Acute pain management: operative or medical procedures and trauma. Rockville, MD: US Department of Health and Human Services, Agency for Health Care Policy and Research, February 1992.

Chudnofsky CR, Wright SW, Dronen SC, et al. The safety of fentanyl use in the emergency department. *Ann Emerg Med* 1989;18:635–639.

Grabinski PY, Kaiko RF, Rogers AG, et al. Plasma levels and analgesia following deltoid and gluteal injections of methadone and morphine. *J Clin Pharmacol* 1983; 23:48–55.

Onghena P, Van Houdenhove B. Antidepressant-induced analgesia in chronic nonmalignant pain: a meta-analysis of 39 placebo-controlled studies. *Pain* 1992;49: 205–219.

Ward KR, Yealy DM. Systemic analgesia and sedation in managing orthopedic emergencies. *Emerg Med Clin North Am* 2000;18:141–166.

42. HYPOTHERMIA, COLD INJURY, AND DROWNING

Samuel A. Tisherman

I. **Introduction. Hypothermia**, defined as a body temperature of <35°C, occurs in up to half the victims of major trauma. It is associated with significantly increased morbidity and mortality. **Hypothermia in trauma patients**, which occurs secondary to injury, shock, fluid resuscitation, anesthesia, and alcohol or drug intoxication, must be differentiated from **exposure hypothermia** secondary to medical conditions (e.g., thyroid or adrenal insufficiency, alcohol intoxication). Uncontrolled, accidental hypothermia in these situations must also be differentiated from controlled, therapeutic hypothermia (as used in cardiac surgery and in neurologic injury treatment) with induction of poikilothermia and prevention of shivering.

A. **Classification of hypothermia.** The severity of hypothermia is classified primarily by the patient's core temperature:

Mild: 32°C to 35°C—physiologic findings subtle

Moderate: 28°C to 32°C—signs and symptoms present, but variable

Severe: Below 28°C—central nervous system (CNS) and hemodynamic alterations impending or present (often extreme)

B. **Core temperature must be measured**, which requires special probes that measure low temperatures. Rectal, bladder catheter, central venous, and esophageal thermistors offer the best temperature data. Rectal probes are preferred because of safety and ease of insertion.

II. **Physiology of hypothermia**

A. **Maintenance of temperature** within a narrow range, despite widely varying environmental temperatures, is critical for homeothermic (warm-blooded) animals, such as humans. The normal response to a cold environment is simultaneous minimization of heat loss and increase in heat production.

1. **Heat loss** occurs via radiation, conduction, convection, and evaporation. Hypothermic patients can minimize heat loss by behavioral responses (moving to a warmer environment), use of warm clothing, and cutaneous vasoconstriction.

2. **Increased physical activity, shivering, increased feeding, and nonshivering thermogenesis can increase heat production**. Shivering causes an increase in oxygen consumption for which the patient may not be able to compensate physiologically, vasodilation that can cause more heat loss, and metabolic acidosis. The need for pharmacologic (neuromuscular blockade) treatment of the shivering is controversial.

B. **Clinical effects of hypothermia**. A progression of changes occurs in all physiologic parameters as temperature decreases, with subtle and inconsistent findings seen in mild hypothermia and more predictable abnormalities seen in severe hypothermia.

1. **Metabolic**. The body initially attempts to conserve body heat via increased metabolic activity and shivering in mild hypothermia, which can cause a metabolic acidosis. These responses are lost as hypothermia progresses, with an eventual decrease in metabolism, which can be protective.

2. **Respiratory**. Initially, tachypnea may be seen; with further cooling, however, the respiratory rate slows, eventually leading to apnea. Arterial oxygenation is usually maintained, but tissue oxygenation may be impaired because of intense vasoconstriction and leftward shift in the hemoglobin dissociation curve. Hypothermia alters the measured arterial pH, P_{CO_2}, and P_{O_2}, tempting some to suggest "correcting" blood gas values for the patient's temperature before treating. This is unnecessary because blood gas determinations are performed with the sam-

ple warmed to 37°C; in addition, **use of the "corrected" values has not proved beneficial.**

3. **Hemodynamic.** Tachycardia is common in early or mild hypothermia, but bradycardia is seen with more severe hypothermia. On the ECG, prolonged PR, QRS, and QT intervals; J (Osborn) waves; sinus bradycardia; atrial flutter or fibrillation; and ventricular dysrhythmias can be seen in moderate to severe hypothermia. Below 28°C exists a high risk of ventricular fibrillation (VF), heart block, or asystole. Pulses often are not palpable because of vasoconstriction, even if cardiac function continues and tissue perfusion is adequate for that temperature level. In addition to the cardiac rhythm changes, vasodilation occurs with early hypothermia and shivering, causing further heat loss and predisposing the patient to hypotension. Vasoconstriction occurs as the temperature decreases.

4. **Neurologic.** Changes with mild to moderate hypothermia are often similar to signs of closed head injury (e.g., apathy, confusion, loss of coordination). Despite this, do not attribute an abnormal sensorium in a trauma patient at risk for hypothermia solely to hypothermia; consider closed head injuries, hypovolemia, and alcohol or drug intoxication. With severe hypothermia, coma occurs, often with electroencephalogram silence, although normal neurologic recovery is still likely.

5. **Coagulation.** Hypothermia has important effects on coagulation parameters. One of the most frequent findings is thrombocytopenia caused by platelet sequestration. This is further complicated by abnormal platelet function, leading to prolonged bleeding times. Impairment of the coagulation cascade occurs secondary to decreased enzyme function. Increased plasma fibrinolytic activity can also occur.

6. **Renal.** Hypothermia decreases the ability of the kidney to reabsorb fluid and electrolytes. Consequently, an inappropriate "cold" diuresis often occurs, further increasing the risk of hypotension. As temperature declines further, urine output decreases. Consequently, urine output has limited utility as a marker of adequate organ perfusion.

III. **Hypothermia in trauma**

A. **Predisposition to hypothermia.** In trauma patients, the incidence and severity of hypothermia correlate directly with injury severity. Between 21% and 50% of severely injured trauma patients become hypothermic. Inciting factors include:

1. **Exposure** in the field with inadequate or wet clothing
2. **Blood loss** and shock
3. **Common standard treatments**, including removal of all clothing, rapid infusion of cool fluids, and opening of body cavities
4. **Limited heat production** capabilities caused by injury and hemorrhagic shock; analgesic, sedative, and anesthetic agents; or alcohol and other drugs taken by the patient. General anesthesia can decrease heat production by 20%.

B. **Clinical studies** often have shown higher mortality in trauma patients who become hypothermic. Hypothermia can contribute to complications or simply be a marker of severe injury. As a result of severe trauma and resuscitation attempts, the patient is often hypothermic, coagulopathic, and acidotic. The "damage control" abbreviated laparotomy (rapid control of active arterial bleeding, rapid control of contamination, packing the abdomen, rewarming in the intensive care unit [ICU], and delayed definitive procedures) has been used successfully to break the cycle of bleeding, transfusion, worsening coagulopathy, worsening hypothermia, and more bleeding.

C. **Animal studies** have shown a protective role for **controlled** hypothermia during hemorrhagic shock. In theory, hypothermia can protect organs that are ischemic or are vulnerable to ischemia (especially the brain and heart) and improve outcome. The mechanisms of the beneficial effects of hypothermia include decreased metabolic demands and other poorly understood effects. Based on current understanding of the effects of **unplanned** hypothermia, rapid rewarming of trauma patients is recommended, particularly if they are coagulopathic. Additional studies regarding therapeutic hypothermia are needed.

IV. Treatment

A. **Prevention**. Awareness of the potential for hypothermia in trauma patients is critical. Initiate measures to prevent hypothermia in the field and continue in the emergency department (ED), operating room (OR), and ICU. These include:

1. **Warming the environment** in the transport vehicle, ED, OR, and ICU. Room temperature is a critical determinant of heat loss because it dictates the rate of heat loss by radiation, convection, and evaporation from skin and operative sites.

2. Use of **warm, humidified oxygen.**

3. **Infusion of warmed intravenous (i.v.)** fluids and blood.

4. **Minimization of exposure**. Radiant heat lights can help.

5. **Application of a heating blanket** or other heat-conserving device.

B. **Standard treatment** begins with standard resuscitation efforts (Table 42.1 and Fig. 42.1).

1. **Airway and breathing**. Patients who maintain a patent airway and have some spontaneous ventilation generally do not require urgent intubation. However, endotracheal intubation is indicated for the patient who is apneic or who has lost protective reflexes.

2. **Circulation**. Initiate external chest compressions for all patients with VF or asystole. If a severely hypothermic patient has no pulse but is breathing spontaneously and has evidence of an organized cardiac rhythm on the ECG, cardiac output should be sufficient to maintain the viability

Table 42.1 Treatment of hypothermia

Handle the patient gently

Prevent further heat loss

Evaluate ABC:
–A—Airway
–B—Breathing
–C—Circulation

For the patient in coma, consider empiric treatments:
–D50
–Naloxone
–Thiamine

Options
–Passive external rewarming
–Insulating blanket
–Warm room
–Active external rewarming
–Heating blankets (Bair Hugger)
–Heating lamps
–Immersion
–Active internal rewarming
–Warm intravenous fluids
–Warm, humidified oxygen
–Gastric, colonic, bladder lavage
–Peritoneal, pleural, mediastinal lavage
–Continuous arteriovenous rewarming
–Hemodialysis
–Cardiopulmonary bypass

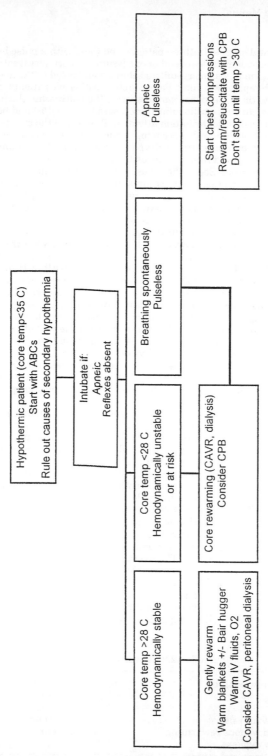

FIG. 42.1. Management of the hypothermic patient. CAVR, continuous arteriovenous rewarming; CPB, cardiopulmonary bypass.

of vital organs. In these patients and those with a pulse but with hypotension or evidence of end-organ dysfunction, primary treatment involves infusion of warm crystalloid solutions and blood (39°C to 40°C) coupled with rapid rewarming. For severely hypothermic patients in VF, attempt up to three electrical countershocks. If unsuccessful, the patient should have ongoing cardiopulmonary resuscitation (CPR) and be warmed before further defibrillation attempts. To improve the chances for successful defibrillation at these temperatures, bretylium is thought to be more effective than lidocaine. Hypovolemia, caused by capillary leak, "cold diuresis," and injuries, needs to be corrected.

3. **Neurologic.** Seek other causes of coma, especially those that are easily reversed (e.g., head trauma, hypoglycemia, electrolyte abnormalities, drug overdose) and treat using dextrose 50%, naloxone, flumazenil, or thiamine, as appropriate. Additionally, provide spinal immobilization if any risk exists of torso or head injury.

C. **Procedures, patient handling, and VF.** As the core temperature decreases to 28°C and below, the risk of **spontaneous VF** increases. This risk can be enhanced by physical stimuli, although a causal relationship has not been proved. It seems prudent to **gently handle all patients with moderate to severe hypothermia.** Perform only those procedures absolutely necessary. On the other hand, **do not withhold intubation in apneic patients or those unable to maintain airway patency,** but perform it with care. Prophylactic bretylium and topical anesthesia may be considered, but are of uncertain benefit. Because of the risk of precipitating VF, withhold naso- and orogastric tubes, urinary bladder catheters, central venous cannulae, and dramatic physical repositioning or movement of the patient with severe hypothermia until the core temperature increases to mild to moderate hypothermia levels. Patients with mild hypothermia have a negligible risk of VF and should have procedures and transport in the usual fashion.

D. **Drug therapy.** Avoid nonessential drugs in hypothermic patients because of unpredictable metabolism, which can lead to toxicity as the patient rewarms.

E. **Signs of irreversibility.** Hypothermic patients may appear dead. Nonetheless, start resuscitative efforts and persist until moderate to severe hypothermia is completely reversed (i.e., the patient is nearly normothermic). The only exceptions are for those patients who have sustained other injuries incompatible with life or when hypothermia is the natural result of the poikilothermic state created with prolonged cardiac arrest in initially normothermic patients. Initial metabolic parameters (e.g., a pH <6.8 or a potassium >7.0 mEq/L) are **relative** markers of irreversibility.

V. **Rewarming.** In hypothermic trauma patients, after the primary survey has been completed and the ABCs (airway, breathing, circulation) have been addressed, initiate rewarming. The average warming rates of commonly used rewarming techniques are listed in Table 42.2.

A. **Mild hypothermia (32°C to 35°C).** Treat patients with **mild hypothermia** with passive, external rewarming methods (e.g., insulating blankets, or active, external rewarming methods such as heating blankets or convective air warmers) (Bair Hugger, Augustine Medical, Inc., Eden Prairie, MN).

Table 42.2 Rewarming rates

Passive external rewarming	0.5°C to 2°C/hour
Shivering	3°C to 4°C/hour
Heated O$_2$	1°C to 2.5°C/hour
Peritoneal lavage/dialysis	1°C to 2.5°C/hour
Continuous arteriovenous rewarming	2°C to 3°C/hour
Cardiopulmonary bypass	10°C/hour

B. Moderate hypothermia (28°C to 32°C). External rewarming alone of moderately to severely hypothermic patients can lead to "after-drop," a decrease in core temperature partly caused by cold peripheral blood flowing to the core as peripheral vasodilation occurs. Patients with **moderate hypothermia** need more active, internal rewarming methods (e.g., warm i.v. fluids and warm inspired gas). Gastric, colonic, or bladder lavage; peritoneal, pleural, or mediastinal lavage; or hemodialysis may be indicated. Continuous arteriovenous rewarming (CAVR) recently has been described for use in hypothermic patients. A heparin-bonded extracorporeal circuit with a countercurrent warming device is attached to cannulas placed in the femoral artery and vein. Venovenous rewarming also can be used in a similar fashion by adding a roller pump.

C. Severe hypothermia (<28°C). The **severely hypothermic** patient is at very high risk of cardiac arrest, particularly if dysrhythmias are already present. Use of cardiopulmonary bypass (CPB), initiated via the femoral vessels or the chest, is the treatment of choice, because CPB is the most efficient rewarming method and its additional benefit is that it can support circulation in the event of cardiac arrest. If hemodynamics are adequate and dysrhythmias have not occurred, active, internal rewarming may be appropriate as long as CPB is available should the patient's condition deteriorate.

VI. Special situations

A. Exposure hypothermia (without trauma) causes ~100,000 deaths worldwide each year. To enhance survival, it is essential (*a*) to recognize patients who are at risk; (*b*) accurately identify the condition using core temperature measurements; and (*c*) initiate appropriate therapy early.

1. **Risk factors**
   a. Extremes of age (the elderly and neonates/infants)
   b. Alcohol, sedative, or illicit drug use
   c. Concomitant neurologic disease or injury, especially stroke and spinal cord lesions
   d. Dermal disruption, including burns
   e. Certain medications, including adrenergic blockers, antipsychotics, and antidepressants
   f. Endocrinologic diseases (e.g., hypothyroidism and hypoadrenalism)
   g. Submersion and immersion

2. **The cause of hypothermia may not be exposure alone.** Clinical clues of the presence of an underlying cause of hypothermia include absence of bradycardia; inability to increase temperature with routine measures; abnormal mental status, stupor, or coma after rewarming to >32°C in the absence of head trauma, or a period of cardiac arrest.

B. Drowning, defined as suffocation from submersion in a liquid medium, is a common cause of accidental death, particularly in children. Risk factors for drowning and near drowning (submersion with recovery) include hypothermia, inability to swim, diving accidents, alcohol and drug ingestion, and exhaustion. Submersion rapidly leads to hypothermia.

1. **Pulmonary failure** is common after drowning unless aspiration is prevented by laryngospasm, which occurs in 10% to 20% of victims. Freshwater aspiration causes pulmonary damage because of washout of surfactant and reflex mechanisms that cause increased airway resistance. Saltwater aspiration causes pulmonary damage via an osmotic gradient leading to shifts of protein-rich fluid into the alveoli. The fluid shifts caused by both types of aspiration generally do not cause significant serum electrolyte imbalances. Water contaminants add to the damage from either type of aspiration.

2. **CNS damage** caused by cerebral hypoxia occurs in 12% to 27% of survivors. Cold water temperature can decrease brain temperature to protective levels before cardiac arrest occurs. No adjuvant therapies have been proved to be effective.

3. **Cervical spine** injuries from diving accidents are common and should be sought.
4. **Shock** is uncommon in near drowning, and its presence should prompt a search for other causes.
5. **Treatment** is based on the standard ABCs. Pay attention to the possible need for ventilatory support, even if the initial chest x-ray study is normal. No role exists for prophylactic antibiotics or steroids.
6. **Cold submersion victims** may appear dead. If the patient has been immersed <1 hour, resuscitative efforts are indicated, at least until the core temperature is >30°C.

C. **Frostbite**
1. **Pathophysiology.** The local complication of hypothermia to external organs (digits, appendages such as the nose or ear) is termed **frostbite**. Frostbite involves tissue freezing and microvascular occlusion leading to cellular ischemia and death. The extent of tissue injury varies from hyperemia and edema to vesicle formation to full-thickness necrosis.
2. **Treatment.** Limiting cold exposure is the best way to minimize injury progression. Rapidly rewarm affected extremities by immersion in warm water (38°C to 41°C). Elevate the extremity to minimize edema and administer tetanus toxoid. Escharotomy may be needed if vascular compromise occurs. Delay surgical debridement or amputation until a clear demarcation has occurred, unless wound sepsis has intervened.

Axioms

- All trauma patients are at risk for developing hypothermia in the field, ED, OR, and ICU. The core temperature must be recorded early. Hypothermia often requires using a low-reading thermometer.
- Prevention of secondary hypothermia during resuscitation is important. Using warmed fluids and blankets, removing wet clothing, and ensuring a warm treatment in the room are important in the management of all trauma patients.
- Moderately and severely hypothermic patients need active core rewarming.
- Severely hypothermic patients can present in cardiac arrest. Unless obvious injuries incompatible with life are present, patients should not be declared dead until they have been warmed.

Bibliography

Gentilello LM, Jurkovich GJ, Stark MS, et al. Is hypothermia in the victim of major trauma protective or harmful? *Ann Surg* 1997;226:439–447.

Gregory JS, Flancbaum L, Townsend MC, et al. Incidence and timing of hypothermia in trauma patients undergoing operations. *J Trauma* 1991;31:795–800.

Jurkovich GJ, Greiser WB, Luterman A, et al. Hypothermia in trauma victims: an ominous predictor of survival. *J Trauma* 1987;27:1019–1024.

Luna GK, Maier RV, Pavlin EG, et al. Incidence and effect of hypothermia in seriously injured patients. *J Trauma* 1987;27:1014–1018.

Splittgerber FH, Talbert JG, Sweezer WP, et al. Partial cardiopulmonary bypass for core rewarming in profound accidental hypothermia. *Am Surg* 1986;52:407–412.

Steinemann S, Shackford SR, Davis JW. Implications of admission hypothermia in trauma patients. *J Trauma* 1990;30:200–202.

Takasu A, Carrillo P, Stezoski SW, et al. Mild or moderate hypothermia, but not increased oxygen breathing, prolongs survival during lethal uncontrolled hemorrhagic shock in rats, with measurement of visceral dysoxia. *Crit Care Med* 1999; 27:1557–1564.

Tisherman SA, Safar P, Rodriguez A. Therapeutic hypothermia in traumatology. *Surg Clin North Am* 1999;79:1269–1289.

43. BLOOD TRANSFUSION AND COMPLICATIONS

Ajai K. Malhortra, Heidi L. Frankel, and C. William Schwab

I. **Indications for transfusion in the traumatized patient**
   - Restoration of circulating blood volume and oxygen-carrying capacity
   - Correction of coagulation abnormalities
   - Whole blood is collected with anticoagulant and then separated into components. Component therapy is used to maximize resources.
   A. **Packed red blood cells (PRBC)**. Normal blood volume is 7% to 8% of ideal body weight (70–80 mL/kg). The normal hematocrit (Hct) is 42% to 48%, corresponding to a hemoglobin (Hgb) of 14 to 16 g/dL.
      1. Acute blood loss usually requires transfusion for grade III or IV shock, or if the patient has ongoing blood loss.
      2. The patient's age and overall condition determine the Hgb–Hct endpoint of resuscitation. A Hgb of 6 g/dL (Hct 18% to 21%) is often well tolerated by the young patient with single-system injury. However, patients who have coronary artery disease, are severely stressed, or have multiple injuries, a Hgb of 10 to 12 g/dL (Hct 30% to 35%) may be required to maintain adequate oxygen delivery and not increase cardiac work. On the other hand, recent studies suggest that a Hgb lower than 10 to 12 g/dL can be tolerated, even in critically ill patients without increased mortality. In a hemodynamically stable patient, 1 U of PRBC will increase Hgb by ~1 g/dL and Hct by 2% to 4%.
      3. **Administration**
         a. **Blood typing and crossmatching**. Blood typing identifies red cell surface ABO and Rh antigens and screens for antibodies to other surface antigens. Crossmatching involves actual mixing of the patient's plasma with donor red cells to lessen the risk of a transfusion reaction from undetected antibodies. Blood typing requires 5 to 10 minutes, and full crossmatching requires 20 to 30 minutes. Therefore, for emergent situations, have 2 to 6 U of **universal donor (O)** blood available immediately within the resuscitation area in all trauma centers at the time of patient arrival. (Administer O negative blood to women of childbearing age.) On patient arrival, have a blood sample drawn (preferably before large amounts of type O blood have been administered), labeled, and sent to the blood bank for processing. In less urgent situations, type-specific blood can be administered before fully crossmatched blood becomes available.
            (1) If no blood components are needed, the patient can have a "type and hold" performed so that the blood type is known, but the labor and cost of crossmatching are avoided.
            (2) If massive transfusion is required, request multiple units of platelets and fresh-frozen plasma as well as 10 to 20 U of PRBC, be prepared and delivered promptly. If >4 U of O blood are given to a patient of a non-O blood type, repeat the crossmatch before transfusion with blood of the original type (unless the change involved Rh incompatibility only).
         b. **Infusion**. PRBC are reconstituted with isotonic fluid without glucose (characteristically normal saline) or can be administered undiluted through rapid-infusion systems with inline warming technology. Mixing with warmed saline decreases viscosity, and warms the blood (Fig. 43.1). Do not warm blood in a microwave.
   B. **Platelets**. The normal platelet count is 150,000 to 500,000/mm³. In nontrauma patients, spontaneous bleeding occurs with platelet counts of <20,000/mm³. In an injured patient, especially with evidence of ongoing

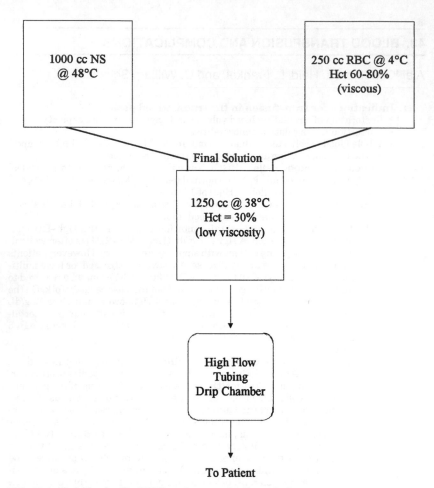

FIG. 43.1. Red blood cells (RBC) and warmed saline admixture.

bleeding, maintain the platelet above 50,000/mm³. **Bleeding time** measures the interaction of platelets with injured vessel to form initial plug (normal <5 minutes-Ivy method). Abnormal bleeding time is usually caused by decreased platelet count (thrombocytopenia) or function (thrombocytopathia).

1. The most common cause for nonsurgical bleeding in the trauma patient is dilutional thrombocytopenia. A linear inverse relationship exists between the number of PRBC units infused and the platelet count. Of patients, 50% have platelet counts of <50,000/mm³ after a two-blood volume (20 U of PRBC) transfusion. Heparin can also cause thrombocytopenia.

2. Thrombocytopathia may be seen in patients who are hypothermic, hypocalcemic, in renal failure, or are on certain medications (aspirin, nonsteroidal anti-inflammatory drugs [NSAID]). Thrombocytopathia caused by hypothermia is not corrected by platelet transfusion.

3. Platelets are stored at 4°C. One unit of platelets increases the platelet count by 5,000 to 10,000/mm³ and contains ~70 mL of plasma.

4. **Indications for transfusion**:
   - Platelet count <20,000/mm^3
   - Massive transfusion, especially after 15 U of PRBC
   - Platelet count <50,000/mm^3 in patients at high risk of hemorrhage (e.g., solid visceral injury [liver, spleen]) being managed nonoperatively or major pelvic fracture; or in patients in whom the consequences of hemorrhage will be disastrous (e.g., intracranial hemorrhage)
   - Evidence of impaired platelet function (e.g., increased bleeding time)
   a. Prophylactic administration of platelets has not been demonstrated to diminish transfusion requirements in the multiply transfused patient; however, hemostasis often is not possible once microvascular bleeding develops.

C. **Coagulation factors** are usually transfused as **fresh frozen plasma** (**FFP**—provides most factors), and **cryoprecipitate** (provides fibrinogen, factors VIII and XIII, and von Willebrand factor). The commonly used tests of coagulation are prothrombin time (**PT**—measures the extrinsic system: normal 10–14 seconds), and partial thromboplastin time (**PTT**—measures the intrinsic system: normal 25–37 seconds). The levels of individual factors (except fibrinogen) in plasma are measured in units of activity. This is compared with activity in normal pooled plasma. The result is expressed as percentage of normal activity. Fibrinogen is measured in milligram/100 mL plasma (normal 150–350 mg/100 mL plasma). The goal is to have adequate levels of factors to provide normal hemostasis. This usually requires factor activity of >50% of normal. In life-threatening situations, factor activity of up to 80% of normal may be necessary.

   1. Coagulopathy can present as hematuria, oozing from the surgical field or venipuncture sites, and mucosal bleeding.
   2. Coagulopathy can result from actual loss (by consumption or bleeding) of clotting factors, or dysfunction of the clotting cascade in a hypothermic environment. Tests of coagulation done at 37°C will underestimate coagulopathy caused by hypothermia, which cannot be corrected by transfusion. It is best to prevent hypothermia in a trauma patient, and if it develops to reverse it as rapidly as possible.
   3. PT prolongation, because of dilution and the lability of factors V and VIII in banked blood, occurs in 70% of patients after a 10-U PRBC transfusion and in nearly 100% after 12 U.
   4. Transfusion of **FFP**
      a. FFP is produced by separating plasma from fresh whole blood and rapidly freezing it. FFP requires 20 to 40 minutes to thaw; therefore, to prevent coagulopathy from developing, anticipate the requirement for FFP.
      b. **Dose**. In a coagulopathic patient, initially administer 10 to 15 mL/kg of FFP, followed by repeat evaluation of coagulation parameters.
      c. **Indications for transfusion**:
         - Ongoing bleeding caused by coagulopathy (documented or presumed).
         - PT or PTT prolongation in face of intracranial hemorrhage, major pelvic fracture, or solid visceral injury.
         - Expected need for >10- to 15-U PRBC transfusion.
   5. Transfusion of **Cryoprecipitate**
      a. Cryoprecipitate is produced by thawing FFP, removing the precipitate, and adding 10 mL plasma. It is rich in fibrinogen (at least 150 mg), factors VIII and XIII, and von Willebrand factor.
      b. **Indication for transfusion:**
         - Hypofibrinogenemia, (<100 mg/100 mL), often seen with massive transfusions
         - Treatment of von Willebrand disease

II. **Massive transfusion (MT)**
   A. **Definition**. The transfusion of at least one blood volume (5 L of whole blood or 10 U PRBC in a 70-kg man) within 24 hours. With rapid transfusion devices

and advances in blood banking, several times the patient's blood volume, can safely be transfused.

B. Because of the mathematical properties of hemodilution, a one-blood volume transfusion replaces 70% to 75% of the patient's original blood; a two-volume transfusion replaces 90% of the patient's original blood.

C. Early identification of the patient who may require MT is important because this allows the best use of resources, alteration of resuscitation strategies, and recognition and treatment of the complications of MT. Common injuries requiring MT are a high-grade liver injury, torso vascular injury (e.g., from a gunshot wound), an unstable pelvic fracture, or multiple intra- and extracavitary blunt injuries.

D. Outcome. In general, outcome is worsened by the following: preexisting disease (particularly cirrhosis), advanced age, hypothermia, closed head injury, coagulopathy, prolonged shock, and, until recently, a blunt mechanism of injury. Trauma patients with blunt and penetrating injuries who require MT now have comparable survival rates (50%). Currently, penetrating trauma patients require MT more often than blunt trauma patients. The outcome in patients requiring MT is improved by shortening prehospital time, minimizing resuscitation time, rapid surgical control of cavitary hemorrhage, and employing "damage control" techniques, where appropriate (Chapter 29).

III. Disseminated intravascular coagulopathy (DIC) occurs by activation of the coagulation cascade within the vasculature. It continues by ongoing, simultaneous thrombosis and thrombolysis. Rapid consumption of the available coagulation factors results. DIC can be initiated by any situation in which tissue thromboplastin like substances(s) is released into the blood stream. In the trauma patient, DIC can be seen after massive transfusion, transfusion reaction, or surgical tissue injury, especially severe closed head injury, and in severe infection. DIC results in a fibrinogen level <100 mg/dL, a platelet count <50,000/mm^3, and a D-dimer level >500 g/L. (Coagulopathy that develops with massive transfusion is rarely DIC.)

A. Treatment

1. Treat the inciting event.

2. Support all failing organ systems (including the coagulation system).

IV. Bleeding and coagulopathy in the patient with premorbid disease. Coagulopathy can be caused by certain disease states or from medications (Table 43.1).

A. Evaluation

1. Obtaining a good history is the most important initial step.

2. The laboratory tests depend on the level of suspicion, based on the history. Usually PT, PTT, and platelet count are sufficient. Occasionally, the activity of individual factors, bleeding time, and platelet function tests are needed.

B. Treatment depends on the problem identified in the evaluation.

1. Platelet deficiency. Both thrombocytopenia and thrombocytopathia (except from hypothermia) can be treated by platelet transfusion. Prolonged bleeding time with normal platelet count suggests thrombocytopathia. This is often seen with uremia, and can be treated by infusion of desamino-8-D-arginine-vasopressin (DDAVP) 0.3 µg/kg every 6–12 hours.

2. Factor deficiency. All factor deficiencies have been described. Deficiency of factor VIII (hemophilia A) is the most common. The principles of treatment are similar for all individual factor deficiencies.

a. Hemophilia A. An x-linked inherited abnormality resulting in >95% reduction in factor VIII levels. Diagnosed by prolonged PTT (normal PT), and a low level of factor VIII activity. Treat by administering factor VIII. Recombinant DNA factor VIII has no infection risk but is expensive. Monoclonal factor VIII has a small (<1%) infection risk but is less expensive; FFP and cryoprecipitate are also effective. Factor VIII has a short half-life; frequent infusions are

Table 43.1 Common comorbid conditions
and medications that affect bleeding and coagulation

Comorbid conditions	Medications/effect
Hypertension	↓Platelets by thiazides, furosemide, alpha-methyldopa Platelet dysfunction by diltiazem, propanolol, verapamil
Atherosclerotic cardio- vascular disease	↓Platelets by quinidine ↑PT by warfarin; platelet dysfunction by aspirin, isosorbide
Congestive heart failure	↓Platelets by furosemide
Alcoholism or liver disease	↓Platelets, ↑PT and PTT, ↓fibrinogen
Renal insufficiency	Platelet dysfunction
Malignancy	↓Platelets in lymphoma, leukemia, myeloma, and from radiation therapy ↑PT and PTT in liver metastasis Platelet dysfunction in polycythemia vera and from chemotherapy (e.g., daunorubicin, plicamycin)
Chronic disease states (e.g. CMV, TB, lupus)	↓Platelets
Other medications Methicillin, dilantin, heparin	↓Platelets
Nonsteroidal anti- inflammatory agents	Platelet dysfunction

PT, prothrombin time; PTT, partial thromboplastin time; CMV, cytomegalovirus; TB, tuberculosis

needed. Bring levels to 30% of normal (>50% with major trauma) to ensure adequate hemostasis.

  b. **von Willebrand's disease** is an autosomal dominant inherited abnormality causing defective factor VIII production, resulting in poor platelet adhesion. It is diagnosed by special tests for platelet adhesiveness. Treat by administering cryoprecipitate or FFP. Some forms of the disease respond to DDAVP.

  c. **Liver disease and vitamin K deficiency.** Deficiency of vitamin K, seen in patients on prolonged antibiotic or warfarin therapy, can cause deficiency of vitamin K-dependent factors (II, VII, IX, X). Treat by administering vitamin K (subcutaneous or intravenous) and discontinuing warfarin. In urgent situations, FFP may be necessary to rapidly achieve normal hemostasis. The situation with liver disease can be much worse, as the liver plays a central role in the production of most factors. In patients with advanced liver dysfunction, vitamin K, FFP, cryoprecipitate, and platelets may all be required.

C. **Hypercoagulable states.** Deficiency of factor V, antithrombin III, protein C, and protein S can cause a hypercoagulable state. Protein C and S are vitamin K-dependent. Treat in acute situations by administering FFP to provide the deficient factors.

V. **Complications of transfusion**

  A. Immunologic reactions

  1. **Intravascular hemolytic transfusion reaction**

  a. **Pathophysiology.** Seen when incompatible blood (usually ABO incompatibility; rarely, incompatibility of Duffy, Kell, Kidd, and Lewis antigens) is transfused. This reaction is almost always caused by clerical errors (misidentification of blood sample or unit), and is rare in modern blood banking.

    b. Manifestation: anaphylactoid (non—IgE-mediated anaphylaxis-like syndrome) shock is seen soon after starting the transfusion. Features include those of a generalized immunologic reaction (fever, nausea, vomiting, diarrhea, loin pain), vasomotor collapse (hypotension, angina, dyspnea), and coagulopathy (bleeding from operative sites, hematuria). Death occurs in 10% from vasomotor collapse.

    c. Diagnosis can be confirmed by positive direct Coombs' test (a sample of the transfused unit and the patient's blood showing hemolysis).

    d. Treatment. Stop the transfusion, treat coagulopathy, promote adequate perfusion with volume (may require vasopressors), and forced diuresis (consider mannitol and alkalinization). Send a sample of the patient's blood and the transfused unit back to the blood bank.

2. Extravascular hemolytic transfusion reaction

    a. Pathophysiology. This is an immunologic response to previous sensitization to one or more of the minor antigens (Duffy, Kell, Kidd, and Lewis; rarely, Rh) by prior transfusion or pregnancy. Sensitization risk is 1% to 1.5% per unit transfused.

    b. Manifestations: jaundice, fever, anemia; rarely, hemoglobinuria, occurring days to weeks after the transfusion

    c. Diagnosis. Positive direct Coombs' test

    d. Treatment. Avoid unnecessary transfusions.

3. Febrile transfusion reaction

    a. Pathophysiology. Represents 75% of all transfusion reactions and is caused by preformed antibodies to leukocyte antigens.

    b. Manifestations: fever, chills, urticaria, headache; rarely, hypotension, tachycardia, dyspnea, vomiting

    c. Diagnosis is generally one of exclusion.

    d. Treatment. Provide symptomatic relief with antipyretics, and antihistamines. In cases of severe reactions, consider a future transfusion with buffy-poor blood.

4. Allergic transfusion reaction

    a. Pathophysiology. Secondary to antibodies against plasma proteins

    b. Manifestations: urticaria; rarely, anaphylaxis (seen in patients with IgA deficiency)

    c. Diagnosis is generally one of exclusion.

    d. Treatment. Symptomatic

B. Infectious complications

1. Human immunodeficiency virus (HIV). Transmission through blood transfusion has been diminished with routine testing of all donated blood since 1985. Despite negative testing, transmission of the virus by transfusion is still possible; a delay of 8 weeks to 8 months between exposure to the virus and seroconversion can occur. Current risk of infection is 1 of 493,000 to 680,000 units of transfusion.

2. Transfusion-associated hepatitis

    a. Hepatitis B represents ~10% of transfusion-associated hepatitis. Incidence has been reduced by 90% by donor screening for hepatitis B surface antigen and the phasing out of professional donors; current risk is 1 of 63,000 units of transfusion.

    b. Hepatitis C. Formerly called non-A, non-B hepatitis, the risk is 1 of 100,000 units of transfusion. Represents ~90% of transfusion-associated hepatitis. Results in chronic hepatitis in 50% and cirrhosis in 20%. Hepatocellular carcinoma can develop. Donor screening with alanine amino transferase (ALT) and core antigen (performed since 1989) has reduced the risk.

    c. Type D (delta) hepatitis. This viral particle can only exist in conjunction with hepatitis B. No commercial screening test is available. Some donor units that are hepatitis B positive, but escape detection by HBsAg testing, are positive for hepatitis D.

3. **Cytomegalovirus (CMV)** is a herpesvirus that can cause mononucleosis-like symptoms. Most individuals are CMV Ab positive from environmental exposure. Severe illness can cause patients to be Ab negative or immunocompromised, if they are given CMV positive blood. Hence, CMV negative blood should be given to neonates, pregnant women, and immunocompromised individuals.
4. **Epstein-Barr virus (EBV)** is readily transmissible through transfusion, yet rarely causes clinical symptoms.
5. **Other**
   a. Malaria, syphilis, brucellosis, and other organisms, all extremely rare.
   b. Approximately 2% of all blood units can have bacterial contaminants; most are *Klebsiella* or *Pseudomonas*,, resulting in fever, hypotension, and abdominal pain, but usually no long-term sequelae result if the patient has a normal immune system.
C. **Complications of MT**. Some complications of transfusion are unique to MT because the preservative solutions and changes in blood associated with storage (Table 43.2) are significant only when a large volume of stored blood is transfused.
   1. **Hypothermia** (Chapter 42)
      a. Occurs in the setting of severe injury or MT. Blood is stored at 4°C and, unless warmed to body temperature before transfusion, adds significantly to the heat loss.
      b. Results in decreased hepatic metabolism of citrate, impaired activity of thrombin and plasmin, decreased platelet function, diminished synthesis of clotting factors, and left shift of the oxygen dissociation curve.
   2. **Bleeding and coagulopathy** (see above) results from dilution of platelets, consumption of coagulation factors, hypothermia, acidosis, and ongoing bleeding.
   3. **Citrate toxicity**. Citrate is used as an anticoagulant (acts by chelating Ca^{2+}) in banked blood. If blood is given more rapidly than 1 U every 5 minutes, then the citrate can reduce serum Ca^{2+} and Mg^{2+} levels and affect cardiac function and the coagulation cascade.
      a. **Manifestations**: decreased blood pressure, decreased cardiac contractility, QT interval prolongation, dysrhythmias
      b. **Diagnosis**. Diminished total and ionized serum calcium and magnesium. Ionized calcium and magnesium determinations can be made rapidly from microanalysis of whole blood. A 56% incidence of hypocalcemia was noted in a recent MT series of patients receiving one blood volume transfusion in 24 hours.
      c. **Treatment**. Some authors recommend prophylactic administration of 1 g calcium (as chloride solution) per 6 U of transfusion, if PRBC

Table 43.2 Characteristics of a red blood cell unit during storage (4°C) over time (average storage time of transfused blood)

Day 1	Day 14	Day 30
210 mL PRBC	210 mL PRBC	210 mL PRBC
40–90 mL plasma	40–90 mL plasma	40–90 mL plasma
pH = 6.6–7.0	pH = 6.6–7.0	pH = 6.6–7.0
K^+ = 10–40 mEq	K^+ = 20–40 mEq	K^+ = 30–40 mEq
Citrate = 2–5 mg/mL	Citrate = 2–5 mg/mL	Citrate = 2–5 mg/mL
2,3-DPG 100%	2,3-DPG 40%	2,3-DPG 5%
ATP 95%	ATP 90%	ATP 70%

PRBC, packed red blood cells; 2-3-DPG, 2-3 Diphosphoglycerate; ATP, adenosine triphosphate.

are given rapidly. Basing treatment on a measured ionized calcium may be safer. Hypomagnesemia potentiates hypocalcemia. Hence, repletion of magnesium may be necessary (magnesium sulfate solution, 1.0 g = 8 mEq).

4. Acidosis
   a. **Pathophysiology**. The pH of stored blood is 6.6 to 7.0. The normal metabolic response to the transfusion of packed cells in the absence of shock is alkalosis, which favors hypokalemia. Acidosis with MT results from lactic acidosis caused by inadequate tissue perfusion and inadequate clearance of citric acid by the hypoperfused liver.
   b. **Manifestations**: hypotension, decreased urine output, increased pulse, and other signs of shock
   c. **Diagnosis**. Presence of anion gap lactic acidosis
   d. **Treatment**. Maintain adequate tissue perfusion with fluids and inotropic agents, if indicated.

5. Potassium abnormalities
   a. **Pathophysiology**. Hyperkalemia can occur, especially with very rapid transfusion (secondary to 10–40 mEq potassium per unit of packed cells; more with old blood). This is rarely a clinical problem because the potassium load is cleared by renal excretion, red cell uptake, and the conversion of citrate to bicarbonate (favoring cellular shifts of potassium, thereby minimizing hyperkalemia and commonly resulting in hypokalemia). In one series of patients receiving MT, 25% were hypokalemic, 15% hyperkalemic, and 60% had a normal serum K^+.
   b. **Manifestations**: high peaked T waves, widened QRS complex, and depressed ST segments are seen initially. Disappearance of T waves, heart block, and diastolic cardiac arrest can be seen with increasing potassium levels.
   c. **Diagnosis**. Serum determination of potassium
   d. **Treatment**. Maintain adequate urine output and replace observed deficits for hypokalemia.

6. Decreased adenosine triphosphate (ATP)
   a. **Pathophysiology**. Decreased availability of phosphate secondary to volume shifts in MT is a feature of "old" blood (>50 days).
   b. **Manifestations**: diminished red cell deformability secondary to loss of biconcave shape
   c. **Treatment**. Usually none. In patients with hypophosphatemia, replete phosphate losses in intravenous fluids, provide adequate FIO_2.

7. Decreased 2,3-DPG (2,3-diphosphoglycerate).2,3-DPG is a component of the red cell membrane that facilitates oxygen off-loading in the tissues.
   a. **Pathophysiology**. Citrate anticoagulation decreases 2,3-DPG levels over time (Table 43.2).
   b. **Manifestations**: decreased oxygen delivery to the tissues.
   c. **Treatment**. None. In situations where oxygen delivery may be a problem, use the freshest available blood.

VI. The future
   A. **Modified whole blood** may be an option to whole blood. After sterile separation of PRBC, platelets, plasma, and cryoprecipitate from the donor unit, the plasma and RBC components are recombined. The product lacks platelets, and factors V and VIII, yet provides adequate levels of other factors. Its use can reduce the donor exposure in patients requiring multiple transfusions and, thus, reduce the chances of disease transmission.
   B. **Solvent and detergent (SD)-treated plasma**. Pooled plasma is treated with TNBP (tri-N-butyl phosphate) and 1% Triton-100, followed by extraction to remove the SD agents. This eliminates the risk of viral disease transmission.
   C. Prolonging shelf life. Attempts are being made to prolong shelf life by changing the anticoagulant mixture used. Also technology is being developed to

rapidly freeze the blood, thus giving it an indefinite storage life. Indefinite storage life can be helpful for rare blood types.
D. Blood substitutes. Solutions based on stroma-free Hgb or on synthetic oxygen-carrying compounds such as perfluorocarbons are being developed. These will give all the advantages of blood without the risk of adverse effects.

Axioms
* **All** injured patients require volume restoration, **some** require RBC, and a **few** need clotting factor replacement.
* The major goals of volume resuscitation are restoration of intravascular volume and red cell mass.
* Of patients, 50% have platelet counts <50,000/mm3 after 20 U of PRBC.
* Prophylactic administration of platelets or FFP does not alter outcome in the multiply transfused patient. However, these deficiencies must be corrected rapidly to avoid microvascular bleeding.

Bibliography
AuBuchon JP, Birkmeyer JD, Busch MP. Safety of blood supply in the United States: opportunities and controversies. *Ann Intern Med* 1997;127:904–909.
Edna TH, Bjerkeset T. Association between blood transfusion and infection in injured patients. *J Trauma* 1992;33(5):659–661.
Frykberg ER, Dennis JW, Butcher JL. Massive transfusion: history, pathophysiology, and management. *Trauma Quarterly* 1993;10(1):12–31.
Gubler KD, Genitello LM, Hassantasha SA, et al. The impact of hypothermia on dilutional coagulopathy. *J Trauma* 1994;36(6):847–851.
Hebert PC, et al. A multicenter, randomized controlled clinical trial of transfusion requirements in critical care. *N Engl J Med* 1999;340:409–417.
Labadie LL. Transfusion therapy in the emergency department. *Emerg Clin North Am* 1993;11(2):379–406.
Lauer GM, Walker BD: Hepatitis C virus infection. *N Engl J Med* 2001;345:41–52.
Schreiber GB, Busch MP, Kleinman SH, et al. The risk of transfusion-related viral infections. *N Engl J Med* 1996;334:1685–1690.
Simon TL, et al. Practice parameters for the use of red blood cell transfusions. *Arch Pathol Lab Med* 1998;122:130–138.
Wilson RF, Dulchavsky SA, Soullier G, et al. Problems with 20 or more blood transfusions in 24 hours. *Am Surg* 1987;53(7):410–417.
Wudel JH, Morris JA, Yates K, et al. Massive transfusions: outcome in blunt trauma patients. *J Trauma* 1991;31(1):1–7.

44. NUTRITION/METABOLISM IN THE TRAUMA PATIENT

Gayle Minard

I. **Introduction**. Nutrition is required in the trauma patient to maintain homeostasis, and prevent catabolism of lean body stores. Early enteral nutrition has been shown to decrease the rate of infectious complications and decrease the length of stay. The harmful effects of moderate to severe malnutrition after trauma include death, compromised immunity, decreased wound healing, and other morbidity associated with reduced mobility, poor cough strength, and so on. The rapidity with which malnutrition develops in a patient correlates with extent of injury, reduction in circulating hormones (insulinlike growth factors and growth hormone), and accelerated release of catecholamines, glucagon, cortisol, prolactin, cytokines, oxygen radicals, and other inflammatory mediators. The overall health and nutritional status of the patient before the injury are key factors. The loss of a significant proportion of lean mass can occur quickly in the multiply injured patient.

II. **Initial patient assessment**. Evaluate the patient to determine the need for nutritional support and, if so, how it should be delivered.
   A. **Is the patient malnourished?**
      1. **Types**
         a. Marasmus, which is characterized by wasting of fat and muscle, is caused by inadequate intake of protein and calories. Examples include patients with acquired immunodeficiency syndrome (AIDS), advanced renal failure, and the elderly.
         b. Kwashiorkor, which is caused by inadequate intake of protein, is characterized by edema and fatty infiltration of liver. Examples include patients on fad diets and those with chronic alcohol abuse.
      2. **Assessment**
         a. Many common markers of nutritional deficiency are not useful in trauma patients because of massive fluid shifts.
            (1) Current weight
            (2) Anthropometric measurements (triceps skinfold thickness, midarm circumference)
            (3) Albumin, transferrin, retinol-binding protein levels—more a reflection of stress than nutritional status
         b. Better markers in trauma populations
            (1) "Normal" weight—can be obtained from the patient, family, driver's license
            (2) History of unintentional weight loss (>10% in last 6 months)
            (3) Comorbid conditions (e.g., cancer, chronic obstructive pulmonary disease [COPD], AIDS, diabetes, liver disease, kidney disease, alcoholism)
            (4) Visual assessment of muscle wasting: thenar and temporalis muscle wasting
            (5) Prealbumin level may be helpful as the patient recovers; much shorter half life than albumin (Table 44.1).
   B. **Is the patient at high risk for malnutrition and infectious complications?** Early feeding via the enteral route decreases the rate of infectious complications. Groups at high risk:
      1. Severe closed head injury (Glascow Coma Scale (GCS) score ≤9)
      2. Abdominal Trauma Index (ATI) ≥15
      3. Injury Severity Score (ISS) ≥20
      4. Burn ≥10%
      5. Current infection or sepsis

Table 44.1 Prealbumin (mg/dL)

Normal	>15
Mild depletion	10–15
Moderate depletion	7–10
Severe depletion	<7

6. Prolonged ventilator requirements: (e.g., head injury, airway injury, pulmonary contusion, adult respiratory distress syndrome [ARDS])
7. Extremes of age

C. How long will the patient be unable to eat? Most uncomplicated trauma patients resume oral feeding within the first 4 to 5 days after injury. Patients unable to eat for 5 to 7 days will need nutritional support. In patients at high risk, began feeding as soon as stable and able to tolerate feedings.

D. Route of feeding. The gut is preferred because of ease of use and lower cost. Obviously, a functional gastrointestinal (GI) tract and enteral access are required to do this. However, do not use the GI tract if the patient is hypoperfused or on vasopressors because of the risk of **massive small bowel necrosis**.

1. **Enteral**
   a. If the GI tract is fully functional, enteral feeding through a naso- or orogastric tube is preferred.
   b. Patients having laparotomy should have a transgastric jejunostomy, jejunostomy, or nasojejunal tube inserted if they are at high risk (see above).
   c. Most patients can be fed transgastrically. Patients with a gastric ileus, but an otherwise functional GI tract and not requiring laparotomy, should have a nasojejunal tube placed.
2. **Parenteral.** Useful when enteral feeding is contraindicated because of any of the following: hemodynamic instability; ongoing fluid resuscitation; peritonitis; significant doses of vasopressors (renal dose dopamine not included); bowel obstruction (unless a feeding tube has been inserted distally to the point of obstruction); proximal or high output GI fistulas; and bowel ischemia.

III. Initial dietary prescription
  A. Determine caloric requirements. Most methods are based on ideal body weight (IBW).
   1. **IBW**
      a. Female = 45 kg/5 feet plus 2.3 kg/inch
      b. Male = 50 kg/5 feet plus 2.3 kg/inch
      c. Obese (>1.3 × IBW) = 0.25 (actual body weight − IBW) + IBW
   2. Kcal/kg/day method
      a. Simplest method to use (Table 44.2)
   3. Equations; many are available but Harris-Benedict used frequently
      a. **BEE (males) = 66 + (13.7 × wt.) + (5 × ht [cm]) − (6.8 × age)**
      b. **BEE (females) = 655 + (9.6 × wt.) + (1.7 × ht.) − (4.7 × age)**
      c. Multiply by activity and injury factors (Table 44.3).
   4. Indirect calorimetry measures the patient's oxygen consumption and CO_2 production. It is a better monitoring method than guide to initiate feeding. It is labor intensive and the patient must be on a ventilator (see section IV.)
  B. Estimate protein requirements.
   1. Protein is required to reduce catabolism of lean muscle mass. Excess protein can be reflected as increased blood urea nitrogen (BUN). Insufficient protein delivery will prolong negative nitrogen balance. Protein provides 4 kcal/g. The amount of nitrogen (grams) is calculated by dividing the

BEE (basal energy expenditure), wt. (kg), ht. (cm), age (years)

Table 44.2 Nutritional requirements (kcal/kg/day)

Maintenance	20–25
Minor infection	25–30
Major surgery, sepsis	35
Severe thermal injury	40

amount of protein (grams) by 6.25. The amount of protein in total parenteral nutrition (TPN) solution can be calculated by multiplying the percent amino acids by the volume; for example, 500 mL of a 5% amino acid solution would be 0.05 × 500 mL = 25 grams of protein (Table 44.4).

C. **Evaluate nonprotein calories to protein ratio (NPC:N) ratio.** Severely injured trauma patients usually require more protein than a nontrauma patient. Patients with renal failure require less protein, particularly if hemodialysis has not been initiated (Table 44.5).

D. **Carbohydrates**
   1. A minimum of 75 to 100 g/day are necessary for carbohydrate-dependent cells. Usually, 50% to 80% of daily calories is supplied as carbohydrates. Carbohydrates provide 3.4 kcal/gram.
   2. The maximal infusion of glucose is ~5 mg/kg/minute or 7.2 g/kg/day. Excessive carbohydrate delivery can contribute to liver steatosis, increased CO_2 production, hyperosmolarity, and hyperglycemia.
   3. The amount of glucose in TPN solution is calculated by multiplying the percent glucose by the volume; for example, 500 mL of D50 would provide 0.50 × 500 mL = 250 g of glucose. Caloric content would be 250 g × 3.4 kcal/gram or 850 kcal.

E. **Lipid**
   1. Absolute requirements are minimal, about 1 to 1.5 g/kg/day.
   2. Fatty acid deficiencies can be avoided during parenteral feeding by supplying 500 mL of 20% lipid emulsion two to three times per week. Parenteral infusion rate: 500 mL 20% emulsion over 16 to 20 hours.
   3. Adequate fat is present in most enteral formulas.
   4. Fat provides 9.0 kcal/gram. The amount of calories in standard intravenous (i.v.) lipid formulas can be calculated by multiplying the percent lipid by the volume; for example, 500 mL of 10% Intralipid (Pharmacin & Upjohn. Peapack, NJ) would provide 0.10 × 500 mL = 50 g of lipid. Caloric content would be 50 g × 9.0 kcal/gram or 450 kcal.

F. **Electrolytes**
   1. Parental nutrition formulae require addition of electrolytes. Monitor serum electrolytes and adjust parenteral nutrition accordingly; avoid fine tuning electrolyte abnormalities (Table 44.6).
   2. Anionic supplementation, which is tailored to equal cations, uses chloride (useful if chloride-responsive metabolic alkalosis is present) or acetate (if bicarbonate deficit is present).

Table 44.3 Activity/injury factors

Activity	1.25
Minor operation	1.05–1.15
Sepsis	1.2–1.4
Closed head injury	1.3
Multiple trauma	1.4
Systemic inflammatory response syndrome	1.5
Severe thermal injury	2.0

Table 44.4 Protein (g/kg/day)

Maintenance	1.0
Moderate stress or repletion	1.2–1.5
Severe stress	1.5–2.0
Renal failure	<1.0

G. Multivitamins

1. Multivitamins are included in enteral formulas but are usually added daily to parenteral nutrition fluids. Example from MVI-12 (Astra, Westborough, MA): vitamin C (100 mg), vitamin A (1 mg), vitamin D (5 µg), thiamine (3 mg), riboflavin (3.6 mg), pyridoxine (4 mg), niacinamide (40 mg), dexpanthenol (15 mg), vitamin E (10 mg), biotin (60 mg), folic acid (400 µg), vitamin B_{12} (5 µg). Additional amounts of some vitamins may be useful in stress i.e., vitamin A (systemic 10,000 U/day), vitamin E (400–1,000 IU/day), vitamin C (1 g/day), thiamine (5 mg), and riboflavin (10 mg/day).

H. Trace elements. TPN additive per day

1. Example from MTE-5 (Lymphomed, Deerfield, IL): zinc (1 mg), copper (0.4 mg), manganese (0.1 mg), chromium (4 µg), selenium (20 µg). These amounts may be insufficient to meet the needs of a patient in stress. Additional amounts include Zn (10–30 mg), Cu (1–3 mg), Se (50–80 µg), Cr (50–150 µg), and Mn (25–50 mg).

I. Other possible additives to TPN

1. Vitamin K: 1 mg/day, as indicated
2. Insulin. Do not use in initial TPN order. Add if hyperglycemia develops that is not easily controlled by a sliding scale. The insulin required is highly variable and should be used only to provide a foundation for glucose control; final adjustment should be attained with other methods. Insulin supplemented in TPN requires adjustment and close correlation with blood glucose determinations.
3. Histamine$_2$ blockers for GI stress prophylaxis. Be aware that the patient may not receive adequate doses if TPN is turned off or reduced.

J. Enteral formulas

1. Enteral dietary plans are established and adjusted as described for parenteral nutrition. Many commercial products are available and can be grouped into categories (Table 44.7).

IV. Assessment during feeding

The initial nutrition plan represents a "best approximation" of the patient's nitrogen and caloric needs. Base continuation and adjustment of nutritional supplementation on continued metabolic demand (fever, infection, and so on) or decreasing metabolic needs (patient recovers).

A. Nitrogen (N) balance = $N_{in} - N_{out}$.

Nitrogen losses, which correlate with severity of injury or stress, can be high. Positive nitrogen balance is rarely attained in severe injury; the practical goal is minimizing the nitrogen deficit.

1. Nitrogen intake (N_{in}) is determined by dietary plan:
   N_{in}= grams protein intake × 0.16 g nitrogen/gram protein

Table 44.5 Nonprotein calories to protein ratio (NPC:N RATIO)

Maintenance	150:1
Stress	90–120:1
Acute renal failure without dialysis	250–300:1
Acute renal failure with dialysis	200:1

Table 44.6 Standard electrolyte composition of TPN

Sodium (chloride or acetate)	30–130 mEq/L
Potassium (chloride or acetate)	30–40 mEq/L
Calcium	5 mEq/L
Phosphate (sodium or potassium)	15 mmol/L
Magnesium sulfate	8–12 mEq/L

TPN, total parenteral nutrition.

For example, a patient receiving a standard TPN infusion of 500 mL of 5% amino acid solution mixed with 500 mL of D20W at 100 mL/hour (2,400 mL/day), the N_{in} would be:

1,200 mL amino acids $\times$ 5% $\times$ 0.16 = 9.6 g nitrogen

  2. Nitrogen output is usually estimated by 3-, 12-, or 24-hour urinary urea nitrogen (UUN), converted to 24-hour UUN.

   a. Not all nitrogen from catabolism is lost via urine; nitrogen is lost via stool, skin, exudation, wounds, and so on. Urea usually accounts for 80% to 90% of urinary nitrogen but may account for only 65% in severely stressed patients. Because of these factors, the estimate of UUN is modified by an additional 3 to 6 g, based on estimated injury, stress severity, or extraneous losses; hence UUN + (3 to 6) = N_{out}.

   b. UUN can be a falsely high estimate of catabolically induced nitrogen loss if other noncatabolic sources of nitrogen are present (e.g., resolving hematomas, GI blood loss, severe crush or burns).

   c. UUN can underestimate important nitrogen losses if significant proteinuria is present. Order total urinary nitrogen (TUN) to determine N_{out}.

 B. **Visceral proteins**

  1. Measurement of some proteins made by the liver (e.g., albumin, transferrin, insulinlike growth factor 1, retinol-binding protein, and prealbumin) can become useful as acute stress responses decline. Albumin has too long a half-life to be useful. In reality, most of the others are used for research purposes and only prealbumin is clinically applicable (see section II for interpretation).

 C. **Indirect calorimetry**

  1. Direct measurement of oxygen consumption (Vo_2) and CO_2 production (Vco_2) estimates resting energy expenditure (REE).

   REE kcal = (3.9 $\times$ Vo$_2$ + 1.1 $\times$ Vco$_2$) $\times$ 1.44

  2. The **respiratory quotient (RQ)** is also calculated by Vco_2/Vo_2. Variations in RQ can be useful in adjustment of the dietary plan (Table 44.8).

 D. **Serum triglycerides**

  1. Hypertriglyceridemia can cause dysfunction of macrophages. A serum level >350 mg/dL should lead to reduction in lipid intake. This has become an increasing problem with the use of propofol for sedation.

 V. **Complications of nutritional support.** Although provision of nutrients can prevent the onset of malnutrition and other complications, it carries some risk. Some problems can occur regardless of route of nutrition; however, many are route specific.

 A. **General complications**

  1. **Refeeding syndrome.** Starting nutritional repletion too aggressively in severely malnourished patients can precipitate the refeeding syndrome (hypophosphatemia, hypokalemia, hyperglycemia, thiamine deficiency, hypomagnesemia, and congestive heart failure). This is uncommon but should be considered in patients with a history of anorexia or chronic alcoholism.

Table 44.7 Commercial enteral formulas

Type	Osmolarity (mOsm/ kg water)	Caloric density (kcal/mL)	Protein (g/L)	Fats	Benefits	Use
General purpose	Isotonic 250–350	1	35–45	MCT LCT	Easily absorbed, cost effective	Most patients; some can be oral supplements
High calorie	Hypertonic 400–700	1.5–2	30–85	Various	Low volume required to meet needs	CHF, severe reflux
High nitrogen	Iso-hypertonic 300–650	1	50–85	MCT LCT	Increased amount of protein	Critical illness (burns, trauma, sepsis)
Elemental and semielemental	Iso-hypertonic 250–650	1	Amino acids, peptides 20–100	Low fat MCT	May enhance absorption	Malabsorption
Fiber-containing	Iso-hypertonic 300–650	1–1.5	40–70	MCT LCT	May reduce diarrhea	Most patients
Hepatic	Hypertonic 450–600	1–1.5	Branched chain amino acids 40–50	Low fat	May reduce encephalopathy	Encephalopathic patients
Renal	Hypertonic 550–700	2	70–80	MCT LCT	Lower K Phosphate, Mg	Renal failure
Pulmonary	Hyperosmolar 450–650	1.5	60–80	MCT LCT	High fat, therefore lower CO_2 production	Severe COPD, CO_2 retention
Diabetic	Iso-hypertonic 300–450	1	40–65	MCT LCT	High fiber, low fat and carbohydrates	Diabetics
Immune enhancing	Iso-hypertonic 350–500	1–1.5	Arginine, glutamine, nucleic acids branched chain 50–80	Omega-3 fatty acids	Enhanced immunity	Severely injured patients (i.e.,) ATI > 25, ISS > 20

MCT, medium chain triglycerides; LCT, long chain triglycerides; CHF, congestive heart failure; COPD, chronic obstructive pulmonary disease; ATI, Adult Trauma Index; ISS, injury severity score.

Table 44.8 Interpretation of respiratory quotient (RQ)

Substrate	RQ
Carbohydrate	1.0
Mixed substrate (normal)	0.8
Lipid	0.7
Overfeeding (lipogenesis)	>1.0
Underfeeding (lipolysis)	<0.7

   2. **Metabolic.** About 60% of patients develop at least one metabolic change secondary to feeding. The most common metabolic complications are:
      a. Hyperglycemia and hyperosmolarity
      b. Electrolyte changes: hyponatremia, hypophosphatemia, and so on
      c. Hyperchloremic normal-anion gap acidosis
B. **Complications associated with TPN**
   1. Central line complications: infection (including line sepsis), pneumothorax, hemothorax, arterial puncture, brachial plexus injury, thoracic duct injury, deep venous thrombosis, and so on.
   2. Liver enzyme or functional abnormalities occur in 25% to 90% of patients receiving TPN; may be manifested by steatosis, intrahepatic cholestasis, inflammation, or fibrosis. These abnormalities are usually associated with excessive carbohydrates in the dietary plan. The carbohydrates that exceed the oxidative capability of the liver will precipitate intrahepatic triglyceride accumulation. Other potential causes of liver changes include higher NPC:N ratios; inadequate nitrogen intake; hepatotoxins from bacterial translocation; reduced biliary, pancreatic, intestinal secretions; and the primary effects of amino acids or changes caused by selected amino acid deficiency. If it occurs, try cycling the feeds or reducing the amount of carbohydrates and substituting fat.
C. **Complications associated with enteral feeding**
   1. Feeding tube complications: sinusitis, infection, bleeding, tube occlusion, tube malposition.
   2. Aspiration. Feeding distal to the ligament of Treitz may alleviate this problem, but this is controversial.
   3. Massive small bowel necrosis
   4. Diarrhea and abdominal distension is common with both enteral and parenteral feeding, but the cause may be unclear.
      a. Causes of diarrhea
         (1) Infectious etiologies: *Clostridium difficile* or other bacteria
         (2) Hyperosmolar medication, particularly those mixed with sorbitol (e.g., aminophylline)
         (3) Promotility agents (e.g., metoclopramide)
         (4) Other medications (e.g., guaifenesin)
         (5) Fecal impaction
         (6) Hyperosmolarity of feedings; this was a more common problem when formulas were very hyperosmolar (i.e., >100 mOsm/liter). Occasionally, the hyperosmolarity of full-strength jejunal feeding causes diarrhea, so diluting the formula may help control diarrhea.
         (7) Feeding of complex nutrients after bowel rest. It is suggested that polypeptidases and polysaccharidases decrease in the GI luminal brush border after 10 days of bowel rest (no GI nutrients). Histologic changes also occur as villi become hypotrophic and flattened. Refeeding with formulas that have complex protein and carbohydrate sources that cannot be metabolized or

absorbed by the brush border can contribute to diarrhea. Consider use of an elemental formula if diarrhea occurs.

b. Treatment of diarrhea

(1) Alter fiber content, usually by changing to a formula containing higher quantities of fiber. At times, actually eliminating fiber can reduce diarrhea.

(2) Review patient's medications for those with diarrhea as a side effect (e.g., antibiotics).

(3) Suspend feeding or reduce infusion rate.

(4) Consider adding lactobacillus.

(5) Antimotility agents: tincture of opium, paregoric, or bismuth can be used but are recommended only when other causes, particularly infectious, have been sought.

Axioims

- Properly timed and titrated nutritional support can reduce comorbidity following trauma.
- Enteral nutrition is preferred over parenteral nutrition. "If the gut works, use it."
- Feeding should be started as soon as possible after initial stabilization from injury.
- Estimate the initial quantity of nutrition using body size.
- Titrate subsequent adjustments to the nutritional plan against physiologic and laboratory parameters that reflect the degree of ongoing catabolism.
- Overfeeding is as harmful as underfeeding the patient.

Bibliography

The ASPEN nutrition support practice manual 1998. American Society for Parenteral and Enteral Nutrition, Silver Spring, MD 1998.

Grahm TW, Zadrozny DB, Harrington T. The benefits of early jejunal hyperalimentation in the head-injured patient. *Neurosurgery* 1989;25(5):729–735.

Kudsk KA, Croce MA, Fabian TC, et al. Enteral versus parenteral feeding. Effects on septic morbidity after blunt and penetrating abdominal trauma. *Ann Surg* 1992; 215:503–513.

Kudsk KA, Minard G, Croce MA, et al. A randomized trial of isonitrogenous enteral diets after severe trauma. An immune-enhancing diet reduces septic complications. *Ann Surg* 1996;224(4):531–543.

Minard G. Enteral access. *Nutr Clin Pract* 1994;9(5):172–184.

Minard G, Kudsk KA. Is early feeding beneficial? How early is early? *New Horizons* 1994;2(2):156–163.

Moore FA, Feliciano DV, Andrassy RJ, et al. Early enteral feeding, compared with parenteral, reduces postoperative septic complications. *Ann Surg* 1992;216(2):173–183.

Moore EE, Jones TN. Benefits of immediate jejunostomy feeding after major abdominal trauma—a prospective, randomized study. *J Trauma* 1986;26(10):874–881.

Moore FA, Moore EE, Jones TN, et al. TEN versus TPN following major abdominal trauma-reduced septic morbidity. *J Trauma* 1989;29(7):916–924.

Young B, Ott L, Twyman D, et al. The effect of nutritional support on outcome from severe head injury. *J Neurosurg* 1987;67:668–676.

45. SUPPORT OF THE ORGAN DONOR

Juan B. Ochoa and Patrick M. Reilly

I. **Introduction.** Organ availability remains the major limitation to the widespread use of organ transplantation in many diseases. In the past decade, the number of people awaiting organ transplantation has doubled, whereas available organ supply has increased one third. As a result, median waiting times for transplants have increased dramatically over the last decade. More people die waiting for organs than ever receive an organ transplant.

A. Organs that can be transplanted include vascularized organs: heart, lung, liver, kidney, pancreas, and small bowel. Other tissues that can be transplanted include bone marrow, bone, fascia, cartilage, cornea, skin, and heart valves.

B. Trauma patients with severe head injuries are the most common organ donors, currently providing one half of the transplanted organs. The number of annual potential organ donors in the United States is estimated to be as high as 27,000. Of these, at a maximum, 15% to 20% of patients become actual donors. **Therefore, strategies aimed at increasing the percent of actual donors could result in an increase in organ availability.**

C. Failure to procure potential organs is multifactorial, including family refusal, lack of awareness by the physician, and inadequate resuscitation of the brain-dead organ donor (Table 45.1). The trauma physician plays a key role in identifying potential donors, contacting the organ procurement organization (OPO), and maintaining homeostasis in the brain-dead patient awaiting harvesting. The OPO should be notified of all potential donors; the OPO and transplant surgeons assess suitability of a potential donor, not the trauma staff. In addition, the OPO is skilled in approaching the family of potential donors and is well versed in brain death. Contact the OPO early in the evaluation of a potential donor.

II. **The potential organ donor**

A. Consider all patients identified to have a fatal or irreversible disease process as potential organ donors. Maximal support of the head trauma victim before brain death guarantees the best chance of organ protection. Exceptions to donation include:
   1. Human immunodeficiency virus (HIV) infection
   2. Viral hepatitis (hepatitis-positive patients can donate to hepatitis-positive patients)
   3. Tuberculosis
   4. Untreated septicemia
   5. Extracranial malignancies
   6. Intravenous drug abuse

B. Over the past 30 years, the definition of death changed from one of cessation of cardiorespiratory functions to that of irreversible damage to the brain. An official change in the attitude toward the diagnosis of death was reflected in the publication of the Uniform Anatomical Gift Act in 1968. In 1981, the President's Commission for the Study of Ethical Problems in Medicine and Biomedical and Behavioral Research published the Uniform Determination of Death Act, which provides the legal basis for the declaration of death. It states:

An individual who has sustained either (1) irreversible cessation of circulatory and respiratory functions, or (2) irreversible cessation of all functions of the entire brain, including the brainstem, is dead. State statutes dictate the mechanism for determination of brain death.

C. **The organ donation process** (Table 45.2)
   1. In trauma victims, lethality of brain injury can often be determined soon after arrival of the patient (especially penetrating head injury).

Table 45.1 Failure to donate: causes and remedial strategies

Causes	Remedial strategies
Failure to recognize potential organ donors	Continuous education Develop a hospital-based organ donation team (social workers, ministers, OPO, ICU staff)
Family refusal –Family approached by primary care team	Call OPO to approach family
–Family informed of death and approached about organ donation at the same time	Primary service informs family of death Temporally separate, telling the family of patient's brain death and approaching the family for organ donation
–Low acceptability of organ donation by minorities	Understand cultural diversity
Failure to expedite diagnosis of brain death	Create clear guidelines for the diagnosis of brain death
Failure to maintain organ homeostasis	Optimize organ perfusion (volume and pressors) Diagnose and treat endocrine abnormalities

OPO, organ procurement organization; ICU, intensive care unit.

Once recognized, contact the OPO to evaluate the patient as a potential organ donor. Inform the family of the severity of brain injury and the potential progression to brain death.
   2. Failure to expedite the determination of brain death results in increased cost to families and the loss of organ donors because of irreversible deterioration of organ function. Brain death is a clinical diagnosis. Confirmation of brain death may require use of diagnostic tests (see below).
III. **Clinical diagnosis of brain death**
   A. Practical determination of brain death varies between institutions. The usual criteria, largely determined by the state, are listed below (see Appendix C).
      1. Documentation of coma
      2. No motor response to painful stimuli
      3. No brainstem reflexes
         a. Pupils are nonreactive to a bright light
         b. Ocular movements—no response to head turning or tympanic caloric testing with ice water
         c. Absence of corneal reflexes
         d. Absence of laryngeal and tracheal reflexes

Table 45.2 Steps in the organ donation process

1. Determine severity of head trauma
2. Determine likely irreversibility of disease process
3. Notify organ procurement organization (OPO)
4. Inform family
5. Optimize organ function, perfusion, and oxygen transport
6. Determine irreversibility of brain injury. First brain death clinical examination
7. Family approached by OPO on the possibility of organ donation
8. Second brain death clinical examination and laboratory evaluation
9. Consent
10. Organ procurement

 4. Apnea—absence of respiratory movements with an increase in $PaCO_2$ >60 mmHg (Table 45.3)
 5. No increase in heart rate following intravenous (i.v.) administration of 2 mg atropine
 B. In addition to a clinical evaluation, intracranial catastrophe must be documented. Most patients will have a neuroimaging procedure (computed tomography [CT] scan or magnetic resonance imaging [MRI]) confirming the clinical impression.
 C. A number of tests can aid in confirming the diagnosis of clinical brain death. They are particularly useful for patients in whom the complete clinical evaluation cannot be done (i.e., uremia or encephalopathy, presence of central nervous system (CNS) depressants, patients with severe ocular trauma, or when the cause of the coma is uncertain). The tests include:
 1. Electroencephalography (EEG)
 2. Cerebral angiography
 3. Transcranial Doppler ultrasonography
 4. Nuclear medicine flow study or xenon flow studies
 5. Somatosensory-evoked potentials
 D. The diagnosis of brain death also requires elimination of confounding factors, which include:
 1. Drug intoxication or poisoning (i.e., barbiturates)
 2. Hypothermia (core temperature must be at least 32°C)
 3. Severe electrolyte and acid-base abnormalities
 4. Severe endocrine disturbances
 5. Hemodynamic instability (systolic blood pressure <90 mmHg)
 E. Clinical brain death evaluation should be completed on at least two different occasions (traditionally 2 to 12 hours apart) and by two different qualified physicians who are not part of the transplant team.
 F. Pronouncement of death. After completion of the two clinical examinations and further confirmatory tests, as indicated, have confirmed lack of brain activity, the patient is declared dead. At many institutions, in a patient with obviously devastating brain injury, a single clinical examination and cerebral blood flow study may be sufficient to declare brain death. Two physicians who are not involved with the transplant team must sign the death certificate. The coroner's permission is required for removal of organs for transplantation, but

Table 45.3 Apnea test

Prerequisites
–Core temperature > 36.5°C
–Systolic blood pressure (SBP) > 90 mmHg
–Euvolemia
–Normal $PaCO_2$
–Normal PaO_2

Connect pulse oximeter and disconnect ventilator

Deliver 100% oxygen, 6 L/min, into the trachea

Look closely for respiratory movements

Measure arterial PO_2, PCO_2, and pH after ~8 minutes and reconnect to the ventilator

If respiratory movements are absent and $PaCO_2$ increases to ≥ 60 mmHg or $PaCO_2$ increases 20 mmHg above baseline, the apnea test is positive and supports the diagnosis of brain death

If respiratory movements are seen, the apnea test is negative

Abort the test if
–Hemodynamic instability (i.e., decrease in SBP < 90 mmHg) or ventricular arrhythmia
–Oxygen desaturation

he or she is not required to sign the death certificate. Permission must be obtained from next of kin.

G. Referral to the local OPO is expedited if the following patient data are available: patient history, diagnosis and date of admission, patient height and weight, ABO group, hemodynamic data, urinalysis, laboratory data, current medications, and culture results.

H. A possible solution to the shortage of organ donors is the use of non–heart-beating cadaveric donors (NHBCD). These are patients who have been declared dead by the traditional cardiopulmonary parameters rather than by brain death criteria. The limiting factor in this situation is warm ischemia time.

IV. **Care of the potential organ donor** (Table 45.4). Physiologic alterations of multiple organ functions are common after brain death. Cardiopulmonary arrest generally follows brain death within hours. The main goal is to maintain organ function while preventing end-organ damage.

A. **Circulatory**. Hemodynamic instability is secondary to myocardial dysfunction, loss of vasomotor tone, and alterations in intravascular volume.

1. Approximately 30% of donor referrals for cardiac transplantation are refused secondary to poor hemodynamic function. Adequate support can minimize poor organ preservation. The goal is to maintain adequate systolic blood pressure and filling pressures to ensure organ perfusion. This is obtained initially by restoration of intravascular volume followed by use of moderate amounts of inotropic support, if needed (see Table 45.4). Blood should be transfused to optimize oxygen delivery. Urine output should be maintained at >0.5 to 1 mL/kg/hour. Excessive use of vasoconstrictive drugs can exacerbate organ hypoperfusion and contribute to myocardial deterioration. Invasive monitoring is often required (arterial and central venous access) to optimize organ perfusion.

2. Dysrhythmias are common. In the absence of hypotension, bradydysrhythmias require no treatment. The patient should be resuscitated if cardiac arrest occurs; solid organ procurement can often still proceed. Cardiac arrest is not a contraindication to solid organ donation.

B. **Respiratory system**. Simple measures should be instituted to prevent accumulation of secretions and atelectasis. Ventilator settings should minimize oxygen toxicity and barotrauma; achieve a PaO_2 of 80 to 100 mmHg with the lowest FIO_2 and positive end-expiratory pressure (PEEP) possible. A PaO_2/FIO_2 <250 and peak inspiratory pressures of >30 cm H_2O are indicative of poor probability of function of the lungs as transplanted organs. Normocarbia and

Table 45.4 Physiologic goals in the organ donor

Cardiocirculatory
–Systolic blood pressure >100 mmHg
–Central venous pressure 10–15 cmH$_2$O
–Inotropic support—dopamine (ideally <10 mg/kg/min)
  —Volume load the patient to wean or minimize vasopressors
  —Avoid alpha-adrenergic agents

Pulmonary
–Arterial O_2 saturation >95%
–FIO_2 < 60%
–PIP < 30 mm H_2O
–PEEP—minimum necessary to attain PaO_2 > 80 mmHg

Fluid and electrolyte management
–Avoid hypernatremia and hypokalemia
–Urinary output between 100 and 250 mL/h

PIP, peak inspiratory pressure; PEEP, positive end-expiratory pressure.

a normal pH should be maintained. Use of excessive amounts of i.v. fluids can cause impaired pulmonary function and affect the suitability of the lungs for organ donation.

C. Fluid and electrolyte therapy. Diabetes insipidus (DI), with concomitant loss of free water, occurs in most brain-dead patients. **Clinical diagnosis is confirmed by the presence of increased urinary output, low urinary osmolality, and hypernatremia.** Desmopressin acetate (DDAVP 0.3 mg/kg i.v.) may be required to treat DI. Adequate volume replacement is essential. Monitor serum electrolytes and correct, as necessary. Hyperglycemia, with the resulting osmotic diuresis, should be avoided.

Axioms
- Trauma victims constitute the largest population of organ donors.
- An extreme shortage of organs exists. The population of patients who actually donate could be increased by early recognition of potential donors, appropriate and timely diagnosis of brain death, and adequate physiologic care of the organ donor.
- The trauma physician plays an essential role in organ donation.
- Brain death is diagnosed using a set of clinical criteria and confirmatory tests.
- Preservation of organ homeostasis requires the understanding that physiologic changes are occurring in each organ after brain death ensues. Maintaining homeostasis increases the chances for a successful function of each transplanted organ

Bibliography
Evans RW, Orians CE, Ascher NL. The potential supply of organ donors. *JAMA* 1992; 267(2):239–246.

Gram HJ, Meinhold H, Bickel U, et al. Acute endocrine failure after brain death? *Transplantation* 1992;54(5):851–857.

Grenvik A, Darby JM, Broznick BA. Organ transplantation: an overview of problems and concerns. In: Civetta JM, ed. *Critical care.* Philadelphia: JB Lippincott, 1992: 803–813.

Jenkins DH, Reilly PM, Schwab W. Improving the approach to organ donation: a review. *World J Surg* 1999;23:644–649.

Kennedy AP, West JC, Kelley SE, et al. Utilization of trauma-related deaths for organ and tissue harvesting. *J Trauma* 1992;33(4):516–520.

Klufas ChI, Powner DJ, Darby JM, et al. Organ donor categories and management. In: Shoemaker WC, Ayres S, Grenvik A, et al., eds. *Textbook of critical care.* Philadelphia: WB Saunders, 1994:1604–1617.

Lee PP, Kissner P. Organ donation and the Uniform Anatomical Gift Act. *Surgery* 1986;100(5):867–875.

Peitzman AB, Udekwu AO, Darby JM. Organ procurement and transplantation. In: Feliciano DV, Moore EE, Mattox KL, eds. *Trauma.* Norwalk, CT: Appleton & Lange, 1996:989–997.

Pennefather SH, Dark JH, Bullock RE. Haemodynamic responses to surgery in brain-dead organ donors. *Anaesthesia* 1993;48:1034–1038.

Powner DJ, Darby JM, Grenvik A. Controversies in brain death certification. In: Shoemaker W, ed. *Textbook of critical care,* 2nd ed. Philadelphia: WB Saunders, 1994: 1579–1582.

Report of the Quality Standards Subcommittee of the American Academy of Neurology. Practice parameters for determining brain death in adults. *Neurology* 1995;45: 1012–1014.

Wheeldon DR, Potter CDO, Dunning J, et al. Hemodynamic correction in multiorgan donation. *Lancet* 1992;339:1175.

46. BURNS/INHALATION

Kevin Farrell and Linwood R. Haith, Jr.

I. **Introduction**
   A. **Epidemiology**
      1. Annually, ~75,000 people in the United States require hospitalization for burn or inhalation injury, with a 10% mortality rate.
      2. Most burn deaths each year occur in residential fires caused by heating unit failure, kitchen accidents, arson, and smoking.
      3. Child abuse must be suspected for unusual burns in children (Chapter 47).
      4. One third of burn patients have other injuries.
   B. **Transfer to burn center**
      1. Approximately one third of hospitalized patients require treatment in a burn center.
      2. American Burn Association (ABA) criteria for considering transfer:
         a. **Second and third degree burns**
            • >10% [1]BSA in ages <10 years and <50 years
            • >20% BSA
            • Face, eyes, ears, hands, feet, genitalia, perineum, major joints
         b. **Third degree >5% BSA**
         c. **Significant electrical and chemical burns**
         d. **Inhalation injury**
         e. **Preexisting illness or associated injuries**
         f. **Children with special needs: social, emotional, rehabilitation, victims of abuse**
II. **Prehospital**
   A. **History**
      1. Time of injury (start time for calculating fluid resuscitation)
      2. Open or closed space (inhalation more likely)
      3. Source: flame, liquid, steam, chemical, explosion
      4. Duration
      5. Presence of toxic materials: plastics, cyanide
      6. Mechanism of injury: motor vehicle crash (MVC), fall, jump
      7. Quantity of prehospital fluid
   B. **Care at scene**
      1. Burn victims are trauma patients and require trauma care.
      2. Remove patient from source of injury.
      3. Remove burning clothing.
      4. Assess for immediate life-threatening injuries.
      5. Cool and rinse wounds with water.
      6. Apply dry dressings.
      7. Provide supplemental oxygen and airway protection.
      8. Initiate rapid transport to hospital.
III. **Initial assessment and resuscitation**
   A. **General**
      1. Burn injury can be dramatic and distract the resuscitation team from associated injuries.
      2. Patients with severe burn injury may appear **deceptively stable on arrival**. A patient may be talking (and even joking) on admission with stable blood pressure and mild tachycardia. Within 24 hours, the patient is frequently critically ill, on a ventilator with respiratory and circulatory failure.

[1] Burn surface area

3. Provide early pain control with frequent small doses of intravenous (i.v.) morphine (e.g., 1–5 mg of morphine sulfate every 5–30 minutes, as needed).
4. Elevate the ambient room temperature to avoid heat loss from the burn wound.
5. Consider gastric decompression for patients with BSA >25% after initial resuscitation of airway, breathing, and circulation.

B. **Airway**
1. **NOTE**: Although urgent endotracheal intubation is sometimes necessary, time usually exists to access the airway and provide a semi-elective intubation, when necessary.
2. Provide supplemental oxygen to all patients. This is sometimes challenging in anxious patients and patients with significant facial burns because of the inability to secure the mask. It may require an assistant to manually hold the oxygen source over the airway.
3. Criteria for intubation are the same as in all trauma patients. The following clinical conditions may require immediate or early intubation in a burn patient.
   a. Apnea, respiratory failure, or profound hypoxia
   b. Patients with severe facial burns may appear initially stable. Consider semi-elective intubation because profound facial and tongue swelling over the next 4 to 8 hours can make intubation very difficult.
   c. Signs and symptoms of inhalation injury
      • History of closed space exposure
      • Singed eyebrows and nasal hair
      • Carbon deposits in oral cavity
      • Carbonaceous sputum
      • Wheezing
      • Apnea, cherry red color
   d. Upper airway obstruction frequently occurs in patients with burns of the face and neck. Soft-tissue swelling of the face, oropharynx, glottis, and trachea can be dramatic, precluding safe endotracheal intubation and making tracheostomy more difficult.
4. The proper securing of an endotracheal tube in a patient with severe facial burns is **critical** in initial management. Inadvertent extubation in a patient with severe facial swelling can be a lethal event. Tie tubes in place with tracheal or umbilical tape or secure with Velcro fasteners. It may be necessary to secure the tube with adhesive tape wrapped around the endotracheal tube and stapled to the face.

C. **Breathing**
1. If intubated, ventilate with 100% oxygen (generally with 5–8 cm H_2O of positive end-expiratory pressure [PEEP]) with a goal of avoiding high airway pressures and maintaining patient comfort. Perform arterial blood gas (ABG) to assure adequate oxygenation, ventilation, and clearance of acidosis.
2. Perform chest radiograph to look for associated trauma, signs of inhalation lung injury, and position of tubes (e.g., endotracheal, nasogastric, central line).
3. Bronchoscopy may be necessary to access inhalation injury.
4. Circumferential chest burns with high airway pressures (>40 cm H_2O) may require escharotomy. **Note**: Patients without complete circumferential chest burns may also require escharotomy to provide adequate ventilation.

D. **Circulation**
1. **Intravenous access** is ideally obtained with large-bore (14–16 gauge in adults) peripheral catheters placed through unburned tissue. In severe burns (>25% BSA), it is optimal to obtain central access early before massive swelling and edema occur. Placement through burned tissue is acceptable if the only option.

2. **Initial fluid resuscitation**
   a. Start with a **nonglucose**-containing crystalloid (**Ringers lactate (RL)** preferred by most).
   b. **How to use the Parkland formula (4 mL/kg/%BSA)**
      - Hang 1,000 mL of RL wide open until time is available to calculate the rate.
      - The formula is **only a guide** to get started and set a general expectation for fluid requirement in the **first 24 hours**.
      - Only partial and full-thickness burns (**second and third degree**) are included in BSA.
      - **BSA** is determined by the **rule of nines** (Fig. 46.1).
      - Start at a rate that would give **one half of the calculated** 24-hour **requirement** in the **first 8 hours**. Conceptually, the second half is given in the next 16 hours.
      - The **first 8 hours begins at the time of burn**, not at the time the patient is first seen.

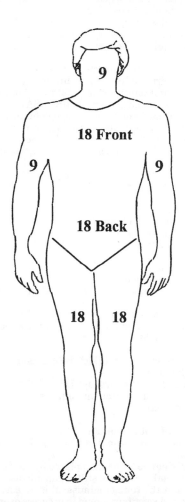
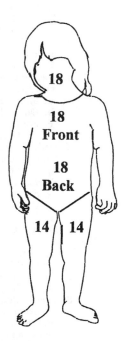

FIG. 46.1. Rule of nines

- Include the fluid given to the patient (even before seen) in the first 8-hour calculation.
- Once started, use **urinary output** to guide the fluid rate to obtain a **minimum of 0.5 mL/kg/hour** in the adult.
- An automated infusion pump is usually necessary to provide the required fluid.
- In the second 24-hours postburn, give crystalloid at a rate of 1 mL/kg/%BSA burn/24 hours. If the patient requires additional crystalloid, use RL or NS (Normal saline). Avoid hyponatremia (Na+ <130 mEq/L). D5NS, D5 1/2 NS, and D5W can be used. Ultimately, after resuscitation, sodium-containing fluids should be minimized.

   c. A subset of patients (**inhalation injury, high voltage electrical, delayed resuscitation, massive deep burns**) may require additional fluid over that recommended by formulas (e.g., chronic diuretic therapy, ileostomies). The presence of hemoconcentration (i.e., hematocrit >55%) may indicate total body fluid deficit, which may require initial fluid beyond that which yields urinary output of 50 mL/hour.

   d. Any patient who does not respond with adequate urine output during the first few hours of resuscitation, is elderly, or has a history of cardiopulmonary disease may require pulmonary artery catheter or ultrasound guided fluid management.

   e. **Colloid** administration (5% albumin, hetastarch, and so on) is recommended by many experts to start at **8 hours postburn** at a rate of **0.5 mL/kg/%BSA/24 hours** and continued from 36 to 48 hours postburn. This is usually reserved for large burns (>40% BSA).

   f. **Discolored urine** can occur from hemolysis or myoglobinuria, which should prompt a **goal urinary output of 100 mL/hour.** If urine does not clear promptly, give 12.5 g of **mannitol**, which can be subsequently added to each 1 L of RL, and search for compartment syndrome.

  E. Pediatric fluid resuscitation (infants and toddlers) (Chapter 47)

    1. The head is a much larger proportion of calculated BSA than in adults (see Table 7, Chapter 47).

    2. Careful fluid resuscitation is necessary to avoid:
      a. Pulmonary edema from excessive fluid administration
      b. Cerebral edema associated with hyponatremia

    3. Formula for estimated fluid = maintenance + 3 mL/Kg/% BSA/24hours with RL
      a. Maintenance prorated over 24 hours
      b. One half of burn component in first 8 hours
      c. For children <age 1, maintenance component is given as D5RL and the burn component as RL.

    4. Colloid (5% albumin) at 0.5 mL/kg/% BSA/24hours is started after 8 hours, continued to 36 hours postburn, and then stopped or tapered up to 48 hours postburn (for patients >20% BSA burn).

    5. Second 24 hours
      a. Start D5 and 1/2 NS at maintenance + 0.8 mL/kg/%BSA/24hours
      b. Goal is urine output of 1 mL/kg/hour
      c. If serum sodium (Na) <130 mEq/L at 24 hours, use D5 and NS

    6. Do not use D5W to resuscitate burned children and infants.

IV. Initial wound assessment and management

  A. Assessment

    1. BSA >10% is best assessed by the **rule of nines** (Fig. 46.1)

    2. Smaller burns or noncontiguous burns are estimated by using the surface of the patients **palm** as 1% BSA.

    3. Terminology for burn depth using **"degree"** is being replaced by the description of **"thickness"**, although both terms are still commonly used (Fig. 46.2). Classification of depth at the time of admission is an estimate and may be inaccurate because deeper burns tend to progress over time from the effect of edema on the microcirculation.

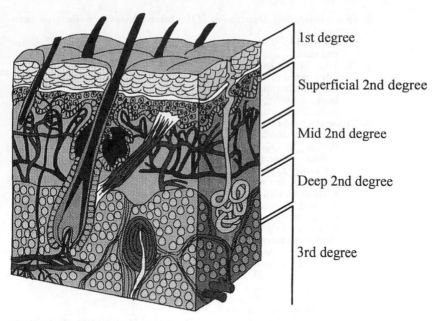

1st degree

Superficial 2nd degree

Mid 2nd degree

Deep 2nd degree

3rd degree

FIG. 46.2. Burn wound depth

4. **Burn depth**
   a. **Superficial** (first degree, sunburn)
      • Confined to epidermis with minimal tissue damage
      • Mild erythema, pain resolving in 48 to 72 hours
      • Epidermis may peel in small scales without scarring
   b. **Partial thickness** (second degree)
      • Entire epidermis with variable layers of dermis
      1) Superficial
         • Painful, red, edematous, and blistered
         • Large number of viable dermal skin appendages
         • Spontaneous healing in 7 to 14 days
      2) Deep
         • Red, extensive weeping, without blisters, less pain
         • Few viable dermal skin appendages
         • Prolonged healing, usually with scarring
   c. **Full thickness** (third degree)
      • Entire epidermis and dermis destroyed
      • Relatively **painless**, leathery, waxy, or charred with **thrombosed vessels**
      • Will not heal without excision and grafting
B. **Initial burn wound management**
   1. In the emergency department before transport to a burn center.
      a. Wash gently with gauze soaked in saline or 4% chlorhexidine.
      b. Remove any obviously loose skin.
      c. Apply **topical agents** (see below) **only** if anticipated **delay in transfer** because removal of the agent at the burn center can prolong the initial cleansing and debridement.
      d. Irrigate debris from the anesthetized eye, if time permits.
      e. Cover wounds with dry sterile dressings.

2. In the emergency department of the **burn center** or **definitive care hospital**.
   a. Burns <10% BSA can be cleansed, debrided, and covered with a topical agent.
   b. Treat **larger burns** by placing the patient in a special gurney (usually located in the burn unit), which allows for total exposure, overhead heating, rapid burn wound debridement by a specially trained team, cleansing using gentle hose spray, provision of adequate analgesia, and continuous monitoring of vital signs.
3. **Topical agents**
   a. **Silver sulfadiazine 1% cream** (Silvadene, Hoechst Marion Roussel, Inc. Kansas City, MO)
      - Most common topical agent used on burn wounds
      - Usually applied daily or twice daily in a thin layer, using a sterile glove or tongue depressor
      - This followed by wrapping loosely with sterile gauze
      - Broad-spectrum bacteriostatic, relatively painless
      - Transitory neutropenia (sulfa effect) can occur
      - Caution in pregnancy and very small infant (<2 months)
   b. **Mafenide acetate 10% cream** (Sulfamyalon, Dista Products and Eli Lilly, Indianapolis)
      - Usually indicated for deep ear burns to prevent otochondritis
      - Penetrates eschar, somewhat painful
      - Mild metabolic acidosis (carbonic anhydrase inhibitor)
      - Broad-spectrum bacteriostatic
   c. **Bacitracin ointment**
      - Ointment (not cream) usually applied to small superficial burns and surfaces difficult to cover with gauze (e.g., face)
      - May require several applications per day because of inadvertent removal owing to exposure
      - Primarily bacteriostatic against gram-positive organisms
      - Neosporin, polysporin, or gentamicin ointments can be substituted for broader bacterial coverage.
   d. **Acticoat**
      - Silver impregnated membrane
      - Left in place on wound for 2 to 3 days
      - Useful for outpatient of small wounds
   e. **Silver nitrate 0.1%**
      - Use only when other broad-spectrum agents contraindicated
      - Costly, messy, electrolyte abnormalities (e.g., hyponatremia)
4. **Escharotomy**
   a. Circumferential **full-thickness** burns of the **chest** or **extremities** can cause a compartment syndrome.
   b. High airway pressures (>40 cm H_2O) in a circumferential torso burn
   c. Markedly diminished or absent distal pulse in a circumferential extremity burn
   d. May be required early in burn wound management
   e. Technique (Fig. 46.3)
      - In theory, bloodless and painless (usually not the case)
      - Provide analgesia and sedation.
      - Perform with electrocautery, when available.
      - Include the skin eschar only, not the fascia.
      - Requires snug (not tight) wrapping to minimize blood loss
      - Inadequate hemostasis with multiple escharotomies can result in significant blood loss, which can be troublesome if the patient is going to be transferred subsequent to the procedure.
V. **Inhalation injury**
   A. **Overview**
      1. Results from **direct thermal injury** (inhalation of superheated air or water vapor), **toxic chemicals** in inhaled smoke, or a combination of both.

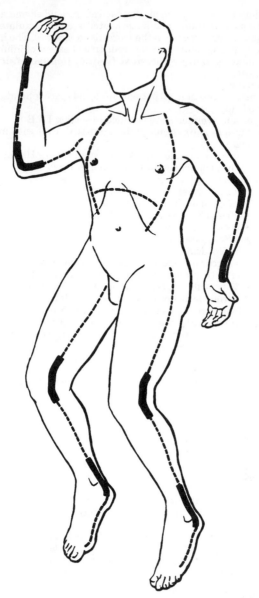

FIG. 46.3. Preferred sites for escharotomy. (From Martin RR, Becker WK, Cioffi, et al. In: Wilson RF, ed. *Management of trauma. Pitfalls and practice.* Baltimore: Williams & Wilkins, 1996, with permission.)

   2. Injury to the proximal airway can cause rapid edema and obstruction.
   3. Chemical irritants and superheated steam stimulate an intense inflammatory response in the more distal airways. The history of the environment of injury may be predictive of extent of injury.
   4. Inhalation injury is the **most frequent cause of death** in thermal injuries.
B. Evaluation
   1. Consider present in all patients in closed space inhalation injuries, until ruled out.
   2. Signs and symptoms are outlined in section **III.B**
   3. Obtain a **carboxyhemoglobin (CO-Hb)** level with initial laboratory studies.
      a. Carbon monoxide has 240 times affinity for Hb than does oxygen
      b. Arterial or venous specimen (heparinized)
      c. Levels
         • <5%, normal
         • <20%, may be asymptomatic
         • 20% to 30%, headache and nausea
         • 30% to 40%, confusion
         • 40% to 60%, coma
         • >60%, death
      d. Can occur as isolated carbon monoxide poisoning in the absence of thermal exposure. However, in the presence of thermal injury, an elevated CO-Hb suggests an associated inhalation injury.
      e. A normal level does not rule out inhalation injury.
      f. **Note**: Patients who have sustained chronic exposure to CO may be obtunded or have significant neurologic deficits at CO-Hb levels considerably lower than those associated with such symptoms after acute exposure.
   4. Initial chest radiograph may be normal.
   5. Bronchoscopy
      a. Usually delayed until initial resuscitation underway and patient is hemodynamically stable
      b. If the patient is not intubated, thread an endotracheal tube onto the scope so that definitive airway can be obtained if bronchoscopic findings warrant.
      c. Findings include erythema, edema, ulcerations, carbonaceous material, and edematous cords.
      d. Irrigation with saline is indicated for copious carbonaceous debris.
   6. Spirometry may reveal a flattened flow volume loop.
C. Treatment
   1. Administer 100% oxygen to all patients until the CO-Hb is <5%.
   2. Early intubation and mechanical ventilation is recommended for symptomatic patients.
   3. In stable patients with symptoms of CO poisoning, hyperbaric oxygen may mitigate against long-term neurologic sequelae of CO exposure, especially if instituted within 6 hours of exposure. However, hyperbaric oxygen may be helpful even if the CO-Hb level is normal at the time of initiation.
VI. Electrical injury
   A. Overview
      1. Electrical injuries are uncommon and frequently present a diagnostic challenge because of the myriad of clinical presentations. Small skin wounds can hide substantial underlying muscle and bony destruction.
      2. Generally, electrical injuries are classified into **low-voltage (<1,000 volts) and high-voltage (≥1,000 volts)**.
      3. Severity of injury to tissues depends on the **amperage** (the amount of current passing through the tissues). Amperage = voltage/resistance.
      4. Resistance of the tissues is dependent on the water content. The tissues with the greatest resistance tend to sustain the most heat damage. The resistance in decreasing order is:

    a. Bone → fat → tendon → skin → muscle → vessel → nerve. (Bone can suffer the greatest heat damage, whereas nerve tissue has little resistance to the current.)

    b. Wet skin has much less resistance than dry skin.

  5. Pathway of current is unpredictable, but generally passes from the point of entry through the body to a grounded site (site with the lowest resistance). However, with high voltage, the pathway may be indiscriminate, exiting at multiple sites.

  6. In general, alternating current (AC) is more dangerous than direct current (DC).

  7. Electrical injuries commonly have associated major traumatic injuries (e.g., falls).

  8. Tetanic contractures associated with alternating current can cause fractures and dislocations.

B. Low-voltage injury

  1. Usually occurs in the household (e.g., hair dryer in bathtub)

  2. Cardiac dysrhythmia is most common, particularly ventricular fibrillation, the cause of which is not clear.

  3. Tetanic contractions (AC household current) can cause fractures and respiratory asphyxia.

  4. Central nervous system (CNS) abnormalities are the result of any associated hypoxia rather than current conduction through the CNS tissues.

  5. Admit for electrocardiographic (ECG) monitoring, unless admitting ECG is normal.

  6. Oral burns in children

    a. Small children sucking on an electrical cord

    b. Can involve all oral structures, but most commonly the **lip**

    c. Treatment includes:

- Hospitalize because of the risk of **delayed bleeding**
- Feed by straw or syringe
- Delay debridement 1 week
- Intraoral splint may be necessary
- Tetanus prophylaxis
- Antibiotic prophylaxis usually not indicated

C. High-voltage injury

  1. The extent of tissue damage is usually **underestimated** because of the unpredictable path of injury. These are usually **devastating** injuries.

  2. Entrance and exit sites are pathognomonic of the injury, but may not be obvious. Entrance wounds are usually at points of contact and exit wounds are usually at points of grounding.

  3. An associated flash skin burn is not uncommon and can distract from the more devastating electrical injury to the deeper and remote tissues.

  4. The subcutaneous or deep injury is characterized by intense **patchy myonecrosis**, especially along the deeper tissues adjacent to bone (high resistance area).Vessel thrombosis and compartment syndrome (both early and delayed) are common sequelae.

  5. Fluid management

    a. Anticipate need >4 mL/kg/% BSA/24 hours

    b. If myoglobin present

- Urine output >1 mL/kg/hour
- Mannitol, 25 g i.v. every 4 to 6 hours
- Sodium bicarbonate to i.v. solution if urine pH <7

  6. Wound management

    a. Early aggressive and repetitive wound debridement

    b. Extremity fasciotomy frequently required

    c. Because of the uneven and patchy nature of tissue necrosis, amputation of a devitalized extremity may be necessary (even in the presence of adequate blood supply).

7. General management
   a. Tetanus prophylaxis
   b. Effective pain management
   c. Local antibiotics to thermal injury
   d. Avoid broad-spectrum system antibiotics early without specific indication.
   e. Anticipate the need for ventilatory support and probable organ dysfunction.
8. After initial resuscitation, most patients with high-voltage injury should be referred to a burn center because **experience** with these injuries is essential.

VII. Chemical burns
A. Overview
1. Most burns are from acids, alkalies, and petroleum.
2. The extent of injury depends on the **concentration** of agent and **duration** of contact.
3. Tissue damage is frequently underestimated.
4. Alkali burns are generally the most severe.

B. Treatment
1. Remove all garments and brush off any dry powder.
2. In the field and on arrival, irrigate with **tap water**.
   a. Acid burns: 1 hour
   b. Alkali burns: 2 hours
3. Irrigate the eyes and obtain ophthalmology consult.
4. **No specific antidote** is available for most chemical burns, except hydrofluoric acid.

C. Hydrofluoric acid burn
1. Highly toxic and painful
2. Can cause hypocalcemia and dysrhythmia with systemic absorption
3. Concentration >40% can be lethal if >2% BSA
4. Treatment
   a. Copious irrigation with water
   b. Apply 2.5% **calcium gluconate** gel
   c. Soft-tissue injection of calcium gluconate (1 g/10 mL) can be done in small areas in cases of persistent pain. Infuse calcium gluconate intraarterially for finger and hand burns in cases of limited tissue space for injection and appropriate expertise exists.
   d. Indications for intraarterial infusion of calcium include severe pain, evidence of tissue necrosis, and pain not improving with calcium gluconate gel.
   e. Method for intraarterial calcium gluconate infusion:
      • Place a brachial artery catheter and perform angiogram to assure adequacy of perfusion to involved fingers (a high brachial artery bifurcation is not uncommon). This procedure is usually performed by interventional radiology.
      • Alternatively, a radial artery catheter can be used if only the thumb, index finger, or both are involved.
      • Infuse calcium gluconate (2 g) in D5W (100 mL) over 4 hours.
      • Repeat every 4 hours until pain is markedly decreased.
      • Infuse heparin (200 U/hour) in between calcium gluconate infusion.
   f. Immobilize arm with brachial artery catheter and keep immobilized for 6 hours after removal.
   g. Monitor ionized calcium and serum magnesium.

VIII. Definitive care of the burn patient
A. Burn wound
1. The depth of the burn wound may be obvious early, but several days may be required to differentiate between superficial and deep partial-thickness wounds.
2. The best diagnostic tools are the eyes of a surgeon experienced in burn wound care.

3. Superficial (first degree) wounds require only cleansing and analgesia.
4. Superficial partial-thickness (second degree) wounds can heal spontaneously with cleansing and topical antibiotic cream (e.g., silver sulfadine).
   a. The appearance of epithelial "budding" is a useful predictor of primary healing.
   b. Several weeks are usually required for epithelization.
5. Deep partial-thickness (second degree) and full-thickness (third degree) wounds usually require excision and grafting to provide coverage and healing.
6. Topical agents are applied once or twice daily. When mafenide acetate (Sulfamylon, Dista Products and Eli Lilly, Indianapolis, IN) is used alternating with silver sulfadine, in extensive deep burns, a twice-daily application is used. Silver sulfadine is frequently used with a single daily application, but can be used twice daily.

B. **Excision**
   1. Small wounds (<5% BSA) can be excised and covered with a split-thickness skin graft (STSG) as soon as the patient is stable.
   2. Larger wounds (>10% BSA) usually require sequential excisions and placement of either temporary or permanent wound coverage.
   3. To avoid excessive blood loss and hypothermia, excise no more that 10% to 15% BSA at an operative session for large surface area burns (>25%).
   4. A variety of dermatome and free hand knives are available for excision.
   5. **Tangential** excision (most common) attempts to remove only devitalized tissue and retain as many dermal elements as possible.
      a. Variable amounts of subcutaneous fat may be visible.
      b. Although fat can decrease the likelihood of graft success, it helps maintain cosmesis.
   6. **Excision to fascia** may be necessary in full-thickness burns with underlying fat necrosis.
      a. Although faster and with less blood loss, the cosmetic deficit is substantial.

C. **Coverage**
   1. The best **permanent** coverage for most burn wounds is a **split-thickness skin graft** (0.010–0.014 in) and meshed at a ratio of 1.5:1.
   2. The graft must be secured to the wound (staples or sutures) and covered with a nonadherent dressing and padding to protect from sheering.
   3. Protective positioning of the patient (e.g., prone) may be necessary to protect the graft.
   4. The graft is usually inspected at 4 to 6 days, unless signs of infection prompt an earlier evaluation.
   5. **Temporary coverage** of the excised burn wound with **cadaver skin**, **pigskin**, or synthetic materials such as Biobrane (Dew Hickam, Inc. Sugarland, TX) and Trancyte (Advanced Tissue Sciences, LaJolla, CA) may be helpful in the following clinical circumstances:
      a. Inadequate autologous donor skin
      b. Uncertainty of the viability of the wound (e.g., potential need for further excision)
      c. Need to reduce fluid and heat loss and the metabolic demand from the wound
      d. Provide patient comfort
      e. **Integra** (Life Sciences Holding Corp. San Diego, CA) and **Allo-Derm** (Life Cell-HealthCare. Branchburg, NJ) are emerging as useful permanent dermal substitutes.
   6. Cultured epithelial cells, although fragile, have been used to provide epithelial coverage in massive burn wounds where no permanent alternatives are available.
   7. Severe burns to the face and hands usually require special techniques and the expertise of a burn unit.

D. Critical care
 1. Most critical care management and organ protection parallels that of the trauma patient (Chapter 38).
 2. Intensive care unit issues more specific to the burn patient include:
    a. Prophylactic antibiotics are not indicated, unless signs of infection are present (e.g., burn wound biopsy/culture).
    b. The presence of inhalation, and face and neck burns require a more conservative approach to weaning and extubation than most trauma patients.
    c. In large burns (>25%BSA), the analgesia and logistic needs of twice-daily dressing changes and sequential operative excisions in the operating room may require heavy sedation and continued ventilatory support.
    d. A **warm environment** is needed to prevent heat loss from wounds.
    e. The burn patient has a very high metabolic rate (until the wounds are fully covered), requiring ~2,000 kcal/m^2 with a protein load of 1.5 to 2.0 g/kg/day.
    f. Enteral nutrition is superior to parenteral support in improving outcome, but frequently both are needed to meet the needs of the patient.
    g. Fever is common in burn patients, but does not necessarily mean an infection exists.
    h. Ionized hypocalcemia is common in burn patients, especially in initial resuscitation.
    i. Patients with major burns commonly develop inability to concentrate their urine and may have an obligatory urinary output. This usually occurs in the critical care phase of care and can be a misleading parameter of adequate perfusion.
E. Burn wound sepsis
 1. In general, significant bacterial colonization of the wound does not occur for several days after injury because of the intact eschar. However, soon thereafter, colonization occurs, primarily with endogenous organisms.
 2. The most common organisms recovered from burn wounds include staphylococcus (85%), B-hemolytic streptococcus (5%), *Pseudomonas aeruginosa* (25%), *Escherichia coli* (40%), enterococcus (55%), and *Candida albicans* (49%).
 3. Invasive infection (versus colonization) is best determined by a burn wound biopsy and quantitative bacteriology demonstrating >10^5 organisms/gram of tissue.
    a. Early burn wound sepsis (first week) is usually caused by *Staphylococcus aureus*, which is characterized by a slow onset, high fever and white blood cell (WBC) count, disorientation and loss of granulation tissue (mortality = 5%).
    b. Later burn wound sepsis (7–10 days) is usually caused by *P. aeruginosa* and is characterized by a rapid onset (12–36 hours), marked hemodynamic instability, high or low temperature and adnormal WBC count and a patchy black surface necrosis. (Mortality = 20% to 30%).
    c. *Candida albicans* is another cause of later burn wound sepsis with a slower onset. The systemic and wound changes may be less marked than bacterial infection, but the mortality ranges from 30% to 50%.
 4. The best prevention and treatment is application of topical antibiotics as described above, combined with early excision of the wound. Early systemic antibiotics are not effective because of the poor tissue blood flow of the burn wound. However, targeted antimicrobial therapy is indicated for invasive wound sepsis diagnosed by clinical examination and wound biopsy with quantitative culture.
F. Rehabilitation
 1. Rehabilitation of the burn patient is one of the most challenging clinical issues in modern medicine because the process is lifelong and the scars are permanent.

   2. Rehabilitation should begin with admission and include the following
   components:
      a. Early wound closure
      b. Exercise
      c. Positioning and splinting
      d. Skin care
      e. Thermoregulation
      f. Psychological support
      g. Restoration of function
   3. See Chapter 50

Axioms

- After initial resuscitation, burn patients meeting ABA burn center criteria should be strongly considered for transfer.
- Burns often present as spectacular injuries; therefore, it is imperative to perform primary and secondary surveys to assess for associated trauma.
- Burn injuries occurring in a closed space (e.g., building, car) should be considered to have an inhalation injury until proved otherwise.
- Early intubation should be considered for patients with facial burns because of the high likelihood of inhalation injury and progressive orofacial edema can impede intubation.
- Document the time of burn injury and the amount of fluid infused before arrival at a hospital or burn center.
- Formulas for fluid requirements are only guides to initiate resuscitation; adequate urine output is the best clinical measure of adequate volume resuscitation.
- Patients with associated inhalation injuries or electrical injuries usually require more resuscitation fluid than those without.
- The initial calculation of BSA, using the "rule of nines," is designed to be an estimate of partial- and full-thickness burns.
- Inhalation of toxic smoke is the most frequent cause of death in burn injuries.
- The severity of high-voltage electrical injuries is often underestimated. This is usually a devastating injury requiring aggressive resuscitation and surgery.
- Definitive care of the partial- and full-thickness burn wound usually requires excision and grafting with a split-thickness skin graft. Apply temporary coverage with nonautologous skin or synthetic materials during the process of permanent coverage.

Bibliography

American Burn Association. *Advanced burn life support manual*. American Burn Association. Chicago. 1998.
American College of Surgeons Committee on Trauma. *Advanced trauma life support manual*. Chicago: American College of Surgeons, 2001.
Demling RH. Thermal injury. In: Wilmore DW, ed. *Scientific American surgery: care of the surgical patient*. New York: Scientific American, 1999;1:III.
Martin RR, Becker WK, Cioffi WG, et al. Thermal injuries. In: Wilson RF, ed. *Management of trauma. Pitfalls and practice*. Baltimore: Williams & Wilkins, 1996:760–771.
Wolfe S, Herndon DN, eds. *Burn care*. Austin, Texas: Landes Bio-Science, 1999.

47. PEDIATRIC TRAUMA

Michael G. Scheidler, James M. Lynch, and Henri R. Ford

I. **Incidence**
   A. Trauma is the leading cause of mortality in children between the ages of 1 and 14 years in the United States; more children succumb to injuries and their sequelae than all other childhood diseases combined. Nearly 16,000,000 children visit emergency departments for injuries each year. Of those, 15,000 die and 20,000 are temporarily disabled. The long-term disability is estimated to be more than three times the mortality rate, and is primarily the result of brain injury. As in adults, boys are more frequently injured than girls by a factor of 2:1.

II. **Mechanisms of injury (Fig. 47.1)**
   A. **Blunt** trauma accounts for nearly 90% of pediatric injuries.
      1. Motor vehicle collisions (MVC) are the most common cause of injury and death in children.
   B. **Penetrating** trauma accounts for 10% of pediatric injuries.

III. **Overview**: difference between children and adults
   A. **General body differences (Table 47.1)**
   B. Organ system differences (see below)

IV. **Resuscitation.** The basic principles of trauma resuscitation apply to children. Specific considerations are outlined below.
   A. **Airway**
      1. **Assessment**
         a. A child's ability to speak, cry, and breathe spontaneously suggests a patent airway. Stridor can result from laryngeal spasm, the presence of nasopharyngeal or oropharyngeal secretions, or a foreign object. Wheezing may indicate bronchial spasm, which is more common in children with small airways.
         b. Nasal flaring or sternal retraction can indicate respiratory compromise.
         c. In children with altered mental status, consider early intubation.
      2. **Management**
         a. Oropharyngeal obstruction can be managed initially with oral suctioning and head positioning. Tongue obstruction, a common cause of airway compromise, can be managed with the jaw thrust maneuver, or by placing the chin in the "sniffing" position with a cervical collar in place, while maintaining cervical spine stabilization.
         b. In most cases, bag valve mask (BVM) ventilation provides adequate oxygenation for pediatric patients. Keep the neck in the neutral position to optimize airway diameter. Maintain cervical spine precautions at all times.
         c. Patients with compromised airway who do not respond to conservative measures—(a) or (b), above—or patients with severe head injury (Glasgow Coma Scale [GCS] score <8) require orotracheal intubation after adequate preoxygenation with BVM ventilation.
      3. Considerations during orotracheal intubation
         a. Preoxygenate, but do not hyperventilate.
         b. The larynx is more anterior and sits higher in the neck at the level of the third cervical vertebra.
         c. The epiglottis is omega shaped.
         d. The trachea is short, therefore, right mainstem intubation occurs more frequently than in adults **(Table 47.2)**.
      4. Nasotracheal intubation is **not** recommended because of the sharp angle between the nasopharynx and the oropharynx and the small

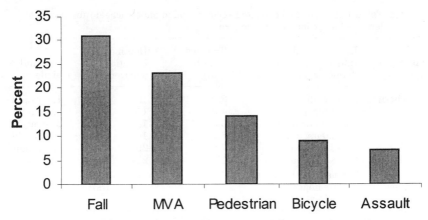

FIG. 47.1. Distribution of the most common causes of pediatric trauma: fall, motor vehicle crash (MVC), pedestrian, bicycle-related, and assault as a percent of all causes of pediatric trauma. Data supplied by the National Pediatric Trauma Registry, 1999.

Table 47.1 General body differences: children versus adults

Factor	Difference
Size and shape	• Less fat and connective tissue available for protection. • Energy is transferred and dispersed over a smaller body surface area. • Internal organs are in relatively close proximity, which predisposes to multiorgan injuries. • Solid organs are larger compared with the rest of the abdomen. • Rib cage is higher, affording less protection to abdominal organs. • The infant's head is disproportionately larger compared with the adult and subjected to a high incidence of shear injuries.
Skeleton	• Incomplete ossification of bones causes them to be more pliable and thus less likely to fracture. As a result, pulmonary contusions and splenic lacerations often occur without rib fractures. • A different array of partial fractures (e.g., greenstick, torus, and buckle fractures). • Injuries to the growth plates during the various stages of childhood development result in a specific pattern of fractures.
Surface area	• Large surface area to weight ratio results in a greater predisposition to heat loss (3 times greater) and hypothermia.
Psychological development	• Children often regress to a previous developmental stage during stressful and anxiety-provoking situations.
Long-term effects of injury	• Splenectomy in children places them at life-long risk for overwhelming postsplenectomy sepsis (OPSS).

Table 47.2 Size of trachea and recommended endotracheal tube size, length of insertion, and blade size

Age (years)	Endotracheal tube internal diameter (mm)	Trachea length (cm)	Depth of insertion (cm from lips)	Size and blade
Newborn	3.0 uncuffed	3.0	10	1, straight
1	3.5–4.0 uncuffed	4.3	11	2, straight
3	4.0–4.5 uncuffed	5.3	13	2, straight
5	4.5–5.0 uncuffed	5.7	16	3, straight
7–10	6.0–6.5 cuffed	7.0	20	3, straight/
Adult	7.0–8.0 cuffed	10.0+	22+	curve
General rules	Diameter of the child's little finger or (16 + age in years)/4		Age (in years) + 10	

(From the Children's Hospital of Pittsburgh, Benedum Pediatric Trauma Program, Pediatric Field Reference, October 1997, with permission.)

diameter of endotracheal tube that can be placed through the child's nares.

5. A surgical airway, which is rarely indicated, is associated with high complication rate, especially in younger children (<8 years). In older children (>12 years), options include surgical cricothyroidotomy or translaryngeal jet (needle) ventilation. **Remember**, BVM ventilation is often effective and, in most cases, allows sufficient time to perform tracheostomy "safely" in the operating room.

6. Pharmacologic management during endotracheal intubation (**Fig. 47.2**).

B. **Breathing**

1. Auscultate in axillary area to reduce noise from opposite chest.

2. Check for symmetric chest wall rise with every breath.

3. Respiratory rate (RR) and tidal volume (TV) vary with age (**Table 47.3**).

4. Increased lung compliance permits easy lung expansion and ventilation. Therefore, vigorous assisted ventilation with large TV can cause barotrauma, leading to bronchial rupture.

5. Hypoventilation and hypoxia are common causes of cardiorespiratory arrest in pediatric trauma patients.

6. Inability to ventilate both lung fields after endotracheal intubation should raise concern about right mainstem intubation or pneumothorax. Early chest x-ray study is recommended.

7. If tension pneumothorax is suspected, perform immediate needle decompression (see section V.C) followed by chest tube insertion. If hemothorax or pneumothorax is found on chest x-ray, insert chest tube (**Table 47.4**).

C. **Circulation**

1. Vital signs are age-related and the response to shock differs in children (**Table 47.5**).

2. Heart rate (HR) is the most important early indicator of hypovolemic shock in pediatric trauma patients.

3. Blood pressure is an inadequate measure of volume status or resuscitation endpoint. Children can maintain their blood pressure until significant volume loss (≥45% of blood volume) has occurred. Stroke volume is relatively fixed in infants and young children and depends on venous return. Therefore, the response to hypovolemia is to increase HR

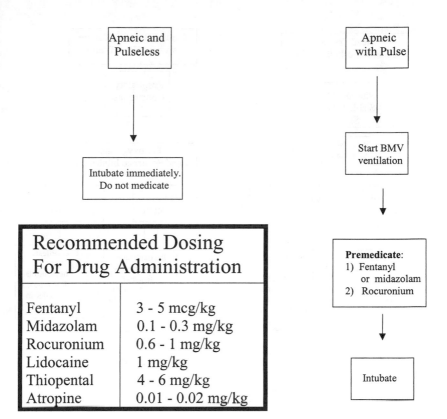

FIG. 47.2A. Protocol for airway management for (**A**) apneic patients and (**B**) those breathing spontaneously with or without associated head trauma. Insert contains current recommendations for appropriate medication doses.

to maintain blood pressure. Hypotension reflects loss of >45% of blood volume or failure of adaptive mechanisms.

4. Fluid resuscitation
   a. Blood volume is estimated at 80 mL/kg. Consider hypovolemic shock if:
      (1) Heart rate is >10% of value calculated for age.
      (2) Blood pressure is <5th percentile (70 + 2× age in years).
   b. Begin fluid bolus with 20 mL/kg of Ringer's lactate, which can be repeated up to three times. If no improvement, transfuse O negative packed red blood cells (PRBC) (10 mL/kg).
   c. Basic fluid requirements (maintenance IVF) can be calculated using the following approaches:
      (1) 100 mL/kg/day for the first 10 kg, plus 50 mL/kg/day for the next 5 kg, plus 20 mL/kg/day for each kg over 16 kg.
      (2) 4 mL/kg/hour for the first 10 kg; between 10 kg and 20 kg, 40 mL/hour plus 2 mL/kg/hour for every kilogram over 10; >20 kg, 60 mL/hour plus 1 mL/kg/hour for every kilogram over 20.
   d. The resuscitation fluid of choice is Ringer's lactate or normal saline. Dextrose-containing solutions are not indicated during the

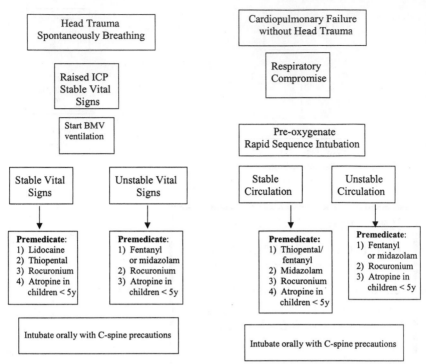

FIG. 47.2B. *Continued.*

resuscitation period because of hyperglycemia from the elevated catecholamine response of traumatic stress.

5. Intravenous access (i.v.)
   a. Place largest size i.v. possible, one on each side of the patient, in upper or lower extremities.
   b. In the hypotensive child (<6 years) with difficult i.v. access, insert an intraosseous (i.o.) line before venous cutdown to initiate fluid

Table 47.3 Age-specific vital signs

Age (years)	Weight (kg)	Pulse per min)	Systolic blood pressure (mmHg)	Respiratory rate	Tidal volume (mL)
Newborn	3	160	70	60	240
1	9	130	85	40	700
3	15	120	89	30	1,200
6	24	110	94	25	2,000
10	35	90	100	20	2,800
Adults	75	70	120	15–20	5,000

(From the Children's Hospital of Pittsburgh, Benedum Pediatric Trauma Program, Pediatric Field Reference, October 1997, with permission.)

Table 47.4 Age appropriate chest tube, nasogastric tube, and Foley catheter sizes

| Age (years) | NG Tube (F) | Foley catheter (F) | Chest tube (F) | |
			Hemothorax	Pneumothorax
Newborn	5	5 feeding	10	10 or pigtail
1	10	8	10–12	small or pigtail
3	10	10	16–20	small or pigtail
6	12	10	20–24	small or pigtail
Adults	16	16	28–32	28–32

resuscitation (see below). In older children in whom venous access cannot be obtained otherwise, cutdown may be necessary. If necessary, preferred venous cutdown sites include:

    (1) Greater saphenous vein anterior to the medial malleolus at the ankle, or proximal thigh below junction with femoral vein

    (2) Basilic and cephalic veins of the antecubital fossa

  6. In children <6 years, i.o. line is a useful method for administering resuscitation fluid (crystalloid or blood) or medication.

    a. Place the i.o. line 1 cm inferior and medial to the tibial tuberosity.

    b. For children 0 to 1 years of age, use an 18- to 20-gauge spinal needle. A 13- to 16-gauge bone marrow needle is required for children >1 year of age.

    c. Contraindications include fracture in the same leg, pelvic fractures, or a conscious child.

    d. Remove the i.o. line within 4 hours to decrease risk of osteomyelitis.

D. Disability: neurologic evaluation

  1. Quick assessment:

    a. GCS score modified for pediatric patients **(Table 47.6)**.

  2. Goal is to minimize secondary brain injury. Secondary injuries can be prevented by maximizing **cerebral perfusion pressure** (mean arterial

Table 47.5 Systemic response to hypovolemic shock in children

System	<25% Blood volume loss	25% to 45% Blood volume loss	>45% Blood volume loss
Cardiac	Weak, thready pulse; increased heart rate	Increased heart rate	Hypotension, tachycardia to bradycardia
Central nervous system	Lethargic, irritable, confused	Change in level of consciousness, dulled response to pain	Comatose
Skin	Cool, clammy	Cyanotic, decreased capillary refill, cold extremities	Pale, cold
Kidneys	Minimal decrease in urinary output, increased specific gravity	Minimal urine output	No urinary output

Table 47.6 Glasgow Coma Scale score

Infant		Child	
Eye opening			
4	Spontaneously	4	Spontaneously
3	To speech	3	To command
2	To pain	2	To pain
1	No response	1	No response
Best verbal response			
5	Coos, babbles, smiles	5	Oriented
4	Irritable, crying	4	Confused
3	Cries, screams to pain	3	Inappropriate words
2	Moans, grunts	2	Incomprehensible
1	No response	1	No response
Best motor response			
6	Spontaneously	6	Spontaneously
5	Withdraws from touch	5	Withdraws from touch
4	Withdraws from pain	4	Withdraws from pain
3	Flexion (decorticate)	3	Flexion (decorticate)
2	Extension (decerebrate)	2	Extension (decerebrate)
1	No response	1	No response

(From the Children's Hospital of Pittsburgh, Benedum Pediatric Trauma, Program, Pediatric Field Reference, October 1997, with permission.)

pressure [MAP] intracranial pressure [ICP] by adhering to basic principles of resuscitation.). **Avoid the following**:
   a. Hypoxemia: keep oxygen saturation >98%.
   b. Hypercapnia or hypocapnia: maintain $Paco_2$ between 32 and 35 mmHg.
   c. Hypotension: maintain blood pressure around 50th percentile for age; 80 + 2× age in years.
   d. Hypertension: monitor fluid resuscitation; avoid excessive hydration. Antihypertensive drugs are rarely required.
3. Indications for intracranial pressure (ICP) monitoring in the child with closed head injury:
   a. GCS <8
   b. Inability to monitor clinical examination
4. Manifestation of head injuries in children:
   a. Seizures: use a short-acting benzodiazepine. Posttraumatic seizures are usually brief and treatment with anticonvulsants is unnecessary.
   b. Vomiting: treat symptomatically, ensuring that significant intra-abdominal trauma has not occurred. During periods of emesis, maintain cervical spine precautions and avoid aspiration of vomitus.
   E. **Exposure**: avoid hypothermia in infants and children.
V. **Secondary survey and management**
   A. **Head**
      1. Of pediatric traumatic deaths, 75% result from head injury.
      2. Computed tomography (CT) is the most sensitive and specific modality to evaluate children with suspected head injury. Children with an altered mental status or loss of consciousness (with GCS 14 or 15), GCS ≤13, or posttraumatic seizures or emesis require a CT of the head. No role exists for skull films.
      3. Scalp lacerations can cause significant blood loss, especially in a child. Examine lacerations for underlying skull fractures.

4. The fontanelle and sutures are open in children <18 months of age.
5. Intracranial lesions
  a. Concussion
  b. Diffuse axonal injury
  c. Intracranial bleed
    (1) Epidural hematomas are more prevalent in children than subdural hematomas.
    (2) Intracranial hematomas can be managed nonoperatively when focal defects are absent and the child is awake and oriented. Operative intervention is required for expanding lesions or those that cause a mass effect or produce neurologic deficits.
    (3) Blood loss can be substantial with an intracranial hemorrhage, and may necessitate blood transfusion.
    (4) Temporal bone fractures are in close proximity to the middle meningeal artery, which accounts for a high proportion of epidural bleeds with this fracture. Intracranial hematomas and contusions generally are much less common in children than adults.
  d. Skull fractures
    (1) Linear, complex, depressed
    (2) Skull fractures are relatively common, with most occurring in the parietal bone. A 10-fold increased risk of intracranial hematoma exists when a skull fracture is present.
    (3) Operative intervention is required in cases of an overlying scalp laceration; underlying intracranial lesion, which requires surgery; or depression greater than the thickness of the skull.
    (4) Controversy exists regarding the long-term consequence of head injuries in children. In general, outcomes in pediatric patients are better than in adults.
B. Neck
  1. Major anatomic differences in children:
    a. Shorter neck with a proportionately heavy head promoting flexion of the neck
    b. Laxity of the ligaments and decreased muscle support
    c. Anterior wedging of the vertebral bodies
    d. Horizontally oriented facet joints of C1–C4
  2. Cervical spine injuries
    a. **Cervical spine fractures**: most (>85%) cervical spine fractures in children <8 years occur between C1 and C3. In children >10 years of age, the cervical spine is similar to, and the pattern of injury resembles, that seen in adults (C4–C7).
    b. **Pseudosubluxation** of C3 on C2 occurs in 40% of children <7 years as a normal variant.
    c. **Subluxations** occur in ~ 10% to 20% of cervical spine injuries alone or in conjunction with associated fractures.
    d. **Spinal cord injury without radiological abnormality (SCIWORA)** occurs predominantly in children and is responsible for 4% to 21% of cervical spine injuries. Transient or permanent neurologic defects occur without any radiologic evidence.
    e. **Altanto-occipital dislocation** (AOD) is the separation of the cranium from the cervical spinal column producing proximal spinal cord injury. This injury results predominately from the laxity of the transverse ligament in children. Mortality is nearly 100%.
C. Chest: (85% blunt; 15% penetrating)
  1. Immediate life-threatening injuries
    a. Tension pneumothorax: air trapped under pressure in the pleural space shifts the relatively mobile mediastinum in children to the opposite side of the chest, obstructing venous blood return to the heart.

         (1) Midaxillary line (MAL) is the optimal place for needle decompression in infants and small children. Insertion via the second interspace, midclavicular line can injure the pulmonary artery

         (2) For infants and young children, an 18-gauge or 20-gauge needle is recommended for decompression.

  b. Cardiac tamponade: treatment is similar to that for adults.

  c. Hemothorax: initial drainage >20% of blood volume or continued bleeding of 1 to 2 mL/kg/hour are indications for thoracotomy.

  d. Tracheobronchial injuries are more common in children than in adults.

         (1) Most laryngeal injuries occur at or above the fourth tracheal ring.

         (2) After securing the airway, early operative exploration and repair is indicated.

  e. Penetrating injuries to the chest are managed in similar manner as in adults.

         (1) Children sustain many chest injuries by air-powered rifles (BB or pellet guns).

         (2) These potentially lethal injuries warrant a high index of suspicion, with 33% to 50% of patients requiring operative intervention.

2. Potentially life-threatening injuries

  a. Pneumothorax: air trapped in the pleural space.

         (1) Requires urgent chest tube decompression

         (2) Place all chest tubes laterally in the MAL.

         (3) Enter the pleural cavity with a hemostat, not a trocar, to avoid damage to the lung.

  b. Rib fractures are uncommon and indicate severe injury.

         (1) Rib fractures represent significant transmission of energy and are associated with a 10% mortality rate from concomitant injuries.

         (2) Rib fractures are related to child abuse in 20% of the cases.

  c. Pulmonary contusion

         (1) Pulmonary contusion is the most common injury to the chest.

         (2) Responds to conservative management with aggressive pulmonary physiotherapy and oxygenation.

         (3) Fewer than 5% of all children with pulmonary contusion require intubation (Chapter 26a).

  d. Traumatic asphyxia

         (1) Sudden compression of the abdomen or chest against a closed glottis

         (2) A sudden increase in intrathoracic pressure that is transmitted to the superior vena cava

         (3) Seizures, mental status change, and respiratory failure ensue and petechiae develop in the face.

  e. Cardiac contusion

         (1) Cardiac contusion does not produce arrhythmias as in adults; however, cardiac monitoring is appropriate for 24 hours.

D. Abdomen

  1. Up to 60% of children with intraabdominal injuries have concomitant head injury.

  2. Gastric distension from swallowing air during the act of crying is the most common cause of abdominal distension. If severe, abdominal distension can interfere with respiratory effort. In such cases, nasogastric decompression is indicated.

  3. Upper abdominal organs are susceptible to injury from minimal forces because of the lack of protection from underdeveloped rib cage and musculature.

4. Evaluation
   a. Inspect, auscultate, and palpate.
   b. Radiographic studies
      (1) Computed tomography is the most sensitive study to evaluate intraabdominal injuries.
      (2) Focused abdominal sonography for trauma (FAST) is useful to detect free intraperitoneal fluid but its role in pediatric trauma is still evolving.
   c. Laboratory tests
      (1) Amylase or lipase
      (2) Aspartate aminotransferase (AST) and alanine aminotransferase (ALT)
      (3) Hemoglobin and hematocrit: type and crossmatch or type and screen.
      (4) Urine analysis
      (5) Prothrombin time (PT) or partial thromboplastin time (PTT) in patients with suspected head injury
5. Specific injuries
   a. **Spleen**
      (1) The most frequently injured abdominal organ in children (40%)
      (2) Patients present with abdominal or shoulder pain (Kehr's sign) or shortness of breath.
      (3) Of patients, 30% to 40% will have associated abdominal injuries.
      (4) CT scan is 98% sensitive and the modality of choice for diagnosis.
      (5) Most pediatric patients are hemodynamically stable on presentation; 95% can be managed nonoperatively, often without blood transfusion.
      (6) Hemodynamic instability, clinical deterioration, or associated hollow viscus injury mandates operation.
         (a) Fewer than 5% to 10% of patients will require blood transfusion.
      (7) Overwhelming postsplenectomy sepsis (OPSS)
         (a) Lifetime risk is 0.026%
         (b) Mortality rate for those who develop OPSS is 50%.
         (c) Prophylaxis with penicillin until the age of 18 years (controversial)
         (d) Vaccination against pneumococcus, *Haemophilus influenza*, and meningococcus.
      (8) Long-term management
         (a) Repeat radiologic studies are not necessary.
         (b) Contact sports or vigorous exercise should be restricted for a period that consists of CT grade plus 2 weeks, although some authors recommend up to 3 months.
   b. **Seatbelt complex**
      (1) Consists of abdominal wall ecchymosis above the anterior iliac spine, intestinal injury, and fracture of the lumbar vertebral body (Chance fracture)
         (a) A rapid deceleration results in flexion of the upper body around the seatbelt, compression of the abdominal viscera, and a sudden increase in intraluminal pressure.
         (b) Injuries occur at points of fixation of intestines with the jejunum, descending and sigmoid colon being most commonly injured.
      (2) Only 60% of radiographic studies will be diagnostic; delayed diagnosis occurs in 10% of cases.
      (3) Between 50% and 70% are associated with a Chance fracture of L1–L3 vertebrae.

c. Liver
   (1) Injuries to the liver are common (15% to 30%) and require operative repair more often than splenic injuries in children
   (2) Of patients, 10% will arrive in shock; 30% of children will have associated injuries.
   (3) Most injuries (60% to 78%) occur in the right lobe.
   (4) Indications for operative intervention are similar to splenic injuries.
      (a) Management in children is similar to adults, with major liver resection used sparingly.
      (b) Mortality rate is 25%.

d. Pancreas
   (1) Represents 1% to 3% of all blunt abdominal injuries in children; epigastric pain is most common symptom.
   (2) Most common mechanism of pancreatic injuries involves blunt force to the abdomen from the handlebar of a bicycle.
   (3) Pancreatic injuries include duct transection and contusion.
      (a) Pancreatic contusions can be treated nonoperatively.
      (b) Early operative intervention of major ductal injuries results in shorter hospitalization, earlier return to enteral feeding, and fewer complications than nonoperative management.
   (4) Differentiation between transection and contusion can be difficult.
      (a) Serum amylase <200 U/mL, and lipase <1,800 U/mL combined with the physical examination (epigastric or abdominal tenderness) correlate with pancreatic transection or major ductal injury.
      (b) CT evaluation: 72% sensitive and 99% specific

e. Duodenum
   (1) Although uncommon, duodenal injuries are associated with serious complications.
   (2) Of duodenal injuries, 20% are related to child abuse.
   (3) Mortality (6% to 25%) and morbidity (33% to 60%) resulting from duodenal perforation is directly related to time of diagnosis and definitive treatment; mortality increases fourfold when diagnosis is delayed by 24 hours.
      (a) Abdominal pain is the most common symptom (80% to 100%) followed by bilious vomiting (80%).
      (b) CT is diagnostic in only 60% of the cases: retroperitoneal air behind the duodenum and right colon.
   (4) Duodenal hematoma: extrinsic compression of the lumen by a hematoma in the bowel wall causes complete obstruction of the duodenum.
      (a) Nonaccidental trauma is associated in 50% of cases.
      (b) Most will resolve with conservative treatment, including nasogastric tube decompression and hyperalimentation.
      (c) Duodenal obstruction from hematoma can take 3 weeks to resolve. Failure to resolve can require operative evacuation.

f. Small bowel
   (1) Injuries to the small bowel usually involve rupture along the antimesenteric border (jejunum).
      (a) The small bowel is fixed at the ligament of Treitz and the cecum.
      (b) The mesentery of the small bowel contains less fat and is more friable in children.
   (2) Resection and primary anastomosis can be performed in most cases.

E. Pelvic fractures
  1. Of children with pelvic fractures, 20% also sustain abdominal injuries. Unless displaced, these fractures are treated nonoperatively.
  2. Associated urethral injuries are rare.
F. Genitourinary (GU) tract injury
  1. The GU tract is injured in 10% of pediatric trauma patients; 98% from blunt trauma (85% from MVC).
  2. The degree of hematuria does not correlate with the severity of injury to the GU tract. Conversely, a normal urinalysis does not preclude the possibility of a GU tract injury.
    a. Renal injuries: kidneys are relatively larger in children and assume a lower position in the abdomen.
      (1) Of pediatric trauma patients, 10% sustain significant renal injuries.
      (2) Renal injuries occur more frequently in children than in adults. The renal capsule (Gerota's fascia) is less developed in children than in adults.
      (3) Children typically present with abdominal pain and either microscopic or gross hematuria.
      (4) CT of the abdomen with i.v. contrast and delayed images is highly specific and sensitive. An angiogram is unnecessary in most cases.
      (5) Fewer than 5% of children with renal injuries require operative repair.
      (6) Hypertension can develop 6 months to 15 years after injury to the renovascular pedicle; blood pressure must be monitored regularly following major renal injury.
    b. Bladder: the narrow and small pelvis of a child allows the bladder to assume an intraabdominal location.
      (1) The dome of the bladder is mobile and distensible.
      (2) Of bladder injuries, 50% are associated with other abdominal injuries and 75% to 95% are associated with pelvic fractures.
      (3) Conventional CT misses 33% of bladder injuries; a cystogram is required in all patients with gross hematuria.
      (4) Bladder size varies with age
        (a) Children <2 years: bladder volume = 7 mL/kg.
        (b) Children between the ages of 2 and 11 years: bladder volume = 2 (age in years) × 30 mL.
    c. Straddle injury: compression of the soft tissue of the perineum against the bony pelvis.
      (1) Injuries are sustained from falls, bicycle-related crashes, and activities associated with playground equipment.
      (2) Patients present with a history of bleeding from the perineum (50%).
      (3) Examine under anesthesia with visualization of the vaginal vault.
      (4) Missed injuries can lead to late complications, including urethral and vaginal strictures.
G. Musculoskeletal injury
  1. Specific injuries in children
    a. Epiphyseal fractures
    b. Shaft fractures
    c. Dislocations
  2. Complications common after musculoskeletal injury in children
    a. Early ischemia
    b. Growth centers during stages of childhood
    c. Growth disturbances
    d. Vascular necrosis
    e. Joint instability

3. Treatment
   a. Traction and splinting
   b. Reestablished circulation before fracture stabilization.

VI. Burns (Chapter 46)
   A. Burns resulting from house fires are the leading cause of accidental death in the home for children <14 years.
   B. Of burned children, 20% are victims of abuse.
      1. Most burn injuries occur in children <4 years.
      2. Scald burns are the most common form of burn injury.
   C. Ringer's lactated is the fluid of choice in the first 24 hours, with the quantity guided by the Parkland formula:
      1. Resuscitate all patients with burns >15% to 20% body surface area (BSA) using the Parkland formula as a guideline **(Table 47.7)**.
      2. Estimated amount of fluid in first 24 hours = 4 mL × %BSA burn × wt (kg).
   D. Fluids during the second 24 hours
      1. Compensates for evaporative loss and maintenance.
      2. Add colloid and D5¼ NS; prevent **hyponatremia** and **hypoglycemia**.
      3. The amount of albumin required can be calculated by the formula: 0.3 mL/kg of a 5% albumin solution for burns with a BSA of 30% to 50%.

VII. Child abuse and nonaccidental trauma
   A. Legality
      1. Any professional is required to report suspected child abuse to civil authorities.
      2. This requirement supersedes doctor-patient relationships, carries penalties for failure to report, and provides immunity if reported in good faith.
      3. Abuse can consist of neglect, physical abuse, sexual abuse, or emotional abuse.
      4. Sexual abuse occurs in all levels of society.
   B. Incidence
      1. Annually, 1 to 1.5 million children are abused; 60,000 with serious or life-threatening injuries; 1,000 to 2,000 die (usually <5 years of age).
      2. One of every 10 children treated in the emergency department for injury has sustained intentional injury.
   C. History
      1. Evasive parent or caregiver
      2. Changing story of the event
      3. Unwitnessed injury in young child

Table 47.7 Pediatric burn "rule of nines"

	Age (years)				
	0	1	5	10	Adult
Head	19	17	13	11	7
Neck	2	2	2	2	2
Anterior trunk	13	13	13	13	13
Posterior trunk	13	13	13	13	13
Buttocks	2.5	2.5	2.5	2.5	2.5
Genitalia	1	1	1	1	1
Upper arm	2.5	2.5	2.5	2.5	2.5
Lower arm	3	3	3	3	3
Hand	2.5	2.5	2.5	2.5	2.5
Thigh	5.5	6.5	8	8.5	9.5
Leg	5	5	5.5	6	7
Foot	3.5	3.5	3.5	3.5	3.5

   4. Delay in seeking care for the child, often several hours or days
   5. Child endowed with physical powers beyond chronologic or physical
      development
   6. History of the incident and degree of injury do not agree
   7. Multiple emergency department or physician visits
   D. Patterns of injury associated with physical abuse
      1. Soft-tissue injuries: most injuries are to soft tissue.
         a. Bruising on normally nonbrusied areas or in various stages of healing
         b. Marks of objects (e.g., cigarettes, belt buckles, whips)
         c. Traumatic hair loss
      2. Musculoskeletal: second most common system affected
         a. Spiral fractures attributed to a "fall"
         b. Subperiosteal calcification with no history of injury
         c. Multiple fractures in various stages of healing
         d. "Bucket-handle" or epiphyseal-metaphyseal separation from shaking
            or jerking
      3. Intracranial: third most commonly injured area, but most common cause
         of death
         a. Chronic or bilateral subdural hematoma
         b. Shaken baby syndrome: petechial hemorrhage throughout brain
            parenchyma. May demonstrate retinal hemorrhage (or detachment)
            in children <3 years of age.
      4. Visceral injuries: fourth most common area injured
      5. Evaluation
         a. CT of head and abdomen, skeletal survey, optical examination for
            those <3 years of age, and laboratory studies (blood count, liver func-
            tion, amylase, and lipase)
VIII. **Pediatric scoring**
   A. Pediatric Trauma Score (PTS) **(Table 47.8)**
      1. The most common scoring system applied to pediatric trauma patients
         is the PTS.
      2. The PTS is an index used to predict outcome. It is based on anatomic
         and physiologic parameters and injuries sustained. Values are assigned
         to six components and range from −2 to +2. A combined score of ≤8 is
         associated with a poor outcome.
   B. Age-specific pediatric trauma score **(Table 47.9)**
      1. Current scoring systems used in pediatric trauma are not age specific.
      2. The Age-Specific Pediatric Trauma Score (ASPTS) incorporates age-
         specific values for systolic blood pressure, pulse, and respiratory rate in
         addition to the GCS.
      3. Values are assigned from 0 to 3 for each parameter.
   C. Other common scoring systems include the Injury Severity Score (ISS) and
      the Abbreviated Injury Score (AIS), both of which also correlate injury with
      outcome.

Table 47.8 Pediatric trauma score

Component	+ 2	+ 1	− 1
Airway	Normal	Maintainable	Unmaintainable
Central nervous system	Awake	Obtunded	Comatose
Weight	>20 kg	10–20 kg	<10 kg
Systolic blood pressure	>90 mmHg	50–90 mmHg	<50 mmHg
Open wounds	None	Minor	Major or penetrating
Fractures	None	Closed	Opened or multiple

(From the Children's Hospital of Pittsburgh, Benedum Pediatric Trauma Program, Pediatric Field
Reference, October 1997, with permission.)

Table 47.9 Age-specific pediatric trauma score (ASPTS)

GCS	Systolic blood pressure (SBP)	Pulse	Respiratory rate (RR)	Coded score
14–15	Normal	Normal	Normal	3
10–13	Mild-moderate hypotension (SBP < mean – 3 SD)	Tachycardia (pulse > mean – SD)	Tachypnea (RR > Mean + SD)	2
4–9	Severe hypotension (SBP < Mean – 3 SD)	Bradycardia (pulse >mean – SD)	Hypoventilation (RR > mean – SD)	1
3	0	0	0 or intubated	0

Age-specific variables (SBP, pulse, and RR) and GCS were stratified by degree of severity, and coded values (0–3) were assigned to each variable. The ASPTS is the sum total of coded values for all four variables.
GCS, Glasgow Coma Scale score; SD, standard deviation.

Bibliography

Black TL, Snyder CL, Miller JP, et al. Significance of chest trauma in children. *South Med J* 1996;89(5):494–496.

Kurkchubasche AG, Fendya DG, Tracy TF Jr., et al. Blunt intestinal injury in children: diagnostic and therapeutic considerations. *Arch Surg* 1997;132(6):652–658.

Luerssen TG, Klauber MR, Marshall LF. Outcome from head injury related to patient's age: a longitudinal prospective study of adult and pediatric head injury. *J Neurosurg* 1988;68:409.

Mutabagani KH, et al. Preliminary experience with focused abdominal sonography for trauma (FAST) in children: is it useful? *J Pediatr Surg* 1999;34:48–52.

Nadler EP, Gardner Mc Schall LC, et al. Management of blunt pancreatic injury in children. *J Trauma* 1999;47(6):1098–1103.

Potoka DA, Schall LC, Ford, HR. Development of a novel age-specific pediatric trauma score. *J Pediatr Surg* 2001;36:106–112.

Sarihan H, Abes M, Akyazici R, et al. Traumatic asphyxia in children. *J Cardiovasc Surg* 1997;38:93–95.

Stylianos S. Evidence-based guidelines for resource utilization in children with isolated spleen or liver injury. The APSA Trauma Committee. *J Pediatr Surg* 2000; 35:164.

Tso EL, Beaver BL, Haller A. Abdominal injuries in restrained pediatric passengers. *J Pediatr Surg* 1993;28(7):915–919.

48. CARE OF THE PREGNANT TRAUMA PATIENT

Glen Tinkoff

I. **Introduction**. Injury occurs in 6% to 7% of all pregnancies and is the leading nonobstetric cause of maternal death. Furthermore, maternal compromise and injury severity are the principal factors in trauma-related fetal demise. Accordingly, optimal early management of the pregnant trauma victim yields the best possible outcome for the fetus; thus, the tenet, "save the mother, save the fetus." Although initial treatment priorities remain the same, anatomic and physiologic changes that accompany pregnancy are important modifiers of trauma care in all settings.

II. **Anatomic changes and potential clinical consequences**
   A. Uterus
      1. Increased size (7 cm/70 g → 36 cm/1,100 g)
      2. Intraabdominal location after 12th week (Fig. 48.1)
      3. Thinning of muscular wall
      4. Increased blood flow (60 mL/minute → 600 mL/minute)
      5. Potential clinical consequences
         a. Increased susceptibility to injury
         b. Increased bleeding
         c. Compression of inferior vena cava in supine position (supine hypotension syndrome)
   B. Placenta
      1. Lack of elasticity
      2. Catecholamine sensitivity
      3. Potential clinical consequences
         a. Prone to separation from uterus wall (abruption)
         b. Decreased placental blood flow, with stress leading to fetal compromise
   C. Pelvis
      1. Venous engorgement
      2. Ligamentous relaxation
      3. Potential clinical consequences
         a. Increased severity of hemorrhage
         b. Gait instability and increased risk of falls
         c. Altered radiologic appearance and misdiagnosis
   D. Genitourinary
      1. Dilated collecting system
      2. Displaced bladder → intraabdominal
      3. Potential clinical consequences
         a. Altered radiologic appearance and misdiagnosis
         b. Increased risk for injury
   E. Gastrointestinal
      1. Intestinal displacement into upper quadrant
      2. Alteration in gastroesophageal junction
      3. Peritoneal "stretching"
      4. Potential clinical consequences
         a. Altered injury pattern
         b. Decreased peritoneal sensitivity and misleading physical examination
         c. Increased risk for reflux and aspiration
   F. Diaphragm
      1. Elevated (4 cm)
      2. Increased excursion (1–2 cm)
      3. Potential clinical consequence
         a. Altered anatomic landmark (e.g., misplaced chest tube)
         b. Decreased functional residual capacity (FRC)

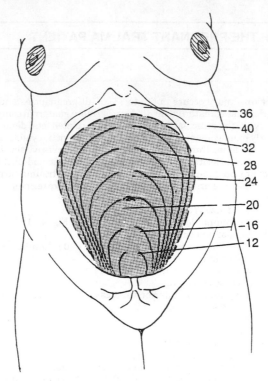

FIG. 48.1. Uterine size. (From Knudson MM. Trauma in pregnancy. In: Blaisdell FW, Trunkey DD, eds. *Abdominal trauma*, 2nd ed. New York: Thieme, 1993:326, with permission.)

    G. Heart
        1. Displaced cephalad
        2. Potential clinical consequences
            a. Electrocardiographic (ECG) changes—left axis deviation; T-wave flattening, or inversion in leads III and AVF
    H. Pituitary
        1. Enlarged by 135%
        2. Increased blood flow demands
        3. Potential clinical consequences
            a. Shock can cause necrosis of the interior pituitary gland, resulting in pituitary insufficiency (Sheehan's syndrome).
III. Physiologic changes or potential clinical consequences
    A. Cardiovascular
        1. Increased cardiac output
        2. Increased heart rate
        3. Increased blood pressure (second trimester)
        4. Decreased central venous pressure
        5. Decreased peripheral vascular resistance
        6. Increased ectopy
        7. Potential clinical consequences
            a. Altered vital signs
            b. Preexisting hyperdynamic condition

B. Hematologic
    1. Increased blood volume predominantly caused by increased plasma volume
    2. Decreased hematocrit (32% to 36%) caused by an increase in plasma greater than red blood cell (RBC) volume
    3. Increased white blood cell (WBC) count (18–25 WBC/mm^3)
    4. Increased factor I, VII, VIII, IX, and X
    5. Decreased plasminogen activator levels
    6. Potential clinical consequence
        a. Altered hematologic parameters
        b. Physiologic "anemia"; physiologic "hypervolemia"
        c. Signs of ongoing hemorrhage delayed; one third of the mother's blood volume can be lost without change in heart rate or blood pressure.
        d. Increased volume requirement with hemorrhage
        e. Hypercoagulability; increased risk for venothromboembolism
C. Respiratory
    1. Increased minute ventilation
    2. Increased tidal volume
    3. Decreased functional residual capacity
    4. Potential clinical consequence
        a. Chronic respiratory alkalosis
        b. Decreased respiratory buffering capacity
        c. Altered response to inhalation, anesthetics
        d. Propensity for rapid oxygen desaturation
        e. Decreased tolerance of hypoxemia
D. Renal
    1. Increased renal blood flow
    2. Increased creatinine clearance
    3. Increased glomerular filtration rate
    4. Decreased glucose resorption
    5. Potential clinical consequences
        a. Decreased blood urea nitrogen
        b. Decreased serum creatinine
        c. Glucosuria
E. Gastrointestinal
    1. Decreased gastric emptying
    2. Increased gastric acid production
    3. Impaired gallbladder contraction
    4. Potential clinical consequence
        a. Increased risk for acid reflux or aspiration
        b. Bile stasis or increased gallstone formation
F. Endocrine
    1. Increased placental lactogen
    2. Increased progesterone
    3. Increased estrogen
    4. Increased parathormone
    5. Increased calcitonin
        a. Insulin resistance or pregnancy-induced diabetes
        b. Lower esophageal sphincter relaxation
        c. Delayed gastric emptying
        d. Increased calcium absorption
G. Neurologic
    1. Pregnancy-induced hypertension (eclampsia)
        a. Increased risk for intracranial hemorrhage
        b. Increased risk for seizures
        c. Mimics head injury
IV. Mechanisms of injury
  A. Blunt
    1. Motor vehicle collisions (MVC) >falls >assaults
    2. MVC are the leading nonobstetric cause of maternal and fetal mortality.

3. Placental abruption is the most common cause of fetal death when the mother survives.
4. Pelvic fractures are the most common maternal injury associated with fetal death.
5. The most common fetal injury is skull fracture, with intracranial hemorrhage.
6. Uterine rupture is associated with ejection from the vehicle and presents with maternal shock and uterine tenderness.
7. Utilization and proper application of seatbelt is the most important factor in preventing maternal injury and associated fetal death.
8. Pelvic ligamentous laxity and the protuberant abdomen contribute to gait instability and increased incidents of falls in pregnancy.

B. Penetrating
1. Gunshot wounds (GSW) >stab wounds
2. Often associated with domestic violence
3. Risk of uterine injury is increased in the second and third trimester.
4. Fetal injury associated with uterine injury is common and carries a high mortality rate (40% to 65%).
5. Maternal mortality is rare.
6. Upper abdominal penetrating injury is often associated with extensive gastrointestinal and vascular injuries.

V. Management
A. General considerations
1. Consider the potential for pregnancy in all female trauma victims of appropriate age. Routinely perform beta-human growth hormone (hCG) testing.
2. Although two patients are being managed, the initial treatment priorities remain the same (i.e., Advanced Trauma Life Support [ATLS] protocol). The best early treatment of the fetus is optimal resuscitation of the mother.
3. Early obstetric consultation and fetal assessment is mandatory. Subsequent care may require neonatal specialists.

B. Prehospital
1. As the fetus is exquisitely sensitive to hypoxia and hypovolemia, prehospital management of the pregnant trauma victim should include administration of supplemental oxygen and intravenous fluid as soon as possible.
2. In late pregnancy, extrication, immobilization, and transport can be complicated by anatomic factors. Supine hypotension syndrome can be prevented by positioning the pregnant patient to avoid uterine compression of the inferior vena cava, such as, left lateral decubitus position, or with the right hip elevated and the uterus manually displaced. If a spinal injury is suspected, immobilize the gravid patient on a long backboard, which is tilted 15° to the left.
3. The pneumatic antishock garments (PASG) can be used to stabilize fractures or control hemorrhage. However, inflation of the abdominal compartment of the PASG is contraindicated because the increased intraabdominal pressure further compromises venous return.
4. Field triage and interhospital transfer protocols must account for pregnancy. Assuming comparable transport times, transport pregnant patients to the facility best equipped to deal with the patient's injuries and simultaneously provide obstetric and neonatology expertise. Notify the receiving facility as early as possible to allow for timely preparation and response.
5. Do not attempt fetal assessment in the field. Rapid extrication, proper immobilization, and prompt transport are the best measures applied to safeguard mother and child.

C. Hospital
1. Primary survey

    a. Simultaneous resuscitation of vital signs, and identification and management of life-threatening injuries are the same as for other trauma patients

    b. Consider early intubation and mechanical ventilation in any pregnant trauma patient with marginal airway or ventilatory status to avoid fetal hypoxia.

    c. Because of "physiologic hypervolemia," the pregnant trauma patient can lose a significant amount of blood volume (1,500 mL) without manifesting any signs of hypovolemia. **Even if the mother's vital signs are normal, the fetus can inadequately be perfused.**

    d. Venous access in the upper extremities is preferred. Initiate prompt and vigorous volume resuscitation. Consider early red blood cell transfusion. Use type O, Rh-negative red blood cell transfusions to avoid Rh isoimmunization. Vasopressors reduce placental blood flow and should be avoided as an initial measure to correct maternal hypotension.

2. Secondary survey

    a. Obstetric history

        (1) Date of last menstrual period

        (2) Expected date of delivery

        (3) First perception of fetal movement

        (4) Status of current and previous pregnancies

    b. Determine uterine size (Fig 48.1) by assessing fundal height as measured in centimeters from the symphysis pubis, which provides a rapid measure of fetal age (1 cm = 1 week of gestational age).

    c. Examination of the gravid abdomen must include assessment of uterine tenderness and consistency, presence of contractions, and determination of fetal lie and movement. Perform internal pelvic examination with special attention to the presence of vaginal blood or amniotic fluid, and to cervical effacement, dilation, and fetal station. The presence of amniotic fluid (pH = 7) can be confirmed by the change in Nitrazine paper from blue-green to deep blue. (Normal amniotic fluid has a pH >7; normal vaginal fluid has a pH of 5.)

3. Fetal assessment

    a. Beyond 20 weeks gestation, fetal heart tones can be auscultated with a fetoscope or stethoscope to determine fetal heart rate. The normal range is from 120 to 160 beats/minute. Fetal bradycardia is indicative of fetal distress.

    b. Institute continuous electronic fetal monitoring for gravid patients at or beyond 20 to 24 weeks as the fetus may be viable if delivered. Obstetric personnel experienced in cardiotocography must be available to interpret fetal heart rate tracings for signs of fetal distress. These signs include an abnormal baseline rate, repetitive decelerations, especially after uterine contractions; and absence of accelerations or beat-to-beat variability.

    c. High-resolution, real-time ultrasonography is excellent for evaluating the fetus for gestational age, cardiac activity, and movement. As with cardiotocography, properly trained and credentialed personnel must be available to perform and interpret this study.

4. Diagnostic modalities

    a. Perform essential radiologic studies, including computed tomography. Whenever possible, shield the lower abdomen with a lead apron and avoid duplicating studies.

    b. Radiation exposure to the preimplantation embryo (<3 weeks) is lethal. During organogenesis (2–7 wks), the embryo is most sensitive to the teratogenic, growth retarding and postnatal neoplastic effects of radiation. Radiation exposure of <0.1 Gy is generally safe (Table 48.1).

Table 48.1 Absorbed radiation doses from radiation study

Radiographic study	Absorbed dose (rads)
Cervical spine series	0.0005
Anteroposterior chest	0.0025
Thoracic spine series	0.01
Anteroposterior pelvis	0.2
Lumbosacral spine series	0.75–1.0
Head CT scan	0.05
Chest CT scan	<1.0
Abdomen CT scan (including pelvis)	3.0–9.0
Limited upper abdomen CT scan	<3.0

CT, computed tomography.

     c. Indications for diagnostic peritoneal lavage (DPL) or focused abdominal sonography for trauma (FAST) are the same as for the nonpregnant patient. For patients in their second or third trimester, perform DPL above the umbilicus and in an open manner.

     d. FAST can be a helpful, noninvasive method of determining the presence of free fluid in the abdomen after trauma. Location of the transducer must be changed to allow for the anatomic displacement of structures.

  5. Definitive care

     a. Proceed with urgent operative intervention as dictated by physical findings and diagnostic studies.

     b. Pregnant trauma patients who are critically ill should be managed in the appropriate surgical or trauma intensive care unit. Onsite obstetric care and bedside fetal monitoring must be available.

     c. Stable gravid trauma patients requiring hospitalization should be obstetrically observed for 24 to 48 hours. Those patients whose fetus is beyond 20 to 24 weeks' gestation should have continuous cardiotocographic monitoring (CTM). A minimum of 24 hours is recommended for patients who present with frequent uterine activity (more than five contractions per hour), abdominal or uterine tenderness, vaginal bleeding, rupture of amniotic membranes, or hypotension.

     d. Asymptomatic gravid patients whose fetus is >20 to 24 weeks gestation with minor injuries not requiring hospitalization with normal findings on CTM of at least 4 hours' duration can be released with appropriate instructions and follow-up care.

VI. Cesarean section and trauma

  A. Indications

    1. Fetal factors

     a. Risk of fetal distress exceeds risk of prematurity

     b. Placental abruption

     c. Uterine rupture

     d. Fetal malposition with premature labor

     e. Severe pelvic or lumbosacral spine fractures

    2. Maternal factors

     a. Inadequate exposure for control of other injuries

     b. Disseminated intravascular coagulation (DIC)

  B. Perimortem cesarean section can be considered in situations of fetal gestational age ≥26 weeks, and the interval between maternal death and delivery can be minimized (<15 minutes). Maternal cardiopulmonary resuscitation must be continued throughout cesarean section and neonatal intensive care support should be immediately available.

C. Technique
   1. Vertical midline abdominal incision
   2. Incise the uterus vertically.
   3. Expose the infant's head, and suction oropharynx with a bulb syringe.
   4. Deliver the infant.
   5. Clamp and divide the umbilical cord.
   6. Manually remove the placenta.
   7. Inspect the endometrial surface to ensure removal of all membranes.
   8. Close the uterus in layers with absorbable suture.
   9. Administer oxytocin (usual dosage = 20 U intravenously) to treat post-partum uterine bleeding.
D. Cesarean section prolongs operative time and increases blood loss by at least 1,000 mL.

VII. Specific problems unique to pregnancy
   A. Placental abruption (*abruptio placenta*) is the most common cause of fetal death with maternal survival. In late pregnancy, even minor injury can be associated with abruption. Placental separation from the uterine wall of >50% generally results in fetal death. Clinical findings include abdominal pain, vaginal bleeding, leakage of amniotic fluid, uterine tenderness and rigidity, expanding fundal height, and maternal shock. Minor degrees of placental separation are compatible with fetal survival *in utero* and should be carefully followed by serial ultrasound, external fetal monitoring, and observation for fetomaternal transfusion (see VII.C).
   B. Disseminated intravascular coagulation is caused by either the release of thromboplastic substances during placental abruption or amniotic fluid embolism. Maternal shock and death can occur precipitously. Treatment includes emergency evacuation of the uterus and blood component therapy to reverse the coagulopathy.
   C. Fetomaternal transfusion, fetal hemorrhage into the maternal circulation, is common after trauma (~26%). Fetomaternal transfusion can result in fetal anemia and death, as well as isoimmunization of an Rh-negative mother. The Kleihauer-Betke (K-B) test measures fetomaternal hemorrhage. This test has been used to determine the need for Rh immunoglobulin in Rh-negative mothers and as an indicator of placental abruption. However, the amount of fetomaternal transfusion sufficient to sensitize Rh-negative mothers is far below the sensitivity of the K-B test. Therefore, it is recommended to treat all Rh-negative mothers who present with abdominal trauma with Rh immune globulin (50 µg if <16 weeks' gestation; 300 µg if >16 weeks). Furthermore, use cardiographic monitoring and high-resolution, real-time ultrasound in patients suspected of abruption, rather than relying on the K-B test.
   D. Premature labor, defined as onset of uterine contractions before 36 weeks' gestation that are forceful enough to cause cervical dilation and effacement, is a common complication of maternal trauma. Most of these premature contractions stop without tocolysis. Tocolytics (usually β-adrenergic agonist or magnesium sulfate) are generally used to allow adequate time for complete evaluation of the preterm fetus. Administer these agents under the direction of an obstetrician and experienced personnel. Tocolysis is contraindicated with fetal distress, vaginal bleeding, suspected placental abruption, maternal shock or hypotension, cervical dilation >4 cm, or maternal comorbidities (e.g. diabetes, pregnancy-induced hypertension, cardiac disease, maternal hyperthyroidism).
   E. Intrauterine fetal death does not necessitate immediate operative intervention. Labor usually ensues within 48 hours. Monitor coagulation studies closely if observation is entertained, as once DIC develops maternal shock and death can occur precipitously as mentioned above.
VIII. Medications in pregnancy
   A. Analgesics
   1. Administer **narcotics** (fetal respiratory depression) and nonsteroidal anti-inflammatory drugs (NSAID; prostaglandin and platelet inhibition) with caution (lower dosing and appropriate monitoring).

  B. Antibiotics
    1. Penicillins, cephalosporins, erythromycin, and clindamycin are safe.
    2. Administer aminoglycoside (fetal ototoxicity), sulfonamide (neonatal kernicterus), quinolone, and metronidazole with caution.
    3. Chloramphenicol (maternal and fetal bone marrow toxicity), and tetracycline (inhibition of fetal bone growth) are contraindicated.
  C. Anticoagulants (Chapter 51)
    1. Heparin is indicated as it does not cross the placenta, has a short half-life, and is immediately reversible with protamine. Low molecular weight heparin is also considered safe for use in pregnancy.
    2. Warfarin is contraindicated as it crosses the placenta, and has a long half-life and takes significant time to reverse.
  D. Anticonvulsants
    1. Administer **benzodiazepines and barbiturates** (fetal respiratory depression) with caution.
    2. Phenytoin (teratogenic) is contraindicated.
  E. Antiemetics
    1. Metoclopramide and prochlorperazine are safe.
  F. Because local anesthetics cross the placenta, administer them with caution and avoid large doses.
  G. General anesthesia and neuromuscular blockers are considered safe.
  H. Stress prophylaxis
    1. Sucralfate is safe.
    2. Use H_2 blockers with caution
  I. Administer **tetanus prophylaxis** according to the standard guidelines.

Axioms

- "Save the mother, save the fetus."
- Perform a routine beta-HCG test on all women of childbearing age.
- In transporting trauma patients in late pregnancy, take measures to displace the uterus to the left side.
- The fetus can be in jeopardy, even with apparent minor maternal injury.
- Although two patients are being managed, the initial treatment priorities remain the same.
- The best early treatment of the fetus is optimal resuscitation of the mother.
- Significant blood loss can occur in the pregnant patient without change in vital signs.
- Placental abruption is the leading cause of fetal death in patients where the mother survives.
- Fetal death is not an indication for cesarean section.
- Under no circumstances should maintaining a pregnancy compromise the management of maternal wounds.

Bibliography

Knudson MH. Trauma in pregnancy. In: Blaisdell FW, Trunkey DD, eds. *Abdominal trauma*. New York: Thieme, 1993:324–339.

Rozyck GS, Knudson MM. Reproductive system trauma In: Feliciano DV, Moore EE, Mattox KL, eds. *Trauma*. Stamford: Appleton & Lange; 1996:695–709.

Trauma in women. In: Subcommittee on Advanced Life Support of the American College of Surgeons Committee on Trauma. Advanced Trauma Life Support for Doctors. Chicago: American College of Surgeons, 1997:315–332.

Vaizey CJ, Jacobsen MJ, Cross FW. Trauma in pregnancy. *Br J Surg* 1994;81: 1406–1415.

Wilson RF, Vincent C. Gynecologic and obstetric trauma. In: Wilson RF, Walt AS, eds. *Management of trauma's pitfalls and practice*. Baltimore: Williams & Wilkins 1996: 21–640.

49. GERIATRIC TRAUMA

Donald R. Kauder

I. **Demographics and epidemiology**
   A. In 1990, 30.9 million people in the United States were >65 years of age, accounting for 12.5% of the total population. By the year 2020, this segment of the population is projected to increase to 52 million, 6.7 million of whom will be >85 years of age. By the year 2040, persons >65 years of age will make up 20% of the populace.
   B. The elderly are living longer and in better health than in past years partly because of advances in healthcare, improved social support, and heightened awareness of the complex medical and socioeconomic issues germane to this age group. These older adults continue to participate in many of the same pursuits as their younger counterparts and, therefore, are subject to a similar, and, in some instances, increased risk of injury.
   C. The 12.5% of our population >65 years of age accounts for almost one third of the deaths from injury. Furthermore, this group incurs higher population-based death rates than any other age group.
II. **Physiology of aging**
   A. **Cardiovascular system**
      1. Progressive stiffening of the myocardium caused by increasing fibrosis leads to diminished pump function and lower cardiac output.
      2. Decreasing sensitivity to endogenous and exogenous catecholamines causes an inability to mount an appropriate tachycardia and, thus, a decreased ability to augment cardiac output in response to hypovolemia, pain, and stress.
      3. Peripheral atherosclerotic disease predisposes to:
         a. Reduced flow to vital organs and diminished physiologic reserve
         b. Baseline diminution in peripheral pulses, potentially leading to a misinterpretation of the character of the pulse, thus, leading to the initiation of inappropriate therapy
      4. The use of commonly prescribed medications (e.g., beta-blockers, calcium channel blockers, and digoxin) can mask or blunt the normal physiologic response to injury and stress. In some cases, the ingestion of prescription medications can directly exacerbate a patient's injuries (e.g., coumadin).
   B. **Respiratory system**
      1. Decreased lung elasticity and progressive stiffening of the chest wall lead to diminished pulmonary compliance and alteration in the ability to mount an effective cough.
      2. Coalescence of alveoli and reduction of small airways support lead to a decrease in surface area for gas exchange.
      3. Atrophy of pseudociliated epithelium lining the bronchi contributes to a decrease in clearance of particulate foreign matter and bacteria.
      4. Chronic colonization of the upper airway with enteric gram-negative bacteria and *Haemophilus* species predisposes to pneumonia.
   C. **Nervous system**
      1. **The brain undergoes progressive atrophy** beginning in the fourth decade; by age 70 years, a 10% reduction in brain size occurs.
         a. The distance between the brain surface and the skull thus increases, putting the dural bridging veins on stretch and making them more susceptible to disruption and bleeding.
         b. The reduction in brain size results in increased intracranial "potential space." Thus, a significant amount of intracranial bleeding can be masked before symptoms of increased intracranial pressure

occur. The initially asymptomatic elderly patient suffering a mechanism of injury that might predispose to an intracranial injury can suffer rapid deterioration from an insidious closed head injury.

2. **Functional deterioration** occurs, increasing the predisposition to injury.
   a. **Cognition**
      (1) Poor memory
      (2) Impaired judgment
      (3) Deficient data acquisition
   b. **Hearing**
      (1) Decreased auditory acuity, especially to high-frequency sounds
      (2) Lack of adequate hearing aids because of financial constraints or limited access to healthcare
   c. **Eyesight**
      (1) Decreased peripheral vision
      (2) Decreased visual acuity
      (3) Decreased tolerance to glare
      (4) Inadequate or inappropriate eyeglasses prescription
   d. **Proprioception and coordination**
      (1) Tendency toward imbalance
      (2) Altered "righting" reflex

D. **Renal**
   1. A decline in renal mass occurs. By age 65 years, a 30% to 40% loss is common.
   2. The nephrons that remain show changes of aging and deterioration in the tubules and glomeruli.
   3. A normal serum creatinine does not imply normal renal function. An estimate of function can be calculated using the following formula for creatinine clearance (C_{cr}):
      C_{cr} (mL/min) = (140 − age) × weight (kg)/serum creatinine × 72
   4. **Exercise caution and good judgment** in the use of potentially nephrotoxic agents, including:
      a. Iodinated contrast solutions
      b. Aminoglycoside
      c. Diuretics
      d. Vasopressors

E. **Musculoskeletal system**
   1. **Osteoporosis** predisposes to fractures with relatively minor energy transfer.
   2. **Diminution in vertebral body height** and osteoarthritis contribute to significant changes in the spine.
      a. **Kyphoscoliosis** leads to decreased mobility and difficulty looking upward, and in twisting and turning the head, predisposing to decreased obstacle avoidance and increased risk of injury.
      b. **Spinal stenosis caused by osteoarthritis** renders the spinal cord more susceptible to injury, especially with cervical extension. Central cord syndrome can occur in this setting.
   3. **Decrease in muscle mass** and progressive fibrosis lead to diminished strength and agility. This predisposes to poor obstacle avoidance and the inability to avoid serious injury, especially when falling (the altered "righting" reflex).

III. **Influence of comorbid conditions**
   A. In addition to the typical changes that occur with aging, the common development of significant disease states can have a profound impact on an elderly person's response to injury and stress. Knowledge of concurrent disease states is critical to the appropriate management of the injured elderly, and an aggressive search for such information is vital. This information will influence resuscitation strategies, as well as assist in planning care once the trauma patient is admitted to the hospital. A helpful listing of the more common conditions encountered and how to quantify them is found in Table 49.1.

Table 49.1 Premorbid illness criteria

Cardiac disease
–History of cardiac surgery
–Any cardiac medication
–Myocardial infarction within 12 months of admission
–Myocardial infarction more that 12 months before admission

Diabetes mellitus
–Insulin-dependent
–Non–insulin-dependent

Liver disease
–Bilirubin >2 mg/dL (on admission)
–Cirrhosis

Malignancy
–Documented history

Pulmonary disease, chronic (asthma, chronic obstructive pulmonary disease, others)
–Bronchodilator therapy
–No bronchodilator therapy

Obesity
–Female >200 lb
–Male >250 lb

Renal disease
–Serum creatinine >2 mg/dL (on admission)

Neurologic (cerebrovascular accident)
–Documented prior history

Hypertension
–Any antihypertensive medication
–Documented prior history

IV. Mechanisms of injury
A. Falls
1. Falls are the most frequent cause of accidental injury in people >75 years of age and the second most common cause of injury sustained by those between the ages of 65 and 74 years.
2. While frequently resulting in isolated orthopedic injury, falls in conjunction with significant energy transfer (e.g., down a flight of stairs or off a ladder or a roof) can be devastating.
3. The reason for the fall must be investigated carefully. Falls caused by the aging process are frequent, and postural instability, poor balance, altered gait, and decreased muscular strength and coordination can all be implicated. However, consider acute or chronic comorbid conditions (e.g., syncope, drop attacks, cardiac dysrhythmias, hypoglycemia, anemia, and transient cerebral ischemia) as possible causes. In the anticoagulated patient, a seemingly minor fall can have devastating consequences.

B. Motor vehicle crashes
1. People >65 years of age account for 13% of licensed drivers. As population demographics change, this percentage will increase. The elderly have a very high crash rate, second only to persons in the age group 16 to 25 years. Further, those aged ≥75 years have a higher rate of fatal crashes than any other age group.
2. Whereas falls are a more frequent mechanism of injury, a motor vehicle crash is the most common reason for an elderly individual to present to a trauma center. Most crashes take place in the daylight hours, in good weather, and close to home. Alcohol ingestion is encountered far

less frequently than in younger populations. As in any mechanism of injury, the events leading to the incident must be elucidated. Physiologic decreases in musculoskeletal coordination and reaction time, visual impairment, alterations in auditory processing, and deficits in cognition function may contribute to the high incidence of crashes. Antecedent medical conditions also must be sought as a cause.

C. Pedestrian-automobile impact
1. Pedestrian-automobile impact seen in the elderly, can produce devastating consequences. Those >65 years of age account for almost a quarter of fatalities caused by this mechanism in the United States each year. As in other mechanisms of injury, the effects of aging are frequently implicated as causative factors.
   a. **Osteoarthritis of the spine** and progressive kyphosis lead to a stooped posture, thus making it more difficult to lift the head so that traffic signals can be seen and onrushing vehicles identified and avoided.
   b. **Changes in gait** combined with a slower pace make it difficult to clear an intersection before the traffic signal changes, whereas decreased strength, agility, and reaction time make it difficult to effect a rapid change in direction critical to avoid a collision.
   c. **Alterations in hearing and vision** and poor judgment, cognition, and memory also may be implicated as contributing factors.

D. Injuries related to violence
1. Injuries resulting from shooting, stabbing, and blunt assault account for 4% to 14% of elderly trauma admissions. Those same changes of aging that predispose to falls and motor vehicle-related injury make older individuals easy prey for the criminal element. Decreased strength and agility alter the ability to fight or flee. Poor vision and hearing and cognitive changes leading to poor judgment also contribute to the potential for victimization. Suicide is the most common reason for gun-related death in older individuals. The elderly account for almost 25% of all deaths ascribed to suicide and <3% of homicides annually.
2. **Domestic abuse of the elderly** is a problem that is gaining more recognition. In excess of 240,000 cases are reported annually, but likely represent only 10% of cases that actually occur. As with young children, a high index of suspicion must be maintained, and telltale signs must be sought. Frequent visits to the emergency department for "minor" injuries, multiple bruises in various stages of healing, poor nutrition, an unkempt appearance, and poor personal hygiene can all be warning signs for the physician to consult the appropriate social services agency to assist in an inquiry.

E. Burns
1. Burns account for ~8% of injury-related deaths in the elderly. When compared with a younger population, the elderly suffer larger and deeper burns and have a significantly higher mortality rate. The elderly are at risk for burn injury from a variety of factors.
   a. **Altered mobility.** Limitations in muscular strength and coordination, poor balance, and altered gait make escaping a fire more difficult.
   b. **Neurosensory changes.** Diminution of auditory and visual cues can make recognition of a fire less likely. Alterations in sensation because of peripheral neuropathy or ischemic peripheral vascular disease can lead to prolonged heat exposure (e.g., burns from scalding bath water). Further, poor judgment regarding safety issues (e.g., the unsupervised use of kerosene heaters) make the elderly more likely to be involved in a fire.
   c. **Skin changes.** Thinning of the skin caused by decreased epidermal cell proliferation makes the elderly more likely to suffer a serious burn than a younger individual given the same thermal exposure.

V. Resuscitation and initial assessment. Initiate early, aggressive efforts to resuscitate the elderly trauma patient while efforts are being made to contact family members and to clearly delineate the patient's preinjury level of function, state of health, comorbid conditions, and presence of a "living will" or other "predetermination" documents.

A. ABCDEs. The initial assessment of trauma victims, as outlined in Chapter 13, is the appropriate starting point for the evaluation of the geriatric trauma patient. However, an awareness of the physiology of aging and the presence of comorbid disease must be taken into account and the resuscitative effort modified as appropriate.

1. **Airway**. Early control of the airway is critical. A lack of pulmonary reserve, combined with a high likelihood that a patient may have underlying cardiovascular disease, can drastically alter the consequences of seemingly "minimal" hypoxemia. A patient who develops a significant tachycardia to compensate for injuries and who then develops myocardial ischemia as a result may be better served with early intubation.

2. **Breathing**

   a. A thorough search for serious chest injuries is vital in ensuring adequate levels of oxygenation. Initial assessment protocols for identification and treatment of immediately life-threatening injuries (e.g., tension pneumothorax, massive hemothorax) must be followed. Flail chest, particularly anterior flail chest, may not be obvious in the elderly patient. A hallmark of excellent treatment is adequate pain control. Although fractured ribs and chest wall contusions are not considered immediately life threatening, these exquisitely painful injuries in the setting of poor chest wall compliance, chronic obstructive pulmonary disease (COPD), and bacterial colonization of the oropharynx can be lethal if good pulmonary toilet is not ensured.

   b. Early use of epidural analgesia can be beneficial in this setting. Do not delay intubation and ventilatory support—another viable option. Delay in initiation of ventilatory support can result in an increased work of breathing and increased myocardial oxygen demand.

3. **Circulation**

   a. Restoring the elderly trauma victim to a normal volume status can present some unique challenges. Preexisting disease and senescence can lead to an inappropriate response to hypovolemia, depriving the physician of the usual signs (e.g., tachycardia and low blood pressure). Delayed capillary refill in the lower extremities secondary to peripheral vascular disease can be misinterpreted as a sign of volume contraction, leading to overzealous fluid administration, a significant problem in a patient with marginal cardiac reserve.

   b. **Fluid resuscitation should be judicious.** Give early consideration to transfusion with packed red blood cells to augment oxygen-carrying capacity and oxygen delivery, thereby lessening the need for the compensatory tachycardia necessary to augment cardiac output.

   c. In many elderly patients, the volume status cannot be determined accurately. The early use of invasive monitoring with pulmonary artery and intraarterial blood pressure catheters can be helpful and should be performed as part of the resuscitation. This information may uncover treatable and previously unrecognized hypovolemia or cardiac dysfunction.

4. **Disability**

   a. **Early and accurate assessment of the neurologic status** of the geriatric trauma patient is important and frequently difficult to accomplish. The history of preexisting mental dysfunction (e.g., senile dementia, Alzheimer's disease) or prior cerebrovascular accidents is frequently lacking or may be denied by the patient or family. If chronic disease states are misinterpreted as being acute, harmful overtreatment can occur. Conversely, a patient with a "normal" mental status following a blow to the head may be harboring a potentially lethal intracranial injury that simply has not had time to manifest itself because of the presence of extensive cerebral atrophy.

  b. Early, liberal use of head computed tomography (CT) scanning must be part of the evaluation of the elderly trauma victim with any suspicion of potentially serious head injury.

5. **Expose**

  a. As in any trauma patient, the elderly must be fully disrobed and carefully examined anteriorly as well as posteriorly. Large quantities of blood can be lost into the elastic soft tissues of elderly patients. Give special attention to the search for signs of prior surgical intervention, because this may provide a clue as to a patient's antecedent medical history. The presence of a median sternotomy incision or signs of peripheral vascular surgery should alert one to the presence of systemic arteriosclerotic disease. Failure to recognize a well-healed abdominal incision can lead to subsequent misinterpretation of abdominal CT scan or to a suboptimal therapeutic maneuver (e.g., diagnostic peritoneal lavage).

B. Secondary survey

1. **As in the initial assessment**, examine the patient in a systematic fashion to search for serious injuries (Chapter 13). However, pay special attention to the history preceding the injury. Failure to do so can lead to inappropriate therapy or contribute to the recurrence of a potentially preventable event. Investigate the following issues.

  a. Did the crash involve a single vehicle during "normal" driving conditions? This scenario suggests that an antecedent medical condition may have been involved (e.g., a transient ischemic attack or cardiac dysrhythmia).

  b. Is this one of several falls or motor vehicle crashes that have occurred in the last year? Clustering of events such as this also can be a clue that an untreated medical condition may be a contributing factor.

  c. Has the trauma victim begun a new medication or had a recent change in dosage of an old prescription? A newly diagnosed diabetics can have difficulty regulating blood sugar, whereas some antihypertensive medications can cause dizziness or orthostatic hypotension.

VI. Issues unique to the severely injured geriatric patient

A. Outcome

1. **Mortality rates** are higher for comparable injuries and injury severity scores when comparing elderly patients with younger patients.

2. Assessment of disability and functional outcome can be more meaningful measures of therapeutic success than mortality alone, but studies in these areas are lacking. It is clear that many elderly trauma victims can return to a preinjury level of function or at least return to some level of functional independence. To regard a patient's age as a sole determinant and predictor of return to the premorbid state would be naive. A multidisciplinary approach to the treatment and rehabilitation of the injured elderly that begins at the time of admission to the hospital is important.

3. **Appropriateness of resuscitation**

  a. Moral and ethical issues surrounding the care of the injured elderly are difficult. It is appropriate to begin aggressive resuscitative efforts and to sustain them at least until some insight can be gained into the patient's and family's wishes. It is uncommon for people to have "living wills" or "predetermination" documents on their person at the time of a serious injury, but early contact with a family member or personal physician can yield crucial information that can influence medical decision-making. It is equally important to help family members interpret such documents, especially with regard to the specifics of medical therapy. To illustrate, a well-meaning family can misinterpret mechanical ventilation that is being used as a bridge to recovery as being counter to a patient's request not to "end up on a ventilator."

B. Early involvement of social services, chaplaincy services, and, occasionally, an expert in medical ethics can be helpful. The need for frank and open discussion between the physician and the family regarding prognosis and expectations for meaningful recovery is essential. Only then can rational decisions be made regarding the appropriateness of care.

C. Family support
1. An assessment of the accident victim's family dynamics and early involvement of the family in discussions of acute care problems and long-term issues are paramount. It is not unusual for the children of the injured elderly to be elderly themselves. As such, they may not have the physical stamina or the economic resources to actively participate in the rehabilitation and final disposition of the patient. As mentioned, early involvement of the family can also serve to clarify issues of appropriateness of care.

VII. An age-related approach to patient care
A. As the response to injury and illness changes with increasing age, a number of treatment axioms have been developed to serve as guidelines to the care of the injured elderly.
1. **Age 55 through 64 years**
   a. Assume some mild decrease in physiologic reserve.
   b. Suspect the presence of some common diseases of middle age (diabetes mellitus, arteriosclerotic cardiovascular disease, hypertension, previous surgery, history of transfusion).
   c. Suspect the use of prescription or nonprescription medications.
   d. Assume that the patient is competent to provide an accurate medical history.
   e. Look for subtle signs of organ dysfunction, especially cardiovascular and respiratory systems. Arterial blood gas measurement and an electrocardiogram (ECG) may be necessary.
   f. With a history of loss of consciousness or abnormalities in cognitive function or personality, presume a serious brain injury is present. CT scan is essential; magnetic resonance imaging (MRI) can be a useful adjunct, especially in evaluating the spine.
   g. Proceed with standard diagnostic and management schemes, unless contraindicated by information collected during history.
2. **Age 65 through 74 years**
   a. Accept the presence of age-related and acquired disease-induced physiologic alteration of organ systems.
   b. Accept the presence of acquired disease and medications to correct or control them. Assume a higher incidence of previous surgery and transfusion.
   c. Decide if the patient is competent to give a reliable medical history. Review the history as soon as possible with the patient's relatives or personal physician.
   d. Aggressively monitor the patient and control physiology to optimize cardiac performance and oxygen metabolism.
   e. Assume that any alteration in mental status or cognitive or sensory function indicates the presence of a brain injury. Imaging of the brain is mandatory in the patient with abnormal mental status.
   f. Proceed with standard diagnostic and management schemes, including early aggressive operative management.
   g. Be aware of poor outcome, especially with severe injury to the central nervous system (CNS) or marked physiologic deterioration secondary to injury. Check for advance directives.
3. **Age 75 years and older**
   a. Proceed as in **a** through **f** in the preceding section.
   b. Assume a poor outcome with moderately severe injury, especially with the CNS injury or any injury causing physiologic dysfunction.

c. After aggressive initial resuscitation and diagnostic maneuvers, reassess the magnitude of the patient's injuries and discuss appropriateness of care with the patient (if competent) and family members.
d. Be humane, and recognize the legal and ethical controversies involved. Consider early consultation with experts in ethics and social
services to help the family and medical team with difficult decisions.

Axioms

- An accurate history is essential.
- Err on the side of early intubation.
- Epidural analgesia to relieve thoracic pain can be lifesaving.
- Early, open discussions with the family are critical.
- Early, proactive involvement by physical medicine and rehabilitation, physical ther-
apy, occupational therapy, social services, and discharge planning is paramount.
- A normal serum creatinine is **not** normal renal function.
- Normal heart rate and blood pressure **do not** imply normovolemia.
- Never underestimate a chest injury.
- A "minor" head injury is a massive subdural hematoma in evolution until proved
otherwise.
- Geriatric trauma victims cannot tolerate any error; consider invasive monitoring.

Bibliography

Committee on Trauma, American College of Surgeons: *Advanced trauma life support
student manual.* Chicago: American College of Surgeons, 1997.
McMahon DJ, Shapiro MB, Kauder DR. Geriatric in the intensive care unit. *Surg Clin
North Am* 2000;80(3):1005–1020.
Milzman DP, Boulanger BR, Rodriguez A, et al. Pre-existing disease in trauma pa-
tients: a predictor of fate independent of age and ISS. *J Trauma* 1992;32(2):236–244.
Scalea TM, Simon HM, Duncan AO, et al. Geriatric blunt multiple trauma: improved
survival with early invasive monitoring. *J Trauma* 1990;30(2):129–136.
Schwab CW, Kauder DR. Trauma in the geriatric patient. *Arch Surg* 1992;127(6):
701–706.
Schwab CW, Shapiro MB, Kauder DR. Injury in aging adults: patterns, care and out-
comes. In: Mattox KL, Feliciano DV, Moore EE, eds. *Trauma*, 4th ed. Stamford:
Appleton & Lange, 2000:1099–1113.
Smith PC, Enderson BL, Maull KI. Trauma in the elderly: determinants of outcome.
South Med J 1990;78:171–177.
van Aalst JA, Morris JA Jr, Yates HK, et al. Severely injured geriatric patients return
to independent living: a study of factors influencing function and independence.
J Trauma 1991;31(8):1096–102.

50. REHABILITATION

Louis E. Penrod, Gary Goldberg, and John A. Horton, III

Trauma results in an acute decrement in the ability of the individual to function. Resulting pathology often leaves individuals with permanent impairments that affect their ability to care for themselves, to fulfill expected social roles, and to return to a pattern of daily activity associated with a meaningful and gratifying existence. Certain injuries (e.g., spinal cord or traumatic brain injury) affect numerous physiologic, psychological, social, and vocational functions to the degree that the individual loses functional independence. The rehabilitation team is responsible for providing services that optimize function, maximize the return to independence, and enable the person to reestablish a meaningful existence. Interventions can involve direct treatment of the patient; education of family members; and recommending equipment and environmental modification to accommodate residual limitations. The rehabilitation team should be involved in the early stages of hospital care; such involvement has been shown to optimize outcome for the trauma patient. Attention to the prevention of disabling complications during the acute phase of treatment can minimize required interventions during the rehabilitation phase of treatment.

I. **Secondary disabilities** are decrements of function that follow the impairments that result from trauma, most often because of prolonged immobilization of the patient. Although rarely life-threatening, they can limit eventual function and contribute as much to the total healthcare cost of trauma as the acute care costs.
   A. **Cardiovascular deconditioning** occurs rapidly with any period of inactivity when the heart and peripheral vascular mechanisms lose the capacity to respond to stressors. With certain types of trauma (e.g., spinal cord injury with its associated loss of sympathetic nervous system control), the inability to maintain perfusion pressure with changes in posture can limit attempts to mobilize the patient. The most important approach is to minimize immobility and begin to have the patient in an upright position as soon as possible. Additional benefits from this emphasis on early mobilization include improved respiratory functioning, with decreased atelectasis and attendant complications.
      1. Prolonged recumbency causes a progressive rise in the resting heart rate of 0.5 beats per minute per day. In addition, as the heart becomes deconditioned, it responds to demands by a greater rise in rate than preinjury. The combined effect of these changes is resting tachycardia and reduced ability to meet oxygen demands with activity; this persists for 26 to 72 days after return to activity.
      2. **Peripheral factors**, including decreases in vascular volume, loss of adaptive baroreceptor reflex responses to the upright posture, and increased pooling of blood in lower limb veins, contribute to the intolerance of the patient to an upright posture after immobility.
         a. **In healthy individuals**, the adaptation response to the upright position can be totally lost after 3 weeks of complete bedrest; it can take up to 72 days to restore proper function of this response after remobilization.
         b. **Older individuals** lose this capacity to respond more quickly, and they return to baseline more slowly. Concomitant disease (e.g., cerebrovascular or cardiovascular lesions) makes older individuals less tolerant of this postural drop in blood pressure.
         c. **Minimization of immobility** is the single most important management technique. Increasing periods of sitting in a chair with the feet dependent helps reconditioning for those who are unable to stand.

      (1) **In severe cases**, a tilt table can be used to gradually place the person in an upright position while blood pressure is monitored.

      (2) **Compressive garments**, full-length elastic stockings, and abdominal binders are also useful to limit venous pooling.

      (3) **Proper nutrition** to maintain plasma protein levels, immune system function, and proper hydration are also important.

      (4) In severe cases, increase salt intake and use of sympathomimetic agents (pseudoephedrine, ephedrine, midodrine or phenylephrine) or mineralocorticoids (fludrocortisone).

B. Contractures result when a joint is not subjected to frequent range of motion, either actively or passively. The formation of contractures is most often a consequence of untreated muscular spasticity because of upper motor neuron impairment, which causes sustained, uncontrolled muscle tension. Muscular tension becomes unbalanced across joints and, therefore, effectively reduces the mobility of the affected joint. The contracture produces a loss of joint range because of shortening and increased stiffness of the soft tissue around the joint. When the limitation of joint range persists, the soft tissues of the joint itself can also become contracted. Remodeling of the connective tissue around the joint contributes to decreased elasticity.

    1. Contractures contribute to increased morbidity.

      a. Difficulties in positioning the patient can lead to the formation of decubitus ulcers.

      b. Hygiene, particularly in the perineum, palms of the hands, and axillae, can be difficult.

      c. Contractures also can limit function as motor control is regained. This leads to prolonged rehabilitation and, thus, higher cost.

      d. Contractures should be prevented.

    2. Contractures can be prevented in most cases by fully ranging all joints twice a day. Active ranging by the patient is preferred, if possible, because it also helps to maintain strength and motor control. If weak but voluntary muscle power is present, use active assisted range of motion. In cases of paralysis or coma, passive range of motion must be used.

      a. After ranging, positioning the patient can help reinforce the gains of therapy. Prone lying provides a prolonged stretch for hip flexion contractures. Splinting of the wrists, hands, and ankles is also useful. Use splints intermittently to avoid skin breakdown. Other physical modalities, in conjunction with range of motion, allow a greater stretch.

        (1) **Superficial heat** can cause reflex relaxation.

        (2) **Deep heat** using ultrasound can increase the elasticity of collagen.

        (3) **Cooling** of the muscle decreases the activity of the muscle spindle mechanism, decreasing muscle tone.

      b. Motor point blocks using neurolytic agents (e.g., phenol) or neuromuscular blocking agents (e.g., botulinum toxin) are useful for temporarily reducing muscular tone in cases where abnormalities of muscle tone prevent maintenance of full range at a joint.

      c. Serial casting of an extremity is useful to provide a prolonged stretch. After adequate padding of bony prominences, a plaster or fiberglass cast is applied. Stretch is maintained as the cast solidifies. The cast is typically left in place for 3 to 5 days before removal. The cast can then be bivalved and used as a resting splint.

      d. Use antispasticity medication to reduce joint immobilization caused by tonic muscular contractions from hyperreactivity of the skeletal muscle. This phenomenon is common, although usually delayed in onset, in the head-injured patient as well as those patients with cerebral vascular accident or spinal cord injury. Common medications used include baclofen, tizanidine, diazepam, and dantrolene sodium. (Dantrolene is generally limited to brain injury).

C. Decubitus ulcers are potentially preventable but common complications of trauma. **Pressure is the major factor in the development of an ulcer.** Ulcers occur over bony prominences when the pressure of body weight is unrelieved for prolonged periods, causing ischemic damage to the skin and underlying soft tissues. Higher pressures cause breakdown in a shorter time than lower pressures.

   1. Shear either between the skin and supporting surfaces or within the soft tissues causes ischemia at lower pressures than when shear is not present.

   2. Anemia, excessive skin moisture from perspiration or urine, infection, poor nutrition, contractures, and lack of sensation contribute to development of pressure ulcers. An ulcer will not occur without prolonged, excessive pressure.

   3. Prevention of ulceration should be the goal.

     a. Careful attention to positioning of the patient. Frequent turning, initially on a schedule of every 2 hours, is essential. Pay particular attention to the occiput, scapulae, sacrum, ischial tuberosities, greater trochanters, malleoli, and heels. Pillows and foam blocks can be used to relieve pressure or distribute it to other areas.

     b. Inspect the skin regularly. If signs of breakdown are seen, avoid pressure to the area to the extent possible. The earliest sign of damage is an area of nonblanching erythema. Palpation may reveal induration of the underlying soft tissue.

     c. Management of urinary and bowel incontinence to prevent prolonged contact between the skin and urine or feces is important in preventing skin irritation and infection.

     d. For patients at high risk, consider use of specialized mattresses and seating surfaces, which have been shown to be a cost effective component of a decubitus prevention program.

D. Heterotopic ossification is a pathologic process; new bone is formed within periarticular soft tissue. It should be distinguished from traumatic myositis ossificans, in which bone is formed within traumatized muscles, often because of ossification of intramuscular hematoma.

   1. Following spinal cord injury or traumatic brain injury, incidence is from 11% to 79%.

   2. The pathophysiology is not well understood. Histologically normal bone develops in the soft tissues.

   3. Different distribution of ossification and time course occurs in spinal cord versus brain injury. In both cases, the lesions develop below the level of the neurologic injury around major joints. The process appears to be more aggressive in limbs with greater spasticity-related muscular tone.

     a. Upper extremity involvement is more common in brain injury. Most patients with brain injury show a pattern of gradual neurologic recovery rather than the static picture following spinal cord injury. Heterotopic ossification tends to be more extensive and persistent following spinal cord injury.

     b. Earliest manifestation of heterotopic ossification is painful loss of range of motion. Otherwise, a striking similarity is seen to the clinical presentation of deep venous thrombosis, with a warm, swollen, erythematous limb.

     c. Triple-phase bone scan, which can be useful to confirm the diagnosis, is the earliest, most specific test. The first and second phases are abnormal in heterotopic ossification. The level of alkaline phosphatase can be used to track the relative activity of new bone formation, although elevation of this enzyme tends to be nonspecific.

     d. Consequences of this process include painful loss of range of motion and compression of vascular or neurologic structures, which can lead to secondary venous thrombosis. When peripheral nerves are being actively damaged by compression, immediate surgical resection may be required. The bony mass also can lead to development of pressure ulceration of the overlying skin.

4. Mainstay of treatment is vigorous range of motion. When sensation is preserved (traumatic brain injury), ranging can be painful, leading to increased agitation. Proper pharmacologic treatment and analgesia can permit appropriate physical therapy.

   a. **Heterotopic ossification** is treated with disodium etidronate (Didronel) 20 mg/kg for 1 to 3 months, followed by 10 mg/kg for 3 months. Indomethacin also has been used in treatment, but the evidence for its effectiveness is more convincing following total hip replacement than in trauma.

   b. **Radiation**, both as prophylaxis and as treatment, seems to be effective. When early surgical resection is required to reduce compressive phenomenon, radiation early after surgery is useful to prevent recurrence.

   c. **Surgical resection** to improve range of motion is useful, particularly when the joint has ankylosed. Surgery is usually delayed 12 to 18 months after trauma, or until repeat three-phase bone scanning shows no active ossification. With good neurologic recovery, surgery usually provides a good result. Ossification tends to recur in cases of poor neurologic recovery or with resection while ossification is active. Postoperative radiation can be helpful in reducing the risk of recurrence.

II. **Musculoskeletal response to immobilization.** Just as exercise leads to strengthening, immobility leads to weakness of both muscles and bone. **Complete bedrest results in loss of 10% to 15% of muscle strength per week.**

   A. Particularly in type I (slow twitch) muscle fibers, which predominate in antigravity muscles. This reduction of type I capacity, combined with cardiovascular deconditioning, leads to poor endurance when the patient is eventually remobilized.

   B. Relative sparing of type II (fast twitch) fibers and the anaerobic nature of strength-type tasks. The result is that in retraining, strength returns rapidly (weeks), whereas endurance requires much longer to return (months).

   C. When a patient is immobilized for any length of time, maintain strength as much as possible through therapeutic exercise. Even when range of motion is not possible, isometric exercises can prevent weakness. When a patient is awake and cooperative, opportunities for regular upper and lower body exercise can be facilitated by an overhead trapeze and special color-coded bands made from elastic latex sheets with specific thickness (Thera-Band), which can provide controlled resistance exercise for the patient while in bed or sitting in a wheelchair.

      1. Daily contractions of 20% to 30% of maximal voluntary contraction for several seconds are sufficient to maintain strength. Use exercise that includes motion (isotonic or isokinetic), when possible, because joint motion and motor control can be maintained as well.

   D. Skeletal strength is dependent on the forces of gravity and muscle pull acting on the bones. With inactivity, osteoclastic activity predominates with the breakdown of both cortical and trabecular bone. This breakdown can be particularly profound in acute tetraplegia of adolescent boys, resulting in markedly elevated calcium excretion with stone formation or hypercalcemia.

      1. Voluntary muscle activity and weight-bearing exercise are important in reversing this **disuse osteoporosis.** Once activity is resumed, it can take years to return to baseline bone density. Disuse osteoporosis is particularly problematic in individuals with preexisting osteoporosis from other reasons (postmenopausal women).

      2. Adequate hydration and vigilance for the clinical manifestations of immobilization hypercalcemia are important in preventing the adverse effects of this condition.

3. Prophylactic use of agents that inhibit either osteoblastic or osteoclastic activity in at-risk patients is being investigated and shows promise in limiting the degree of disuse osteoporosis.

III. **Frequently encountered functional deficits**
   A. **Agitation following recovery from traumatic brain injury** can lead to further injury to the patient (e.g., self-extubation, falls out of bed, dislodgment of vascular catheters). These potential dangers lead to significant pressure on the medical staff to stop this behavior. It is convenient to sedate or physically restrain the patient, but this approach also can put the patient at additional risk. Attempt to understand the cause of the agitation and control the situation through the least intervention possible. First, exclude causes (e.g., hypoxemia, hypotension, hypoglycemia) from the etiology of the agitation.

   1. Agitation is often a response to a specific stimulus or inability of the individual to sort out overwhelming stimuli. Following brain injury, the individual is often presented with both external and internal stimuli that are distorted by altered perception and difficult to interpret. Additionally, impairments of expression can prevent the individual from expressing needs. This leads to frustration and poorly controlled motor responses.

      a. Seek and eliminate irritating internal stimuli such as pain (undiagnosed fractures, pressure ulcers), a full bowel or bladder, or difficulty with breathing.

      b. Minimization of environmental stimuli should be the first approach. To the extent possible, present a single stimulus, allowing adequate time for cognitive processing and response. Noise should be reduced. Lighting should be subdued. Verbal stimuli should be calm and simple in content. Careful observation usually detects when the patient is beginning to lose concentration; perseveration and reduced accuracy of responses are typical clues to this problem.

         (1) Modification of the environment may be sufficient to control the situation and minimize risk to the patient.

         (2) Defusing the emotional response of the staff to the patient's behavior is often part of the environmental control necessary.

   2. The goal of treatment when pharmacologic restraint is necessary is to minimize both the intervention so that the individual can participate in recovery as much as possible and the side effects of treatment.

      a. Short-acting benzodiazepines are useful for episodes of acute agitation.

      b. If agitation occurs in a specific and reproducible daily pattern, attention to correcting sleep-wake cycle disturbance may also help to alleviate the agitation. For example, a patient who becomes agitated in the evening and stays awake through the night would benefit from sedating medication such as trazodone given at bedtime to help induce sleep and limit nighttime agitation.

      c. Mild tranquilizers, antidepressants, and beta-blockers have been used when agitation is frequent or persistent. In using tranquilizers, start with a low dose and slowly titrate; individuals with traumatic brain injury can have greater response to a given dose than do psychiatric patients. Some of the newer serotonergic antidepressants can be particularly effective if the agitation is a manifestation of an underlying psychiatric disorder.

      d. Haloperidol, which is used frequently, is effective to control agitation, but avoid using it, if possible, in cases of traumatic brain injury. Haloperidol can retard the rate of recovery from injury. Restrict its use to patients in whom all other measures fail. The use of neuroleptic antipsychotic agents in traumatic brain injury is associated with an increased risk of posttraumatic seizures and neuroleptic malignant syndrome.

   3. Physical restraints may be necessary, but caution is required. Cases of injury and death resulting from use of either vest or extremity restraints

have been reported. In addition, the restraint is an irritating stimulus that can exacerbate agitation.

B. **Autonomic dysreflexia**, a life-threatening emergency that can occur following spinal cord injury, is the result of pathologic sympathetic reflex activity in response to a noxious stimulus below the level of injury. Interruption of descending pathways allows an uncontrolled sympathetic outflow, leading to a profound increase in blood pressure, piloerection, and diaphoresis.

1. **Symptoms** include severe pounding headache, nasal congestion, general malaise, sustained penile erection, and paresthesias, in addition to the diaphoresis and piloerection. The uncontrolled hypertension can lead to cardiac ischemia, stroke, or fatal intracerebral hemorrhage.

2. The baroreceptors of the great vessels and vagal outflow are still intact; associated bradycardia usually results.

3. Because reflex activity is necessary to cause autonomic dysreflexia, it is rarely seen early after injury when spinal shock is present. Typically, autonomic dysreflexia is seen in lesions above T6 and is more common at higher levels. With spinal cord injury at lower levels, the intact descending sympathetic control minimizes or prevents the syndrome.

4. **Treatment**. Because this syndrome occurs in response to a noxious stimulus, identify and remove the stimulus. Most common cause is an overdistended bladder or overdistended bowel. Relief of this distension is often the only treatment required, with rapid return of the blood pressure to normal.

   a. **Other causes** include fractures, infected decubiti, ingrown toenails, constricting clothing, intraabdominal emergencies, bowel program stimulation, dysmenorrhea, and onset of labor in pregnancy.

   b. In cases in which the cause is not readily identified and corrected, the blood pressure must be brought under control pharmacologically. Sublingual nifedipine (10 mg) is usually effective, but can cause a precipitous drop in blood pressure or cardiac arrhythmia. This is to be repeated in 15 to 20 minutes, if necessary. Sublingual nitroglycerine also has been used. Applied to the skin, it can also provide a more controlled reduction in blood pressure because removing the medication eliminates the effect of the transdermally absorbed nitroglycerine. This can be useful when elimination of the noxious-driving stimulus results in hypotension from the residual drug-related vasodilatation. In refractory cases, intravenous nitroprusside or spinal anesthesia can be used.

   c. In cases where the daily bowel or bladder management activities produce dysreflexia, use of topical anesthetic agents (lidocaine gel or alternatives) limits the cutaneous stimuli and, thus, the risk of developing these symptoms. Use lidocaine lubricating gel when attempting to disimpact a patient's bowel to minimize the noxious stimulus of this procedure. In recurrent cases (such as with bowel routines), oral guanethidine, starting with 5 mg daily, can be used prophylactically. Mecamylamine, starting with 2.5 mg twice daily and titrating up to a total dose of 25 mg daily, is an alternative agent.

   d. Monitor blood pressure closely. With concomitant relief of the noxious stimulus and the administration of a vasodilating agent, the danger exists of lowering the pressure too drastically.

C. **Neurogenic bladder** is one of the most serious alterations of physiologic function following neurologic trauma. In spinal cord injury, the most frequent cause of death (after initial survival) until recently was renal failure. Renal failure was caused by frequent infections combined with reflux and subsequent pyelonephritis. Renal failure is now rare, because of aggressive management of neurogenic bladder function. Coordinated function of sensory, reflex, and voluntary motor pathways allows normal elimination. The pathways include both autonomic (sympathetic and parasympathetic) and somatic motor tracts. Classification of the bladder dysfunction requires detailed knowledge of these pathways and is beyond the scope of this chapter. What is presented is a protocol of care for acute management of neurogenic bladder in spinal cord injury. This protocol allows safe management of the situation while other acute problems are addressed. For proper management of neurogenic bladder, further workup is necessary.

1. Maintaining a high degree of suspicion is the single most important factor in diagnosis and management of neurogenic bladder. Any process that can affect balanced control of the bladder (traumatic brain injury, spinal cord injury, lumbosacral plexus injury, stroke) has the potential to cause neurogenic bladder. Remember, the patient with neurologic injury may maintain good urine output with a bladder that is operating at a very high residual volume, which induces a high risk of infection. Postvoid residual volumes must be checked to ensure that the bladder is emptying properly. Several postvoid volumes of >75 to 100 mL indicate that bladder function requires further attention. The protocol that follows for spinal cord injury also will suffice in the acute phase of management with other types of trauma.

   a. **Discontinue Foley or suprapubic catheter** unless mandated by coexisting urethral or bladder injury, diabetes insipidus, pharmacologic diuresis, large fluid loads, or other conditions where a high urine volume is expected.

   b. **Institute an intermittent catheterization program** as soon as possible after injury, unless contraindicated. Catheterization should be sterile when not performed by the patient. When performed by the patient, the technique can be "clean only." Use a 14 F Bard, Mentor, or MMG Nelaton-type PVC catheter. For intermittent self-catheterization, the catheter should be cleaned with warm water after use, dried, and stored dry in the package. It can be used for up to 1 month.

   c. Urinary volumes obtained by catheterization should not exceed 300 mL. Adjust frequency of catheterization according to the patient's typical output pattern. Record all output volumes and incontinent episodes on a frequency and volume chart.

   d. Restrict patient fluid intake when on intermittent catheterization so that the total urine output is <1,500 mL/24-hour period.

   e. Perform a **fluorourodynamic study** when the patient's bladder is out of spinal shock or at least by 6 months after injury. With lower urinary tract dysfunction as evidenced by detrusor function (incontinence) or autonomic dysreflexia, perform this testing sooner. Repeat testing 1 to 3 months after the initiation of any intervention as a result of the initial urodynamic study, to evaluate the efficacy of the intervention. Conduct this examination on a yearly basis for the first 5 to 10 years after injury and continue on a biennial basis thereafter for optimal monitoring of the lower urinary tracts.

   f. Perform a **baseline upper-tract radiologic evaluation** when the patient's bladder is out of spinal shock or at least by 6 months after injury. Renal ultrasound is recommended to evaluate structural abnormalities. Renal scans using intravenous radioisotopes evaluate function and can be quantified to provide an estimate of glomerular flow rate or effective renal plasma flow. Computerized tomography is essential in evaluating detected structural abnormalities. Plain abdominal x-ray (KUB) can be useful when renal or bladder stones are suspected. Intravenous pyelogram (IVP) does evaluate both function and structure; however, the attendant risks of adverse reaction to the contrast (allergic and nephrotoxic reactions), radiation exposure, and necessity for colonic bowel preparation all decrease the utility of this test as a screening examination for first-line evaluation. Carry out follow-up imaging at the urodynamic assessment intervals noted above.

    g. Carry out **baseline flexible cystoscopy** at the time of the initial urodynamic assessment and repeat at least yearly. With a suspicion of stones or anatomic anomalies, evaluate earlier.

    h. Obtain **urine cultures** as a baseline and repeat only as suspicion of infection occurs or yearly in asymptomatic patients. Do not administer prophylactic antibiotics or urinary antiseptics unless a **complicated** urinary tract infection is documented. Complicated urinary tract infection is indicated by symptoms that can include:
- Fever not attributable to other pathology
- Increasing spasticity
- Autonomic dysreflexia
- Urinary retention or incontinence as a deviation from established patterns
- Hematuria
- More than 50 white blood cells per high-power field on microscopic evaluation
- Evidence of stone disease
- Bacteruria—>10^2 colonies in specimen obtained by intermittent catheterization, or any growth in samples obtained from indwelling catheters

    Existence of a "positive" bacterial culture alone is insufficient to prompt treatment in absence of any of the attendant symptoms described above

    i. Give **pharmacotherapy** to modify bladder function, as appropriate **based on CMG (cystometrogram) findings**.

D. Neurogenic bowel usually coexists in patients in whom neurogenic bladder is present; control of pathways for fecal elimination are similar to those for bladder control. The goal of a bowel program is to provide controlled fecal elimination with intervening periods of relative continence so that the individual can participate in daily activities. Because the individual with spinal cord injury usually has impaired or absent rectal and perineal sensation, symptoms are usually absent or vague. Lack of appetite or nonspecific malaise may be the only indication that the problem of retained feces exists.

    1. In the initial period after spinal cord injury, an ileus typically exists. Once the ileus subsides, the bowel program should be initiated on a routine basis. Initially this should be administered daily. Once the bowel program is producing predictable results, the schedule can be modified if desired. The patient's preinjury bowel pattern is the best guide to modification of timing. Individuals who had routine, daily bowel movements usually will continue with this pattern after injury. Individuals who had less frequent bowel movements may require a less frequent bowel program.

    2. Frequent liquid stools can indicate bowel motility is too great or inspissated feces are blocking the rectum or descending colon. Liquid stool from above passes around this blockage and leaks from the anus. It may be possible to detect a full colon on examination, but the most reliable method of detection is to obtain a KUB (flat plate x-ray study of the abdomen). The proper approach to this problem is to evacuate the colon and then institute a routine and reliable bowel program.

    3. Classify neurogenic bowel as either an upper motor neuron or lower motor neuron injury.

        a. In cases of upper motor neuron injury (tetraplegia), the sacral reflex arcs are intact. Presence of these reflexes is useful in initiating bowel evacuation. In some cases, the individual can initiate evacuation with digital stimulation (stretch) of the anal sphincter or use of a suppository.

        b. In lower motor neuron lesions (*conus medullaris* or *cauda equina* injuries), the local reflexes are lost. This situation is much more difficult to control, often requiring digital disimpaction on a routine basis.

4. The following bowel program for individuals with spinal cord injury also can be initiated for other clinical entities in which bowel control is a problem.

   a. Start the bowel program once the postinjury ileus has resolved and the patient has resumed eating or tube feedings. The goal of the initial management is to start routine bowel management that leads to predictable continence.

   b. A typical bowel management protocol consists of a stool softener titrated to the patient's needs and a mild, orally administered stimulant laxative coordinated with a laxative enema (suppository in selected patients). Initially, this is done on a daily schedule so that evacuation occurs at a time convenient for the patient and nursing staff. Protocol for evening evacuation is Colace (100 mg) twice daily, two tablets of Senokot (Purdue Frederick, Norwalk, CT) at noon, with a Fleets (Fleet, Lynchburg, VA) bisacodyl enema or Dulcolax (Ciba, Woodbridge, NJ) suppository, in combination with digital stimulation of the rectum, in the evening. If morning evacuation is desired, the Senokot is given at bedtime.

IV. The scope of rehabilitation following trauma

  A. Rehabilitation of patients after trauma occurs in several stages, each with a corresponding venue.

    1. Inpatient rehabilitation is required when patients, for either physical or cognitive reasons, are unable to manage their own basic self-care or mobility needs because of physical limitations. The goal of inpatient rehabilitation is to reestablish capability for basic routines of daily living so that the patient can function safely in the community, with a minimal amount of physical assistance or supervision. Ideally, patients are restored to the point where they are both physically and cognitively independent, although, this is not always possible. Rehabilitation interventions are directed toward minimizing the amount of physical or cognitive assistance that a patient will require on return to the community.

    2. Initial phases of **outpatient rehabilitation** are directed toward enhancing the ability of the patient to return to active participation in the community outside of the home, and to improving the patient's ability to manage more complex instrumental activities of daily living (e.g., cooking, laundry, managing finances, home maintenance). These tasks involve more complex organizational and executive skills that are frequently affected in brain injury. Patients may also require assistance with behavioral problems that affect their interpersonal relationships. Residual deficits that limit mobility in the community can also be addressed along with continuing cognitive limitations. This phase of rehabilitation is sometimes referred to as "community reentry."

    3. The final phase of rehabilitation involves helping the affected individual (now often referred to as a "client" rather than a "patient") to return to some form of competitive employment. Referred to as **vocational rehabilitation**, this involves the training of skills that enable an individual to return to the workplace. It can also involve the provision of some assistive services (e.g., job placement and job coaching) as well as trial placements in voluntary positions in the community.

Bibliography

Berrol S, Kraft GH, eds. Traumatic brain injury. *Phys Med Rehabil Clin N Am* 1992;3:2.

Cope N, Hall K. Head injury rehabilitation: benefit of early intervention. *Arch Phys Med Rehabil* 1982;63:433–437.

DeLisa JA, Gans BM, eds. *Rehabilitation medicine: principles and practice,* 3d ed. Philadelphia: JB Lippincott, 1999.

Goldberg G. Symposium on care after neurologic injury. What happens after brain injury? *Postgrad Med* 1998;104:91–105.

Linsenmeyer, TA, Culkin, D. APS recommendations for the urological evaluation of patients with spinal cord injury. *J Spinal Cord Med* 1999;22(2):139–142.

Mackay LE, Bernstein BA, Chapman PE, et al. Early intervention in severe head injury: long-term benefits of a formalized program. *Arch Phys Med Rehabil* 1992;73:635–641.

MacKenzie EJ, Shapiro S, Siegel JH. The economic impact of traumatic injuries. *JAMA* 1988;260(22):3290–3296.

NIDRR Consensus Statement. The prevention and management of urinary tract infections among people with spinal cord injuries. *Journal of the American Paraplegia Society* 1992;15:194–204.

Penrod LE. Medico-legal issues in traumatic brain injury. In: Horn LE, Zasler ND, eds. *Medical rehabilitation of traumatic brain injury*. Philadelphia: Hanley and Belfus (*in press*).

Sandel ME, Robinson KM, Goldberg G, et al. Neurorehabilitation. In: Cruz EJ. *Neurological and neurosurgical emergencies*. Philadelphia: WB Saunders, 1998:503–546.

Staas WE Jr, Ditunno JF Jr, Kraft GH, eds. Traumatic spinal cord injury. *Phys Med Rehabil Clin N Am* 1992;3:4.

51. VENOUS THROMBOEMBOLISM

Jon W. Johnson and Patrick M. Reilly

Deep Venous Thrombosis and Prophylaxis

I. **Definition.** Deep venous thrombosis (DVT) is clinically thought of as an intraluminal blood clot obstructing flow of the iliac or femoral venous system. In fact, DVT refers to any clot (obstructing or nonobstructing) in any deep venous system, including the upper extremity and the calf.

II. **Incidence.** DVT affects > 2.5 million people each year in the United States. This is likely an underestimate of the actual incidence, as many cases go unrecognized by patient and physician. Series have shown the incidence of DVT to be as high as 65% in the untreated major trauma patient. One of the complications of DVT, pulmonary embolism (PE), accounts for as many as 200,000 deaths per year.

   A. **Risk factors, in general,** include advanced age, **immobilization, general anesthesia, major surgery,** estrogen therapy, pregnancy, prior DVT, congestive heart failure, malignancy, hypercoagulable state, and tissue trauma.

   B. **Risk factors specific to trauma** include advanced age, multiple blood transfusions, surgery, fracture of the femur or tibia, complex pelvic fracture, venous injury, immobility, and spinal cord injury. For trauma patients, scoring systems and rank tables have been devised to assess risk factors and better estimate the risk of DVT or PE (Table 51.1).

III. **Complications.** DVT is a major cause of morbidity and mortality; superficial venous thrombosis is usually a benign self-limiting disease. Although DVT may be associated with a number of serious local complications (e.g., phlegmasia cerulea dolens), these are usually infrequent. Most of the morbidity is related to PE and the postphlebitic syndrome.

   A. **Pulmonary embolism.** The incidence of PE in all trauma patients reportedly is 0.3%; in high-risk patients this incidence can increase to 5%, even with DVT prophylaxis. The mortality rate for PE that is diagnosed and treated remains approximately 10%; it may be higher in the high-risk trauma patient. Long-term morbidity can result from PE and includes crippling pulmonary hypertension.

   B. **Postphlebitic syndrome.** Pathophysiologically, venous valves in the lower extremities are destroyed by clot formation when DVT occurs. After the clot dissolves, valvular competence is permanently lost in the affected segment of vein. As a result, nonpitting edema, swelling, discoloration, and pain frequently occur, which can progress to venous hypertension and venous stasis ulceration. Serious disability can result from these changes. Even with prompt heparin therapy after a diagnosis of DVT, the postphlebitic syndrome occurs in up to 90% of patients, with severe sequelae in nearly 6%. As the changes associated with postphlebitic syndrome often take years to become evident, these numbers may actually be underestimated.

IV. **Prophylaxis.** Contemporary forms of prophylaxis for DVT include early ambulation, graded compression stockings, sequential compression devices and foot pumps, and low-dose anticoagulation. A preventative technique against DVT is early ambulation. This routine activity, which simply represents good patient care, may not be as attractive as sequential compression devices or low molecular weight heparin, but is less expensive and likely as effective as the other commonly prescribed methods. Prophylaxis has proved to decrease the incidence of DVT after elective general surgery, but its utility in trauma patients remains less clear. However, because of the reported high incidence of DVT after major trauma and the minimal morbidity associated with most prophylactic regimens, some form of prophylaxis should be used for all trauma patients **at risk** (Fig. 51.1).

Table 51.1 DVT risk factor categories

Risk factors
–Age 40 years
–Injury severity score (ISS) >9
–Blood transfusion
–Surgical procedure ≥2 hours
–Lower extremity fracture
–Pelvis fracture
–Spinal cord injury (SCI)
–Immobilization
–Pregnancy
–Estrogen therapy
–History of deep venous thrombosis or pulmonary embolism
–Malignancy
–Hypercoaguable state (e.g., AT III [Antithrombin III] deficiency)
–Extensive soft tissue trauma
–Congestive heart failure

High risk factors
–Age >50 years
–ISS ≥16
–Femoral central venous catheter in trauma resuscitation
–Abbreviated injury score (AIS) ≥3 (any body region)
–Glasgow Coma Scale (GCS) score ≤8
–SCI
–Pelvis fracture
–Femur or tibia fracture
–Venous injury

Very high risk factors
–SCI
–AIS—head/neck ≥3 + long bone fracture (upper or lower)
–Severe pelvic fracture (posterior element) + long bone fracture (upper or lower)
–Multiple (≥3) long bone fractures

A. **Sequential compression devices (SCD).** Intermittent external pneumatic compression of the legs (or arms) minimizes venous stasis and also systemically activates the body's fibrinolytic system. This latter effect is thought to explain the apparent efficacy of SCD in preventing thrombus formation when applied to a site(s) remote from a deep venous system at risk. The use of SCD does not result in an increase in hemorrhagic side effects. Therefore, it is ideal for patients who have sustained neurologic trauma. The use of these devices is contraindicated in patients with arterial insufficiency or trauma of the lower extremity, although they can be placed on the upper extremity, as mentioned. Improper application of the devices (as often as 50% on some general care units) can be a frequent reason for failure of SCD.

B. **AV foot pumps.** The discovery of a venous pump on the plantar aspect of the foot in 1983 led to the development of a device to reproduce this action. Clinical trials using these devices are primarily in the orthopedic literature. The most attractive aspect of the AV foot pump is its utilization in the multiply injured patient with a contraindication to anticoagulation coupled with the inability to place SCD because of extremity trauma or external fixation devices. Recent evidence suggests that they may be less effective than more traditional methods of DVT prophylaxis in the trauma population.

C. **Subcutaneous heparin.** Low-dose, unfractionated heparin (5,000 U subcutaneously every 8–12 hours) may represent adequate prophylaxis in the

DVT Prophylaxis

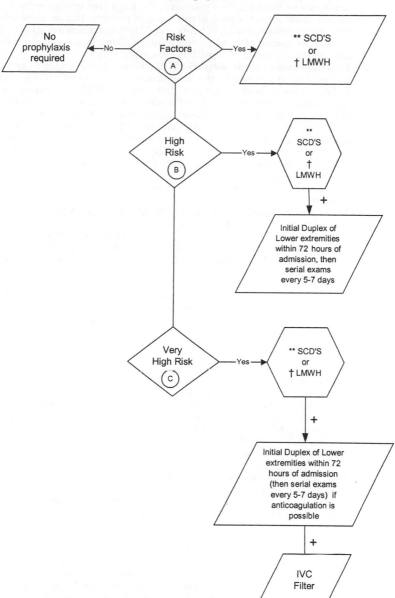

Modified from Clinical Management Guidelines, Deep Venous Thrombosis Prophylaxis. Division of Trauma and Surgical Critical Care. Hospital of the University of Pennsylvania. Philadelphia, PA, 2000.

FIG. 51.1. Algorithm for deep venous thrombosis and pulmonary embolism prophylaxis. **Sequential compression devices (SCD) are indicated when access to both lower extremities is available. Otherwise, low molecular weight heparin (LMWH) will be utilized. LMWH is contraindicated in patients with an epidural catheter in place.

low risk trauma patient. Convincing evidence indicates unfractionated heparin may be no better than placebo in the **high risk** trauma patient and, therefore, should not be used in this group of patients. Hemorrhagic side effects are uncommon (~2%), but care should be taken when using heparin in patients suspected of head or spine injury. Heparin-induced thrombocytopenia can also occur, even with low-dose heparin.

D. **Low molecular weight heparin (LMWH)** is gaining popularity as a prophylactic agent of choice for the trauma patient. The longer half-life of some LMWH compounds allows for once-daily dosing. LMWH also has a reduced hemorrhagic-to-antithrombotic ratio when compared with standard heparin. Accumulating clinical studies suggest that LMWH is superior to other forms of prophylaxis after major trauma and may well be the preferred agent. The standard dose used for prophylaxis is 30 mg subcutaneously every 12 hours of enoxaparin. Of note, The US Food and Drug Administration has warned about placement of epidural catheters in patients receiving LMWH (bleeding complications). In addition, the use of LMWH as prophylaxis in the neurotrauma population (bleeding complications) is poorly studied.

E. **Low-dose warfarin** (international normalized ratio [INR] ~1.5) is preferred for some patients with lower extremity or pelvic fractures. The risk of bleeding is small, but higher than the risk with low-dose heparin. For this reason, warfarin use is not routinely recommended for patients who have sustained neurotrauma, have large pulmonary contusions, or are being managed nonoperatively for an intraabdominal solid viscus injury.

F. **Graded compression stocking** use is aimed at minimizing venous stasis in the deep venous system by the compressive shunting of blood from the superficial venous system. Although graded compression stockings can provide adequate prophylaxis for patients at very low risk for DVT, their use as a sole means of DVT prophylaxis in the trauma patient is not recommended.

V. **Diagnosis.** The symptoms and signs of DVT are nonspecific or often nonexistent. They can be mimicked or obscured by a number of other conditions. Objective testing is necessary to confirm the diagnosis before a prolonged course of anticoagulation (or other invasive therapy) is undertaken in a trauma patient.

A. **Clinical examination.** Physical examination is unreliable in the diagnosis of DVT. More than 50% of documented DVT can be clinically silent. Even when the patient has lower extremity symptoms, fewer than one third have the classic syndrome of calf discomfort, edema, venous distension, and pain on dorsiflexion of the foot (Homans' sign).

B. **Duplex ultrasound.** Ultrasound imaging can be used to assess both the superficial and deep venous systems of the upper and lower extremities. Duplex scanning combines hemodynamic (flow velocity) and imaging modalities. Inability to compress the vein, the actual presence of thrombus on the ultrasound image, and dilation of the vein are duplex characteristics of thrombosis. The methodology is noninvasive and portable. It is an effective screening tool. The sensitivity and specificity of this method (when compared with venography) is approximately 95%. The ability of duplex ultrasonography to evaluate the pelvic veins for thrombus is limited.

C. **Impedance plethysmography (IPG)** uses a large thigh cuff to obstruct venous return while allowing arterial inflow. Venous capacitance and maximal venous outflow are measured when the cuff is deflated. Limited capacitance and a delayed maximal venous outflow are suggestive of DVT. IPG has a sensitivity and specificity of nearly 90%, but is insensitive to nonobstructing or infrapopliteal thrombi. In addition, its sensitivity in the trauma population has been questioned.

D. **Venogram** is the most accurate diagnostic modality for detecting DVT. However, it is invasive, often painful, and can cause allergic reactions. It also involves a contrast load, and must be performed in the radiology suite. The role of venography as a screening tool is limited, and its routine use has been largely replaced by noninvasive diagnostic methods.

E. **Spiral computed tomography (CT) scan and magnetic resonance imaging (MRI).** Computed tomography can detect DVT in the abdomen and pelvis, and is considered superior to venography in imaging these great veins. MRI also has a superior sensitivity and specificity in diagnosing proximal DVT. However, both techniques are expensive and require patient transport for performance. Their use in the trauma population, especially as screening tools, is therefore limited. Occasionally, an unsuspected DVT is identified on imaging of the abdomen and pelvis, which warrants treatment as for symptomatic DVT (see below).

F. **D-Dimer.** The measurement of D-dimer, a fibrin breakdown product, has the potential to greatly alter the current diagnostic approach to venous thromboembolism. The assay is highly nonspecific, being positive in a multitude of fibrin deposition phenomena. A negative result, however, reliably excludes clinically significant clot. Simplified laboratory assays are necessary and they are rapidly becoming available. The ultimate role of the D-dimer assay in the management of venous thromboembolism is yet to be elucidated.

G. **Intensive care unit (ICU) screening.** Many groups have begun the practice of routine surveillance screening of the lower extremity veins of patients in the ICU. Duplex ultrasonography is usually the diagnostic method selected for this population. A reasonable approach is a baseline ultrasound examination within 72 hours of admission and then serial ultrasound examination every 5 to 7 days, especially when the patient is in the ICU.

VI. **Definitive treatment.** The goals of definitive treatment of DVT include preventing clot propagation, reducing the risk of PE, facilitating clot lysis, preserving valve function, reducing swelling, alleviating pain, and preventing recurrence.

A. **Anticoagulation.** Provided no contraindications to anticoagulation exist, heparin and subsequently warfarin are the hallmarks of therapy for DVT (Table 51.2). Tight control of heparin is very labor intensive, but both over- and undercoagulation can have devastating consequences. Warfarin can be

Table 51.2 Heparin dosing guidelines

Initial order
–**Bolus** 70 units/kg
–**Infusion** 18 units/kg/h
Monitor efficacy—6–8 hours after initial bolus or change in dosing
–Check partial thromboplastin time (PTT) Therapeutic range 51–68 seconds

Heparin adjustment

–PTT	Adjustment
–<41 sec	REBOLUS 35 units/kg INCREASE infusion 3 units/kg/h
–41–50 sec	INCREASE infusion 2 units/kg/h
–51–68 sec	No Change
–69–96 sec	DECREASE infusion 1 unit/kg/h
–96–120 sec	HOLD infusion 30 minutes DECREASE infusion 2 units/kg/h
–>120 sec	HOLD infusion 90 minutes DECREASE infusion 3 units/kg/h

Concomitant orders
–Complete blood cell count with platelet count every other day while on heparin
–No intramuscular injections
–Check all stool for occult blood

(Modified from Heparin dosing protocol. Philadelphia: Hospital of the University of Pennsylvania, 2002, with permission.)

started after a therapeutic partial thromboplastin time (PTT) has been reached (provided no need for reversal of anticoagulation is foreseen). An INR between 2 and 3 is desirable when following the prothrombin time (PT). The course of therapeutic anticoagulation generally ranges from 3 to 6 months. Shorter lengths of therapy can increase the incidence of recurrent DVT, whereas a longer period of treatment yields an unfavorable risk-to-benefit ratio. Recent studies suggest that outpatient therapy for DVT with LMWH can result in significant cost savings with comparable efficacy. For therapeutic anticoagulation, the dose of enoxaparin is 1 mg/kg subcutaneously every 12 hours. Generally, no laboratory studies are necessary to monitor anticoagulation with this dosing regimen.

    B. Other measures. Bedrest is recommended for patients diagnosed with DVT, but ambulation is allowed once a therapeutic PTT has been reached. Elevation of the leg and graded compression stockings are also recommended to minimize lower extremity swelling.

    C. Lytic therapy. Although lytic therapy is used to decrease the incidence of the postphlebitic syndrome, the risk of bleeding in the trauma patient generally precludes its use.

    D. Vena caval filters. Vena caval interruption is indicated to prevent PE in patients with a proximal lower extremity DVT who cannot be safely anticoagulated. Another absolute indication for placement of a vena caval filter would be PE, despite adequate anticoagulation. Relative indications for vena caval filters include proximal iliac DVT, recurrent DVT or PE, and presence of a DVT in a patient with minimal respiratory reserve. Of note, vena caval filters do not treat the underlying DVT and, if possible, these patients require full anticoagulation.

VII. DVT can occur in other sites beside the ileofemoral system. Significant morbidity and mortality can result from these less common sites.

    A. Calf vein thrombosis. Untreated calf DVT can propagate proximally (in 5% to 23% of calf DVT). Untreated calf DVT can also resolve without complications, therefore, making therapy of calf DVT controversial. If no therapy is undertaken, follow-up studies (e.g., duplex ultrasound) are necessary to ensure that the clot has not propagated and that the initial thrombus has resolved. If therapeutic anticoagulation is undertaken, a full 3-month course is warranted to prevent recurrence.

    B. Upper extremity. The most common cause of upper extremity DVT is subclavian vein catheterization. When clinically suspected, duplex ultrasonography is used to confirm the diagnosis. Once the diagnosis is made, remove any offending catheter and start lytic therapy or systemic anticoagulation. The incidence of PE from upper extremity DVT is ~12%. With this clinical entity, PE can occur during anticoagulation treatment.

    C. Pelvic veins. Ileofemoral thrombosis generally requires full anticoagulation.

    D. Other. With a PE and no identified source, consider mural thrombi of the heart, which are diagnosed by echocardiography.

VIII. Pulmonary embolism. Despite an improved understanding of the pathogenesis, diagnosis, and management of PE, it remains a frequent and often fatal disorder. As with DVT, the cornerstone of management is prevention.

    A. Incidence. More than 500,000 cases of PE occur annually in the United States. The incidence of PE in the trauma population is estimated as 0.3%. In trauma patients at high risk (Table 51.1), the incidence increases.

    B. Prophylaxis—vena caval filters. Despite the routine use of mechanical or pharmacologic prophylaxis, the risk of DVT and PE in severely injured trauma patients is significant. For this reason, patients with specific injury complexes (e.g., complex bony injury, spinal cord injury) may benefit from prophylactically placed vena caval filters. With the routine use of prophylactic vena caval filters, the incidence of PE has decreased (compared with historical controls) in these patients at high risk. Once a patient with a prophylactic inferior vena cava (IVC) filter is considered an acceptable candidate for anticoagulation, perform a surveillance ultrasound weekly. Treatment of subsequent DVT decreases the development of postphlebitic syndrome. Prospective studies of prophylactic vena caval filters are ongoing. The long-term consequences of vena caval filters are unknown, particularly in the young or pregnant trauma patient. The recent introduction of absorbable or retractable filters may allay these concerns.

C. **The diagnosis** of PE in the trauma patient is often clouded by a number of other medical and surgical problems. Not infrequently, patients who have had a PE may have an "impending sense of doom". Dyspnea and pleuritic chest pain, the two most common symptoms of PE, are frequently present in patients who have sustained thoracic trauma. Signs and symptoms of PE often suggest a differential diagnosis that includes many common conditions (e.g., pneumonia, atelectasis, myocardial ischemia). Often, more sophisticated means of diagnosis are necessary.

1. **Physical examination**. Tachypnea and tachycardia are the most frequent physical signs associated with PE. However, these and other physical signs are nonspecific. Cyanosis and hypotension occur infrequently, and only with massive PE. Consider patients on a ventilator who have an increase in A-a gradient (shunt) without a corresponding decrease in lung compliance at substantial risk for having sustained a PE.

2. **Laboratory tests**. An arterial blood gas (ABG) is the most useful laboratory test to confirm the clinical suspicion of a PE. Only 10% of patients with a PE have a PaO_2 on room air of >80 mmHg. Hypocarbia and mild hypoxemia (PaO_2 between 60 and 80 mmHg) are the most common ABG findings in patients with PE. Sudden decreases in PaO_2 without explanation are highly suggestive of PE. As mentioned, measuring a D-dimer can be helpful. A negative result appears to reliably exclude clinically significant clot. The ultimate role of the D-dimer assay in the management of venous thromboembolism is yet to be elucidated.

3. **Chest x-ray (CXR) study**. More than one-half of patients with PE have an abnormal CXR. These changes are most often nonspecific. However, the CXR is important to exclude other pulmonary problems (e.g. pneumonia, atelectasis) that can mimic PE.

4. **Electrocardiography (ECG)** changes, although common, are nonspecific. The classic $S_1Q_3T_3$, RBBB, and right ventricle axis deviation are uncommonly seen.

5. **Ventilation and perfusion (V-Q) scan** can help in diagnosing PE. However, other pulmonary abnormalities can limit its usefulness. A high probability scan, which demonstrates ventilation without perfusion (V-Q mismatch), has a positive predictive value for PE of 87%. In addition, a normal scan generally rules out PE. Intermediate and low probability scans leave the diagnosis in doubt. A pulmonary angiogram may be warranted to confirm the diagnosis.

6. **Dynamic-enhanced (spiral) computed tomography**. Recent data suggest that contrast-enhanced spiral CT can play an increasing role in the evaluation of patients with suspected PE. In addition to demonstrating clot, the study can also demonstrate other reasons for a worsening A-a gradient in a critically ill patient. The test is readily available in most institutions, although protocols for the timing of dye injection and image acquisition must be in place. Its sensitivity for proximal emboli is ~85% but declines significantly when more peripheral emboli are present (not uncommon). Recent studies suggest this sensitivity is improving as technology advances. The amount of contrast necessary is similar to that for the gold standard pulmonary angiogram. The exact role of spiral CT in the diagnosis of PE continues to be defined and debated.

7. **Pulmonary arteriography**. The diagnostic standard for PE is pulmonary angiography. Central venous, right ventricle, and pulmonary artery pressures can be obtained during the study and provide important diagnostic information. The mortality rate of pulmonary arteriography is

0.5%, occurring most commonly in patients with pulmonary hypertension. Perform additional interventional techniques (e.g., placement of vena caval filters or suction embolectomy) at the time of diagnosis, if indicated.

8. **Transesophageal echocardiography (TEE).** Although transthoracic echocardiography can yield indirect evidence of PE (e.g., right ventricular strain), TEE possesses a sensitivity and specificity of >90% in demonstrating clot. It is a useful test in those patients too ill to transport to the radiology suite or those allergic to radiocontrast media. TEE also aids in determining other pathology that may present as PE.

D. **Treatment or uncomplicated PE** (simple) PE is similar to that for DVT.

1. **Anticoagulation** with heparin and warfarin is the therapy of choice for most PE. A PTT of 2× normal and an INR of 2 to 3 are the therapeutic goals. Therapy should be for 3 to 6 months.

2. **Vena caval filter.** As discussed, vena caval interruption can be warranted in patients who have sustained a PE and cannot be anticoagulated (e.g., recent neurotrauma patients) or have developed PE while on therapeutic anticoagulation. Although the filter will not treat the PE already present, it does prevent 95% of recurrent PE. Patients with **septic** PE may require vena caval interruption rather than simple filter placement.

E. **Treatment of complicated PE** (complex, life-threatening) PE, which cause hemodynamic instability and may require life support, can mandate urgent intervention in addition to standard anticoagulation.

1. **Lytic therapy.** Patients who sustain a massive PE with hemodynamic instability may be candidates for lytic therapy. A marked improvement in oxygenation and hemodynamics may be seen with resolution of the thrombus. The risk of bleeding with thrombolytic therapy is significant, making it usually not applicable to the trauma patient.

2. **Suction embolectomy.** If hemodynamic instability persists despite thrombolytic therapy, or if thrombolytics are contraindicated in a patient with a massive central PE, suction embolectomy may be warranted. Although the risks of such heroic procedures are significant, the high mortality rate of untreated, massive PE does make embolectomy a viable option in these critically ill patients. The ability to perform this procedure at the time of angiographic diagnosis and without the use of cardiopulmonary bypass makes it advantageous over surgical embolectomy.

3. **Surgical embolectomy** may be the only viable option in the patient with massive, hemodynamically significant PE. This technique generally requires cardiopulmonary bypass. When this procedure is performed on a patient in full cardiopulmonary arrest (i.e., cardiopulmonary resuscitation) the prognosis is dismal.

Axioms

- The incidence of DVT after major trauma remains significant.
- Patients should be evaluated for risk of venous thromboembolism after injury, and treated accordingly.
- Duplex ultrasound is a rapid, portable, and noninvasive technique to diagnose DVT.
- Pulmonary embolism should always be considered with unexplained hypoxia, hypocarbia, or an impending sense of doom.
- Prophylactic IVC filter placement may be indicated in the trauma patient with excessive risk.

Bibliography

Geerts WH, Code KI, Jay RM, et al. A prospective study of venous thromboembolism after major trauma. *N Engl J Med* 1994;331:1601–1606.

Geerts WH, Jay RM, Code KI, et al. A comparison of low-dose heparin with low molecular weight heparin as prophylaxis against venous thromboembolism after major trauma. *N Engl J Med* 1996;335:701–707.

Knudson MM, Morabito D, Paiemont GD, et al. Use of low molecular weight heparin in preventing thromboembolism in trauma patients. *J Trauma* 1996;41:446–459.

Levine MN, Raskob G, Landefeld S, et al. Hemorrhagic complications of anticoagulant treatment. Fifth ACCP Consensus Conference on Antithrombotic Therapy. *Chest* 1998;114:511s–523s.

Lipchick RJ, Goodman LR. Spiral computed tomography in the evaluation of pulmonary embolism. *Clin Chest Med* 1999;20(4):731–738.

Owings JT, Gosselin RC, Batttistella FD, et al. Whole blood D-dimer assay: an effective noninvasive method to rule out pulmonary embolism. *J Trauma* 2000;48: 795–800.

Philbrick JT, Becker DM. Calf deep venous thrombosis—a wolf in sheep's clothing? *Arch Intern Med* 1988;148:2131–2138.

Raskob GE, Hull RD. Diagnosis of pulmonary embolism. *Curr Opin Hematol* 1999; 6(5):280–284.

Rogers FB. Venous thromboembolism in trauma patients. *Surg Clin North Am* 1995; 75:279–291.

Rogers FB, Shackford SR, Ricci MA, et al. Routine prophylactic vena cava filter insertion in severely injured trauma patients decreases the incidence of pulmonary embolism. *J Am Coll Surg* 1995;180:641–647.

Tuttle-Newhall JE, Rutledge R, Hultman CS, et al. Statewide, population-based, time series analysis of the frequency and outcome of pulmonary embolus in 318,554 trauma patients. *J Trauma* 1997;42:90–99.

Velmahos GC, Kern J, Chan LS, et al. Prevention of venous thromboembolism after injury: an evidence-based report. Part II: analysis of risk factors and evaluation of the role of vena cava filters. *J Trauma* 2000;49:140–144.

Winchell RJ, Hoyt DB, Walsh JC, et al. Risk factors associated with pulmonary embolism despite routine prophylaxis: implications for improved protection. *J Trauma* 1994;37:600–606.

52. INJURY PREVENTION

Therese S. Richmond

I. **Introduction**. Injury remains among the top ten causes of death in the United States. The composite of unintentional, suicide, and homicide deaths was the leading cause of death in those from 1 to 44 year of age (data from the Centers for Disease Control and Prevention, Atlanta, GA). Unintentional injury alone is the fifth leading cause of death for all age groups and, when combined with suicides, is the fourth leading cause of death. In 1997, 146,400 injury-related deaths were documented. The top four causes of injury deaths in the United States were:
- Motor vehicle traffic (42,473)
- Firearm-related (32,436)
- Poisoning (17,692)
- Falls (12,555)

The injury epidemic is not restricted to the United States. Worldwide, it is estimated that 5.8 million people died from injuries in 1998; a rate of 97.9/100,000 population. Around the world, almost 16,000 individuals die daily from injury; 1 of 10 deaths is from injury. In all age groups, injury is a significant cause of death. In 1998, in high-income countries (which includes the United States), road traffic injuries were the leading cause of death for those aged 5 to 44 years. In these same countries, road traffic injuries, self-inflicted injuries, and interpersonal violence were the top three causes of death in the 15 to 44 years of age group.

Mortality alone does not characterize adequately the profound physical, psychosocial, and economic effects of injury. Injury most commonly affects individuals early in their productive life (i.e., young adults). The years of productive life lost from all injuries >3.5 million, outranking diseases such as cancer, heart disease, and human immunodeficiency virus (HIV) for which each has <2 million years of productive life lost. More recently, disability-adjusted life years (DALY) methodology has been used to indicate the burden of injury. DALY combine the number of years of life loss from premature death with the loss of health and presence of disability in survivors of injury. Simplistically, 1 DALY is equivalent to 1 lost year of healthy and productive life. According to the World Health Organization (WHO) using the DALY methodology, 16% of the world's burden of disease in 1998 was attributed to injury. The main injury-related causes of DALY are road traffic injuries, falls, interpersonal violence, and self-inflicted injuries. WHO projects that injuries will impose an even greater burden by the year 2020.

Physicians typically focus on the resuscitation and definitive treatment of injuries. Yet, once the burden of injury is thoroughly recognized and the fact that as many as 50% of deaths take place at the scene of the injury or within minutes of the event, the mission of trauma care must expand to include injury prevention.

II. **Responsibility for injury prevention**. Prevention is the ideal way to relieve the burden of injury. Prevention of all types of injury is a priority and an expectation of personnel in hospitals, both trauma centers and those that are not. The Committee on Trauma (COT) of the American College of Surgeons mandates that trauma center personnel educate people about injury as a public health epidemic. Physicians are natural leaders in expanding trauma care to include the primary prevention of injury. The COT indicates that physicians move beyond public education to activities that include surveillance, epidemiology, intervention research, and evaluation of prevention program effectiveness.

III. **The science of injury prevention**. Knowledge of successful strategies to reduce injury for specific injuries has increased. The decline in incidence of motor vehicle injuries is a case in point. Although motor vehicle injuries continue to be the leading cause of injury death in the United States, rates have declined considerably over the past 25 years. (Fig. 52.1). This decrease is the result of systematic and multifaceted prevention efforts that include attainment of adequate surveillance data (via the Fatality Analysis Reporting System), implementation of policy and regulation, introduction of active and passive safety devices, improved roadway design, and public advocacy cultivating behavioral change.

This success has not extended to all mechanisms of injury, as can be seen in the concurrent increase in firearm injury fatality during the same time period that motor vehicle injury fatalities decreased (Fig. 52.1). However, the precedents and steps used in reducing motor vehicle injuries can be used to address other major injuries (e.g., firearm injuries, falls in the elderly).

Injury prevention is multifaceted, including the development of public policy, federal and state regulation, and changing individual behavioral components. Injury is not a random event. Methodically building the science of injury deterrence is best founded on the surveillance and epidemiology of specific injuries, with strategies designed, tested, and implemented and then systematically evaluated. The following four steps can be taken to more fully understand the epidemiology of injury and to reduce those injuries.

A. **Determine the magnitude, scope, and characteristics of the problem.** National surveillance data provide a global indication of the scope of injury in the United States. Such systems as the Fatality Analysis Reporting System, a surveillance system for motor vehicle fatalities and the National Electronic Injury Surveillance System (NEISS), a stratified sample of US emergency departments, are illustrations of nationally available data that assist with prevention efforts. National and state level data can assist in identifying trends and allocating resources to address priority regional problems, but it is most important to gain an understanding of injury in the local community. The Emergency Medical Services Data, Hospital Discharge Data, hospital-based trauma registry, and medical examiners' information can be used to study injury specific to the local community.

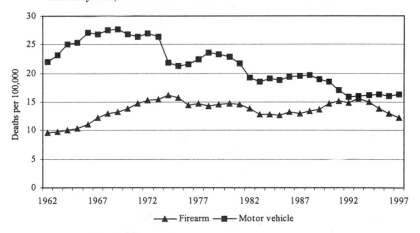

Mortality Rate, 1962-1997: *Firearm & Motor Vehicle-Related Death*

Source: National Center for Injury Prevention and Control, Centers for Disease Control and Prevention

FIG. 52.1. Firearm and motor vehicle-related death rates. (From National Center for Injury Prevention and Control, Centers for Disease Control and Prevention, with permission.)

B. Identify factors increasing the risk of injury and determine which of those factors are potentially modifiable. The public health model supplies a helpful framework to identify and tackle the modifiable risk factors for injury (Fig. 52.2). The components are:
- **Host** (individuals and contributing behaviors)
- **Agent** (automobiles, motorcycles, firearms, knives)
- **Environment** (physical [e.g., road design, throw rugs, poor lighting]; economic [e.g., high unemployment]; social [e.g., access to and use of drugs and alcohol]; temporal [e.g., season or time of day])

By categorizing injury risk into the host, agent, and environment, a comprehensive profile of specific injuries can be constructed that highlights the complexity of the causal chain of events leading to injury. Analysis of these factors is an important step in identifying modifiable risk factors. Because of the complex causes of injury, it is helpful to work within an interdisciplinary team, embracing such diverse disciplines as other healthcare providers, epidemiologists, health services and public policy scientists, economists, and behavioral scientists, to grasp a strong understanding of the factors leading to injury and better design interventions.

C. Evaluate the effectiveness of strategies to reduce injury. All trauma centers are required to participate in trauma prevention. It is important for trauma centers to take the lead in examining the effectiveness of implementing interventions at the local level. In the absence of a program of prevention research, trauma centers can take interventions shown to be effective in other communities and examine if these same interventions can be transferred to their local community. Indicators of successful transplantation of intervention strategies include, but are not limited to (*a*) evidence of public support for prevention activities, (*b*) commitment from local community and political leaders, (*c*) media buy-in for prevention priorities, and (*d*) changes in monitored behaviors. Strategies can best be judged if they are linked to specific outcomes (e.g., decrease in the incidence of injuries, reduced mortality).

D. Implement and evaluate the most promising strategies. Some strategies, known to be effective, can form the foundation of an ongoing prevention program. Such strategies as seatbelt use, child restraints, separate storage and locking of ammunition and weapons, and designated driver programs are tested interventions that can be implemented in all communities.

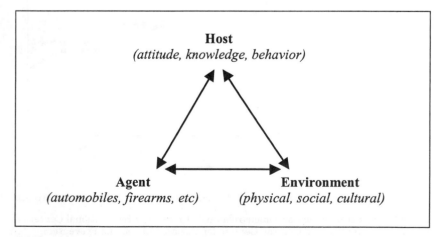

FIG. 52.2. Public health model

IV. Responsibilities of physicians. Prevention of injury is an important obligation, and physicians have two main roles: to spearhead trauma prevention at the community level and to incorporate patient-specific prevention in daily practice.

A. Educate the public that injuries are preventable, nonrandom events. Physicians are respected members of the community and can powerfully advocate for injury prevention. A vital first step is to overcome the traditional view of injury as an accident. It is not random and is rarely accidental. Removing the word "accident" from the vocabulary of all trauma personnel is a key action that helps debunk a dangerous myth and more appropriately places injury on a solid public health footing. Presenting unique profiles of individuals at risk for injury aids in identifying high risk groups and the factors that contribute to the injury.

B. Recruit colleagues and collaborate with key players. Effective prevention efforts require a multitude of skills that extend beyond those typically held by physicians. As leaders of the trauma center and leaders in prevention, physicians can magnify their effectiveness by joining together with other interested parties. For example, involving the hospital media relations department can be key in helping to establish contacts with local media and in framing the messages that need to be communicated. Making connections with community leaders and agency personnel will bring additional ideas, new contacts, and personnel with additional skills and resources to facilitate successful prevention efforts.

C. Identify priority injuries to tackle in the community. Defining the injury problem specific to the local community helps frame efforts and target resources to those injuries having the greatest impact on the local community. It is important to focus on a targeted at-risk population. A good first step is to use data that are retrievable from the Trauma Center's registry. This will provide information on the nature of injuries that reach the Trauma Center. These data can be supplemented by other sources of nonfatal and fatal injuries (e.g., statewide hospital discharge data, coroner or medical examiner, police, and emergency medical systems) to create a community-specific profile. Local data can then be placed in context by comparing them with state and national statistics. These registry data will highlight the injuries of importance to the community served by the Trauma Center. Injuries that should assume importance for prevention activities are those that occur frequently, those with the highest mortality, or those most likely to result in prolonged disability. Data that are specific to the local community are the most persuasive in generating interest and commitment from community leaders.

D. Disseminate injury information of importance to the community. The general public has an understanding of injury in their local community that is shaped by the media, be it local or national. Therefore, their understanding of injury can be skewed, often driven by the most recent high-profile case that has received intense media attention. These high profile cases, however, can be unusual and often do not adequately reflect the nature of the injury problem in a particular community. Further, the general public is constantly exposed to messages that highlight their risk for a variety of ailments, but have limited understanding or knowledge of how to weigh the importance of these various risks to their communities or their own lives. Trauma physicians are in a prime position to communicate the actual profile of injuries and to inform the public of the relative risk of various activities or behaviors.

Decide on the main public health messages to be targeted to the community and educate fellow professionals to be data-driven, passionate spokespeople. It is more effective to have consistent, clear, data-driven messages disseminated by many messengers than to have only one messenger.

E. Secure funding for and implement local projects. In today's healthcare environment, hospitals cannot independently fund or implement prevention activities aimed at the community. Establish an advisory board, composed of community leaders of influence and affluence, who can assist in obtaining modest funds to support community-based interventions.

Although most trauma centers cannot undertake major research agendas in injury prevention, they can utilize established prevention programs. Using established programs that have been tested elsewhere is efficient and can be effective in securing interest and funding from local leaders. Further, the best use of limited resources is to implement and adapt programs that have already been evaluated for effectiveness.

Optimal interventions are thoughtfully planned, specific, and systematically executed. Specificity can be achieved by focusing on a specific mechanism of injury, specific risk factor, a target population, or the mode of intervention. Choosing a specific prevention program is driven both by the data and by the interest and willingness of the community to support and participate. Together with colleagues, advisory board, and community partners, develop an implementation plan that will serve as a specific guide to what needs to be accomplished and who is responsible, and establish a timetable. This implementation plan should be driven by specific objectives, strategies for training personnel who are involved in the prevention efforts, and methods to monitor and adjust the implementation. Evaluation of effectiveness focuses on quality monitoring to ensure that the planned activities are being carried out and proceeding according to plan and outcome evaluation.

F. Help shape reasonable policy decisions. The most effective interventions are those that passively safeguard public health rather than those that require active behavioral change. These passive interventions are often legislated (e.g., road design, air bags, drunk driving laws). Policy makers frequently look to experts in the field to secure information and help shape policy. Thus, physicians can be approached to present testimony before policymaking bodies, giving them the opportunity to present relevant data combined with the human aspects of injury. Development of appropriate and reasonable policies is an important function that trauma centers can perform in the community.

Physicians can also take a more pro-active stance and spearhead efforts to enact legislation that is driven by their data. In this case, it is important to secure the support of one or several key legislators to sponsor the legislation. Establishing relationships with the legislative staff, providing information clearly and succinctly, and working with them to develop legislation is a possible role that physicians can assume. Data are convincing when packaged in such a way that they are understandable and present a fair and balanced portrait of the issue.

G. Work with industry to improve product design and safety. One strategy to reduce the burden of injury is to work directly with industry (either through influence or consultation) to create safer products. Obviously, not all physicians will assume this role. However, this can be an effective intervention to reduce injury. Working with firearm manufacturers to establish standards for load-chamber indicators or changing designs to reduce the ability to conceal a weapon are examples.

H. Incorporate injury prevention practices in daily practice. Physicians can incorporate injury prevention as a core part of daily clinical practice. Trauma patients can be especially receptive to one-on-one prevention counseling from healthcare providers during this time of crisis. A helpful first step is to document risk factors that potentially contributed to the injury episode. Break risk factors into host (e.g., presence of positive drug or alcohol screen, lack of seatbelt or helmet use, contributing comorbidity); agent (e.g., airbag deployment, type of firearm and safety devices); and environment (e.g., loose rugs, dangerous intersections). Documenting specific risk factors will guide potential interventions and lead to appropriate strategies to reduce future injuries. These strategies can include counseling, teaching, and referrals to abuse counselors.

I. Systematize routine screens to identify patients at risk. Physicians should put systematic routine screens in place to identify patients at risk for recidivism. Screens to capture the presence of interpersonal violence (domestic and child abuse); use of illegal drugs (biological screens); elderly falls (physical surroundings, comorbid conditions, medications); and abuse of alcohol (CAGE, biological screens) can help identify patients at high risk. For example, the CAGE screen is one that has proved effective in identifying patients with an alcohol problem. CAGE is a mnemonic of the following four items:
- Have you ever felt you should **C**ut down on your drinking?
- Have people **A**nnoyed you by criticizing your drinking?
- Have you ever felt bad or **G**uilty about your drinking?
- Have you ever had a drink first thing in the morning to steady your nerves or get rid of a hangover (**E**ye-opener)?

A positive reply to any of these questions suggests the need for intervention and a positive response to two or more of these questions should prompt a referral for alcohol treatment.

J. Reduce recidivism by referring patients at high risk to appropriate services. Linking patients identified as high risk with established community services, either through positive routine screens or as indicated by the circumstances surrounding the injury event, allows the routine initiation of appropriate interventions to lessen the potential for recidivism. Such interventions include but are not limited to:
- Individual counseling of at-risk patients (e.g., seatbelt and helmet use, safe firearm storage)
- Group counseling by capable professionals
- Referral to suitable in-hospital services (e.g., substance abuse, psychiatric follow-up)
- Linkages to community-based resources (e.g., domestic abuse hotlines and shelters)

V. Summary. Physicians perform a key role in the prevention of injury. The three core components to successful prevention efforts are:
- Knowledge
- Advocacy
- Research

Individual physicians can focus on one aspect of prevention with a focus that is either clinically oriented or research oriented. The clinically oriented physician who uses tested interventions in clinical practice is as pivotal to a well-rounded program as the research-based physician whose focus is largely in building knowledge about injury prevention. Prevention activities are a rewarding extension of the acute care trauma mission and hold promise of further reducing the magnitude of trauma morbidity and mortality.

Bibliography

Bonnie RJ, Fulco CE, Liverman CT, eds. *Reducing the burden of injury: advancing prevention and treatment*. Washington, DC: Institute of Medicine, National Academy Press, 1999.

Cherpitel CJ. Screening for alcohol problems in the emergency department. *Ann Emerg Med* 1995;26(2):158–166.

Committee on Trauma. *Resources for optimal care of the injured patient: 1999*. Chicago: American College of Surgeons, 1998.

Karlson TA, Hargarten SW. *Reducing firearm injury and death*. New Brunswick, NJ: Rutgers University Press, 1997.

Krug EG, Sharma GK, Lozano R. The global burden of injuries. *Am J Public Health* 2000;90(4):523–526.

Meyer M. Death and disability from injury: a global challenge. *J Trauma* 1998;44(1):1–12.

Murray C, Lopez AD. Alternative projections of mortality and disability by cause 1990–2020: global burden of disease study. *Lancet* 1997;349(9064):1498–1504.

Murray C, Lopez AD. Mortality by cause for eight regions of the world: global burden of disease study. *Lancet* 1997;349(9061):1269–1276.

National Center for Health Statistics. *Latest final mortality statistics available.* Available at: http://www.cdc.gov/nchs/releases/99facts/99sheets/97mortal.htm. Accessed January, 2000.

NCIPC (National Center for Injury Prevention and Control): *Ten leading causes of death, United States, 1997, all races, both sexes* Available at: http://www.cdc.gov/ncipc/osp/states/101c97.htm. Accessed January, 2000.

NCIPC (National Center for Injury Prevention and Control): *Years of potential life lost before age 65 (YPLL) by cause of death, U.S. 1995.* Available at: http://www.cdc.gov/ncipc/images/ypll95.gif. Accessed January, 2000.

Rivera FP, Britt J. *You can do it: a community guide to injury prevention.* Available at: http://www.aast.org/YouCan.html. Accessed August, 2000.

World Health Organization: *Injury: A leading cause of the global burden of disease.* Geneva: World Health Report, 1999.

53. HOUSE STAFF RESPONSIBILITIES

G. Paul Dabrowski and Patrick M. Reilly

The contributions of medical students, residents, and fellows to the delivery of optimal patient care at trauma centers cannot be overstated. They are relied on to remain in house for long hours to fulfill the often unappreciated duty of being the ones immediately available to care for trauma victims in their "golden hour" of need. For this, they are often armed with no more than a growing appreciation of general surgery and the fundamentals of the Advanced Trauma Life Support (ATLS) course. The following are some basic recommendations regarding their input to the service.

I. **General requirements.** House staff responsibilities on a trauma service generally fall under the two broad categories of **patient care** and **teaching**. Their responsibilities should increase with seniority. Students, residents, fellows, and staff are expected to be well groomed, punctual, and attentive to the needs of the patients and their families.

   A. **Attire.** Scrubs are highly recommended for the trauma team throughout the day. At any time, your presence may be required in the resuscitation area, OR, or critical care unit for an injured patient. Replace soiled scrubs and laboratory coats.

   B. **Documentation.** All care rendered to the patient must be documented in the medical record (Chapter 17). If it is not in the medical record, **it did not happen**. In most states, documentation by medical students is not adequate, either medically or legally. Likewise, no procedures, no matter how basic, should be performed by them without supervision. Their work must be corrected and cosigned by a licensed and responsible physician at a minimum, and a house staff addendum note is recommended. All chart entries should be dated and timed.

   C. **Conferences.** Most busy trauma services have a "morning report" or trauma team information meeting daily (see below). This conference is an outstanding forum to blend patient care specifics with house staff education. Attendance at this daily meeting, as well as at weekly and monthly surgery conferences, is usually mandatory.

II. **Inpatient units.** Admission to a specific inpatient trauma unit depends on the level of acuity of a patient's injury. Senior members of the trauma team are responsible for this decision. In all units, clear and concise communication is of critical importance to the appropriate care of patients. At admission or transfer to the unit, **team members need to discuss management plans with the nurses** and allied health professionals responsible, or others responsible for patient care. Written notes in the chart do not obviate this need.

   A. **Intensive care unit (ICU).** Critically ill trauma patients are admitted to the ICU. This unit generally handles the very sick and has the lowest patient-to-nurse ratio (i.e., maximal nursing hours per patient per day). Although most of the day-to-day patient care responsibilities can shift from the trauma team to the house staff assigned to the surgical critical care service, the patient ultimately remains the responsibility of the trauma service. To this end, the trauma residents, fellow, and staff should remain active and involved in the formulation of all management plans. Again, communication between the critical care service and the trauma service, which is crucial to ensure quality patient care, requires a daily face-to-face exchange of information, ideas, and opinions. Once a consensus care plan has been formulated, it is articulated to the nursing staff and others providing care to the patient.

   B. **Step-down unit**, an intermediate-care unit, is used most frequently to care for patients requiring neurologic, cardiac, or vascular monitoring. In addition, the patient-to-nurse ratio is usually lower than that on a general care floor but higher than in the ICU. As a result, nursing assessment and intervention can be performed more frequently than on the general care floor. The brain-injured, debilitated patient, a patient with extensive wound care needs, or a patient who is unable to care for self also can benefit from this increased level of care.

C. **General care unit.** Most trauma patients can be safely cared for on a general trauma care unit. Staff should be familiar with chest tubes, tracheostomies, and other devices commonly used in the trauma patient. Because of a higher patient-to-nurse ratio, nursing assessment is done less frequently. The junior house staff should be a constant presence on this unit.

III. **Daily routine.** Conferences can necessitate some flexibility in the daily routine, but most days should follow a schedule such as the following:

A. **Morning rounds** are to be completed on all patients before morning report (see below). All notes should be written, problems identified, and discharges either planned or executed. Routine orders for the day should be written at this time and management plans formulated. If not already completed, all new patients admitted during the previous 24 hours should have a repeat history and physical examination (tertiary survey) during morning rounds to identify injuries missed during the initial assessment. Any x-ray studies or tests indicated by the tertiary examination should be ordered.

B. **Morning report** is a formal daily session where all new patients encountered during the previous 24 hours is encouraged. Attendance is mandatory. Each patient is presented by the admitting resident or senior resident responsible for his or her care in the resuscitation area. Pertinent x-ray films should be available. Digital camera images may be useful. A list of radiographic or laboratory studies to be reviewed or ordered is summarized. A problem-oriented list of the trauma team's patients that includes all diagnoses, comorbid conditions, medications, complications, consultants, and therapies is helpful and can be generated at this time. In addition to new patients, issues such as planned operations, diagnostic test results, and evolving complications on in-house patients are discussed.

C. **Staff rounds.** Faculty teaching rounds with the trauma service generally follow morning report. Patients are presented to and reexamined with the staff surgeon. Their care is discussed, teaching points made, and care plans endorsed or reformulated.

D. **General care unit work.** Throughout the day, radiograph and laboratory results are obtained, and patient care is altered, as appropriate. Minor procedures are performed (and documented) as needed, always with senior supervision. Three major aspects of floor work merit mention.

1. **Coordination with other services.** Most trauma patients are seen by more than one service. The trauma service is responsible for the coordination of the patient's care. **Daily** communication with consulting services (e.g., orthopedics, critical care, rehabilitation medicine) is necessary to facilitate care. If a problem in communication occurs or any confusion arises, the fellow or staff surgeon should be notified immediately so that the situation may be remedied at the appropriate level.

2. **Transfers.** When appropriate and approved by the staff surgeon, patients can be transferred from the trauma service to another service. This is especially common with blunt-injured patients with multiple fractures who are then transferred to the orthopedic service for continued care of their injuries. All patients should remain on the trauma census and be seen daily by the trauma service until the staff surgeon formally signs off. To facilitate communication and good overall care, it may be necessary to keep multiply injured patients on the trauma service purely to coordinate care among numerous consultants. When transferring a patient to another service, a transfer note summarizing all pertinent information about the care rendered to date is invaluable to the accepting team. In addition, arrange follow-up with the trauma staff.

3. Discharge. Planning for eventual discharge, whether to home or to another facility (e.g., rehabilitation hospital, nursing home), should begin on admission. Case managers, social workers, and other allied health personnel are invaluable in assisting in patient disposition.

    a. Discharge instructions. The process of discharge is a critical event for the patient and family. Discharge instructions need to be both oral and written. Questions must be solicited to ensure a proper understanding by the patient.

    b. Return visits. Appropriate phone numbers and scheduled return visits should be listed for the patient and family. Make sure plans are made for follow-up for all consultants, if necessary.

    c. Prescriptions should be supplied for all medications needed after discharge. Make sure that an adequate amount of pain medication is prescribed and that the patient and family understand the drug being prescribed and how to use it.

    d. Emergencies. Besides routine follow-up with all treating physicians, give the patient a means to contact or reenter the Trauma Center should an urgent or emergent problem arise in the convalescent period.

E. Office visit. Patient follow-up is essential. Continuity of care outside the hospital setting is an important aspect of medical education. In addition, documentation of outpatient care is a requirement of the residency review committee on surgery.

F. Trauma team pages and consults. Although the arrival of a new patient can disrupt the daily routine, the prompt response of the trauma team to the resuscitation area is imperative. The specific roles of the trauma team during evaluation and resuscitation are described in detail in Chapter 13.

G. Operating room assignments for both elective and emergency surgery are made by the fellow or chief resident in conjunction with the staff surgeon.

H. Sign out. New laboratory and radiographic findings and other significant issues should be reviewed with the on-call team each evening. Potential problems should be identified and discussed and management plans formulated.

I. Evening rounds. Each evening, the on-call team should walk through each unit to see select patients, identify those ready for morning discharge, and identify and rectify new problems.

IV. Medical students are welcomed on the trauma service. Their priority, however, remains their general medical education. To this end, all educational conferences and didactic sessions should be attended by students, despite the lure of incoming emergencies and the intensity of the Trauma Center.

A. Patient care. Medical students should be allowed to take an active part in patient care. History and physical examinations and progress notes on rounds should be a requirement and proactively supervised by house staff and staff surgeons. Presentations during attending rounds are encouraged. Data acquisition during work rounds is done at the direction of more senior house staff. In addition, medical students are encouraged to attend trauma resuscitations and assist in operative cases. No matter how basic, patient care rendered by medical students must be supervised. Documentation in the medical record needs to reflect this supervision.

B. Education. Medical students should be familiar with ATLS principles and supplied a manual, if available. In addition, it is recommended that they become familiar with the "trauma" section of one of the major surgical textbooks.

V. PGY I. First-year residents provide most of the direct patient care on the general care unit. Patients often remember the care rendered on the general care unit, as well as the discharge process, more than any other part of the hospitalization. As a result, the junior residents often leave the greatest impression on the patient.

A. Patient care. Interns are expected to have morning rounds completed before morning report. Concise, yet comprehensive, documentation of patient care activities, including histories and physical examinations, daily progress notes, and discharge summaries, is a vital part of good patient care on a busy service. Medical student chart entries are not a substitute for house staff notes and, at a minimum, should be amended and cosigned by a resident. First-year residents play a role in trauma resuscitations and operative cases, contingent on their ability to complete assigned general care unit tasks in a timely and efficient manner.

    B. Education. First-year residents should be certified in ATLS. In addition, they should familiarize themselves with general trauma principles as described in most major surgery textbooks.

VI. PGY II/III. Junior residents function largely in the emergency department and the ICU of the Trauma Center.

    A. Patient care. As part of the trauma service, junior residents assist with rounds each morning. Throughout the day, their major function centers around the evaluation and resuscitation of incoming patients and the care of patients in the ICU. They play an active role as an important member of the trauma team and may function as trauma team leader. They are also responsible for all consults in the emergency department and on the floor. These should be discussed with their senior resident, fellow, or staff, and management plans formulated. Junior residents should also be actively involved in operative cases when intermediate-level procedures are performed.

    B. Education. Junior residents should be ATLS certified. Their knowledge base should be expanding beyond the basics to include the initial management and operative care of complex trauma patients. Trauma texts should be used to supplement general surgery texts. Whenever the opportunity presents itself, especially during on-call time, the junior resident is expected to assist in the teaching of medical students and PGYI.

VII. PGY IV/V. Leadership is the hallmark of the successful resident at the senior level on the trauma service. Good communication is essential to ensure continuity and excellence in patient care. The senior resident is expected to ensure this both within the team and with the consulting services.

    A. Patient care. The senior residents are responsible for all patients on the trauma service. They oversee morning rounds, are responsible for the formulation and implementation of management plans on all patients, and are actively involved with the decision making in the OR. They respond to all trauma resuscitations and function as team leader. They review all consults with the junior resident and are responsible for communication with the attending staff regarding admissions and discharges from the emergency department. Finally, they are responsible for assigning appropriate resident coverage for all elective and emergency operative cases. The senior resident should become comfortable with the operative care of the acutely injured patient as part of his or her rotation on the trauma service.

        1. Coordination with consulting services. One of the most important functions of the senior resident is as a liaison between the trauma service and the multiple consultative services involved in the care of the multiply injured trauma patient. Again, communication is key to excellent patient care.

    B. Education. Senior residents should be ATLS certified. Their reading should center on the care of the complex trauma patient, including options and techniques employed in the OR. To this end, trauma textbooks are liberally used to enhance general surgery texts. Senior residents are also responsible for the ongoing education of medical students and junior residents on the trauma service. Part of this responsibility involves active participation in all teaching and quality improvement conferences. In addition, each senior resident will ideally become involved in a clinical research project while on the trauma service.

VIII. Fellows. If the Trauma Center has fellows, they have both clinical and administrative roles on the trauma service. In addition, they are a valuable educational resource for all levels of house staff. Each institution has its own unique responsibilities for fellows that vary widely from purely research to purely clinical responsibilities at a junior staff level. For the most part, any trauma center administrative duties required of the faculty should involve the fellow as well.

IX. **Staff.** Appropriately trained trauma surgeons, board-certified or eligible in general surgery and ATLS certified, should make up the staff trauma faculty. They should always be available to deliver and supervise the care of every trauma patient.

  A. **Call.** Attending staff surgeons must be available promptly when notified of incoming, severely injured patients. With advanced notification, it is ideal for the trauma surgeon to be present on arrival of the patient to the trauma resuscitation area to help the senior resident or fellow guide the resuscitation.

  B. **Rounds.** The staff surgeon on call runs the morning report and attending rounds. These sessions should be as educational as possible and tailored to meet the needs of all present.

  C. **Conferences.** All staff should attend morning report, if possible, but especially those with call responsibilities. The staff surgeon must be intimately familiar with all patients and their medical and psychosocial problems and oversee all care delivered. In addition, he or she must have a firm grasp of each house officer's capabilities.

Axioms

- Excellent patient care is the most important responsibility of all members of the trauma team.
- Medical student and resident education should encompass all aspects of trauma care.
- Clear communication between members of the trauma team is essential to ensure excellent patient care.
- Coordination with consultative services is key to organized patient care.
- Physical and occupational therapy and rehabilitation medicine should be involved in patient care as soon as the patient is medically stable.
- Discharge planning begins on admission with the help of case managers and other allied health personnel.
- The process of discharge and discharge planning are perhaps the most important parts of the hospital stay for the patient and family.
- Work not documented is work not done.
- Do not abandon patients transferred to another service. They should continue to be followed by the trauma team until those on the attending staff formally sign off the case.

54. LEGAL, ETHICAL, AND FAMILY ISSUES

G. Paul Dabrowski and Harry L. Anderson, III

Although laws governing medical issues pertinent to the care of injured patients differ in scope or interpretation depending on political region and are expected to change over time, their basic underlying intent does not. Physicians are expected to work within the law to deliver ethical medical care to these patients. Guided by such broad principles as "first, do no harm," physicians can occasionally find their treatment plans at odds with individual patient's rights, such as a Jehovah's Witness refusal of blood transfusion after life threatening hemorrhage. Understanding the basis of these conflicts and the resources available to assist healthcare workers in their resolution is imperative to delivering appropriate and legally defensible care in these often emergency situations. This chapter highlights several legal and ethical issues regarding the care of injured patients and suggests helpful resources for when questions arise.

I. Legal issues
   A. Informed consent. The acute nature of trauma often forces physicians into situations in which time to contemplate treatment options is not available. Moreover, head injuries, intoxicants, and shock can further impair effective communication with the patient. These factors do not absolve providers from the need to supply informed consent, discuss treatment options, and consider the wishes of patients with regard to their care.

   Documentation of the informed consent process before surgical procedures is vitally important, regardless of the patients' mental status. Always enter the following information in the chart preoperatively: (*a*) date and time of any discussion; (*b*) participants and their relationship to the patient; (*c*) how or where the discussion took place (e.g., if via telephone, identify the phone number called); (*d*) the nature of the injury requiring the procedure; (*e*) the intended procedure (identity and location of the operative site, if possible); and (*f*) any unanticipated yet commonly related procedures (e.g., colostomy). This information, with the signed consent form, is more than mere legal justification of the proposed treatment. It documents the surgeon's thought processes, records patient and family contacts for future reference, and assists subsequent healthcare providers involved in the patient's care understand the initial care.

   1. **The intoxicated patient**. The patient's use of alcohol or drugs does not automatically signify mental incompetence, even if blood alcohol level exceeds the legal standard for intoxication. Although intoxicated, if a patient is (*a*) capable of making a decision, (*b*) demonstrates awareness of the consequences of choice, and (*c*) the decision does not substantially affect others to whom the patient is responsible, these wishes should be respected. For situations in which a patient adamantly refuses treatment but the above conditions are not met, the surgeon should contact family members, if possible, and consider consulting the hospital's legal representative.

   Furthermore, intoxicated patients can prove to be a risk to themselves or others they encounter, including healthcare personnel. Although it is important to recognize the impaired status, the treatment of their medical condition is always the first priority; the circumstances surrounding the nature of the impairment can be dealt with later. If restraints, either physical or pharmacologic, are required, the medical record should reflect why they were needed. This is particularly important because the detention or treatment of competent patients against their will constitutes assault and battery.

   2. **Surrogate decision-makers**. If an injured patient is unable to participate in decision making because incompetent, unconscious, or another

impediment, a surrogate decision-maker or legal representative must be sought. A legal spouse (currently married and living with the patient) is usually the primary legal representative of an adult patient. Other suitable surrogates might include the patient's parent, sibling, or child. Either a parent or designated legal guardian is a minor's legal representative. If no representative is found and time permits, the court can appoint a temporary guardian.

When life-threatening emergencies exist, appropriate stabilization and care of the patient takes precedence, regardless of the inability to obtain consent. Unconscious or incompetent adult patients, as well as minors who require emergency care but lack parental or legal guardianship, should be treated in a fashion consistent with that which a reasonable person would request.

When the wishes of a patient's family members conflict or a surrogate decision-maker requests treatment that might be considered at odds with the patient's best interest, the physician should consider seeking in-house legal counsel. Such legal issues are complex. A competent adult is within his or her right to refuse any treatment, even though the treatment constitutes the appropriate standard of care, and refusal is likely to result in the patient's death.

   a. Advanced directives. Many adults, wishing not to burden their families with the need to make treatment decisions should they become incapacitated, make their wishes known in the form of advanced directives. Advanced directives are legal and binding documents prepared in anticipation of situations where the patient is incapacitated. They can speak for the patient when the patient cannot. These documents generally express the patient's wishes with regard to limits of medical care to be administered (e.g., cardiopulmonary resuscitation [CPR], endotracheal intubation, feeding tubes, long-term ventilatory care). These directives should be sought, reviewed with the family, and followed explicitly.

B. **Transfers.** A portion of the Consolidated Omnibus Budget Reconciliation Act (COBRA) passed by Congress in 1985 includes legislation to discourage "dumping" of poorly insured or nonpaying patients from private hospitals to public or county medical centers solely because of their inability to pay. Under COBRA, the transferring facility must first provide appropriate care, within its capacity, to minimize health risks to the patient. The receiving hospital must agree to accept the patient and have space and personnel available to care for the patient. Finally, the patient, and all relevant medical records from the transferring facility, must be transported with qualified personnel and equipment. The reasons for transfer from one facility to another should be clearly stated in the medical record. Whenever possible, the referring and receiving physicians should communicate directly to optimize the receiving physician's understanding of the patient's condition and the care provided thus far.

C. **Brain death.** Determination of brain death is usually a complicated algorithm defined by hospital policy or state regulation (Chapter 45). Practitioners should be familiar with the applicable directives in their states or communities. Death, by definition, entails (a) irreversible cessation of function of the entire brain, or (b) irreversible cessation of circulatory and respiratory function. Determination of death by neurologic criteria usually involves consultation by a neurologist or neurosurgeon, with documentation of the absence of brain activity by clinical examination with or without diagnostic confirmation (e.g., absence of blood flow to the brain determined by nuclear medicine scan or cerebral arteriography).

   Determination of brain death is a medical responsibility; it does not require consent by the patient's family. As state laws vary to how and who can declare brain death, trauma centers should draft policies for this process in accordance with the state's statutes. The family should nonetheless be informed and communication maintained throughout the process of determining brain death. Some jurisdictions mandate notification of organ procurement agencies (the state of Pennsylvania requires such action). As "brain death" is synonymous with "death," once it has been established, the patient can be taken off life support without the family's consent.

D. Risk management. The hospital's risk management or legal affairs department is the physician's ally. The expert assistance of the hospital's on-call attorney is particularly welcome when risk of legal action against the hospital (and, consequently, against all healthcare personnel involved in the care of the patient) is perceived. The earlier risk management or legal affairs is notified, the more effective their response can be.

The legal department should be alerted to events such as, but not limited to:

   1. Untoward event in the emergency department, operating room, or patient care area (e.g., medication error, missed diagnosis).
   2. Angry or hostile family, particularly when a verbal threat of legal action is expressed.
   3. Unexpected poor outcomes or complicated hospital course.

II. Ethical issues

A. A myriad of ethical dilemmas arise in the care of the trauma patient. Although common themes exist, each situation presents its own particular variation that needs to be individualized. Situations common after injury include:

   1. Death and dying
   2. Futile care and when to stop care
   3. Care of the uninsured
   4. Quality-of-life
   5. Conflicts between family members or between family and care providers
   6. Issues regarding differences based on nationality or religion

B. Identifying ethical issues. Ethical issues with healthcare personnel and the patient need to be identified early in the patient's course, because all disciplines (e.g., medical, nursing, rehabilitation) have a role in resolving the problem. These issues should be discussed in a closed but multidisciplinary fashion. Once the healthcare team has identified, discussed, and developed a plan, it is necessary to meet with the key family members (or patient) to involve them in the resolution, modify the plan if needed, and answer questions to further enhance communication.

Many hospitals have an ethics committee to assist in resolving these issues. This committee most often is multidisciplinary and composed of individuals not directly involved in the patient's care. Representation from medicine, nursing, social work, pastoral care, hospital administration, and the lay community is recommended. An ethics consult can be initiated by any care provider or even a family member. Some consults can be handled by telephone call, whereas others require the group to assemble, review the chart, examine the patient, and interview key healthcare personnel or family members. The recommendation of the ethics committee is not binding on any party but is designed to be a thoughtful unbiased recommendation by a group familiar with such complex ethical issues. The recommendation can be given to individuals of the healthcare team, the family, or a combination of both in an abbreviated meeting, which also permits questions from all parties involved.

III. Family issues

A. Approaching the family. Family members need to be informed at the first possible opportunity, either by telephone or in person, once a patient arrives in the emergency department after injury. The initial contact is best made by the key physician caring for the patient (attending, trauma fellow, or senior resident) but can be handled by any designated individual who communicates well with families. The communicator must be familiar with the patient's injuries, definitive care plan, and probable outcome. Representatives of the pastoral care service or social service act as an excellent resource to the trauma team in making initial contact with the family of the injured patient, and then coordinating the most important contact with family—the initial meeting.

This meeting is best done in a quiet, comfortable, private space, near but not within the primary treatment area (e.g., an adjoining waiting or consultation room near the emergency department, intensive care unit, or operating room waiting area). Ideally, the initial communicator, if not the trauma team leader, can arrange and attend this meeting and afterward continue to coordinate and direct communication and services for the family. Important information includes:

1. Initiate with a simple overall statement in plain nonmedical terms that gently sets the tone to relieve anxiety (e.g., "Your son was in a car crash and arrived here safely. He is awake and talking to me." Or, "Your grandfather fell down his stairs at home. His heart rate and blood pressure are okay, but he's currently in a coma and not talking to me.").

2. Outline the nature of the injuries, what has been done thus far, and predict the probable course.

3. Delineate the key services involved (e.g., neurosurgery, orthopedics.).

4. Explain the reasoning for the patient's sedation, pharmacologic paralysis, or mechanical ventilation. If necessary, explain indications for any emergency procedures such as chest tubes, peritoneal lavage, or operation.

5. Assure that pain is being relieved.

6. Ask for questions from the family members.

B. The surgeon should communicate all "significant" events (e.g., instability in vital signs, cardiopulmonary arrest, need for additional emergent operative intervention). Lastly, the next likely encounter should be tentatively set (e.g., "I'll see you in the intensive care unit [ICU] waiting area after the computed tomography [CT] scan, or after we finish the operation"). Ensure that the family knows where the meeting will be held and how to contact you if and when questions arise. Again, support persons from pastoral care or social services can help orient the family to the hospital and its services.

Daily encounters (during rounds or preferably after rounds) should be anticipated, encouraged, and utilized to convey information, answer questions, and so on. These encounters should be short, frequent, and limited to a few key family members. For the patient whose stay is prolonged, beyond 2 or 3 weeks, or whose stay has been complicated, it is sometimes useful to have a formal family meeting involving key players from the surgical team, consultants, nursing, social work, rehabilitation, and so forth. These longer meetings are useful to bring the family up to date on current care and the planned or expected course. Always document a family encounter in the medical record, regardless of how brief, with names of everyone involved and content of the conversation.

C. **Delivering bad news**. Inevitably, occasions arise when "unpleasant" information (e.g., complications, iatrogenic problems, mishaps, or even death) needs to be relayed to family members, which should be delivered by the attending surgeon. The family members should be assembled away from the patient care area, and the surgeon should have one or two team members (e.g., nurse, chaplain) in attendance. Use an approach displaying empathy (understanding of the family's feelings), using clear language (e.g., "died," not "passed"), and with a willingness to answer questions afterward.

D. **Information adjuncts** (e.g., brochures about the hospital, the Trauma Center, or community resources along with business cards listing provider names and office phone numbers) are of particular utility to the patient and family members. If physician assistants, clinical practitioners, or service-based case managers are part of the team, they should be included as well. Brief booklets explaining trauma care, with basic definitions of therapies and possible complications, are helpful to families.

Axioms
- Communicate effectively and repetitively with the patient and family to understand their needs.
- Keep the family informed on at least an every-other-day basis.
- Communicate major events to the family, no matter when they occur.
- Clear, consistent, and complete documentation in the progress note is part of appropriate medical care.
- Make a plan for care that takes into consideration both the patient's medical and psychological needs.
- When in doubt whether to treat or not, it is better to treat in accord with the standard of care and sort out medical, legal, or ethical issues later.
- Utilize and involve all hospital resources, especially risk management and legal affairs, early to gain their expertise in the management of difficult medicolegal questions.

Bibliography
Hospital of the University of Pennsylvania. *Policy regarding determination of death by neurologic criteria*. Philadelphia, 1994.
Jurkovich GJ, Pierce B, Pananen L, Rivara FP. Giving bad news: the family perspective. *J Trauma* 2000;48:865–873.
Nisonson I. Update your record-keeping skills: informed consent and refusal. *Bulletin of the American College of Surgeons* 2000;85:18–20.
Peitzman AB, Arnold SA, Boone DC. *University of Pittsburgh Medical Center trauma manual*. Pittsburgh: University of Pittsburgh Medical Center, 1994.
Razek T, Olthoff K, Reilly PM. Issues in potential organ donor management. *Surg Clin North Am* 2000;80:1021–1032.
Sullivan DJ, Hansen-Flaschen J. Termination of life support after major trauma. *Surg Clin North Am* 2000;80:1055–1066.
Weigell CJ II. Medicolegal issues. In: Mattox KL, Feliciano DV, Moore EE, eds. *Trauma*, 4th ed. New York: McGraw-Hill, 2000:1463–1472.

55. MISCELLANEOUS PROCEDURES

Glenn Tinkoff and Michael Rhodes

I. **Urinary catheter**
  A. **Indications**
    1. Patient not following commands
    2. Hemodynamic instability
    3. Obvious indication for operative intervention (i.e., distended abdomen, open fractures)
    4. External signs of major torso trauma
    5. Spinal fractures
  B. **Contraindications**
    1. Stable patient with minimal evidence of trauma
    2. High suspicion of urethral injury in the male
      a. Blood in urethral meatus
      b. Massive scrotal ecchymosis
      c. Boggy prostrate on rectal examination
  C. **Insertion of the urinary catheter in a male patient**
    1. Prepare the head of penis.
    2. Stretch the penis gently and extend upward. Hold the penis with the nondominant hand.
    3. Adequately lubricate urinary catheter (the practice of squirting lubricant into the meatus is not recommended).
    4. Hold the catheter close to the meatus and with the dominant hand, gently insert the catheter with short, frequent 1-cm advances with fingers close to the meatus.
    5. Resistance met at the posterior urethral sphincter can be overcome by stopping the advancement temporarily and applying gentle, forward pressure on the catheter until the sphincter relaxes, which can take several seconds.
    6. Continue with short, frequent, gentle advances of the catheter until urine is obtained. (In a male patient, insert the catheter as far as possible to avoid inflation of the balloon in the urethra). Inflate the balloon, then slightly withdraw the catheter until gently tethered by the balloon. Discard the initial 5 mL of urine and test the second 5 mL for blood with a dipstick. Formal urinalysis is unnecessary in the male (Chapter 31).
    7. With blood in the urethra or a suspected torn urethra, a Foley catheter can be gently inserted through which a urethrogram can be performed (Chapter 31). The urology resident, attending physician, or most experienced team member, if necessary, can advance the catheter to stent the urethra, which can spontaneously pass into the bladder. Avoid forcing passage of the urinary catheter in this setting, as an incomplete urethral tear can be converted to a complete urethral tear.
  D. **Insertion of the urinary catheter in a female patient**
    1. The anatomic position of the female urethra is variable and can be difficult to visualize.
    2. This should be a two-person procedure.
    3. With adequate lighting, prepare the urethra with antiseptic. Have an assistant spread the labial folds with the patient in a frogleg position, when possible.
    4. Place the catheter gently and inflate the balloon return of urine.
    5. Urethral rupture is unusual.
  E. **Pediatric**
    1. Use an appropriately sized catheter for the toddler or infant male (Chapter 47).

        2. Spontaneous voiding around the catheter during insertion is common. Urethral rupture is uncommon. In the infant, a small polyethylene feeding tube can be used, which is then taped in place.

        3. Gentleness is essential.

II. Nasogastric tube

A. Indications

    1. Patient not following commands

    2. Obvious need for operative intervention

    3. Hemodynamic instability

    4. Endotracheally intubated patient

    5. Any child with a distended abdomen

B. Contraindications

    1. Massive mid-face fractures or basilar skull fracture, for which an orogastric route is a reasonable alternative.

C. Technique

    1. Be gentle and explain the procedure to the patient.

    2. Placing the tube on ice allows pre-forming the tube into a gentle curve.

    3. Judicious anesthetic spray into the nose and throat are helpful.

    4. The tube should be well-lubricated.

    5. Place tube gently into nostril, aiming and directing it inferiorly and slowly until it is in the back of the throat. Push in 1- or 2-cm segments with hands and fingers next to the nostril.

    6. Never push in long segments.

    7. Do not advance tube while the patient is talking or actively inhaling. If the patient can cooperate to swallow, push gently as the patient is swallowing. If the patient will not cooperate and is talking, spitting, or not cooperating, wait until the patient stops talking and swallows spontaneously. This can be viewed by carefully observing the patient and with precise timing gently advance the tube as the patient takes a mandatory swallow. The tube can be introduced. Gagging is common, but if the patient loses voice or becomes hoarse or has violent coughing, withdraw the tube slightly to the back of the throat. It is likely that the tube is in the trachea.

    8. After the tube is advanced, auscultation over the stomach is an important step. This should be followed by irrigation of the tube with a plastic Tomey syringe to remove particulate matter. All too frequently, a nasogastric tube is inserted, slightly irrigated, and placed on suction. This can fail to empty the stomach, which could create problems later in computed tomography (CT) scan or surgery. For acute resuscitation, the largest nasogastric tube that will fit is optimal for evacuating the stomach. This is usually a size 18 F for an adult.

III. Chest tube thoracostomy (Chapters 26a, 26b)

  A. Fifth intercostal space to avoid intraabdominal placement

  B. Anterior axillary line to avoid dissecting through muscle

  C. Insert the chest tube without the use of a trocar.

  D. In the conscious patient, use adequate anesthesia with particular attention to anesthetizing the pleura.

  E. Digitally palpate before tube placement to identify the structures and possibly a diaphragmatic rupture on the left side.

  F. Precise placement, aiming posteriorly and cephalad

  G. After placement, rotate the tube 360° to relieve kinks.

  H. Do not place dressing over chest site if patient needs immediate surgery.

IV. Needle decompression of thorax (Chapter 7)

  A. Second intercostal space, mid-clavicular line; or fourth or fifth intercostal space, anterior axillary line. Use a 14-gauge angiocatheter.

  B. Temporary, should be followed by chest tube

V. Traction splint

  A. Minimum, two-person procedure

  B. Prepare the splint before application (i.e., length and straps).

C. Use intravenous (i.v.) analgesia in the awake patient.
D. Assess the distal pulses before applying the splint.
E. Using at least two persons, apply gentle manual traction via the foot strap while raising the leg, followed by rapid and precise positioning of the splint into position. This requires a coordinated and focused effort by the team to avoid unnecessary pain to the patient.
F. The proximal covered rim of the splint should rest against the ischial tuberosity.
G. Then gently and slowly apply traction to the foot strap after affixing the traction hook to the foot strap sling.
H. Leg straps are meant to secure the leg from falling off of the splint; they are not to be tight.
I. Reassess distal pulses after the splint is applied.

VI. **Skeletal traction pin**
   A. Traction pin for temporary use, place tibial pin 1 cm distal to anterior tibial tubercle.
   B. For more prolonged traction (i.e., >1 week) place at distal femur.
   C. Technique for tibial pin placement
      1. Align leg so that one can visualize a straight line from the great toe, through the patella to the anterior iliac spine while standing at the foot of the bed.
      2. Place a pillow or blankets under the lower leg to elevate it from the bed, which allows the drill handle to turn without striking the bed.
      3. Prepare and drape the knee and proximal tibia.
      4. Place local anesthesia on the lateral and medial skin and subcutaneous tissue 1 inch distal to the anterior tibial tubercle and ~1 inch posteriorly from the anterior tibia.
      5. A threaded pin is used for a more permanent placement (e.g., femur). For the tibia, use a nonthreaded Steinman pin or Kirschner wire, which should be affixed to the hand drill using a chuck key.
      6. Most surgeons proceed from lateral to medial, staying parallel to the ground. Make a small skin incision medially and then engage the pin against the bone and drill through both cornices. The pin can then be seen pushing against the medial skin, which is incised with the scalpel. The pin should extend beyond the skin ~1 to 2 inches. A pin cutter is necessary to cut the pin length. The pin edges are usually capped with corks or rubber stoppers to avoid puncture injury to the caregivers.
      7. Then place the pin in either the Steinman or Kirschner bow and attach to the appropriated traction. Dress the pin sites with povidone-iodine and a 2×2 gauze.
      8. The most frequent error in placement is failure to get enough purchase on the bone (i.e., not posterior enough from the anterior tibial edge).

VII. **Bedside tracheostomy**
   A. **Indications**
      1. Airway protection
      2. Pulmonary toilet
      3. Prolonged ventilatory support
      4. Decontamination of oropharynx
      5. Extensive orofacial trauma
   B. **Technical points**
      1. Plan and time a bedside tracheostomy for periods of optimal staffing. Have a checklist of supplies and procedure steps available and review it before the procedure.
      2. Bedside tracheostomy can be done by the open or percutaneous dilational technique.
      3. The patient should intubated, except for emergency conditions.
      4. Have resources for conscious sedation available, including continuous blood pressure, electrocardiography (ECG), and pulse oximetry monitoring.

5. Position the patient to extend the neck, if possible.
6. A person skilled at endotracheal intubation should be positioned at the head of the bed to control the endotracheal tube and reintubate, if necessary.
7. Have an instrument tray allowing for open tracheostomy available, even when using a percutaneous technique.
8. Have surgical lighting available over the patient's neck area. A portable headlight can be helpful.
9. The tracheostomy tube should be opened, tested, and prepared for insertion before beginning the procedure.
10. Bedside tracheostomy is a surgical procedure and the team should wear gown, gloves, cap, mask, and eye protection. The patient should be fully draped. Place equipment on tables, not directly on the bed.
11. Both the open and percutaneous technique should be considered a two-person technique. Have a scrubbed assistant available at the bedside.
12. The bedside nurse should direct full attention to this procedure during its performance.
13. The anterior neck skin is prepared, draped, and usually anesthetized with local anesthesia.
14. Some prefer to use bronchoscopic guidance in performing the percutaneous technique.
15. Have extra tracheostomy tubes, endotracheal tubes, and tracheostomy tray immediately available.
16. A detailed description of both open and percutaneous tracheostomy is beyond the scope of this manual.
17. If a percutaneous endoscopic gastrostomy (PEG) is planned at the same time, it is usually preferable to follow the tracheostomy because the endotracheal tube will have been removed, facilitating endoscopy.

C. **Complications**
1. The most serious complication is **loss of the airway** during the procedure.
   a. Hypoxia and bradycardia
   b. If uncertain about position of the endotracheal tube or tracheostomy tube → reintubate
2. Other complications
   a. Tube misplacement (e.g., pretracheal)
   b. Tracheal laceration
   c. Tube dislodgment
   d. Bleeding
   e. Pneumothorax
   f. Tracheal stenosis

VIII. **Percutaneous endoscopic gastrostomy**
A. The **primary indication** for a PEG in a trauma patient is to provide **long-term** gastric access for either decompression or feeding. In general, if a patient is not expected to survive >30 days or will likely be eating within 30 days, a PEG may not be indicated.
B. Technical points
1. Have the resources to provide and monitor conscious sedation available.
2. If a PEG is to be combined with a tracheostomy, the PEG should be the second procedure.
3. Review a checklist for the proper equipment before starting.
4. In general, plan the procedure at periods of optimal staffing to include the use of gastrointestinal endoscopy nurses, when practical.
5. A remote monitor, in addition to the scope, facilitates coordination of the team performing the procedure.
6. A PEG is generally a two-person procedure, in addition to the person monitoring the conscious sedation.

7. Inspect the esophagus, stomach, and duodenum before beginning placement of the PEG tube.

8. Gastric insufflation, transabdominal illumination, and endoscopic visualization of finger depression of the abdominal wall are essential for proper placement.

9. The detailed technique of the procedure is dependent on the type of PEG tube and is beyond the scope of this manual.

10. Most endoscopists do not routinely reintroduce the endoscope to inspect the stomach after placement.

11. Feeding can usually be started immediately.

C. **Complications**

1. Mild to moderate pneumoperitoneum is common.

2. A mild cellulitis can occur around the tube site. Warm soaks and adjusting the tension on the tube fastener are usually all that is required. Occasionally, a short course (three doses) of a first-generation cephalosporin is helpful.

3. Rarely, tube erosion through the stomach and dislodgment can occur, requiring laparotomy.

IX. **Naso-, orogastric, or jejunal feeding tube**

A. **Indication**

1. A trauma patient requiring nutritional support (Chapter 44); the enteral route is preferred, if feasible.

2. The anticipated length of support is <30 days (PEG or surgical gastrojejunal tube recommended for support extending >30 days).

3. Attain postpyloric access (at or beyond ligament of Treitz) in patients with high risk of aspiration (i.e., head-injured, pharmacologically sedated, diabetic gastroparesis).

4. Postpyloric access has been achieved more frequently with unweighted feeding tubes and the use of metoclopramide (Reglan, AH Robins, Richmond, VA).

B. **Technique for postpyloric insertion of unweighted feeding tube**

1. Equipment
   a. 8,10, or 12F nasoenteric feeding tube (length >100 cm) with Y adapter and stylet
   b. Metoclopramide 10 mg i.v. (adults) or 0.1 mg/kg i.v. (pediatric)
   c. A 60-mL Luer tip syringe
   d. Stethoscope
   e. Examination gloves
   f. Taping materials for securing tube

2. Administer metoclopramide i.v. over 1 to 2 minutes ~10 minutes before tube insertion.

3. Elevate head of bed at least 30°, if possible.

4. With side port of feeding tube closed and stylet in place, flush 5 mL of sterile water through the tube to check for patency or leaks and facilitate stylet withdrawal.

5. Lubricate tip and body of tube.

6. See section II.C, steps 1 through 7 for naso- and orogastric insertion.

7. Once the tube is confirmed in intragastric position, roll the patient to the right lateral decubitus position, if possible.

8. With the stylet still in place, insufflate the stomach with 500 to 1,000 mL of air as rapidly as possible, using the 60-mL regular tip syringe.

9. Advance the feeding tube to a point such that only 10 cm of tubing remains externally.

10. Return the patient to the supine position with stylet in place and tube secured with tape.

11. Assess tube position with chest or abdominal x-ray study.
    a. If tube is transpyloric, flush with 10 mL of sterile water and remove stylet before initiating tube feeds.

      b. If tube is at the pylorus, wait 24 to 48 hours and reassess.

      c. If the tube is looped around the stomach with the tip away from a pylorus, retract it to the centimeter mark estimating gastric placement. Administer repeat dose of metoclopramide and reattempt tube insertion.

  12. When properly positioned, secure tube to patient's nose and cheek and note centimeter marking on the tube at the tip of the patient's nose. If it is unsuccessful in transpyloric passage, arrange for a fluoroscopic or endoscopic manipulation.

X. Fiberoptic bronchoscopy (FOB)

  A. Indications for the trauma patient

    1. Adjunct to endotracheal intubation

    2. Evaluation of posttraumatic hemoptysis, acute inhalation injury, suspected bronchial injury, and injury caused by prolonged intubation

    3. Extraction of foreign bodies

    4. Clearance of secretions and mucous plugs

    5. Diagnosis of nosocomial pneumonia (see D below)

  B. Contraindications

    1. Uncooperative patient

    2. Persistent, marked hypoxemia or hypercarbia

    3. Severe bronchospasm

    4. Severe pulmonary hypertension

    5. Cardiac ischemia

    6. Coagulopathy (relative)

  C. Procedure

    1. Most trauma patients for whom FOB is indicated will have an endotracheal tube in place.

    2. Consider those trauma patients not intubated and for whom FOB is indicated for endotracheal intubation before the procedure.

    3. For patients not intubated, FOB should be performed by the most experienced bronchoscopist available.

    4. Have cardiac and pulse oximetry monitoring and skilled assistance available.

    5. Perform FOB only through a ≥8 mm internal diameter endotracheal or tracheostomy tube.

    6. Maintain 100% FIO_2 throughout the procedure and minimize airway suctioning to avoid reduction in tidal volumes.

    7. Make adjustments to mechanical ventilation before the procedure to maintain adequate minute ventilation and avoid increased inflation pressures.

    8. Use local anesthetics judiciously; 200 to 300 mg of lidocaine (20–30 mL of 1% Lidocaine solution).

    9. Premedication with i.v. analgesics and sedatives as indicated.

    10. Use silicone spray rather than gel lubricant.

    11. Consider use of a swivel adaptor, which minimizes air leak.

  D. Diagnosis of nosocomial pneumonia

    1. Cultures of sputum aspirates or traditional FOB specimens are unreliable because of contamination by upper airway secretions.

    2. Protected brush catheter (PBC)

      a. A PBC is a telescoping double catheter with a recessed sterile brush.

      b. The inner catheter with brush can be advanced into subsegmental bronchi for sampling of focal infiltrates.

      c. Avoid proximal lidocaine administration and suctioning during the procedure.

      d. Postsampling. Retract the inner catheter and brush and remove from the bronchoscope. The brush is severed from the catheter for quantitative cultures ($>10^3$ colonies per milliliter).

3. Bronchoalveolar lavage (BAL)
   a. Bronchoscopic tip is wedged into a subsegmental bronchi.
   b. Instill sterile normal saline solution (NSS; 50–100 mL) and remove via suction.
   c. Take quantitative cultures of the sample (>10^5 colonies per milliliter)

XI. **Insertion of bedside inferior vena caval filter (IVC)**
   A. **Indication**
      1. Recurrent pulmonary embolism despite anticoagulation
      2. Venous thromboembolic disease with contraindication to full anticoagulation
      3. Progression of ileofemoral clot, despite anticoagulation
      4. Large, free-floating thrombus in the iliac vein or IVC
      5. Massive pulmonary embolism (PE) in which recurrent emboli would prove fatal
      6. During or after surgical embolectomy
      7. Prophylaxis in patients who cannot receive anticoagulation because of increased bleeding risk and have high risk injury pattern (e.g., severe closed head injury, spinal cord injury, complex pelvic fractures with associated long bone fracture, or multiple long bone fractures).
   B. **Bedside insertion** of IVC filters can be performed with minimal complications and eliminate the risk associated with intrahospital transport; bedside application of this procedure reduces cost and operating room utilization.
   C. **Technique**
      1. Equipment
         a. Fluoroscopic image intensifier and monitor (Cine-loop and subtraction capabilities preferred)
         b. Fluoroscopic-ready bed
         c. Lead aprons
         d. Sterile barriers, gowns, masks, caps
         e. Introducer kit with guidewire
         f. Intravenous contrast material
         g. Heparinized saline (10 U/mL NSS)
         h. Radiopaque markers for measurements
            Note: Be familiar with introducer system and size restrictions of individual vena cava filters
      2. **Procedure**
         a. Prepare access site with povidone-iodine (solution or chlorhexidine gluconate, right internal jugular or femoral vein approach preferred).
         b. Identify T-12 and all lumbar vertebrae under fluoroscopic guidance.
         c. Gain venous access and advance guidewire under fluoroscopic guidance.
         d. Insert introducer with dilator previously flushed with heparin solution.
         e. Perform venogram (hand-injected or power-injected, if available) to assess for anomalies, venal caval size, and location of renal veins.
         f. Flush introducer with heparinized saline solution and advance filter into infrarenal position.
         g. Deploy filter under fluoroscopic guidance.
         h. Remove introducer and hold pressure at site for 10 minutes or until bleeding stops.
         i. Confirm placement of IVC filter with abdominal x-ray.

Bibliography

Croce MA, Fabian TC, et al. Using bronchoalveolar lavage to distinguish nosocomial pneumonia from systemic inflammatory response syndrome: a prospective analysis. *J Trauma* 1995;39:1134–1138.

Dellinger PR. Fiberoptic bronchoscopy in critical care medicine. In: Shoemaker WC, Ayers SH, Grenvig A, et al., eds. *Textbook of critical care.* Philadelphia: WB Saunders, 1995:761–769.

Lord LM, Weiser-Maimone A, Pulhamus M, et al. Comparison of weighted vs nonweighted enteral feeding tubes for efficiency of transpyloric intubation. *JPEN* 1993;17:271–273.

Rogers, FB, Cipolle MD, et al. Practice management guidelines for the management of venous thromboembolism in trauma patients. Available at http://www.east.org.

Schultz MD, Santatello SA, et al. An improved method for transpyloric placement of nasoenteric feeding tubes. *Int Surg* 1993;78:79–82.

Sing, RF, Smith CH, et al. Preliminary results of bedside interior vena cava filter placement. *Chest* 1998;114:315–316.

Appendix A. INJURY SCALES

Cervical vascular organ injury scale

Grade*	Description of injury	AIS-90
I	Thyroid vein	1–3
	Common facial vein	1–3
	External jugular vein	1–3
	Unnamed arterial or venous branches	1–3
II	External carotid arterial branches (ascending pharyngeal, superior thyroid, lingual, facial, maxillary, occipital, posterior auricular)	1–3
	Thyrocervical trunk or primary branches	1–3
	Internal jugular vein	1–3
III	External carotid artery	2–3
	Subclavian vein	3–4
	Vertebral artery	2–4
IV	Common carotid artery	3–5
	Subclavian artery	3–4
V	Internal carotid artery (extracranial)	3–5

* Increase one grade for multiple grade III or IV injuries involving >50% vessel circumference. Decrease one grade for <25% vessel circumference disruption for grade IV or V.
AIS, Abbreviated Injury Score.

Chest wall injury scale

Grade*	Injury type	Description of injury	AIS-90
I	Contusion	Any size	1
	Laceration	Skin and subcutaneous tissue	1
	Fracture	Fewer than three ribs, closed; nondisplaced clavicle closed	1–2
II	Laceration	Skin, subcutaneous tissue and muscle	1
	Fracture	Three or more adjacent ribs, closed	2–3
		Open or displaced clavicle	2
		Nondisplaced sternum, closed	2
		Scapular body, open or closed	2
III	Laceration	Full thickness, including pleural penetration	2
	Fracture	Open or displaced sternum flail sternum	2
		Unilateral flail segment (<3 ribs)	3–4
IV	Laceration	Avulsion of chest wall tissues with underlying rib fractures	4
	Fracture	Unilateral flail chest (≥3 ribs)	3–4
V	Fracture	Bilateral flail chest (≥3 ribs on both sides)	5

* This scale is confined to the chest wall alone and does not reflect associated internal thoracic or abdominal injuries. Therefore, further delineation of upper versus lower or anterior versus posterior chest wall was not considered, and a grade VI was not warranted. Specifically, thoracic crush was not used as a descriptive term; instead, the geography and extent of fractures and soft-tissue injury were used to define the grade. Advance by one grade for bilateral injuries up to grade III.
AIS, Abbreviated Injury Score.

Heart injury scale

Grade*	Description of injury	AIS-90
I	Blunt cardiac injury with minor electrocardiographic abnormality (nonspecific ST- or T-wave changes, premature atrial or ventricular contraction or persistent sinus tachycardia)	3
	Blunt or penetrating pericardial wound without cardiac injury, cardiac tamponade, or cardiac herniation	
II	Blunt cardiac injury with heart block (right or left bundle branch, left anterior fascicular, or atrioventricular) or ischemic changes (ST- depression or T-wave inversion) without cardiac failure	3
	Penetrating tangential myocardial wound up to, but not extending through endocardium, without tamponade	3
III	Blunt cardiac injury with sustained (≥6 beats/min) or multifocal ventricular contractions	3–4
	Blunt or penetrating cardiac injury with septal rupture, pulmonary or tricuspid valvular incompetence, papillary muscle dysfunction, or distal coronary arterial occlusion without cardiac failure	3–4
	Blunt pericardial laceration with cardiac herniation	
	Blunt cardiac injury with cardiac failure	3–4
	Penetrating tangential myocardial wound up to, but extending through, endocardium, with tamponade	3
IV	Blunt or penetrating cardiac injury with septal rupture, pulmonary or tricuspid valvular incompetence, papillary muscle dysfunction, or distal coronary arterial occlusion producing cardiac failure	3
	Blunt or penetrating cardiac injury with aortic mitral valve incompetence	
	Blunt or penetrating cardiac injury of the right ventricle, right atrium, or left atrium	5
V	Blunt or penetrating cardiac injury with proximal coronary arterial occlusion	5
	Blunt or penetrating left ventricular perforation	5
	Stellate wound with < 50% tissue loss of the right ventricle, right atrium, or left atrium	5
VI	Blunt avulsion of the heart; penetrating wound producing >50% tissue loss of a chamber	6

* Advance one grade for multiple wounds to a single chamber or multiple chamber involvement.
AIS, Abbreviated Injury Score.

Lung injury scale

Grade*	Injury type	Description of injury	AIS-90
I	Contusion	Unilateral, less than one lobe	3
II	Contusion	Unilateral, single lobe	3
	Laceration	Simple pneumothorax	3
III	Confusion	Unilateral more than one lobe	3
	Laceration	Persistent (>72 hours) air leak from distal airway	3–4
	Hematoma	Nonexpanding intraparenchymal	
IV	Laceration	Major (segmental or lobar) air leak	4–5
	Hematoma	Expanding intraparenchymal	
	Vascular	Primary branch intrapulmonary vessel disruption	3–5
V	Vascular	Hilar vessel disruption	4
VI	Vascular	Total uncontained transection of pulmonary hilum	4

* Advance one grade for bilateral injuries up to grade III. Hemothorax is scored under thoracic vascular injury scale.
AIS, Abbreviated Injury Score.

Thoracic vascular injury scale

Grade*	Description of injury	AIS-90
I	Intercostal artery or vein	2–3
	Internal mammary artery or vein	2–3
	Bronchial artery or vein	2–3
	Esophageal artery or vein	2–3
	Hemiazygous vein	2–3
	Unnamed artery or vein	2–3
II	Azygos vein	2–3
	Internal jugular vein	2–3
	Subclavian vein	3–4
	Innominate vein	3–4
III	Carotid artery	3–5
	Innominate artery	3–4
	Subclavian artery	3–4
IV	Thoracic aorta, descending	4–5
	Inferior vena cava (intrathoracic)	3–4
	Pulmonary artery, primary intraparenchymal branch	3
	Pulmonary vein, primary intraparenchymal branch	3
V	Thoracic aorta, ascending and arch	5
	Superior vena cava	3–4
	Pulmonary artery, main trunk	4
	Pulmonary vein, main trunk	4
VI	Uncontained total transection of thoracic aorta or pulmonary hilum	4

* Increase one grade for multiple grade III or IV injuries if > 50% circumference; decrease one grade for grade IV or V injuries if <25% circumference.
AIS, Abbreviated Injury Score.

Diaphragm injury scale

Grade*	Description of injury	AIS-90
I	Contusion	2
II	Laceration <2 cm	3
III	Laceration 2–10 cm	3
IV	Laceration >10 cm with tissue loss $\leq$ 25 cm^2	3
V	Laceration with tissue loss > 25 cm^2	3

* Advance one grade for bilateral injuries up to grade III.
AIS, Abbreviated Injury Score.

Spleen injury scale (1994 revision)

Grade*	Injury type	Description of injury	AIS-90
I	Hematoma	Subcapsular, <10% surface area	2
	Laceration	Capsular tear, <1 cm parenchymal depth	2
II	Hematoma	Subcapsular, 10% to 50% surface area; intraparenchymal, <5 cm in diameter	2
	Laceration	Capsular tear, 1–3 cm parenchymal depth that does not involve a trabecular vessel	2
III	Hematoma	Subcapsular, >50% surface area or expanding; ruptured subcapsular or parenchymal hematoma; intraparenchymal hematoma $\geq$ 5 cm or expanding	3
	Laceration	Parenchymal depth >3 cm or involving trabecular vessels	3
IV	Laceration	Laceration involving segmental or hilar vessels producing major devascularization (>25% of spleen)	4
V	Laceration	Completely shattered spleen	5
	Vascular	Hilar vascular injury that devascularizes spleen	5

* Advance one grade for multiple injuries up to grade III.
AIS, Abbreviated Injury Score.

Liver injury scale (1994 revision)

Grade*	Type of injury	Description of injury	AIS-90
I	Hematoma	Subcapsular, <10% surface area	2
	Laceration	Capsular tear, <1 cm parenchymal depth	2
II	Hematoma	Subcapsular, 10% to 50% surface area; intraparenchymal <10 cm in diameter	2
	Laceration	Capsular tear 1–3 cm parenchymal depth, <10 cm in length	2
III	Hematoma	Subcapsular, >50% surface area or expanding; ruptured subcapsular or parenchymal hematoma; intraparenchymal hematoma >10 cm or expanding	3
	Laceration	Parenchymal depth >3 cm	3
IV	Laceration	Parenchymal disruption involving 25% to 75% hepatic lobe or 1–3 Couinaud's segments	4
V	Laceration	Parenchymal disruption involving >75% of hepatic lobe or >3 Couinaud's segments within a single lobe	5
	Vascular	Juxtahepatic venous injuries (i.e., retrohepatic vena cava/central major hepatic veins)	5
VI	Vascular	Hepatic avulsion	6

* Advance one grade for multiple injuries up to grade III.
AIS, Abbreviated Injury Score.

Extrahepatic biliary tree injury scale (1995 revision)

Grade*	Description of injury	AIS-90
I	Gallbladder contusion/hematoma	2
	Portal triad contusion	2
II	Partial gallbladder avulsion from liver bed; cystic duct intact	2
	Laceration or perforation of the gallbladder	2
III	Complete gallbladder avulsion from liver bed	3
	Cystic duct laceration	3
IV	Partial or complete right hepatic duct laceration	3
	Partial or complete left hepatic duct laceration	3
	Partial common hepatic duct laceration (<50%)	3
	Partial common bile duct laceration (<50%)	3
V	Transection of common hepatic duct (≥50%)	3–4
	Transection of common bile duct (≥50%)	3–4
	Combined right and left hepatic duct injuries	3–4
	Intraduodenal or intrapancreatic bile duct injuries	3–4

* Advance one grade for multiple injuries up to grade III.
AIS, Abbreviated Injury Score.

Pancreas injury scale

Grade*	Type of injury	Description of injury	AIS-90
I	Hematoma	Minor contusion without duct injury	2
	Laceration	Superficial laceration without duct injury	2
II	Hematoma	Major contusion without duct injury or tissue loss	2
	Laceration	Major laceration without duct injury or tissue loss	3
III	Laceration	Distal transection or parenchymal injury with duct injury	3
IV	Laceration	Proximal transection or parenchymal injury involving ampulla†	4
V	Laceration	Massive disruption of pancreatic head	5

* Advance one grade for multiple injuries up to grade III.
† Proximal pancreas is to the patient's right of the superior mesenteric vein.
AIS, Abbreviated Injury Score.

Esophagus injury scale

Grade*	Description of injury	AIS-90
I	Contusion or hematoma	2
	Partial thickness laceration	3
II	Laceration circumference <50%	4
III	Laceration circumference ≥50%	4
IV	Segmental loss or devascularization <2 cm	5
V	Segmental loss or devascularization ≥2 cm	5

* Advance one grade for multiple lesions up to grade III.
AIS, Abbreviated Injury Score.

Stomach injury scale

Grade*	Description of injury	AIS-90
I	Contusion or hematoma	2
	Partial thickness laceration	2
II	Laceration in GE junction or pylorus <2 cm	3
	In proximal one third of stomach <5 cm	3
	In distal two thirds of stomach <10 cm	3
III	Laceration >2 cm in GE junction or pylorus	3
	In proximal one third of stomach ≥5 cm	3
	In distal two thirds of stomach ≥10 cm	3
IV	Tissue loss or devascularization <two thirds of stomach	4
V	Tissue loss or devascularization >two thirds of stomach	4

* Advance one grade for multiple lesions up to grade III.
GE, gastroesophageal.

Duodenum injury scale

Grade*	Type of injury	Description of injury	AIS-90
I	Hematoma	Involving single portion of duodenum	2
	Laceration	Partial thickness, no perforation	3
II	Hematoma	Involving more than one portion	2
	Laceration	Disruption <50% of circumference	4
III	Laceration	Disruption 50% to 75% of circumference of D2	4
		Disruption 50% to 100% of circumference of D1,D3,D4	4
IV	Laceration	Disruption >75% of circumference of D2	5
		Involving ampulla or distal common bile duct	5
V	Laceration	Massive disruption of duodenopancreatic complex	5
	Vascular	Devascularization of duodenum	5

* Advance one grade for multiple injuries up to grade III.
D1, first position of duodenum; D2, second portion of duodenum; D3, third portion of duodenum; D4, fourth portion of duodenum
AIS, Abbreviated Injury Score.

Small bowel injury scale

Grade*	Type of injury	Description of injury	AIS-90
I	Hematoma	Contusion or hematoma without devascularization	2
	Laceration	Partial thickness, no perforation	2
II	Laceration	Laceration <50% of circumference	3
III	Laceration	Laceration ≥ 50% of circumference without transection	3
IV	Laceration	Transection of the small bowel	4
V	Laceration	Transection of the small bowel with segmental tissue loss	4
	Vascular	Devascularized segment	4

* Advance one grade for multiple injuries up to grade III.
AIS, Abbreviated Injury Score.

Colon injury scale

Grade*	Type of injury	Description of injury	AIS-90
I	Hematoma	Contusion or hematoma without devascularization	2
	Laceration	Partial thickness, no perforation	2
II	Laceration	Laceration <50% of circumference	3
III	Laceration	Laceration ≥ 50% of circumference without transection	3
IV	Laceration	Transection of the colon	4
V	Laceration	Transection of the colon with segmental tissue loss	4

* Advance one grade for multiple injuries up to grade III.
AIS, Abbreviated Injury Score.

Rectum injury scale

Grade*	Type of injury	Description of injury	AIS-90
I	Hematoma	Contusion or hematoma without devascularization	2
	Laceration	Partial-thickness laceration	2
II	Laceration	Laceration <50% of circumference	3
III	Laceration	Laceration ≥50% of circumference	4
IV	Laceration	Full-thickness laceration with extension into the perineum	5
V	Vascular	Devascularized segment	5

* Advance one grade for multiple injuries up to grade III.
AIS, Abbreviated Injury Score.

Abdominal vascular injury scale

Grade*	Description of injury	AIS-90
I	Non-named superior mesenteric artery or superior mesenteric vein branches	NS
	Non-named inferior mesenteric artery or inferior mesenteric vein branches	NS
	Phrenic artery or vein	NS
	Lumbar artery or vein	NS
	Gonadal artery or vein	NS
	Ovarian artery or vein	NS
	Other non-named, small arterial or venous structures requiring ligation	NS
II	Right, left, or common hepatic artery	3
	Splenic artery or vein	3
	Right or left gastric arteries	3
	Gastroduodenal artery	3
	Inferior mesenteric artery, or inferior mesenteric vein, trunk	3
	Primary named branches of messenteric artery (e.g., ileocolic artery) or mesenteric vein	3
	Other named abdominal vessels requiring ligation or repair	3
III	Superior mesenteric vein, trunk	3
	Renal artery or vein	3
	Iliac artery or vein	3
	Hypogastric artery or vein	3
	Vena cava, infrarenal	3
IV	Superior mesenteric artery, trunk	3
	Celiac axis proper	3
	Vena cava, suprarenal and infrahepatic	3
	Aorta, infrarenal	4
V	Portal vein	3
	Extraparenchymal hepatic vein	3/5
	Vena cava, retrohepatic or suprahepatic	5
	Aorta suprarenal, subdiaphragmatic	4

* This classification system is applicable to extraparenchymal vascular injuries. If the vessel injury is within 2 cm of the organ parenchyma, refer to specific organ injury scale. Increase one grade for multiple grade III or IV injuries involving > 50% vessel circumference. Downgrade one grade if <25% vessel circumference laceration for grades IV or V.
NS, not scored.
AIS, Abbreviated Injury Score.

Adrenal organ injury scale

Grade*	Description of injury	AIS-90
I	Contusion	1
II	Laceration involving only cortex (<2 cm)	1
III	Laceration extending into medulla (≥ 2 cm)	2
IV	Parenchymal destruction (>50%)	2
V	Total parenchymal destruction (including massive intraparenchymal hemorrhage)	3
	Avulsion from blood supply	3

* Advance one grade for bilateral lesion up to grade V.
AIS, Abbreviated Injury Score.

Kidney injury scale

Grade*	Type of injury	Description of injury	AIS-90
I	Contusion	Microscopic or gross hematuria, urologic studies normal	2
	Hematoma	Subcapsular, nonexpanding without parenchymal laceration	2
II	Hematoma	Nonexpanding perirenal hematoma confined to renal retroperitoneum	2
	Laceration	Parenchymal depth of renal cortex (<1.0 cm) without urinary extravasation	2
III	Laceration	Parenchymal depth of renal cortex (>1.0 cm) without collecting system rupture or urinary extravasation	3
IV	Laceration	Parenchymal laceration extending through the renal cortex, medulla, and collecting system	4
	Vascular	Main renal artery or vein injury with contained hemorrhage	4
V	Laceration	Completely shattered kidney	5
	Vascular	Avulsion of renal hilum which devascularizes kidney	5

* Advance one grade for bilateral injuries up to grade III.
AIS, Abbreviated Injury Score.

Ureter injury scale

Grade*	Type of injury	Description of injury	AIS-90
I	Hematoma	Contusion or hematoma without devascularization	2
II	Laceration	Transecection <50%	2
III	Laceration	Transection ≥50%	3
IV	Laceration	Complete transection with <2 cm devascularization	3
V	Laceration	Avulsion with >2 cm of devascularization	3

* Advance one grade for bilateral lesions up to grade III.
AIS, Abbreviated Injury Score.

Bladder injury scale

Grade*	Injury type	Description of injury	AIS-90
I	Hematoma	Contusion, intramural hematoma	2
	Laceration	Partial thickness	3
II	Laceration	Extraperitoneal bladder wall laceration <2 cm	4
III	Laceration	Extraperitoneal (≥2 cm) or intraperitoneal (<2 cm) bladder wall laceration	4
IV	Laceration	Intraperitoneal bladder wall laceration ≥2 cm	4
V	Laceration	Intraperitoneal or extraperitoneal bladder wall laceration extending into the bladder neck or ureteral orifice (trigone)	4

* Advance one grade for multiple lesions up to grade III.
AIS, Abbreviated Injury Score.

Urethra injury scale

Grade*	Injury type	Description of injury	AIS-90
I	Contusion	Blood at urethral meatus; urethrography normal	2
II	Stretch injury	Elongation of urethra without extravasation on urethrography	2
III	Partial disruption	Extravasation of urethrography contrast at injury site with visualization in the bladder	2
IV	Complete disruption	Extravasation of urethrography contrast at injury site without visualization in the bladder; <2 cm of urethral separation	3
V	Complete disruption	Complete transection with ≥2 cm urethral separation, or extension into the prostate or vagina	4

* Advance one grade for bilateral injuries up to grade III.
AIS, Abbreviated Injury Score.

Uterus (nonpregnant) injury scale

Grade*	Description of injury	AIS-90
I	Contusion or hematoma	2
II	Superficial laceration (<1 cm)	2
III	Deep laceration (≥1 cm)	3
IV	Laceration involving uterine artery	3
V	Avulsion/devascularization	3

* Advance one grade for multiple injuries up to grade III.
AIS, Abbreviated Injury Score.

Uterus (pregnant) injury scale

Grade*	Description of injury	AIS-90
I	Contusion or hematoma (without placental abruption)	2
II	Superficial laceration (<1 cm) or partial placental abruption <25%	3
III	Deep laceration (≥1 cm) occurring in second trimester or placental abruption <25% but <50%	3
	Deep laceration (≥1 cm) in third trimester	4
IV	Laceration involving uterine artery	4
	Deep laceration (≥1 cm) with >50% placental abruption	4
V	Uterine rupture	
	Second trimester	4
	Third trimester	5
	Complete placental abruption	4–5

* Advance one grade for multiple injuries up to grade III.
AIS, Abbreviated Injury Score.

Fallopian tube injury scale

Grade*	Description of injury	AIS-90
I	Hematoma or contusion	2
II	Laceration <50% circumference	2
III	Laceration ≥50% circumference	2
IV	Transection	2
V	Vascular injury; devascularized segment	2

* Advance one grade for bilateral injuries up to grade III.
AIS, Abbreviated Injury Score.

Ovary injury scale

Grade*	Description of injury	AIS-90
I	Contusion or hematoma	1
II	Superficial laceration (depth <0.5 cm)	2
III	Deep laceration (depth ≥ 0.5 cm)	3
IV	Partial disruption of blood supply	3
V	Avulsion or complete parenchymal destruction	3

* Advance one grade for bilateral injuries up to grade III.
AIS, Abbreviated Injury Score.

Vagina injury scale

Grade*	Description of injury	AIS-90
I	Contusion or hematoma	1
II	Laceration, superficial (mucosa only)	1
III	Laceration, deep into fat or muscle	2
IV	Laceration, complex, into cervix or peritoneum	3
V	Injury into adjacent organs (anus, rectum, urethra, bladder)	3

* Advance one grade for multiple injuries up to grade III.
AIS, Abbreviated Injury Score.

Vulva injury scale

Grade*	Description of injury	AIS-90
I	Contusion or hematoma	1
II	Laceration, superficial (skin only)	1
III	Laceration, deep (into fat or muscle)	2
IV	Avulsion: skin, fat or muscle	3
V	Injury into adjacent organs (anus, rectum, urethra, bladder)	3

* Advance one grade for multiple injuries up to grade III.
AIS, Abbreviated Injury Score.

Testis injury scale

Grade*	Description of injury	AIS-90
I	Contusion or hematoma	1
II	Subclinical laceration of tunica albuginea	1
III	Laceration of tunica albuginea with <50% parenchymal loss	2
IV	Major laceration of tunica albuginea with ≥50% parenchymal loss	2
V	Total testicular destruction or avulsion	2

* Advance one grade for bilateral lesions up to grade V.
AIS, Abbreviated Injury Score.

Scrotum injury scale

Grade	Description of injury	AIS-90
I	Contusion	1
II	Laceration of scrotal diameter <25%	1
III	Laceration of scrotal diameter ≥25%	2
IV	Avulsion <50%	2
V	Avulsion ≥50%	2

AIS, Abbreviated Injury Score.

Penis injury scale

Grade*	Description of injury	AIS-90
I	Cutaneous laceration or contusion	1
II	Buck's fascia (cavernosum) laceration without tissue loss	1
III	Cutaneous avulsion	3
	Laceration through glans or meatus	3
	Cavernosal or urethral defect <2 cm	3
IV	Partial penectomy	3
	Cavernosal or urethral defect ≥ 2 cm	3
V	Total penectomy	3

* Advance one grade for multiple injuries up to grade III.
AIS, Abbreviated Injury Score.

Peripheral vascular organ injury scale

Grade*	Description of injury	AIS-90
I	Digital artery or vein	1–3
	Palmar artery or vein	1–3
	Deep palmar artery or vein	1–3
	Dorsalis pedis artery	1–3
	Plantar artery or vein	1–3
	Non-named arterial or venous branches	1–3
II	Basilic or cephalic vein	1–3
	Saphenous vein	1–3
	Radial artery	1–3
	Ulnar artery	1–3
III	Axillary vein	2–3
	Superficial or deep femoral vein	2–3
	Popliteal vein	2–3
	Brachial artery	2–3
	Anterior tibial artery	1–3
	Posterior tibial artery	1–3
	Peroneal artery	1–3
	Tibioperoneal trunk	2–3
IV	Superficial or deep femoral artery	3–4
	Popliteal artery	2–3
V	Axillary artery	2–3
	Common femoral artery	3–4

* Increase one grade for multiple grade III or IV injuries involving >50% vessel circumference.
Decrease one grade for < 25% vessel circumference disruption for grades IV or V.
AIS, Abbreviated Injury Score.

References
Moore EE, Cogbill TH, Jurkovich GJ, et al. Organ injury scaling III: chest wall, abdominal vascular, ureter bladder, and urethra. *J Trauma* 1992;33:337.

Moore EE, Cogbill TH, Jurkovich GJ, et al. Organ injury scaling V: spleen and liver (1994 revision). *J Trauma* 1995;38:323.

Moore EE, Cogbill TH, Malangoni MA, et al. Organ injury scaling. *Surg Clin North Am* 1995;75:293–303.

Moore EE, Cogbill TH, Malangoni MA, et al. Organ injury scaling II: pancreas, duodenum, small bowel, colon, and rectum. *J Trauma* 1990;30:1427.

Moore EE, Dunn EL, Moore JB, et al. Penetrating abdominal trauma index. *J Trauma* 1981;21:439.

Moore EE, Jurkovich GJ, Knudson MM, et al. Organ injury scaling VI: extrahepatic biliary, esophagus, stomach, vulva, vagina, uterus (nonpregnant), uterus (pregnant), fallopian tube, and ovary. *J Trauma* 1995;39:1069–1070.

Moore EE, Malangoni MA, Cogbill TH, et al. Organ injury scaling IV: thoracic vascular, lung, cardiac and diaphragm. *J Trauma* 1994;36:226.

Moore EE, Malangoni MA, Cogbill TH, et al. Organ injury scaling VII: cervical vascular, peripheral vascular, adrenal, penis testis, and scrotum. *J Trauma* 1996;41:523–524.

Moore EE, Shackford SR, Pachter HL, et al. Organ injury scaling: spleen, liver and kidney. *J Trauma* 1989;29:1664.

Appendix B. TETANUS PROPHYLAXIS

Marilyn J. Borst

Tetanus (lockjaw) is a preventable disease that can be lethal to its victims. It is caused by *Clostridium tetani,* a spore-forming anaerobic bacillus. Under ideal wound conditions, the spore is converted to the vegetative form, which produces an exotoxin, tetanospasmin, which acts on the nervous system. The average incubation period for tetanus is 10 days (range, 4 to 21 days). It can appear in 1 to 2 days in severe trauma cases. Attention to tetanus prophylaxis is important in all trauma patients, especially those with multiple injuries or open-extremity trauma.

I. **Prevention**
   The prevention of tetanus has two components: proper wound care and immunization.
II. **Wound characteristics and susceptibility to tetanus.** Traumatic wounds can be classified as tetanus prone or nontetanus prone based on various characteristics of the wound (Table A-1). A wound with one or more of these characteristics is a tetanus-prone wound.
III. **Wound care**
   A. **Aseptic surgical techniques** should be used when caring for any wound. All devitalized tissue and foreign bodies must be removed.
   B. Wounds should be left open if any one of the following is present:
      1. Doubt about the adequacy of debridement
      2. A puncture injury
      3. A tetanus-prone wound
IV. **Agents for tetanus immunization**
   A. **Active immunization** is performed with tetanus toxoid, which can be given as a single or combined agent.
      1. **Types of tetanus toxoid agents**
         a. **Diphtheria and tetanus toxoids and pertussis vaccine adsorbed (DTP or DPT).** This agent is used for patients younger than 7 years of age.
         b. **Diphtheria and tetanus toxoids adsorbed (DT) (pediatric type).** This agent is used for patients younger than 7 years of age and for patients in whom the pertussis vaccine is contraindicated.
         c. **Tetanus and diphtheria toxoids adsorbed (Td) (adult type).** This agent is used in patients 7 years of age or older. This preparation is preferable to tetanus toxoid alone because many adults are susceptible to diphtheria, and the simultaneous administration of diphtheria toxoid will enhance protection against this disease.
         d. **Tetanus toxoid adsorbed (Tt).** This agent is for use only in adults. Tetanus toxoid is a sterile preparation of inactivated toxin. It is available as a fluid or in an adsorbed form. The adsorbed form is preferable because it induces higher antitoxin titers and a longer duration of protection.
      2. **Administration.** Agents containing tetanus toxoid adsorbed are administered intramuscularly (IM) in doses of 0.5 mL.
   B. **Passive immunization**
      1. **Agents**
         a. **Tetanus immune globulin (TIG) (human) (Hyper-Tet).** This agent is preferable. The risk of hypersensitivity reactions is minimal because it is a human preparation. The dose for tetanus prophylaxis is 250 to 500 U IM.
         b. **Tetanus antitoxin equine.** This agent has a significant risk of hypersensitivity reactions and should not be used unless TIG (human)

Table A-1. Wound characteristics and susceptibility to tetanus

Wound characteristics	Tetanus-prone wounds	Nontetanus-prone wounds
Age of wound	>6 hours	≤6 hours
Configuration	Stellate, avulsion, abrasion	Linear
Depth	>1 cm	≤1 cm
Mechanism of injury	Missile, crush, burn, frostbite	Sharp surface (knife, glass)
Signs of infection	Present	Absent
Devitalized tissue	Present	Absent
Contaminants (dirt, feces, grass, saliva)	Present	Absent
Denervated and/or ischemic tissue	Present	Absent

is unavailable and the possibility of tetanus outweighs the potential reactions of horse serum. Tests for sensitivity to equine serum should be performed before the administration of equine serum.

   2. A separate syringe and separate injection site must be used when Tt and TIG are both administered.

V. Immunization guidelines

   A. Active immunization

   1. Infants and children. For children younger than 7 years of age, immunization requires four injections of DTP or DT. A booster injection (fifth dose) is administered at 4 to 6 years of age (not necessary if fourth dose is given on or after the fourth birthday). A routine booster of Td is indicated at 10-year intervals.

   2. Adults. Immunization requires at least three injections of tetanus toxoid. An injection of Td should be repeated every 10 years, provided that no significant reactions to Td have occurred.

   3. Pregnant women. Active immunization of the pregnant mother during the first 6 months of pregnancy will prevent neonatal tetanus. Two injections of Td are given 2 months apart. After delivery and 6 months after the second dose, the mother is given a third dose of Td to complete her active immunization. An injection of Td should be repeated every 10 years, provided that no significant reactions to Td have occurred.

   If a child is born to a nonimmunized mother who had no obstetric care, the infant should receive 250 U of TIG. The mother should also receive active and passive immunization.

   B. Prophylaxis against tetanus in wound management. In patients with wounds, the guidelines illustrated in Table A-2 should be used to determine whether tetanus toxoid with or without TIG administration is necessary.

   The effectiveness of prophylactic antibiotics is unknown. Penicillin delays the onset of tetanus. For patients who need TIG as part of the treatment for tetanus prophylaxis, but TIG is not readily available, penicillin allows a period of 2 days in which to obtain the TIG and begin passive immunization.

VI. Contraindications

   A. Tetanus and diphtheria toxoids

   1. *A history of neurologic or severe hypersensitivity* reaction to a previous dose is the only contraindication in a patient with a wound. Local side effects alone do not necessitate discontinuing the use of these toxoids.

   2. Immunization should be postponed until appropriate skin testing can be performed if a systemic reaction is suspected to represent allergic hypersensitivity.

Table A-2. Prophylaxis against tetanus in wound management

History of adsorbed tetanus toxoid (doses)	Tetanus-prone wounds		Nontetanus-prone wounds	
	Td[a,b]	TIG	Td[a,b]	TIG
Unknown or <3	Yes	Yes	Yes	No
≥3[c]	No[d]	No	No[e]	No

[a] For persons 7 years old or older. Td is preferred to tetanus toxoid alone.

[b] For persons younger than 7 years old, DPT (diphtheria-pertussis-tetanus) (or DT [diphtheria-tetanus] if pertussis vaccine is contraindicated) is preferred to tetanus toxoid alone.

[c] If only three doses of fluid toxoid were received previously, a fourth dose, preferably an adsorbed toxoid, should be given.

[d] Yes, if it has been more than 5 years since last dose (more frequent boosters are not needed and can accentuate side effects)

[e] Yes, if it has been more than 10 years since last dose

Td, tetanus-diphtheria toxoid (adult type); TIG, tetanus immune globulin.

3. **Passive immunization should be considered** for a tetanus-prone wound if a contraindication to the use of tetanus toxoid exists.
B. **Tetanus immune globulin.** If a history of previous systemic reaction to horse serum representing allergic hypersensitivity exists and it is necessary to administer tetanus antitoxin equine, immunization should be withheld until appropriate skin testing is performed.
C. **Pertussis vaccine in DTP.** DT, instead of DTP, should be administered if there was a previous adverse reaction after DTP or a single-antigen pertussis vaccination. Adverse reactions include:
   1. **Immediate anaphylactic reaction**
   2. **Temperature ≥105° within 48 hours**
   3. **Collapse or shocklike state within 48 hours**
   4. **Encephalopathy within 7 days,** including severe alterations in consciousness with generalized or focal neurologic signs persisting for >12 hours
   5. **Persistent, inconsolable crying lasting ≥3 hours**
   6. **High-pitched cry within 48 hours**
   7. **Convulsion with or without fever within 3 days**
VII. **Patient instructions**
A. Written instructions should be given to the patient regarding
   1. Treatment received, including immunizations administered
   2. Follow-up appointments for:
     a. Wound care
     b. Completion of active immunization if necessary
B. Each patient should be given a wallet-size card documenting immunization dosage and date received. The patient should be instructed to carry this card at all times.

Axioms

• Wounds should be classified as tetanus prone or nontetanus prone based on characteristics of the wound. If uncertain, administer active immunization.
• Recognize high-risk groups who may not have had the primary immunization series as children: individuals born outside the United States or populations in this country who are secluded for religious or other reasons.
• Elderly patients may have a diminished response to tetanus toxoid.

References

Agents for immunization. In *Drug evaluations subscription*. Chicago: American Medical Association, 1991.

Committee on Trauma, American College of Surgeons: Resources Document 6: Tetanus immunization. In *Advanced trauma life support course for physicians*. Chicago: American College of Surgeons, 1993.

Furste W, Aguirre A: Tetanus. In Howard RJ, Simmons RL, eds. *Surgical infectious disease, 3rd ed.* Norwalk, CT: Appleton & Lange, 1995.

Ross SE. *Prophylaxis against tetanus in wound management*. Chicago: American College of Surgeons Committee on Trauma, 1995.

Webb KP: Tetanus prophylaxis. In Lopez-Viego MA, ed. *The Parkland trauma handbook*. Philadelphia: Mosby-Year Book, 1994.

Table 1 Check list for clinical diagnosis of brain death

	Clinical Evaluations	
	#1	#2
Cause of Brain Death_____		
Date of Exam	____	____
Time of Exam	____	____
I. Absence of confounding factors		
A. Systolic blood pressure > 90 mmHg	____	____
B. Temperature > 32°C	____	____
C. No CNS depressants (e.g. anesthetics, sedatives, narcotics, alcohol) or neuro-muscular blocking agents	____	____
D. No uremia, meniagoencephalitis, hepatic encephalopathies or other metabolic encephalopaties	____	____
II. Absence of cerebral and brainstem function		
A. Unresponsiveness to painful stimuli (e.g. supraorbital pressure)	____	____
B. No spontaneous muscular movements, posturing, or seizures	____	____
C. Pupils light-fixed	____	____
D. Absent corneal reflexes	____	____
E. Absent response to upper and lower airway stimulation (e.g. pharyngeal and endotracheal suctioning)	____	____
F. Absent oculocephalic reflexes		
G. Absent oculovestibular reflexes (irrigation of the ears with 50 mL of ice water)	____	____
H. No increase in heart rate after IV atropine (2 mg)	____	____
1. Heart rate before atropine	____	____
2. Heart rate after atropine	____	____
I. Apnea (at $Paco_2$ > 60 mmHg)		
1. $Paco_2$ at end of apnea test	____	____
2. Pao_2 at end of apnea test	____	____
III. Confirmatory tests (in selected situations)		
A. An electroencephalogram demonstrating electrocerebral silence	____	
B. Cerebral arteriography showing absent intracranial circulation	____	
C. Cerebral bloodflow study		
IV. Comments: _____		

Certification of death

Having considered the above findings, we hereby certify the death of:

Date_____ Time of Death_____
Physicians' Signatures_____MD _____MD
Names Printed_____MD _____MD

This document must be signed by two physicians licensed by the State of Pennsylvania

(Modified from The University of Pittsburgh Medical Center, Clinical Diagnosis of Brain Death)

UPMC HEALTH SYSTEM

TRAUMA ADMISSION HISTORY AND PHYSICAL

Date: _____

ED Arrival Time: _____

History / Mechanism of Injury: _____

IMPRINT PATIENT IDENTIFICATION HERE

PMH:

PSHX:

Allergies:

Medications:

Initial Trauma Room VS: P_____ BP_____ RESP_____ O2 Saturation_____ T_____

Glasgow Coma Scale (GCS)

Eye	Spontaneous	4
Opening	To Voice	3
	To Pain	2
	None	1
Verbal	Oriented	5
Response	Confused	4
	Inappropriate Words	3
	Incomprehensible Words	2
	None	1
Motor	Obeys Command	6
Response	Localizes Pain	5
	Withdraw (Pain)	4
	Flexion (Pain)	3
	Extension (Pain)	2
	None	1

GCS Total

Revised Trauma Score (RTS)

Glasgow Coma Scale	13 - 15	4
Find a subtotal for GCS. Use this	9 - 12	3
subtotal to obtain a corresponding RTS.	6 - 8	2
Add this value to the scores of the two	4 - 5	1
other categories.	3	0
Respiratory Rate	10 - 29	4
Number of respirations in	> 29	3
15 seconds: multiple by four	6 - 9	2
	1 - 5	1
	0	0
Systolic	> 89	4
Blood Pressure	76 - 89	3
Systolic Cuff Pressure	50 - 75	2
Either arm	1 - 49	1
Palpate or auscultate No Pulse	0	0

RTS Total

Primary Survey

Physical Exam: _____

Airway: _____

Breathing: _____

Circulation: _____

Page 1

1328-01-U   FORM 2233-3670-0799

FIG. 1. Trauma admission history and physical (page 1)

Appendix C. FREQUENTLY USED FORMS